Chromosome Abnormalities
and Genetic Counseling

OXFORD MONOGRAPHS ON MEDICAL GENETICS

General Editors

ARNO G. MOTULSKY   MARTIN BOBROW
PETER S. HARPER   CHARLES SCRIVER

Former Editors

J. A. FRASER ROBERTS   C. O. CARTER

OXFORD MONOGRAPHS ON MEDICAL GENETICS NO. 29

Chromosome Abnormalities and Genetic Counseling

R. J. McKinlay Gardner
Medical Geneticist
Murdoch Institute and Victorian Clinical Genetics Services
Melbourne, Australia

Grant R. Sutherland
Director
Department of Cytogenetics and Molecular Genetics
Women's and Children's Hospital
Adelaide, Australia

New York   Oxford
OXFORD UNIVERSITY PRESS
1996

Oxford University Press

Oxford   New York
Athens   Auckland   Bangkok   Bombay
Calcutta   Cape Town   Dar es Salaam   Delhi
Florence   Hong Kong   Istanbul   Karachi
Kuala Lumpur   Madras   Madrid   Melbourne
Mexico City   Nairobi   Paris   Singapore
Taipei   Tokyo   Toronto

and associated companies in
Berlin   Ibadan

Copyright © 1996 by Oxford University Press, Inc.

Published by Oxford University Press, Inc.,
198 Madison Avenue, New York, New York 10016

Oxford is a registered trademark of Oxford University Press

Library of Congress Cataloging-in-Publication Data
Gardner, R. J. M.
Chromosome abnormalities and genetic counseling/
R.J.M. Gardner, G.R. Sutherland.—2nd ed.
p.   cm.—(Oxford monographs on medical genetics : no. 29)
Includes bibliographical references and index.
ISBN 0-19-510615-6
1. Genetic counseling.
2. Human chromosome abnormalities—Patients—Counseling of.
I. Sutherland, Grant R.
II. Title.   III. Series.
[DNLM: 1. Genetic counseling.   2. Human chromosome abnormalities.
QS 677 G228c   1996]   RB155.7.G37   1996   616'.042—dc20
DNLM/DLC   for Library of Congress   95-52072

9 8 7 6 5 4 3 2 1

Printed in the United States of America
on acid-free paper

This book is dedicated to Jocelyn, Geoffrey, and Craig, their parents, and all other families who seek our ''chromosomal advice''

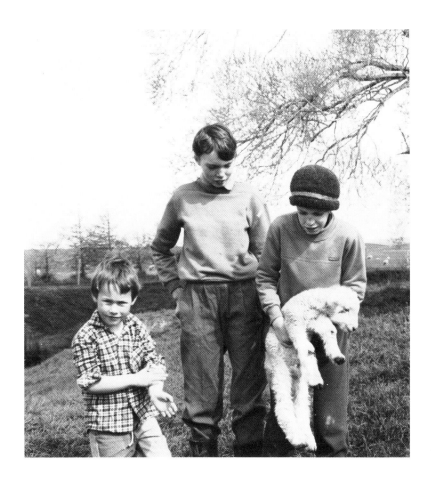

Jocelyn and Geoffrey (with lamb) have a partial trisomy for chromosome 4 long arm, and Craig, the youngest, had a 46,XY result on amniocentesis. Their father is a translocation carrier (see Figure 4-1, lower).

Heredity

Inescapably, this is me—the diagnosis
is cause for anger at those
who brightly say we choose our destinies.

There is no store
of courage, wit or will
can save me from myself and I must face
my children, feeling like
that wicked fairy, uninvited
at the christening, bestowing on my own,
amidst murmurs of apprehension, a most
unwanted gift—that
of a blighted mind. No one
could tell me of this curse when I
was young and dreamt of children
and the graces they would bear. Later,
it seemed that a chill morning
revealed deeper layers
of truth. For my romancing
there is a price to pay—
perhaps my children's children
will pass this tollgate after me.
My grandmothers gaze down from their frames
on my wall, sadly wondering.

                                    Meg Campbell

Contents

REPRODUCTIVE FAILURE

PRENATAL DIAGNOSIS

APPENDIXES

Preface

It is in the nature of a textbook to become outdated; it is the mark of a useful one that its philosophy endures. Clinical cytogenetics has seen much growth in knowledge and understanding since the first edition of this book was published, and we have refined several of the concepts set forth, as well as some of the advice offered. We have treated in greater detail the segregation and risks in reciprocal translocations, X-autosome translocations, inversions, insertions, and prenatal diagnosis. If the reader should fail to find mention of a circumstance they have encountered in the clinic, we can only suppose (not that we are trying to prefabricate excuses) that it must be something that is extraordinarily rare. The deletion syndromes have become more numerous and more precisely defined, and this required treatment. Fluorescence *in situ* hybridization has become a routinely applied methodology, and its use has extended the power, and increased the sophistication, of the discipline of clinical cytogenetics. The Human Genome Project is unraveling the complexity of our genetic inheritance, and the reader will find evidence of its influence on the practicalities of human cytogenetics throughout the book.

Dynamic mutation and genomic imprinting were not mentioned in the first edition but are now important topics. The fragile X syndrome has the status of the prototypical dynamic mutation; we have completely rewritten this chapter, and in its new form it is more of a molecular than a cytogenetic document. The Prader-Willi and Angelman syndromes have become the classic examples of genomic imprinting and uniparental disomy. Compared with the tentative comments on these syndromes in the previous edition, we now offer a rather extensive treatment although the definitive picture is yet to be drawn.

While the subject has become more complicated, our aim remains the same: to furnish a straightforward scientific description that will help readers understand the various chromosome abnormalities encountered in clinical practice, and to provide practical advice that can be passed on to the people who have, or whose families have, these abnormalities. The reader must judge how well we have met this aim.

February 1996   R.J.M.G.
Melbourne, Australia   G.R.S
Adelaide, Australia

Preface to First Edition

We have written this book with two particular categories of reader in mind. The first, and chief, audience is the genetic counselor, the person whose role it is to explain and interpret a chromosomal problem to the individual or family in whom it has been identified. Second, we have considered the needs of cytogenetic laboratory workers, who in addition to possessing the technical skills for chromosomal analysis, should understand the theoretical basis of clinical cytogenetics and be aware of the practical implications of their work.

A pithy definition of counseling is assisting clients to recognize the nature of their problems and to find their own solutions to them. The description applies aptly to the specific case of genetic counseling. One tool the counselor needs to do the job well is accurate information about the nature of the problem. The aim of this book is to provide in convenient form accurate information concerning chromosomal conditions. We address these major questions clients have: How and why did it happen? Could it happen again? If so, how likely would it be to happen again? Most chapters follow the general format of a Biology section, which discusses the first question, and a Genetic Counseling section, which deals with the latter two. (The division is not always clear-cut, and recognizing that readers may at times wish to refer just to the Genetic Counseling section, there is some duplication.) We do not claim, in using the expression ''genetic counseling,'' to encompass all that is involved in this multifaceted process. Rather, we seek to provide information and figures that will assist the client to decide what, for them, would be an appropriate course of action and to provide pointers to assist the counselor in communicating that information.

Chromosomes are not a theoretical concept; they are real things. (In this spirit, it is helpful in counseling sessions to have on hand a real karyotype, preferably from the counselee's own family, for use as a teaching aid.) To be able to give to the concept of chromosomes being passed down from parent to child a sense of reality, the counselor should have a broad and comfortable understanding of the mechanisms of chromosome behavior. Thus, we have gone into considerable detail in describing particular chromosomal situations. Rare conditions are given almost as extensive a hearing as the more common abnormalities. We make these points: First, rare conditions, for the families that have them, are very common. Second, the intellectual exercise of coming to grips with the complexities of a variety of disorders sharpens the reader's thinking.

Is there a risk of the same (or another) chromosomal defect occurring in a future pregnancy, and leading to the birth of an abnormal child? And if such a risk exists, how great is it? The perception of risk is subjective. The fact that in this book we give probabilities to perhaps a fraction of one percent does not allow the counselor the comfort of supposing that interpreting risk to consultands is a neat and tidy business (Pearn, 1977; Bloch et al., 1979; Wertz et al., 1986). Sir William Osler said of clinical medicine that what kind of disease the patient had was not as important as what kind of patient had the disease. In a similar vein, we may remark that what kind of person faces a genetic risk warrants no less consideration than the degree of risk. But of course, a precise estimate does provide a major reference point to assist in making the subsequent decision. It is good to have good figures. Dr. Chapman explores the idea of ''good figures'' in Chapter 3.

Other than peripherally, we do not describe details of karyotype-phenotype correlation (except in Chapter 22, where we directly address the problem of interpreting and managing unexpected chromosome abnormalities discovered in the course of prenatal diagnosis). This aspect of clinical cytogenetics is dealt with well in other texts. We will presume the reader has access to these and will not rework the information they contain.

Likewise, we take it for granted the reader knows that skill in sensitive communication is an absolute requirement for effective genetic counseling. It is a continuing challenge to be able to communicate the gist of a situation in straightforward language, at the client's level of comprehension. We recognize that however well done the cytogenetics and the risk determination, if counselees are not able to absorb this information and to react to it in a way that is most consonant with their own values, aspirations, and interests, the exercise has been less than successful. We do not explore the psychodynamics of counseling or the processes by which people make decisions: these issues are well addressed in other sources (Kelly, 1977; Hsia et al., 1979; Kessler, 1979; Epstein et al., 1979; Reed, 1980; Emery and Pullen, 1984; Reif and Baitsch, 1985; Hsia, 1987). A course couples need to consider when an abnormality is shown at prenatal diagnosis is termination of the pregnancy (''genetic abortion''). We assume the counselor is well aware of the support needed through this most difficult time (Landenburger and Delp, 1987; Magyari et al., 1987; Thomson, 1987).

We have, more than once, taken some liberties of interpretation, and made some statements a little more firmly and less complicatedly than the current state of cytogenetic knowledge might allow. We trust that this will not undermine the validity of the book, bearing in mind its intended purpose—to be of use to both the experienced and the neophyte.

''Families pursue genetic counseling in an effort to demystify the mysterious. They seek answers and information. If they did not want to 'hear it all,' they would not bother with genetic counseling. Families want an honest evaluation of what is known and what is unknown, a clear explanation of all possibilities, both good and bad, and a sensitive exploration of all available information with which they can make knowledgeable decisions about future family planning.'' Thus Bloch et al. (1979) succinctly convey the essence of why people go to the genetic counselor. We hope this book will assist counselors in their task.

January 1989   R.J.M.G.
Dunedin, New Zealand   G.R.S.
Adelaide,Australia

Acknowledgments

We are grateful to cytogenetic colleagues who have allowed us to use examples of their work as illustrative material. We have had the benefit of advice from several colleagues, and owe particular debt to E. Baker, D. F. Callen, J. L. Halliday, J. C. Mulley, R. D. Nicholls, M. D. Pertile, V. Petrovic, R. I. Richards, L. J. Sheffield, A. H. Sinclair, H. R. Slater, A. Smith, and L. E. Voullaire. M. H. Winsor has computer-drawn the new illustrations for this edition. K. V. Gardner and F. A. Keltie assisted in the tasks of manuscript preparation. G. R. S. is an International Research Scholar of the Howard Hughes Medical Institute.

The poem ''Heredity'' is reproduced with the kind permission of Meg Campbell and the editor of the *New Zealand Listener*.

BASIC CONCEPTS

Elements of Medical Cytogenetics

Chromosomes were first seen and named in the 19th century. *Chromosome* is a combination of Greek words meaning "colored body". It was early appreciated that these brightly staining objects appearing in the cell nucleus must be the "stuff of heredity," the very vessels of our genetic inheritance. But not until 1956, following a serendipitous laboratory error (cells washed in an overly hypotonic solution) that had a fortunate technical consequence, was it possible to get a clear look at human chromosomes (Hsu, 1979). Three years later came the first demonstration of a medical application, with Dr. Jérôme Lejeune's discovery of the extra chromosome in Down syndrome (Lejeune et al., 1959), and this was followed shortly by the recognition of the other major aneuploidy syndromes. Thereafter, medical cytogenetics evolved into a practice in its own right, and it is now a well-established and mainstream medical and laboratory discipline.

"Colored bodies" has become, in the late 20th century, an especially apt derivation. New staining techniques can show different parts of chromosomes in many different colors (even computer-generated false colors), and the images produced by this kaleidoscopic karyotyping can be rather beautiful. Black and white photographs are less splendid but usually suffice (Figure 1–1).

Chromosomal Morphology

Chromosomes have a linear appearance: two *arms* that are continuous at the *centromere*. The shorter arm is designated **p** (for petit) and the longer is **q** (next letter in the alphabet). In the early part of the cell cycle, each chromosome is present as a single structure, a chromatid. During the cell cycle (Figure 1–2) the chromosomes replicate, and two *sister chromatids* form. Now the chromosome exists as a double-chromatid entity. Each chromatid contains exactly the same genetic material. This replication is in preparation for cell division so that, after the chromosome has separated into its two component chromatids, each daughter cell receives the full amount of genetic material. It is during mitosis that the

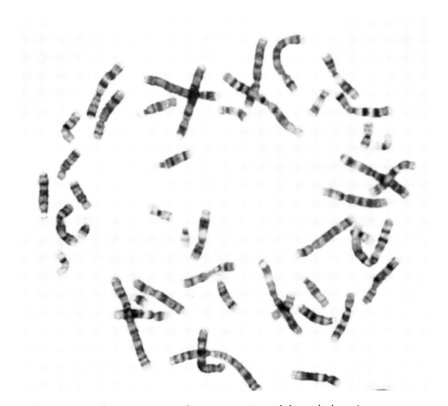

FIGURE 1–1. Chromosomes as they appear viewed through the microscope.

chromosomes contract and become readily distinguishable. (At other times in the cell cycle, chromosomes are attenuated and not analyzable.) Routine cytogenetic analysis is done on mitotic cells, usually obtained from blood. Blood lymphocytes have two convenient properties for the cytogeneticist: they are easily obtained and easily stimulated to go into mitosis. The chromosomes of the small number of lymphocytes studied are taken as representative of the chromosomal constitution of (essentially) every other cell of the body. In the case of prenatal diagnosis, the cells from amniotic fluid or chorionic villi are likewise assumed to represent the fetal chromosomal constitution.

The 46 chromosomes come in 23 matching pairs, and constitute the genome. One of each pair came from the mother, and one from the father. For 22 of the chromosome pairs, each member (each *homolog*) has the same morphology in each sex: these are the *autosomes*. The *sex chromosome* constitution differs: the female has a pair of X chromosomes, and the male has an X and a Y chromosome. The single set of homologs—one of each autosome plus one sex chromosome—is the *haploid* set. The haploid number (n) is 23. The haploid complement exists, as such, only in the gametocytes (ovum and sperm). All other cells in the body—the *soma*—have a double set: the *diploid* complement

(2n) of 46. If there is a difference between a pair of homologs, in the sense of one being structurally rearranged, the person is described as a *heterozygote*.

The chromosomes are distinguishable on the basis of their size, centromere position, and banding pattern. The centromere may be in the middle, off-center, or close to one end—metacentric, submetacentric, and acrocentric, respectively. Originally the chromosomes were assigned to groups A through G according to their general size and the position of the centromere. With banding, each chromosome is individually distinguishable. The diagrammatic representation of the banding pattern is the *ideogram* (Appendix A). The autosomes are numbered from largest to smallest, No. 1 through 22. (To split hairs, this order is not exact; for example, Nos. 10 and 11 are shorter than No. 12, and No. 21 is smaller than No. 22.) Certain parts of some chromosomes may show variation in the population. Increasing precision in banding (high-resolution banding) permits more and more subtle definition of the chromosome (Figure 1–3). Chromosomes are conventionally displayed cut out from a photograph and arranged as a "paste-up" with p arms upward, in their matching pairs. This is a *karyotype* (Figure 1–4). The word karyotype is also used in the general sense of "chromosomal constitution." Cytogeneticists describe karyotypes with a shorthand notation (ISCN 1995); an outline is given in Appendix B.

Chromosomal Structure and Function

The two chemical components of chromatin are DNA and protein. Proteins provide the scaffolding of the chromosome and are divided into histone and nonhistone proteins. Histones are strongly conserved DNA-associated proteins; the fact that they differ little between species such as ourselves and the sweet pea (for example) indicates how fundamentally important their role is in maintaining the integrity of the chromosome. Chromatin exists in differently condensed forms: the less condensed *euchromatin* and the more condensed *heterochromatin*. Euchromatin contains the coding DNA—the genes—while heterochromatin comprises noncoding DNA . Chromosomes are capped at the terminal extremities of their long and short arms by *telomeres*, specialized DNA sequences that can be thought of as sealing the chromatin and preventing its fusion with the chromatin of other chromosomes. The *centromere* is a specialized region of DNA which, at mitosis, provides the site at which the spindle apparatus can be anchored and draw each separated chromatid to opposite poles

   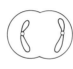 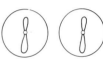

single chromatid chromosome   replication   separation at centromere   segregation of chromosomes   daughter cells

FIGURE 1–2. Outline of chromosome activity during the mitotic cycle.

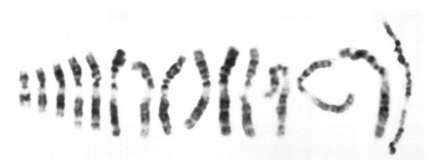

FIGURE 1–3.   Increasing resolution of banding (chromosome 11). (Courtesy D. R. Romain.)

of the dividing cell. Centromeric heterochromatin contains "satellite DNA," so-called because these DNA species have different buoyant densities and produce distinct humps on a density gradient distribution. (These are not to be confused with the satellites on acrocentric chromosomes.) The foregoing is only the barest outline: the interested reader is referred to Therman and Susman (1993) for a detailed treatment.

CHROMOSOME ABNORMALITY

Chromosomes are distributed to each daughter cell during cell division in a very precise process. It is prone to error. From our perspective, the two cell divisions of *meiosis*, during which the gametes are formed, are particularly important. Most of the discipline of medical cytogenetics focuses on the consequences of disordered meiosis having produced a chromosomally abnormal gamete, causing a chromosomal abnormality in the *conceptus*. A chromosome abnormality that is present from conception and involves the entire body is a *constitutional abnormality*. If an additional cell line with a different cytogenetic complement arises before the basis of the body structure is formed (i.e., in embryonic or pre-embryonic life) and becomes an integral part of the organism, *constitutional mosaicism* results. In this book we concern ourselves solely with constitutional abnormalities. Acquired chromosomal abnormality certainly exists, and indeed it is the major initiating cause in most cancers; but this is more the field of study of the molecular pathologist than the genetic counselor.

An incorrect amount of genetic material carried by the conceptus disturbs and distorts its normal growth pattern (from zygote → blastula → embryo → fetus). In *trisomy* there are three of a particular chromosome, instead of the normal two. In *monosomy* only one member of the pair is present. Two of each is the only combination that works properly! It is scarcely surprising that a process as exquisitely complex as the development of the human form should be vulnerable to a confused outflow of genetic instruction from a nucleus with a redundant or incomplete "database."

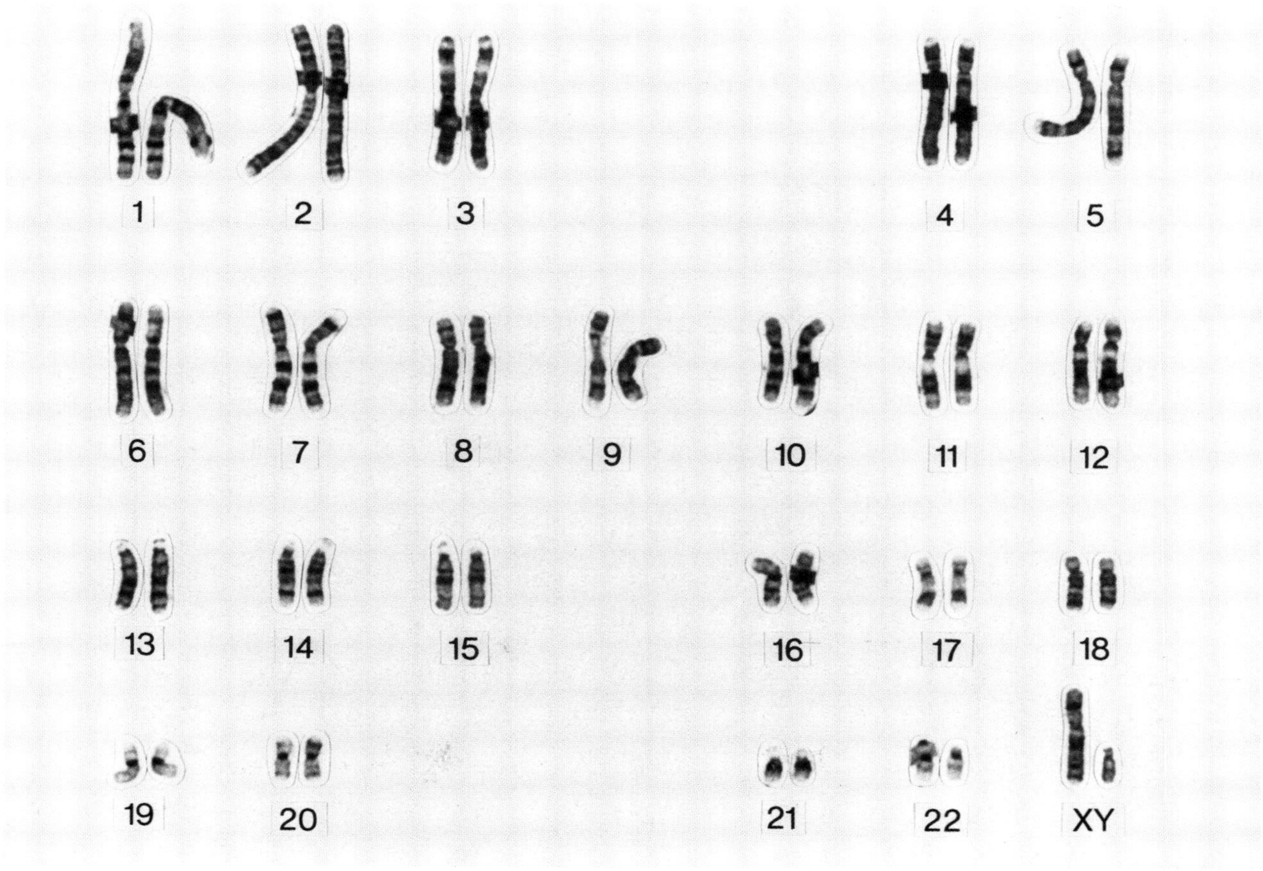

FIGURE 1–4. Chromosomes arranged in formal karyotype.

Table 1—1   The spectrum of effects, in broad outline, resulting from constitutional chromosomal abnormality

1. Devastation of blastogenesis, with transient implantation or nonimplantation of the conceptus
2. Devastation of embryogenesis, with spontaneous abortion, usually in the first trimester
3. Major disruption of normal intrauterine morphogenesis, with stillbirth or early neonatal death
4. Major disruption of normal intrauterine morphogenesis, but with some extrauterine survival
5. Moderate distortion of normal intrauterine development, with substantial extrauterine survival
6. Mild distortion of normal intrauterine development, with substantial extrauterine survival
7. Minimal or no discernible phenotypic effect

Autosomal Imbalance

Structural Imbalance

Imbalance may involve the gain or loss of a whole chromosome—*full* (or *pure*) *aneuploidy*—or of part of a chromosome—*partial aneuploidy*. The abnormality may occur in the nonmosaic or mosaic state. Loss (i.e., monosomy) of chromosomal material generally has a more devastating effect on growth of the conceptus than does an excess of material (i.e., trisomy). Certain imbalances lead to certain abnormal phenotypes. The spectrum is listed in outline in Table 1–1 and in some detail in Table 1–2. Most full autosomal trisomies and virtually all full autosomal monosomies set development of the conceptus so awry that, sooner or later, abortion occurs—the embryo ''self-destructs'' and is expelled from the uterus. This issue is further explored in Chapter 20. A few full trisomies are not necessarily lethal in utero, and many partial chromosomal aneuploidies are associated with survival through to the birth of an infant.

Characteristically, ''survivable imbalances'' produce a phenotype of widespread dysmorphogenesis, and there may be malformation of internal organs and limbs. It is often in the facial appearance (''*facies*'') that the most specific physical abnormality is seen. The most complex organ of all, the brain, is the most vulnerable to a less than optimal genetic constitution; and some compromise of mental and intellectual functioning, usually to the extent of an obvious deficit, is an almost invariable feature. Thus, the central concern of most people seeking genetic counseling for a chromosomal condition is the fear of having a physically and mentally handicapped child.

Functional Imbalance

A correct amount of chromatin does not necessarily mean the phenotype will be normal. Inappropriate inactivation, or activation, of a segment of the genome can distort the genetic message. Some segments of the genome require only monosomic expression, and the homologous segment on the other chromosome is inactivated. If this control fails, both segments can become activated, or both inactivated; and the over- or underexpression of the contained loci can cause phenotypic abnormality. The classic example of this is genomic imprinting according to parent of origin, and we discuss this concept in Chapters 2 and 17. A rather specialized example arises with the X-autosome translocation. A seg-

Table 1—2 The impact of constitutional chromosomal abnormality on human mortality and morbidity[a]

Conceptuses or individuals with:		Proportion with cytogenetic abnormality:
1. "Occult abortion" (early embryonic death in unrecognized pregnancies)		Unknown, perhaps 33–67%
2. Miscarriage (recognized embryonic and fetal death, ≥5 weeks' gestation)		About 30% total. Rate varies from 50% at 8–11 weeks to about 5% in stillbirths (≥28 weeks)
3. Infant and childhood deaths		5–7%
4. Structural congenital malformations		4–8%
5. Congenital heart defects		13%
6. Multiple (3 or more) birth defects and mental retardation		5.5%
7. Mental retardation (excluding fragile X)	IQ < 20	? 3–10%
	IQ 20–49	12–35%
	IQ 50–69	? 3%
8. Other neurodevelopmental disability		? 1–3%
9. Criminality (defined by presence in security setting)	Males in "ordinary" prisons	0.8%
	Psychopaths, retarded criminals (male)	3.0%
	Females in prison	0.4%
10. Male infertility		2% (15% in those with azoospermia)
11. Defect in sexual differentiation (male)		<25%
12. True hermaphroditism		25%
13. Defect in pubertal development (female)		27%
14. Primary ovarian deficiency		65%
15. Multiple miscarriage		2–5%

[a]The contribution of FISH-detected deletions not included.
Source: From Hook (1992).

ment of X chromosome can fail to be inactivated, or X-inactivation can spread into an autosomal segment (Chapter 5).

Sex Chromosomal Abnormality

Sex chromosome imbalance has a much less deleterious effect on the phenotype than does autosomal aneuploidy. In both male and female, one and only one completely active X chromosome is needed. X chromosomes in excess of one are almost wholly inactivated, as the normal 46,XX female exemplifies. With X-chromosome excess or deficiency, a partially successful buffering mechanism exists in which the imbalance is counteracted in an attempt to achieve the effect of a single active X. Excess whole X chromosomes are inactivated; abnormal

X chromosomes are selectively inactivated to leave the normal X as the active one; and if in the female one X is missing, the single X remaining is not subject to inactivation. In X imbalance, the reproductive tract and brain are predominantly affected. The effect may be minimal. As for Y chromosome excess, there is a rather limited phenotypic consequence, because this chromosome is composed largely of constitutively inactive material.

The fragile X syndromes concern, obviously enough, a sex chromosome. They "began life," as their names attest, as cytogenetic abnormalities but are now seen largely as single gene disorders, testable by molecular methodology. Nevertheless, their cytogenetic patrimony is necessary knowledge for the counselor, and it remains perfectly appropriate that we continue to include the fragile X syndromes in this book.

The Frequency and Impact of Cytogenetic Pathology

According to the window of observation, chromosomal disorders make a greater or lesser contribution to human mortality and morbidity. Looking at prenatal existence, chromosomal mortality is very high, and aneuploidy is the major single cause of spontaneous abortion. Perinatal and early infant death has a significant chromosomal component, of which trisomies 18 and 21 are the major contributors. As for morbidity, chromosomal defects are the basis of a substantial fraction of all intellectual deficit, and many of these retarded individuals will also have structural malformations that cause functional physical disability. Adolescence is a period in which many sex chromosome defects come to light, when pubertal change fails to occur; and in young adulthood, chromosomal causes of infertility are recognized. Few new cytogenetic defects come to attention later in adult life, but many retarded children survive well into adulthood and some into old age, and some require life-long care from their families or from the state. This latter group impose a considerable emotional and financial burden. While some parents and carers declare the emotional return they have from looking after these individuals, for others this responsibility may be a source of continuing, if attenuated, unresolved grief.

Hook (1992) has summarized the categories of cytogenetic pathology and their impact, and we have reproduced his synopsis in Table 1–2. In Table 1–3 we set out the birth incidence of the various categories of chromosomal abnormality. Overall, 1 in 120 liveborn babies has a chromosomal abnormality, and about half of these are phenotypically abnormal due to the chromosome defect. If we were to look at 10-day blastocysts, the fraction might be 1 in 4. If we studied a population of 70-year-olds, we could expect to see very few individuals with an unbalanced autosomal karyotype. The finer the cytogenetic focus, the greater the incidence: with the highest resolution banding and the application of molecular methodologies, some previously unrecognized defects would be included (Lamb et al., 1989; Flint et al., 1995).

Table 1—3 The frequency of chromosome abnormality in newborns

Autosomal trisomy	13	0.08‰ ⎫	
	18	0.15 ⎬	1.4‰
	21	1.2 ⎭	
Triploidy			0.02
Sex chromosome aneuploidy, male	XXY	1.2 ⎫	
	XYY	1.2 ⎬	2.5
	other	0.15 ⎭	
Sex chromosome aneuploidy, female	45,X	0.3 ⎫	
	and X/XX	⎬	1.4
	XXX	1.1 ⎭	
Structural rearrangement, unbalanced, $2n=46$			0.3
Extra structurally abnormal chromosome, $2n=47$			0.4
Total unbalanced (averaged for both sexes)			4.0‰
			(1 in 250)
Structural rearrangement, balanced	rcp	2.5‰ ⎫	
	rob	1.0 ⎬	4.3‰
	inv peri	0.8 ⎭	
Total			8.3‰
			(1 in 120)

Source: From Hook (1992) (nonbanded data) and Jacobs et al. (1992) (moderate level banding data). Rates are per thousand.

LOOKING AT CHROMOSOMES

Chromosomes are analyzed in the cytogenetics laboratory under the light microscope at a magnification of about $1000\times$. The chromosomes must be stained to be visible, and many staining techniques are available to demonstrate different features of the chromosome (Holmquist, 1992). Only a small number of these are in routine use. These are the main methods and their uses:

1. *Plain staining.* Many histologic stains, including Giemsa, orcein, and Leishman stains, will stain chromosomes uniformly. Until the early 1970s these were the only stains available. Plain staining continues to have a role and is particularly applicable in the study of fragile sites and deletions of chromosomes with small short arms, notably chromosome 18.

2. *Giemsa or G-banding.* This is the main staining method in use in routine clinical cytogenetics. It allows for precise identification of every chromosome and for the detection and delineation of structural abnormalities. Its precision is increased by manipulations designed to arrest the chromosome in its more elongated state at early metaphase or prometaphase—high-resolution banding. Alternative methods to demonstrate essentially the same morphology are quinacrine or Q-banding (see method 6) and reverse or R-banding. In R-banded chromosomes the palely staining regions seen in G-banding stain darkly, and vice versa.

3. *Centromere or C-banding.* This technique stains constitutive heterochro-

matin—the centromeric heterochromatin, some of the material on the short arms of the acrocentric chromosomes, and the distal part of the long arm of the Y chromosome. Constitutive heterochromatin, by definition, has no phenotypic effect. Variation in the amount of C-band positive material is of no clinical significance.

4. *Replication banding.* This technique is used primarily to identify inactive X chromatin. A nucleotide analog (bromodeoxyuridine, BrdU) is added either as a pulse at the beginning or toward the end of the cell cycle to allow the cytogenetic distinction of chromatin that replicates early from that (for example, the facultative heterochromatin of the inactivated X) which replicates late. It produces a banding pattern similar to that of R-banding.

5. *NOR (silver) staining.* The nucleolar organizing regions (NORs) contain multiple copies of genes coding for rRNA and are sited on the satellite stalks of the acrocentric chromosomes. Those that actively produce rRNA stain black with silver nitrate. Silver (Ag) staining can be used in characterization of small marker chromosomes and in translocations involving the short arms of the acrocentric chromosomes.

6. *Quinacrine or Q-banding.* Chromosomes stained with quinacrine (and with a variety of other fluorochromes) and examined after illumination with ultraviolet (UV) light have a pattern of bands similar to that seen in G-banding. It also has a role in identifying normal variation with respect to differential fluorescence. A particularly significant use is in examining abnormal Y chromosomes, because the long arm of the Y stains intensely with quinacrine. Quinacrine may also be used to identify the Y chromosome(s) in interphase nuclei (equivalent to the Barr body test for X chromatin, described on p. 192). But (like the Barr body test) the technique is not sufficiently precise to determine the sex chromosome complement in the clinical setting.

7. *Distamycin* A/DAPI *staining.* This fluorescent stain identifies the heterochromatin of chromosomes 1, 9, 15, 16, and Y. Its major usefulness is in distinguishing the inverted duplication 15 chromosome (p. 264) from other small marker chromosomes.

8. *Fluorescence in situ hybridization (FISH).* The major cytogenetic advance of the 1990s has been the ability to identify specific chromosomes and parts of chromosomes by in situ hybridization with labeled probes. The hybridization method may be direct or indirect. Direct attachment of a detectable molecule (e.g., a fluorophore) to the probe DNA enables microscopic visualization immediately after its hybridization to the target DNA in the chromosome. The more sensitive indirect procedure requires special modification of the probe with a hapten detectable by affinity cytochemistry. The most popular are the biotin-avidin and digoxigenin systems. By using combinations of biotin-, digoxigenin-, and fluorophor-labeled probes, multiple simultaneous hybridizations can be done to localize different chromosomal regions in one preparation (multicolor FISH). Probes may be prepared from individual chromosome libraries (''paints'') and used to detect complete or partial aneuploidies. Cosmid probes may be prepared from the actual chromosomal regions involved in microdeletions or microduplications.

Chromosomes stained by various techniques are illustrated in Figure 1–5.

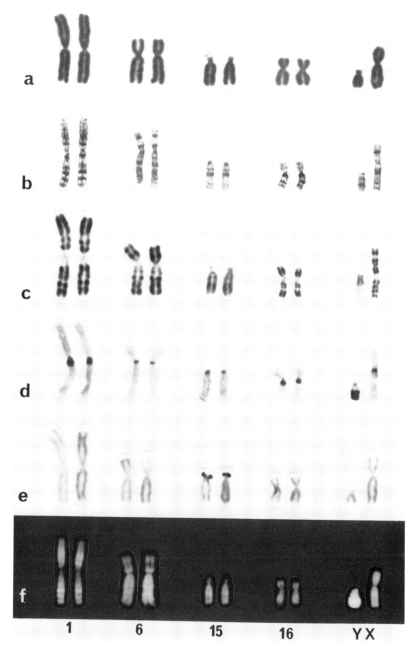

FIGURE 1–5. Chromosome pairs 1, 6, 15, 16, and Y and X stained by various techniques: plain stain *(a)*, G-banding *(b)*, replication banding *(c)*, C-banding *(d)*, Ag-NOR stain *(e)*, and Q-banding *(f)*.

ETHICAL AND COUNSELING ISSUES

Our focus in this book is on the biology of chromosomal defects and the reproductive risks they may, or may not, entail. Certain bioethical issues that are
being more formally defined in the late 20th century, however, demand attention.
Counselors must hold fast to these requirements: that they act beneficently toward their clients, and that they strive to make their services accessible to those
who may need them.

Non-directive Counseling

In a Western ethos, the counselor is required to respect the autonomy of the
client, and this largely translates into the principle that counseling be nondirective. There is a fine line between directive and detached counseling, a point
nicely illustrated in Karp's (1983) deft essay ''The Terrible Question'' (required
reading for every counselor). Ingelfinger (1980) comments, admittedly in a
somewhat different context: ''A physician who merely spreads an array of vend-
ibles in front of the patient and then says, 'Go ahead and choose, it's your life,'
is guilty of shirking his duty, if not of malpractice.'' It is the skill of the counselor that enables clients to reach the (or a) decision that is, for them, the (or
a) right one, and for the clients to feel satisfied that they have done so. In other
societies, the perceived good of the group may carry more weight than the
professed wishes of the individual. The degree to which one society can seek
to influence practice in another is a matter of no little controversy (Lancet editorial, 1995).

"Guilt" in a Carrier

Some chromosomal diagnoses may be made in an older child or even an adult
while the parents will have held for years to the notion that obstetric misadven-
ture, or a virus, or some other blamable event was the cause of the child's
defects. Some people find it upsetting, even devastating, to have to readjust and
to know that they may have been the source of the abnormality. They are likely to use words like ''guilt,'' ''blame,'' and ''fault.'' Helping these people adjust
to the new knowledge is the counselor's challenge.

Mental Retardation and Genetic Abortion

Intellectual deficiency is a defect for which many parents are unwilling to accept
a significant recurrence risk, hardly remarkable since intellectual function is such
an obvious attribute of humanness. The great majority of those who choose to
have prenatal diagnosis opt for pregnancy termination if a chromosomal condition implying major mental defect is identified. In a French series of trisomy
21 diagnosed prenatally and postnatally over 1984–1990 in the Marseille district,
all of the 76 cases of prenatal diagnosis were followed by abortion (Julian-
Reynier et al., 1995). Some for whom abortion is not acceptable may neverthe-

less choose prenatal diagnosis for reassurance, or for the preparedness that certain knowledge can allow. Community views on mental handicap are changing and the late 20th century has seen something of an exodus from institutions and from special schools as the mentally and psychologically disabled join the "mainstream," some more successfully than others. Counselors need to handle the tension inherent in these views and the views of parents who want to avoid having a handicapped child, and the separate conflict that parents experience when a decision is taken to terminate an otherwise wanted pregnancy. As we discuss above, the doctrine of nondirective counseling is a central tenet of modern practice; and it is a test of counselors' professionalism that their own views not unduly influence the advice and counsel that they give. Renaud et al. (1993) canvass issues and implications of genetic termination. Brock (1995) discusses the philosophy of "wrongful handicap," addressing the esoteric issue of whether *not* producing a child who would suffer has harmed that potential child, and enunciates a principle that "individuals are morally required not to let any possible child for whose welfare they are responsible experience serious suffering or limited opportunity if they can act so that, without imposing substantial burdens or costs on themselves or others, any alternative possible child for whose welfare they would be responsible will not experience serious suffering or limited opportunity."

Pregnancy and the Mentally Retarded

One issue that scarcely was an issue at the outset of the discipline, but which now looms quite significantly, is that of the rights of the intellectually handicapped to have children (Elkins et al., 1986a). What of the person with Down syndrome, or some partial trisomy compatible with fertility, in whom a question of procreation arises? Zühlke et al. (1994) give a recent example in describing a man with Down syndrome living in special local authority housing who developed a relationship with a mentally retarded girl living in the same house. She requested removal of an intrauterine contraceptive device, became pregnant, and the normal baby is being brought up by the maternal grandmother. On the one hand, the right of the handicapped person to experience parenthood is debated; and the American Academy of Pediatrics (1990) expressed reservation about the sterilization of intellectually handicapped women on the basis of anticipated hardship to others. On the other hand, Gillon (1987) notes that normal people have the option of being sterilized, and the mentally handicapped should have the same right. The Law Lords in Great Britain concur that sterilization may be in the best interest of the handicapped person herself (Brahams, 1987). Many parents or guardians, not wishing to become "parental grandparents," favor sterilization. Some regard hysterectomy as having the double benefit of ensuring sterility and facilitating personal hygiene; others consider only reversible contraception to be acceptable. The High Court of Australia decided in 1992 that the parents of a handicapped child cannot themselves lawfully allow sterilization, but that a court authorization is required, and noted that this requirement ". . . ensures a hearing from those experienced in different ways in the care of those with intellectual disability and from those with experience of the long term social and psychological effects of sterilization'' (Monahan, 1992).

When a retarded woman with a chromosomal defect is pregnant, or is pregnant by a retarded man, one or other of the couple having an unbalanced karyotype, and the pregnancy is recognized in time, some would propose the grounds for termination to be substantial. The ethical issue arises over the difficulty (or impossibility) of securing the woman's informed consent versus the expressed wishes of her guardians. Martínez et al. (1993) report from Alabama a mother with cri du chat syndrome, who was severely retarded and had no speech, and who was pregnant by an unknown male, and ''although pregnancy termination had been desired by the patient's grandmother, social and legal limitations prevented access to this procedure.'' Some less severely affected persons (if they are able to grasp the issue) may not regard it as undesirable to have a child like themselves; on the other hand, they may have the insight to recognize their own deficiency and not wish to pass it on. We may perhaps read this into the brief report of Bobrow et al. (1992) of a man with Down syndrome fathering a child, the mother having had first-trimester prenatal diagnosis. (The baby was normal.) There is the concept of imagining what a retarded person would want, were they intellectually competent to make a decision; a concept some would regard as paternalistic (and infringing personal autonomy), and which others see as valid. The sociology rather than the biology will exercise the counselor's mettle in this uncommonly encountered situation.

The other party is the child. What of a normal child born, say, to a man mosaic for a dup(10)(p13p14) chromosome and a mother with idiopathic mental defect? How can the interests of the child and of the parents be resolved? This is an actual case that we have seen: it was quite poignant as this mildly retarded man, who had some insight into his own handicap, struggled to understand how best he might be a father to his 46,XX baby, and expressed sadness at the abnormal behavior displayed by his older (nonmosaic) 46,XY,dup(10) child. The capable and willing grandmother stepped into the breach; but when the daughter is older, and assuming she is of normal intelligence, how will the realization of her parents' abnormality affect her? Whether a normal child in this sort of setting has a legal claim for ''dissatisfied life'' (Shaw, 1984) is an intriguing and as yet untested notion.

Testing Children

To state the obvious, familial rearrangements are familial. It is natural that parents would be concerned whether children they already have might be carriers, once an abnormality has been identified in one of them. Children, certainly, need to know their carrier status, sooner or later; it would be unfortunate if a failure to transmit information led to more affected babies unknowingly being born elsewhere in the family. Genetic counselors are attuned to the principle of not taking away a child's right to make, in the fullness of time, their own informed decision to learn about genetic risks they may face: the experience with Huntington disease (HD) has brought these issues into sharp focus. While a translocation is different from an HD gene in that it will have no influence upon a person's physical health other than their reproductive health, there do remain issues of potential damage to a child's self-esteem, distortion of the family's perceptions of the child, and adverse effects upon the child's capacity to form future relationships (Clarke et al., 1994). Clayton (1995) comments that there is the possibility of conflict with parents, as physicians come increasingly to act as advocates for the child's interests, but notes further that "children are generally ill-served if their parents feel they have not been listened to"; she also draws the conclusion that, at least in the American context, this is a medico-ethical rather than a medico-legal issue.

Our own view is that, these issues having been canvassed, acquiescence to a parental request to test a young child may, in some circumstances, be reasonable. (Many, of course, will have had a prenatal karyotype from amniocentesis or chorionic villus sampling; and it may not seem entirely logical to decline to test a postnatal child.) Either the parent's mind is set at rest or they know of the need to raise the issue with the child at a "suitable age," which should be with the assistance of the genetic counseling clinic. The task for the counselor is to assist parents in deciding what age would be suitable for their child, and to convey the information in such a way that concern for the future is kept in perspective, and the child's self-confidence is kept intact. The Genetic Interest Group in the U.K. gently chides the profession in commenting that "the vast majority of people are better able to understand the implications than they are often given credit for", and has enunciated the following principle: "After suit-able counselling, parents have the right to make an informed choice about whether or not to have their children tested for carrier status. Ideally, children should only be tested when of an age to be involved in the decision" (Dalby, 1995a). The debate continues (Michie and Marteau, 1995; Dalby, 1995b).

Family Studies

More widely, the parents' siblings and cousins could be carriers. Grandparental karyotypes may be useful in knowing which branch of a family to follow. The rights of individuals could, potentially, clash with the obligation that flows from belonging to a family: "no man is an island, entire unto himself'', and some may see altruism as a duty. If counselors take pains to provide clear information and to do so sensitively, such studies should proceed without unfortunate con-sequence.

Access to Prenatal Diagnostic Services

It would not, at the present writing, be economically feasible to make prenatal diagnosis available to every pregnant woman. Even among those for whom testing is, in principle, freely available, a fraction will not present, either because they are opposed to abortion or because they have not been informed about or have not understood the issues involved (Halliday et al., 1995a). Those who can afford it and who do not meet criteria (essentially maternal age) for acceptance in the public system may have the privilege of access to private testing. Mass screening methodologies (Chapter 21) may bypass the inequity inherent in the public/private dichotomy. Mehlman et al. (1994) discuss more general issues of accessibility to genetic medicine.

2

The Origins and Consequences of Chromosome Pathology

"What went wrong? And will it happen again?" These are the common questions that bring people from "chromosomal families" to the genetic clinic. We can recast these questions: "Did I, or one of us, produce an abnormal gamete? If so, why? What gamete might be produced next time? Or, if the chromosomes were normal at conception, what went wrong thereafter?" To deal intelligently with the client's questions, the counselor needs a broad knowledge of how gametes form, how chromosomes behave, and how the early conceptus grows. We consider the distinction between abnormality due to structural defect (full or partial aneuploidy) and that due to functional defect (activation or imprinting status). Most of the clinical pathology that counselors see will have arisen from errors during formation of the germ cells, and we focus particularly upon meiosis, the specialized cell division of gametogenesis. Chromosome defects can arise postzygotically, and abnormalities of mitotic cell division in the pre-embryo and embryo can produce chromosome mosaicism. We review the possible consequences of this. We refer in passing to the concept of dynamic mutation, but leave its full discussion for the fragile X chapter.

Firstly, we look at *etiology*. We discuss three chromosomal settings within which genetic abnormality may arise, namely meiosis, mitosis, and genomic imprinting, and we note also the special category of trinucleotide-repeat transmission. Within each, we consider what types of abnormality may occur. In meiosis and mitosis, nondisjunction and anaphase lag can produce aneuploidy for a whole chromosome; and asymmetric segregation of a structural rearrangement produces an incorrect amount of only part of a chromosome (partial aneuploidy). In genomic imprinting, the defect is qualitative, with abnormal expression of what can be a normal amount of chromosome. Sometimes there is overlap: for example, a meiotic error can subsequently lead to an abnormality of imprinting. Sometimes we cannot be sure which is the correct category: a supposed meiotic error, for example, could actually have arisen in a premeiotic mitosis. Nevertheless, this format is not too arbitrary, and provides a useful framework within which the generality of chromosomal abnormality can be appreciated. Secondly, we consider *pathogenesis*: the process by which the underlying genetic defect then leads to phenotypic abnormality. Thirdly, we make some general comments about which categories of abnormality are likely to recur, and those for which sporadic occurrence is the rule.

MECHANISMS THAT PRODUCE GENETIC ABNORMALITY, AND SETTINGS IN WHICH THEY ARISE

MEIOSIS

Meiosis in Chromosomally Normal Persons

The purpose of meiosis is to achieve the reduction from the diploid state of the gonadal stem cell ($2n = 46$) to the haploid complement of the normal gamete ($n = 23$), and to ensure genetic variation in the gametes. The latter requirement is met in that meiosis enables the independent assortment of homologs (the physical basis of Mendel's second law) and provides a setting for recombination between homologs. While we do not dwell on recombination per se, this is a raison d'être of the chromosome to the molecular geneticist: "from the long perspective of evolution, a chromosome is a bird of passage, a temporary association of particular alleles" (Lewin, 1994).

The mature gamete is produced after the two meiotic cell divisions: meiosis I and meiosis II (Figure 2–1). In meiosis I, the primary gametocyte (oocyte or spermatocyte) gives rise to two secondary gametocytes, each with 23 chromosomes. These chromosomes have not divided, and they remain in the double-chromatid state. In meiosis II, the chromosomes of the secondary gametocyte separate into their component chromatids, and the daughter cells produced are either the mature ovum and its polar bodies, or four spermatids, which mature into spermatozoa. Each gamete contains a haploid set of chromosomes. The diploid complement is restored at conception with the union of two haploid gametes (Figure 2–2).

Note that spermatogenesis divides the cytoplasm evenly, so that after meiosis II there are four gametes of equal size. The sperm head that penetrates the ovum comprises virtually entirely nuclear material; the tail is cast off. In oogenesis cytoplasmic division is uneven, producing a secondary oocyte and first polar body after meiosis I and the mature ovum and second polar bodies after meiosis II. The ovum and its polar bodies each contain a haploid chromosome set, but the ovum keeps almost all of the cytoplasm.[1] Another major sex difference concerns the timing of the gamete's maturation. In the female, meiosis is partway through, in the late prophase of meiosis I, by the eighth month of intra-uterine life. At birth, there are around 3,000,000 oocytes. Most of these disappear, but those destined to mature stay in a "frame-freeze" until they enter ovulation, some 10 to 50 years thereafter, and meiosis continues. Testicular stem

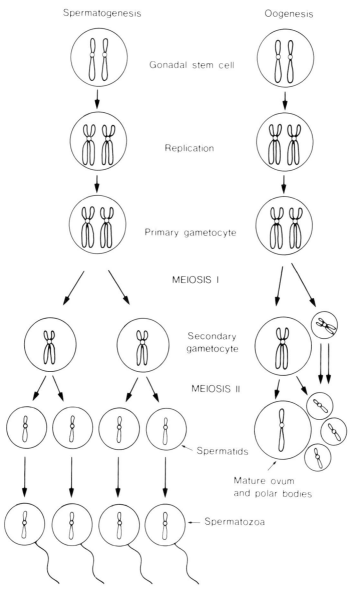

FIGURE 2–1. Outline of chromosomal behavior and distribution during gameto-genesis.

cells, on the other hand, do not begin to enter meiosis until the onset of puberty. Thereafter, millions of mature sperm are continuously produced.

We now examine more closely the details of meiosis. As they enter the mei-otic cell cycle, the homologous pairs of chromosomes have replicated their DNA to change from the single-chromatid to the double-chromatid stage (Figure 2–3a). Then, as meiosis I proceeds to prophase, chromosomes conduct a "ho-

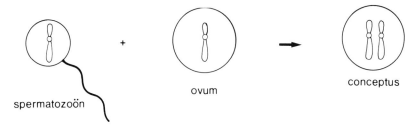

spermatozoön

ovum

conceptus

FIGURE 2–2. Haploid gametes producing the diploid conceptus.

mology search'' and come together and pair, with matching loci alongside each other (Figure 2–3b). It may be that this process is facilitated by special anchor points, such as the *Alu* family of repeats, existing along the lengths of the chromatids, which comprise common sequences of DNA that can attach by mutual recognition (Chandley, 1989). The cell now enters the pachytene phase, and the chromosomes pair more intimately. This is the process of *synapsis*, with the formation of the *synaptonemal complex*. The paired chromosomes themselves are called *bivalents.*[2] Synapsis sets the stage for an exchange of matching chromosome segments[3]: this is the process of *recombination*, or *crossing-over* (Figure 2–3c). Next, desynapsis occurs (the diplotene stage), with dissociation of the synaptonemal complex and the formation of chiasmata. Now, the two homologs *disjoin* and go to opposite poles of the cell. This is the anaphase stage; the orderly movement of chromosomes during this sequence is facilitated if synapsis, recombination, and chiasmata formation have proceeded normally. Finally, the cell divides into the two daughter cells (Figure 2–3d). How the chromosomes are distributed—which chromosome goes to which pole—is called *segregation*. Normally, each daughter cell gets one of each of the pair of chromosomes, and this is referred to as one-to-one (1:1) segregation. Uniquely in this cell division, daughter cells are produced with double-chromatid chromosomes.

These cells then enter meiosis II. In this cycle, the chromosomes do not replicate, because they are already in the double-chromatid state. The chromosomes separate at the centromere, and the resulting single-chromatid chromosomes disjoin, one going to each pole, as in a mitotic division (Figure 2–3e). In oogenesis, meiosis II is completed only after fertilization occurs. Chromosomal pathology arises when these processes of disjunction and segregation go wrong—*non*disjunction and *mal*segregation.

Meiosis in Chromosomally Abnormal Persons

Two main categories fall under this heading. The first, and by far the most important, is the phenotypically normal person heterozygous for a balanced structural rearrangement (translocation, inversion, and insertion being the major forms). Second, there is the rare instance of persons who are themselves chromosomally unbalanced with either a full or a partial aneuploidy, and thus phenotypically abnormal, and who present with questions of their reproductive potential. We will deal in detail with each situation in separate chapters, but consider the broad principles here.

Balanced Carriers

In heterozygotes for some balanced rearrangements involving only small segments, the chromosomes may "ignore" the nonhomologous material they contain and pair ("heterosynapsis") and segregate much as would happen at a normal meiosis. In other balanced rearrangements, the inherent tendency to pairing dictates that homologous segments of rearranged chromosomes will align, as much as is possible ("homosynapsis"). This may require the chromosome to be something of a contortionist, forming complex configurations such as multivalents and reversed loops. According to either scenario, the stage is set for the possibility of unbalanced segregation. The gametes produced—and therefore the conceptuses that arise—are frequently unbalanced. In this context a *partial* aneuploidy is usually involved, that is, a part of a chromosome is present in the trisomic or monosomic state; or, frequently, a combination of

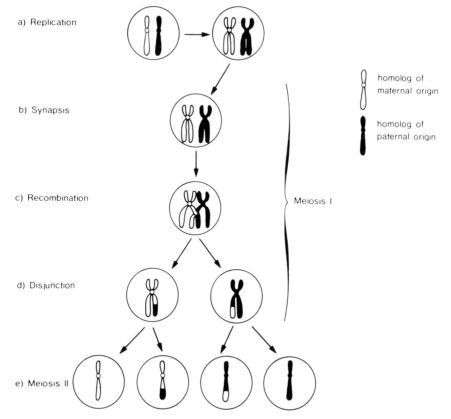

a) Replication

b) Synapsis

c) Recombination

d) Disjunction

e) Meiosis II

Meiosis I

homolog of
maternal origin

homolog of
paternal origin

FIGURE 2–3. Closer detail of chromosomal behavior during meiosis. One crossover has occurred between the long arms of one chromatid of each homolog.

trisomy for one segment and monosomy for another. Partial trisomy and partial monosomy are also referred to as *duplication* and *deletion*, respectively.

In some rearrangements, recombination presents a further hazard. Inversions and insertions may produce a new *recombinant* (rec) chromosome that has a different genetic composition from that of the original rearrangement. A conceptus would inevitably be genetically unbalanced.

> Gametogenesis in the male heterozygote for a balanced rearrangement appears more vulnerable than in the female to the complexities imposed by a chromosomal abnormality, and infertility occasionally results. An important element in this male vulnerability may be the integrity at meiosis of the X–Y bivalent, synapsing and recombining at the pseudoautosomal regions at the tips of Xp and Yp (Hale, 1994). Unpaired autosomal segments, particularly of acrocentric autosomes, might disturb this integrity (Luciani et al., 1987; Johannisson et al., 1987; Guichaoua et al., 1990), leading to disruption of spermatogenesis. Another element may be impaired synapsis of homologous segments in the normal and the rearranged chromosomes (Saadallah and Hultén, 1985; Chandley et al., 1986, 1987; Hale, 1994), which of itself prevents further progress in gametogenesis, and spermatogenesis may be more sensitive than oogenesis to this obstacle. Alternatively, the translocation jeopardizes the process before the gametocyte enters meiosis, and pairing failure is an effect rather than a cause (Mittwoch and Mahadevaiah, 1992).

Aneuploid Persons

In the individual who has a full aneuploidy, and in whom gametogenesis is able to proceed, in theory a trivalent may form, or a bivalent and an "independent" univalent. Either could lead, effectively, to a 2:1 segregation. This appears actually to be the case in trisomy 21, whereas in XXX and XYY, the "third" chromosome is, as it were, disposed of (see p. 193 and 195). In the person with a partial aneuploidy due to an unbalanced rearranged chromosome, whether 46,(abn) or 47,+(abn), the abnormal chromosome may have an even chance to be transmitted in the gamete, but the opportunity to observe such outcomes rather infrequently arises.

MITOSIS AND MOSAICISM

The purpose of a mitotic cell division is faithfully to pass on an intact and complete copy of the genome to the progeny cells. The mitotic cycle consists of the following sequence: gap-1 period (G1) $\rightarrow$ synthesis period (S) $\rightarrow$ gap-2 (G2) $\rightarrow$ cell division. The G1$\rightarrow$S$\rightarrow$G2 segments together comprise the interphase period of the cell cycle. During the S period of interphase the chromosomes replicate their DNA, thus converting from the single-chromatid to the double-chromatid state. (Since a single chromatid can be regarded as a complete chromosome, and each replicated homolog comprises two chromatids, with a pair of each of the 23 homologs, in one sense the cell at G2 has $23 \times 2 \times 2 = 92$ chromosomes.) Genetically active segments of chromosomes replicate earlier during the S period, while inactive segments, which include almost the entire inactivated X chromosome in the female, are late-replicating. The cell division period is further subdivided into prometaphase → metaphase → anaphase → telophase. The chromosomes condense to enter prometaphase, and condensation continues into metaphase. Metaphase chromosomes align on the equatorial plate, and the spindle apparatus becomes attached to the (bipartite) centromere of each chromosome. The chromatids of each chromosome then separate ("disjoin"), are drawn in opposite directions (anaphase), and arrive at the opposite poles of the cell (telophase). Then the nuclear membrane reconstitutes, the cytoplasm constricts and divides, and two daughter cells now exist.

A mitotic error can cause phenotypic abnormality by generating an abnormal cell line at some point during embryogenesis. If we focus on the end result, the feature distinguishing mitotic from meiotic errors is that the former usually produce a mosaic conceptus while meiotic errors produce a nonmosaic abnormality. We define chromosomal mosaicism[4] as the coexistence, within the one conceptus, of two or more distinct cell lines which are genetically identical except for the chromosomal difference between them, these cell lines having been established by the time that embryonic development is complete (the point at which the embryo becomes a fetus). Thus, the different cell lines are fixed in the individual, and are part of his or her chromosomal constitution. The earlier in embryogenesis that mitotic mutations occur the greater the likelihood for a substantial fraction of the soma to be aneuploid, leading to increasing departure from normality of the phenotype. It is probable that many mitotically arising abnormalities lead to cell death, leaving no trace.

Considering the enormous numbers of mitoses that proceed successfully, it is a robust mechanism. Rare instances of mitotic instability indicate the existence of control mechanisms in which error can occur, some at least of which may be genetically determined (Mikkelsen, 1966). Fitzgerald et al. (1986) describe a mother who had three trisomic 21 conceptions. Her own tissues (blood, skin) were mostly 46,XX, but some cells had a variety of aneuploidies (47,+21, 47,+18, 47,XXX), indicating a proneness to chromosome maldistribution apparently operating both in meiosis and mitosis. The fault may lie in premature centromere division (PCD). Miller et al. (1990) karyotyped a child because of major physical and neurodevelopmental defects, and he had cells trisomic and monosomic for almost every chromosome; only about a quarter were 46,XY. Tolmie et al. (1988) report abnormal siblings, one with 47,+18/46,N and the other trisomic for a variety of chromosomes including No. 18. Papi et al. (1989) describe sibs from a consanguineous union who had a range of aneuploidies in about a fifth of lymphocytes and fibroblasts; likewise Kher et al. (1994) report sisters both with 45,X/46,XX Turner syndrome. These several authors propose the existence of mutations in genes controlling cell division, the consequence of which may be the generation of somatic mosaic aneuploidy and recurring gonadal aneuploidy; the differences in the several cases above indicate the existence of numerous such genes. The quite common finding of loss of an X chromosome in an occasional cell in the normal female population (Horsman et al., 1987; Catalán et al., 1995) may reflect "normal" age-related anaphase lag, as may the similar loss of the Y chromosome in males (Kirk et al., 1994).

If we do a chromosome test on any normal person—a routine analysis from a sample of peripheral blood—we would probably get a normal result (46,N). We would conclude from an analysis of a dozen or so cells from one specialized tissue that the rest of the soma is also 46,N. In most of the person's tissue, this will be truly the case. But the body comprises a vast number of cells—a trillion (10^{12}) or so—which required a vast number of mitoses for their generation. The dozen cells checked in the laboratory are only a billionth of one percent (10^{-11}) of all the person's cells, and we routinely (and, for practical purposes, not unreasonably) regard this minute fraction as a valid representative of the remaining 99.999999999%. Notwithstanding, we can surely suppose that one or more errors will have happened, during one or some of the many mitoses, and these will have produced a chromosomally abnormal cell line and the person is really a chromosomal mosaic. It seems plausible to imagine that unrecognized islands of mosaicism, involving a tiny number of cells—only a few thousand or a few dozen, perhaps—could well be a fairly frequent state. Perhaps everyone is a mosaic.

One intriguing suggestion for the *meiotic* generation of mosaicism is a mechanism based on the "half-chromatid mutation" model (Cantu and Ruiz, 1986). A mutation, arising in meiosis, may involve just one DNA strand of a chromatid. This "mosaic chromosome" can be transmitted by the gamete. When it replicates, at the first mitosis of the zygote, it will give rise to daughter chromosomes which are different, and produce constitutional mosaicism.

Somatic Recombination

Genetic exchange can take place, as a normal event, during a mitotic cycle. Sister chromatid exchange is the exchange of homologous segments between the chromatids of one chromosome; the cytogenetic demonstration of this is rather dramatic (Figure 19–2). Exchange of segments can also take place between the pair of homologous chromosomes, as a presumably uncommon event.

NONDISJUNCTION

Nondisjunction in Meiosis

Nondisjunction is the failure of homologous chromosomes to segregate symmetrically at cell division. The classical description of the mechanism of meiotic nondisjunction is as follows. In a chromosomally normal person, if the pair of homologs comprising a bivalent at meiosis I fail to separate (fail to "disjoin"), one daughter cell will have two of the chromosomes and the other will have none. This is 2:0 segregation (Figures 2–4a and 2–5, left). In other words, one cell is disomic for that homolog, and the other is nullisomic. Nondisjunction may occur in meiosis II, meiosis I having proceeded normally: in this case, it is the chromatids that fail to separate (Figure 2–4b). From whichever scenario, at fertilization the conceptus ends up trisomic or monosomic, if the other gamete

a) Nondisjunction at meiosis I

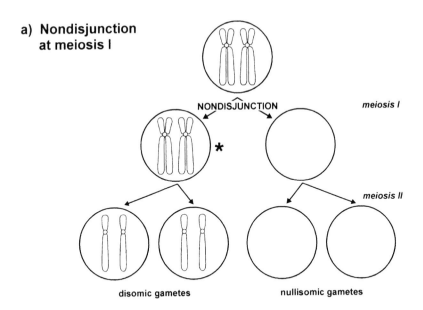

disomic gametes　　　　nullisomic gametes

b) Nondisjunction at meiosis II

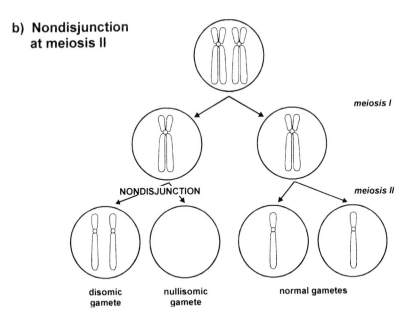

disomic gamete　　nullisomic gamete　　normal gametes

FIGURE 2–4. The classical view of the mechanics of nondisjunction. The asterisked gamete reflects the complement of the oocyte in FIGURE 2–5 (*left*).

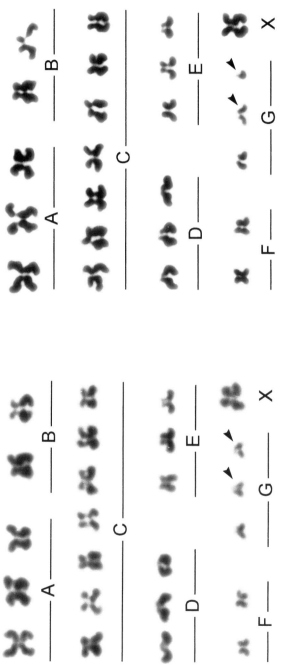

FIGURE 2-5. Oocytes at metaphase of meiosis II, showing nondisjunction of a G-group chromosome. *Left,* oocyte with classical nondisjunctional disomy, showing an additional G-group dyad. Possibly the arrowed pair are No. 21s. *Right,* oocyte with "predivisional" disomy, showing an additional G-group monad. The arrowed pair may be No. 21s. (From Kamiguchi et al., 1993; courtesy Y. Kamiguchi.)

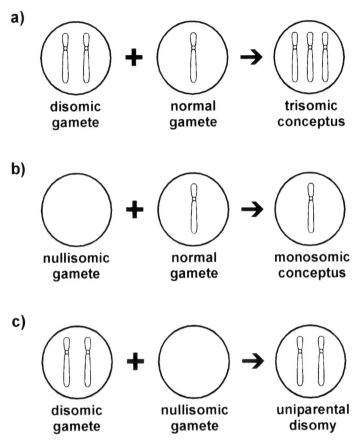

FIGURE 2–6. Aneuploid gametes producing an aneuploid conceptus (a and b), and aneuploid gametes producing uniparental disomy (c).

is normal (Figure 2–6a,b). Trisomy or monosomy in the offspring of normal parents is called primary trisomy or primary monosomy.

> Alternatively, the homologs may never have joined in the first place (and thus could not recombine; Sherman et al., 1991), and they then segregate at random 2:0, 1:1, and 0:2. The imbalance is perpetuated through meiosis II. To be pedantic, if the homologs had never joined together, they cannot disjoin. In that sense, nonconjugation might be a more accurate word than nondisjunction (Sturtevant and Beadle, 1962). If Angell's hypothesis (see below) is correct, predivision may be a proper word. Nonetheless, "nondisjunction" is well entrenched in the genetic lexicon, and its general meaning of "asymmetric segregation of homologous elements" well accepted.

Most meiotic nondisjunction occurs in oogenesis, at the first division. Direct analysis of oocytes suggests each of the 23 chromosome pairs has about an equal chance of undergoing segregation error (Kamiguchi et al., 1993). For the acrocentric chromosomes (Nos. 13–15, 21–22) about 90% of nondisjunctions are of maternal origin, and three-quarters of these arise at meiosis I (Zaragoza et al., 1994); the proportions for X nondisjunction causing 47,XXX are similar (MacDonald et al., 1994). In trisomy 16, the commonest recognized trisomy, maternal meiosis I nondisjunction accounts for all recorded cases (Hassold et al., 1991b). One predisposing mechanism at meiosis I may be an absence of recombination between homologs, with no chiasmata forming; in consequence, the stability of the bivalent on the metaphase plate is compromised, and both members of the bivalent pair may travel to the same pole ("nullichiasmate nondisjunction") (Sherman et al., 1994; MacDonald et al., 1994). Other mechanisms presumably exist. With trisomy 18, maternal meiotic II nondisjunctions are the major contributor (Fisher et al., 1995). Sequential nondisjunctions at both meiotic divisions could lead to tetrasomy, and this is the basis of some X chromosomal polysomy (Hassold et al., 1990; Deng et al., 1991). Simultaneous nondisjunctions of two chromosome pairs can lead to double aneuploidy, such as 48,XXX,+21 (Park et al., 1995). Retention of the polar body of the ovum, effectively a "complete nondisjunction," is one basis for triploidy (Martin et al., 1991).

In spermatogenesis, the 22 autosomes have about an equal likelihood of undergoing nondisjunction; the rate in sex chromosome segregation is greater (Martin and Rademaker, 1990). The second meiotic division is the site for most paternal acrocentric chromosome nondisjunction (Zaragoza et al., 1994) and also (obviously enough) for all nondisjunction that produces 24,YY sperm. About half of 47,XXY is due to nondisjunction in spermatogenesis, and this may have been the consequence of absence of X–Y recombination at meiosis I (MacDonald et al., 1994).

About 3–4% of sperm are aneuploid as a result of nondisjunction (Martin et al., 1991). The fraction in ova remains to be settled; it may be close to 10% (Kamiguchi et al., 1993) or 20% (Martin et al., 1991), or possibly a low rate rather similar to sperm (Hassold et al., 1993). A considerable proportion of human conceptions are aneuploid due to nondisjunction, but in utero selection means the proportion in term babies is much less. For example, as many as 1 in 150 conceptions may be trisomic 21, but the birth incidence is a quarter of this, about 1 in 600 (Sherman et al., 1994).

Angell's hypothesis Angell et al. (Angell, 1991; Angell et al., 1994), having studied "reject" ova which failed to fertilize in vitro, proposed a new mechanism for nondisjunction. It has the merit that it is based on actual observation, not upon theory; it has the shortcoming that the numbers of observations are small, the material observed may be atypical, and the methodology may cause misleading artifact. Three sequential events comprise the gist of this theory (Figure 2–7). Firstly, homologs fail to pair during meiosis I; or, if they do pair (and perhaps recombine), they separate again before meiosis I is complete. In other words, instead of homologous pairs existing as a bivalent in meiosis I, they exist as two separate univalents. Secondly, these univalents are prone to "predivide"—that is, the separation of the two chromatids that should normally occur at meiosis II instead takes place while they are still in the first meiotic cycle. This

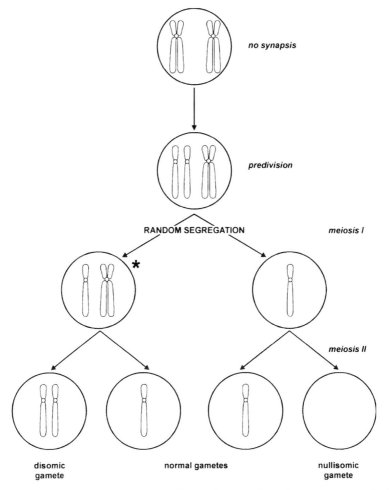

FIGURE 2–7. An alternative view of the mechanics of nondisjunction (Angell's hypothesis, see text). The asterisked gamete reflects the complement of the oocyte in FIGURE 2–5. (*right*).

could happen to both univalents, or just the one. Thirdly, at anaphase of meiosis I, these separated chromatids segregate at random to either the oocyte or to the polar body. A proportion of these segregants will be unbalanced. Univalent chromosomes are seen more frequently in the oocytes of older women (Angell, 1995).

If both gametes are coincidentally abnormal, one disomic and the other nullisomic, one parent will have contributed both members of the homologous pair, and the other none (Figure 2–6c). This is *uniparental disomy* (UPD), due to "gametic complementation." If the disomy in one gamete was due to nondisjunction at meiosis I, the two homologs will be different: uniparental heterodisomy. If the disomy had arisen from a meiosis II nondisjunction, the homologs will be identical (barring the effects of recombination), and this is uniparental isodisomy.

Nondisjunction In Mitosis

Normal Zygote

Mitotic nondisjunction is a major mechanism in the causation of mosaicism. Nondisjunction can occur in an initially normal (46,N) zygote, with the generation of mosaicism for a trisomic and a concomitant monosomic line, as well as the normal line (Figure 2–8a). In autosomal nondisjunction, growth of the monosomic cell line is severely disadvantaged, and it may well die out, leaving just the normal and the trisomic cell lines comprising the individual. Mosaic Down syndrome, with the karyotype 47,+21/46,N, is the classic example. Actually, about 5% of standard, apparently nonmosaic 47,+21 is also due to a mitotic defect (Antonarakis et al., 1993a), with the "third" No. 21 equally likely to be maternal or paternal. Most mosaic 47,+8/46,N is the result of this mechanism (Robinson et al., 1995a). In 3% of apparently non-mosaic 47,XXY and 9% of 47,XXX the error was postzygotic, presumably prior to the formation of the inner cell mass (MacDonald et al., 1994). If there is a nondisjunction of an X chromosome later in embryonic life, both abnormal cell lines may remain; such as, for example, 45,X/46,XX/47,XXX mosaicism, which is presumed to come from an initially 46,XX zygote (Figure 2–8b). More than one mitotic error can happen, separate in time and place; for example, DeBrasi et al. (1995) identified concomitant 45,X and 47,XX,+8 (and 46,X,+8) in a woman with clinical features of both trisomy 8 and Turner syndrome, in whom the molecular study supported the hypothesis of an originally 46,XX conception.

Aneuploid Zygote

Nondisjunction can occur in a postzygotic mitosis in a conceptus that is initially trisomic for an autosome (say, 47,+21). Thus, one copy of the homolog in question is lost; the same result may be due to the mechanism of anaphase lag. (In this latter case, the chromosome fails to connect to the spindle apparatus, or is tardily drawn to its pole, and fails to be included in the reforming nuclear membrane. On its own in the cytoplasm, it will form a micronucleus and soon be lost.) This converts the trisomy in this cell to 46,N. Its descendant cells are 46,N, and the karyotype of the conceptus is, say, 47,+21/46,N (Figure 2–8c). Most mosaic disomy/trisomy 13, 18, 21, and X arises in this way (Robinson et al., 1995a).

   If this conversion—sometimes referred to as "correction" or "rescue"— occurs prior to the formation of the pre-embryo, and if the 46,N line gives rise to the pre-embryo, then the embryo will be nonmosaic 46,N. According to which one of the three chromosomes was lost, normal biparental disomy in the embryo could be restored, or uniparental disomy (UPD) could result (Figure 2–9). This may actually be a more common mechanism to cause UPD than the scenario of coincidental nondisjunctions in both gametes as depicted in Figure 2–6c. Purvis-

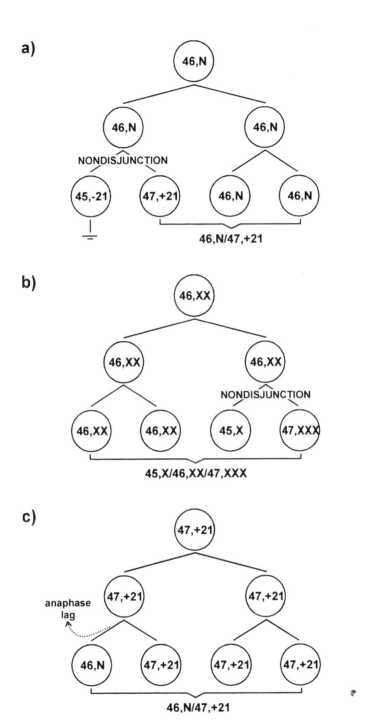

FIGURE 2–8. Generation of mosaicism. (a) Postzygotic nondisjunction in an initially normal conceptus. In this example, one cell line (monosomic 21) is subsequently lost, with the final karyotype 46,N/47,+21. (b) Postzygotic nondisjunction in an initially 46,XX conceptus, resulting in 45,X/46,XX/47,XXX mosaicism. (c) Postzygotic anaphase lag in an initially 47,+21 conceptus.

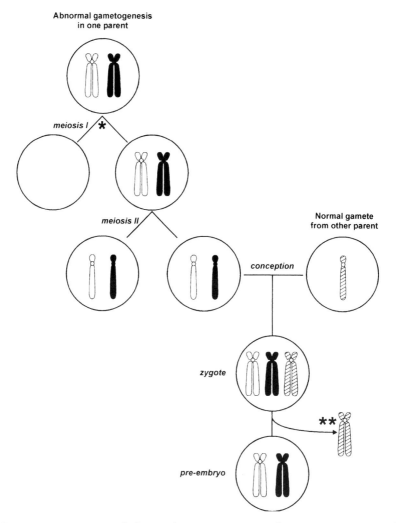

Abnormal gametogenesis
in one parent

meiosis I *

meiosis II

Normal gamete
from other parent

conception

zygote

**

pre-embryo

FIGURE 2–9. Uniparental disomy from "correction" of a trisomic conceptus by loss of a homolog. Nondisjunction* at meiosis I, followed by postzygotic loss** of one homolog, causes uniparental heterodisomy. (If, for example, this were chromosome No. 15, and the meiotic nondisjunction occurred in the mother, the child would have Prader-Willi syndrome.) Nondisjunction at meiosis II would cause uniparental isodisomy.

Smith et al. (1992) and Cassidy et al. (1992) illustrate this mechanism in pregnancies showing 47,+15 at chorionic villus sampling, with conversion to 46,N at amniocentesis; the infants had maternal UPD 15 (which produces the phenotype of Prader-Willi syndrome). If the "correction" occurs after the onset of embryogenesis, 46/47 mosaicism results, and UPD is possible in the euploid cell line. For example, Willatt et al. (1992) describe a 47,XY,+9/46,XY boy, in whose apparently normal cell line both No. 9s are of maternal origin, due to meiosis II nondisjunction; but in another case of trisomy 9 mosaicism, UPD 9 was excluded in the normal 46,XX line (Lindor et al., 1995).

> A very early mitotic nondisjunction in a 46,N conceptus, with both chromatids of one homolog passing to the same pole, could produce trisomy in a cell destined to give rise to the pre-embryo. Subsequent loss of one homolog could restore a disomic karyotype; according to which one, the disomy would be biparental or uniparental. Paternal UPD 15 (producing Angelman syndrome) is characteristically due to this sequence of events (Robinson et al., 1993b).

Sex chromosome aneuploidy may convert to the mosaic state, usually by loss of one of the supernumerary chromosomes, for example 47,XXY → 47,XXY/ 46,XY. A different means to produce X mosaicism is "compensatory" uniparental isodisomy: a 45,X conceptus could convert to 45,X/46,XX in embryonic life by replication of the single X (Schinzel et al., 1993).

STRUCTURAL REARRANGEMENT

We can list the following structural rearrangements: translocations, insertions, inversions, isochromosomes, intrachromosomal and interchromosomal duplications, deletions, and complex rearrangements. All arose de novo at one point: whether with the index case in whom the abnormality was discovered, or in a parent or more distant ancestor, with a balanced (or, rarely, unbalanced) form transmitted thereafter in the family. The "illegitimate" breakage and reunion which produces these rearrangements may be due to the apposition of chromosomal segments containing DNA sequences with a high degree of homology (Giacalone and Francke, 1992). Jacobs (1981) has derived the following mutation rates for the generation of de novo rearrangements: 1.6×10^{-4} for the balanced reciprocal translocation, and 2.9×10^{-4} for unbalanced rearrangements. If the breakpoint in one chromosome were to disrupt a gene, phenotypic defect may be the consequence (Brueton and Winter, 1993); in fact most breakpoints are in nontranscribed DNA. We discuss possible mechanisms of formation in the appropriate chapters.

Setting in Which Rearrangement Occurs

Mutations causing chromosomal rearrangement can occur during both meiosis and mitosis. Classically, meiosis has been considered the mutational setting par excellence; chromosomes are particularly active during meiotic synapsis and recombination, and it is plausible to suppose that error could readily creep in. Spermatogenesis, during which there are great changes in cell size as meiosis proceeds, may be a particularly hazardous environment; and in fact most de novo rearrangements arise in male gametogenesis (Olson and Magenis, 1988; Chandley, 1991; Tommerup, 1993; Batista et al., 1994; Powell et al., 1994). Some of these mutations may have arisen after the second meiotic division is complete, but before the mature sperm has been produced.

Mitosis offers ample opportunity for mutation in terms of the number of individual cell divisions[5], and this would lead to the mosaic state, i.e., 46,N/ 46,rea or 47,+rea/46,N. In fact, mosaicism for a structural rearrangement is infrequently recognized. If a conceptus is initially 46,rea, the abnormal chromosome may be discarded in fetal life, and the remaining homolog replicated (''compensatory isodisomy''), to give a 46,N karyotype at least in some tissues; but if the 46,rea cell line was operative during embryogenesis, the developmental damage it caused is irreversible (Bartsch et al., 1994). In a 46,X,rea(X) or 46,X,rea(Y) conceptus, an abnormal sex chromosome may actually promote embryonic survival, and then be lost to give apparently nonmosaic 45,X; whereas a conceptus that is 45,X ab initio may not survive (Held et al., 1992).

Balanced and Unbalanced Rearrangements

Structural rearrangements can be balanced or unbalanced, with respect to the amount of genetic material per cell. Arguing somewhat circularly, in the phenotypically normal person it is inferred that, although such an individual's genetic material is in a different chromosomal arrangement, it is present in the proper (balanced) amount and functioning properly. (At the cytogenetic level, one can only use the term ''apparently balanced''; even the highest-resolution banding does not reveal a genetic imbalance at the level of kilobases of DNA.) It is irrelevant to the person's health, other than his or her reproductive health. It may be helpful in explaining this to think of the person's genome as a recipe book—a series of instructions for everything that is genetically determined. If an error occurs in the pagination (a translocation), and, say, pages 17 to 24 are inserted between pages 36 and 37, the recipes are all still there; they can still be read, but in a different order. If a sequence of pages is inserted upside down (an inversion), one need only turn the book around to read them. A problem that often cannot be resolved is the instance of a phenotypically abnormal individual who has an ''apparently balanced'' rearrangement. Might it be, at a submicroscopic level, that genetic imbalance really exists? If the (normal) parent has the apparently identical chromosome, the problem becomes thornier. Might there be some parent-of-origin effect, with the same structural chromosome being functionally different? Actually, it is most likely that the phenotypic abnormality is coincidental, and not the result of the karyotypic abnormality.

Cryptic Rearrangement

Similar mechanisms to those outlined above, but only involving relatively tiny segments of chromatin, can be the basis of chromosomal rearrangements not detectable on routine or even the highest resolution cytogenetics. Flint et al. (1995) identified two de novo unbalanced derivative chromosomes in two retarded persons who had previously been regarded as 46,XY and 46,XX. One had a deletion of a tiny subtelomeric segment in 13q, with a fragment from the X-Y pseudoautosomal region inserted in its place, and the other had a deletion of 25 centimorgans (about 10 megabases) of telomeric 22q, with a translocation of subtelomeric 9q to 22q. Each, therefore, had a combination of a partial monosomy and a partial trisomy. Biesecker et al. (1995), using subtelomeric dinucleotide microsatellites, detected a 23–30 centimorgan 22q duplication due to recombination from a parental inversion, which had not been seen on 450-band resolution cytogenetics. These examples beg the question: what fraction of "karyotypically normal" individuals with mental and possibly physical defect actually have a subtle imbalance?

GENOMIC IMPRINTING

Some parts of some chromosomes are subject to *genomic imprinting*, or parent-specific gene expression. Imprinting can lead to a differential activation status of the two alleles of the locus or loci concerned: one is functional, and the other is "silent." At the time of writing, the practical application of genomic imprinting appears to be confined to a very small number of conditions; whether a wider range will come to be subsumed under this heading remains to be seen. In any event, the theoretical interest is considerable, and we must discuss the concept in some detail.

Most of the autosomal genome is not subject to imprinting, and is functionally disomic. That is, with each locus having a pair of alleles, each of the pair is functionally active, contributing more or less equally to the genetic output from that locus. This is *biallelic gene expression*. A minority of the genome requires only one of the pair of alleles to be active, while the other one becomes inactivated: in other words, the locus is functionally monosomic, with a genetic output from only one allele. This is *monoallelic expression*. Which one of the two alleles comes to be inactivated depends upon its parent of origin: that is, whether it had been transmitted in the sperm or in the ovum. If the allele of maternal origin is inactivated, only the allele of paternal origin is functionally active; and vice versa. Following conception, the imprint remains through cycles of postconceptional somatic mitoses: the chromosome "remembers" the sex of the parent who contributed it.

Imprinting is a normal mechanism of gene regulation. It is mediated, in part at least, through an epigenetic process during gametogenesis of methylation of cytosine bases within the gene(s), or in controlling sequences upstream of it. In the "life" of an autosomal allele or chromosomal segment, as it passes from individual to individual down the generations and across the centuries, imprinting will be acquired, maintained, lost ("erased"), reacquired ("reset"), and lost again according to the sexes of the individuals through whom it is transmitted. Throughout, it retains the same DNA sequence.

Mechanisms Whereby Functional Genetic Abnormality Can Arise

We may consider three categories of functional genetic defect concerning a segment or segments of a chromosome subject to imprinting. These are: uniparental disomy with overexpression and/or nonexpression; deletion with nonexpression; and relaxation with overexpression. *(1)* Uniparental disomy will lead to either biallelic expression or to no expression at the locus or loci within the imprintable segment. *(2)* If a deletion removes a chromosomal segment that would otherwise have been "silenced," all that is lost is a nonfunctioning genetic segment, and there is no untoward consequence. On the other hand, if the deletion removes the segment on the active chromosome, the corresponding part of the other homolog is inactive, and so neither chromosome will be genetically functioning in this segment; in a sense, the silent allele is unmasked. *(3)* If, in a chromosomally normal conceptus, a segment which should have been imprinted loses its imprint ("relaxation" of imprinting), the locus or loci contained therein will be operating at double normal capacity.

TRINUCLEOTIDE-REPEAT TRANSMISSION

Runs of trinucleotide sequences ("triplet-repeats") are not uncommon in genes; these sequences may have a role in binding to proteins involved in the control of gene expression. The number of copies can vary considerably in the normal population, but this number on any chromosome is stable, and chromosomes are normally transmitted having the same number of repeats from generation to generation. Instability in the number of repeats—dynamic mutation, or allele expansion—was first observed in 1991 in fragile X syndrome, and has now been seen in a small number of other Mendelian disorders (all of which comprise, in part or in whole, a neurological phenotype). With these disorders, the number of repeats can change as the allele is transmitted from parent to child. Once an increase has reached a critical number, the gene's function is compromised, and the phenotypic abnormality declares itself. The trinucleotide of cytogenetic importance is cytosine-cytosine-guanine (CCG). The rare folate-sensitive fragile sites (p. 233) are most likely due to expansions of these naturally occurring highly polymorphic sequences.

CONSEQUENCES OF GENETIC ABNORMALITY

STRUCTURAL IMBALANCE

An incorrect amount of genetic material in every cell of the conceptus distorts its development to a greater or lesser extent. Large losses or gains almost invariably set early development so awry that abortion occurs. Lesser imbalances may be compatible with continued intrauterine survival, but the child is phenotypically abnormal. Very minor imbalances may cause defects that are not readily detectable in early infancy, and some chromosomal "defects" may be without effect. However, as a first principle, anything but 100% of the normal amount of (at least autosomal) genetic material produces a less than 100% normal phenotype.

How do we determine what is a large or a small degree of genetic imbalance?

First, we can take a quantitative approach—how much material is involved? For autosomal chromatin, the index of measurement is the haploid autosomal length (HAL) (see Appendix A). The largest chromosome, No. 1, comprises 8.4% of the HAL while No. 21, the smallest, is 1.9%. As a very general rule, if the imbalance consists of less than 1% of HAL, the conceptus is often viable in utero, and live birth frequently results. If the excess is greater than 2%, abortion is likely. Imbalance involving *deficiency* (partial monosomy) is generally much less survivable.

Quantitative assessment is rather crude. Of course, different segments of chromatin contain different material. In general, dark G-bands are low in gene content, and light G-bands are gene-rich; telomeric regions have the highest gene density (Bickmore and Sumner, 1989; Bernardi, 1989). Some segments (e.g., 9p, all of 21) appear to have a substantial pre- and postnatal survivability in the trisomic state, while a lesser number of segments (e.g., distal 4p) are sometimes viable when monosomic (Schinzel, 1993b). Chromosome 13 provides the most impressive examples of viability for a large autosomal imbalance. Trisomy for the whole of chromosome 13—fully 3.7% of the HAL—frequently goes through to live birth, and in the 13q− deletion syndrome, monosomy occurs for up to 2.5% of HAL. This may reflect a low gene density on this chromosome. Occasionally, imbalance is so ''small'' that the effect on the child's physical phenotype is only very minor, and intellectual function can remain within the normal range, for example, a duplication of bands q42.11–12 in chromosome 1 (Bortotto et al., 1990). There are some segments which, when duplicated or deleted, appear to cause no abnormality at all, for example, deletion of band p14 in chromosome 5 (Overhauser et al., 1994). Others impart a serious trisomic effect even for a tiny amount of chromatin, and deletion of the single band 17p13.3, for example, causes the severe phenotype of the Miller-Dieker syndrome. The least number of loci that can be removed in a deletion is one: in Rubinstein-Taybi syndrome, for example, the loss of a single gene *CREBBP* within 16p13.3 suffices to produce the phenotype (see p. 281). Thus, a qualitative assessment is necessary to know whether a particular duplication or deficiency is of nil, minor, major, or lethal effect.

Two particular sources provide information on, firstly, viability of a particular segment, and secondly, the clinical features of specific duplications and deficiencies. Stengel-Rutkowski et al. (1988) have gathered data from 1,120 translocation pedigrees, determining, for numerous segments in the partially trisomic and partially monosomic states, the likelihood that a pregnancy would proceed through to live birth. Schinzel (1994) has compiled the Human Cytogenetics Database, a useful resource documenting clinical phenotype in some hundreds of different aneuploid states that are compatible with live birth, many of which are associated with survival to early childhood or beyond.

Sex chromosome imbalances need to be considered separately. Any X chromosomes in excess of one are almost completely genetically inactivated. Thus, indicating the inactivated X in lowercase, normal females are 46,Xx; normal males are 46,XY; Turner females are 45,X; Klinefelter males are 47,XxY;

and other X aneuploidies are 47,Xxx, 48,Xxxx, 48,XxYY, 49,XxxxY, and 49,Xxxxx. As for the Y chromosome, its genetic material is constitutively almost entirely inactive. Thus, in spite of the presence of one or more whole X or Y chromosomes in excess in the $2n = 47$, 48, and 49 states, in utero survival remains possible. Indeed, for 47,XXX, 47,XXY, and 47,XYY, survival is apparently quite uncompromised. Gonadal development in X aneuploid males is particularly affected, and intellectual function is jeopardized to a mild or moderate extent in the $n \geqslant 47$ states in both sexes. 45,X has a high in utero lethality, although the small fraction surviving to term as females with Turner syndrome show, in comparison, a remarkably mild phenotypic effect. These survivors may actually have had a 46th chromosome in early embryonic life, which was subsequently lost (Held et al., 1992).

It is an obvious point, but worth restating: the defect in these aneuploid states involves too much or too little of what is *normal* chromosome material. The "third" chromosome in, for example, standard trisomy 21 is a perfectly normal No. 21 chromosome, with a perfectly normal complement of chromosome 21 genes. How, therefore, could it be that an additional amount of normal genetic message leads to an abnormal reading of that message? This is one of the great remaining unanswered questions of biology, for which molecular studies are now just beginning to offer some glimpses (Korenberg et al., 1990; Epstein, 1993a,b; Fisher and Scambler, 1994; Peterson et al., 1994).

The Mosaic State

Whether mosaicism matters depends on which tissue, and how much of that tissue, is abnormal. If a majority of the soma is chromosomally abnormal, the phenotype is likely to be abnormal, assuming the particular aneuploidy is characteristically associated with clinical defect. If only a tiny fraction of some tissue were involved, in which the aneuploidy would have essentially no effect—if, say, some of the bony tissue of the distal phalanx of the left little toe was trisomic 21, and the rest of the person 46,N—it would never be known. Indeed, as we speculate above, it could be that many people carry a tiny and completely unimportant abnormal cell line somewhere in their soma. A very minor degree of mosaicism could still be important if a crucial tissue carried the imbalance. An abnormal chromosome confined to tissues of, say, a localized area or cell type in one part of the brain could theoretically cause neurological dysfunction; and abnormality involving a gonad ("gonadal mosaicism"), or part of a gonad, could lead to a child being conceived with that aneuploidy. Mosaicism confined to extra-embryonic tissue may be without phenotypic effect, although it certainly raises concern if it produces an abnormal test result at prenatal diagnosis.

Mosaicism for a Full Aneuploidy

As a general principle, an individual with an aneuploid line in only some of their tissues is likely to have a less severe but qualitatively similar phenotype to that of someone with the nonmosaic aneuploidy. The ascertainment of these individuals is biased: those with a more obvious phenotypic defect are, naturally, more likely to be detected. Mosaic Down syndrome—47,+21/46,N—can be less obvious, and with a lesser compromise of intellectual function, than in standard trisomy 21. The existence of 46,N cells in some of the brain tissue can have a moderating effect. Some aneuploidies can only, or almost only, exist in the mosaic state, the nonmosaic form being lethal in utero. Examples of this are 47,+8/46,N and 47,+9/46,N. If the distribution of the aneuploid cell line is asymmetric, body shape may be asymmetric, generally with hypoplasia in regions of aneuploidy. In sex chromosome mosaicism, fertility can exist when otherwise infertility is the rule: for example, in "formes frustes" of Turner syndrome with 45,X/46,XX and of Klinefelter syndrome with 47,XXY/46,XY.

Mosaicism for a Structural Rearrangement

Mosaicism for a *balanced* structural rearrangement would be expected to be without any phenotypic effect. The only practical implication would be if the mosaicism extended into the gonad. With an *unbalanced* karyotype, again the broad rule applies that the mosaic form is likely to be less severe than the nonmosaic. Some imbalances are seen only in the mosaic state, for example, 46,N/47,+i(12p), the nonmosaic 47,+i(12p) state presumably being invariably lethal in utero. One notable and clinically useful phenotypic trait that can characterize this type of mosaicism is hypomelanosis of Ito or similar skin variegation (Ritter et al., 1990; Ohashi et al., 1992). This pigmentary anomaly may be due to disordered melanin production in the chromosomally abnormal epidermal cells (Moss et al., 1993). The distribution of the abnormal cells, and thus of dyspigmentation, follows the lines of Blaschko, and so producing the characteristic streaky distribution ("tiger striping"). Asymmetry is a further clinical pointer (Woods et al., 1994). Mosaicism can in theory be very widespread, and Kingston et al. (1993) describe a fetal study in which several tissues taken posttermination had various fractions of mosaicism for an additional abnormal chromosome, including 88% of brain cells, while only 3% of amniotic fluid cells and no cells from a sample of fetal blood had the abnormal chromosome. On the borderland between cytogenetics and Mendelian genetics, some women who are carriers for Duchenne/Becker muscular dystrophy can show a "cytomolecular deletion" of the dystrophin gene at Xp21 using FISH which, if it is present in only a fraction of blood cells, demonstrates somatic mosaicism for the deletion (Bunyan et al., 1995).

Mosaicism from Somatic Recombination Between Homologs

Probably, in the great majority of instances, and providing the exchange is balanced and does not involve imprintable chromatin, somatic recombination would not adversely influence embryogenesis. If the exchange between two homologs *A* was uneven, a duplication and a deletion cell line could be produced, and the karyotype in consequence 46,dir dup(A)/46,del(A)/46,N (Pescia et al., 1982). Loss of the deletion cell line, if this were to happen, would then bring about mosaicism for a direct duplication (and see also p. 263). The amount and mix of the different cells throughout the soma will influence the extent to which normal morphogenesis is compromised.

Gonadal Mosaicism

It is generally taken that most gametes with a chromosomal abnormality are produced by 46,N parents with chromosomally normal gonads: the abnormality arose at meiosis, and affected only the gametes arising from that meiosis. Indeed, Chandley (1991) suggests many structural rearrangements transmitted by the male may have arisen during a postmeiotic phase of spermatogenesis; obviously, a mutation at this stage would involve just the one single spermatozoon. But if an abnormality had arisen during formation of a germ cell prior to the onset of meiosis, an abnormal cell line can become established and occupy a part of the gonad or gonads. This is gonadal mosaicism.

Cells destined to give rise to gametocytes originate from the yolk sac in early embryogenesis, and migrate to the gonadal ridge on the dorsal wall of the abdominal cavity where, along with the supporting cells, they come to comprise the tissue of the gonad. In doing so, gametocytes must replicate many times, going through about 30 cycles of division. Thirty cycles produces 2^{30} (about 1,000,000,000—a billion) progeny cells, and the potential for error exists at each cell division contributing to this population. These errors could be nondisjunctions or the production of structural rearrangements.

Edwards (1989) offers a startling insight into the actuality of gonadal mosaicism. He points out that, in the male, the total length of seminiferous tubule is about 1 km. If a mutation were to occur in a spermatogonium in, say, the 20th cycle of division, its progeny would then go through 10 more cycles and comprise 2^{10} (about 1000) cells. This would be only a millionth (1000/ 1,000,000,000) of the 1 km of tubule—a mere 1 mm. So a man mosaic in such a way would have a risk of only one in a million of fathering a conception with this particular abnormality. From similar reasoning, a defect arising at the 10th cycle could affect 1 m of tubule, and thus carry a risk of 1 in 1000. Oogonia need go through a lesser number of cycles; but the same principles broadly apply.

Gonadal mosaicism cannot usually be recognized until after the event of two siblings born both with the same "de novo" abnormality. The most direct demonstration would be by karyotyping mature or developing gametes. Brandriff et al. (1988) analyzed sperm from a 46,N man who had fathered two children with del(13)(q22q32), but found no del(13) sperm. In situ hybridization of testicular material is another potential approach (Goldman and Hultén, 1992). Sachs et al. (1990) demonstrated ovarian mosaicism by direct gonadal samplings in a woman who had had one Down syndrome child and three other trisomic pregnancies, whose blood karyotype was 46,N[97%]/47,+21[3%]. Tissue cultured from ovarian biopsies showed almost half the cells in each ovary to be 47,XX,+21.

If the abnormal chromosome had been generated at a mitosis prior to the separation of the germline, a combined somatic-gonadal mosaicism could result. We have seen an extraordinary example of such a thing. A woman presented with a baby having an 18q deletion, the breakpoint at q21.3, and she was checked to see if she might be a translocation carrier. The first two (peripheral blood) cells were 46,XX; on the third cell analyzed, she was 46,XX,t(5; 18)(p15.3;q21.3). A further 997 cells were all 46,XX, as were 200 skin fibroblasts. We assume the balanced reciprocal 5;18 translocation arose in a cell that contributed both to the germline and to the blood-forming tissue, but at least in the latter, to only a very small fraction; and the child was the result of an unbalanced segregation within the translocation-bearing part of the germline. A few other similar cases are on record (Gardner et al., 1994), such as that of Sciorra et al. (1992b), who found a single translocation rcp(7q;14q) cell, the 16th out of 100 blood cells eventually analyzed and with no abnormal cells out of 100 skin fibroblasts, in a man who had had an abnormal child with an unbalanced ''7q+'' chromosome. As a less subtle example, if the abnormal cell line is unbalanced, and comprises a substantial fraction of the soma, the individual may display a partial form of the characteristic phenotype. For example, Zori et al. (1993) describe a woman with 46,del(17)(p11.2p12)/46,N on blood karyotyping who had some features of Smith-Magenis syndrome and whose 46,del(17)(p11.2–12) child had the full syndrome. Moog et al. (1994) describe a mildly retarded woman with the karyotype 46,XX,dir dup(18pter→cen)/46,XX on peripheral blood analysis having a nonmosaic son with 46,XY,dir dup(18pter→cen): in her case, much of the soma and at least some of the germline stock had the unbalanced complement. The 46,N/46,dup(10) father we discuss on p. 16 under Ethical and Counseling Issues is a similar example.

Placental Mosaicism
About 1–2% of placentas can have a different chromosomal constitution from that of the embryo; usually the embryo is normal and the placenta is trisomic. Thus, in 1–2% of chorionic villus samplings, there will be a potentially misleading result. Fortunately, these uncommon instances can, as a rule, be recognized as such.

Amniotic Fluid Cell Mosaicism
True mosaicism is infrequently recognized at amniocentesis. Occasional cells with a chromosomal abnormality, if they are solitary or involving a single clone, are generally regarded as having arisen in vitro (''artifactual mosaicism''). At least most of the time, this is probably the correct interpretation. We consider placental and amniotic fluid cell mosaicism in detail in Chapter 23.

QUALITATIVE IMBALANCE

The idea that abnormality could be due to a correct amount of chromosome material overall, but with unequal parental contributions, seemed most remarkable in 1980 when Engel first made the suggestion and coined the expression ''uniparental disomy.'' A decade later, the concept had progressed from esoteric theory to an important and illuminating practicality (Engel, 1993). The two disorders which, par excellence, exemplify the concept of qualitative imbalance are Prader-Willi syndrome (PWS) and Angelman syndrome (AS). The concept of genomic imprinting, discussed above, is central to an understanding of the etiology. Each syndrome is due to failure of expression of different but closely linked segments within the proximal long arm of chromosome 15. A *"PWS critical region"* is normally expressed from only one chromosome (functional monoallelism), in this case the paternally originating chromosome. The maternal region is normally inactive and alleles in this region are not transcribed. If the paternal PWS region is absent, the maternal one cannot "fill the gap"; and this functional nullisomy is the root cause of PWS. An *"AS critical region"* exists, lying just a little distal from the PWS region. Likewise, it needs only monoallelic expression for normal phenotypic function. In this case, the maternal region is active, and the paternal region, having been imprinted, is inactive. If the maternal region is absent, there can be no genetic activity, and this causes the AS phenotype. Absence of the paternal PWS region or maternal AS region can occur from two major mechanisms. Firstly, in uniparental disomy (UPD), one parent fails to contribute a No. 15 chromosome; and the "correcting" presence of two copies from the other parent cannot restore a proper balance. Secondly, there can be a deletion within proximal 15q that removes a segment of chromatin containing the two regions. We discuss these issues in Chapter 17.

As well as No. 15, UPD for some other chromosomes has been implicated as causative of phenotypic abnormality. Maternal (but not paternal) UPD for No. 7, for example, can produce effects upon growth and intellectual development (Spence et al., 1988; Voss et al., 1989; Höglund et al., 1994). Paternal and maternal UPD for chromosome No. 14 may follow asymmetric segregation in some Robertsonian translocations and be associated with different physical phenotypes with or without intellectual deficit (Temple et al., 1991; Wang et al., 1991; Pentao et al., 1992; Antonarakis et al., 1993b; Donnai, 1993; Healey et al., 1994) or, in one case, with complete normality (Papenhausen et al., 1995). If the homologs in a case of UPD are identical (uniparental isodisomy), any recessive gene the "uniparent" happens to be carrying on that chromosome will be in homozygous state in the child and will produce its characteristic untoward effect (Pentao et al., 1992; Höglund et al., 1994). An extraordinary "double hit" is the child described by Woodage et al. (1994) who had PWS due to UPD 15, and concomitant Bloom syndrome due to isodisomy at distal 15q, wherein lies the Bloom locus. A different route to a similar karyotype is "compensatory" uniparental isodisomy: for example, a conceptus with X monosomy could convert to 45,X/46,XX in embryonic life by replication of the single X (Schinzel et al., 1993).

If both homologs are equally genetically active, regardless of the parent of origin, UPD will have no untoward effect—other than, perhaps, one parent making an undue contribution to the child's phenotype (Engel, 1993)! Some chromosomes (Nos. 13, 21, and 22, at least) appear not to be subject to imprinting, at least from one parent, with no evident untoward effect of UPD (Donnai, 1993; Blouin et al., 1993; Schinzel et al., 1994a; Slater et al., 1994, 1995; Stallard et al., 1995); whether a single case of blighted ovum with UPD 21 (Henderson et al., 1994) represents a causal effect remains to be shown. Syndromes of dysmorphism and intellectual deficit which characteristically occur sporadically are candidates for having UPD as the cause, and it will not be surprising if, by the time this book is in print, the list of UPD syndromes has lengthened somewhat. A deluge may be unlikely, however; in a molecular study of 99 apparently karyotypically normal retarded individuals, two-thirds of whom had dysmorphic features, and using a methodology that would have detected 69% of any UPD that was present, Flint et al. (1995) found no cases. Similarly, Lindor et al. (1995) studied 25 individuals who displayed one or more of these features: nonsyndromic multiple congenital anomalies, short stature, mental retardation, or dysmorphism. Scanning every chromosome, biparental inheritance of at least one locus per chromosome was identified in each case.

Uniparental disomy for the entire chromosome set—"uniparental diploidy"—has a devastating effect on development. If a conceptus has lost its maternal complement, and the paternal complement doubles in an attempt to compensate, no embryo at all forms, and the chorionic villi are grossly abnormal. This is a hydatidiform mole (p. 317). If an ovum attempts a parthenogenetic development, a grossly disorganized mass of embryonic tissue results: an ovarian teratoma (p. 267). If a triple set of chromosomes (triploidy) is present at conception, there is either a diploid maternal set plus a haploid paternal set, or vice versa. These different parental origins determine different abnormal fetal and placental phenotypes (p. 253).

Segmental Uniparental Disomy

A mitotic mechanism that can lead to functional imbalance, if the segments exchanged are in a region subject to imprinting, is somatic recombination. The only example of this causing a dysmorphic syndrome known at present is the segmental paternal uniparental disomy for 11p of some Beckwith-Wiedemann syndrome (BWS) (p. 267), 11p being a segment that is normally maternally imprinted. In the partially UPD cell line, this segment will now be expressing biallelically at distal 11p. The asymmetry of body growth in this syndrome may reflect mosaicism of two tissue types: tissue descendant from the original genotype and tissue descendant from the cell in which the segmental UPD arose.

Relaxation of Imprinting

BWS may exemplify yet another category of imprinting error: that of relaxation (or erasure) of the imprint effect, which may be the consequence of an "epigenetic accident" in early development (p. 290). In some BWS, the *IGF-2* (insulin-like growth factor 2) locus on distal 11p shows biallelic expression; normally, only the paternal allele is functional (Weksberg et al., 1993a). This overexpression of a growth factor could plausibly have a role in the overgrowth that is characteristic of the syndrome.

SPORADIC AND RECURRENT ABNORMALITIES

SPORADIC ABNORMALITIES

Chromosomally normal parents can produce abnormal gametes by nondisjunction or by one of the other mutational mechanisms we have discussed above. The combination of factors that causes these defects in an individual case is unknown. The analysis of trisomic miscarriages in couples (Hassold et al., 1993) suggests randomness rather than individual biological predisposition. While such a thing as, for example, increased maternal age could be suspected to be contributory (but not directly causative) in the case of nondisjunction, most 45-year-old mothers have chromosomally normal babies. We cannot discern any biological differences between 45-year-olds who have a Down syndrome baby from those who do not. The age-related incidence of Down syndrome seems to be substantially similar in different races and in different parts of the world (Hook, 1994). No real case has ever been made for the agency of diet, illness, or chemical exposure in maternal No. 21 meiotic nondisjunction. Stoll et al. (1990) showed no seasonality or clusters in time or space in Strasbourg and the Départment du Bas-Rhin in Eastern France from 1979 to 1987 (the Chernobyl nuclear plant accident notwithstanding). One proposal for the Prader-Willi deletion is a previous paternal exposure to industrial solvents. Whether or not solvents really could damage testes and cause deletions, it is implausible that this would be a universal explanation for the Prader-Willi deletion. This is a question for the reproductive toxicologist (Wyrobek, 1993). More likely, proximal 15q is simply a region of inherent instability that will from time to time be the basis of deletions and other rearrangements (Nicholls, 1993).

Chromosomes are plastic, dynamic entities, and cell division is a complex mechanical process; and these qualities alone may suffice to endow the vulnerability that causes human aneuploidy and rearrangement. Given the assumption that all persons with intact gametogenesis are capable of producing an abnormal gamete, it may simply be that a certain background abnormality rate is intrinsic to the human species, and it is a chance matter whether this or that couple will have the misfortune to conceive the abnormality which, inevitably, someone has to bear. If that view were to be accepted (we are not necessarily saying it should be), we would conclude that essentially no increased recurrence risk applies to chromosomally normal couples possessing chromosomally normal gonads (an impossible state ever to prove) who have had an aneuploid child. The unprovable individual who is truly 46,N throughout the gonad can still have more than one chromosomally abnormal offspring due to unrelated chance de novo events. We would, for example, advise a couple who have had, sequentially, a child with trisomy 18 and a chorionic villus result from the next pregnancy of 47,+i(22q) that these events involved causally different mechanisms and it was simply a case of "bad luck" twice in a row; we might then be tested to overcome their not unnatural skepticism.

RECURRENT ABNORMALITIES

An abnormality has a substantial risk of recurrence if the parent has an abnormality. Persons with balanced rearrangements can produce balanced and unbalanced gametes: thus, a translocation carrier can have a second abnormal child with a partial aneuploidy. Chromosomally unbalanced individuals who are fertile can transmit the same defect; for example, a woman with Down syndrome can

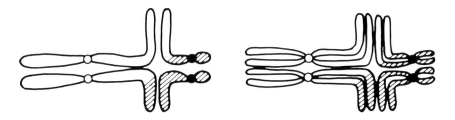

FIGURE 2–10. Chromosomes at synapsis exist as double-chromatid structures (e.g., the reciprocal translocation quadrivalent at *right*). But, for simplicity, we generally represent them with just the one chromatid (*left*).

have a Down syndrome baby. These facts are obvious enough; and the practical implications flowing from them comprise much of what this book is written about. Less readily identified is the person who is karyotypically 46,XX or 46,XY on a blood test but who may be an occult gonadal mosaic to a significant degree. Gamete sampling might be a theoretical means to identify gonadal mosaicism ahead of having a second affected child; but this is scarcely a practicable proposition.

Rarely, specific important predisposing factors can be suspected. An intrinsic fault in one parent in the mechanism of chromosome distribution at cell division could be the basis of recurring defects. Given the complexity of the apparatus and process of cell division, it is logical that error-causing mutants would exist; and we discussed this point above. Whether there might, for example, be milder alleles at these postulated cell-division loci which could be the cause of occasional nondisjunction remains entirely a matter for speculation. Spectacular cases such as that of a couple having sequential +21, +18, and +13 pregnancies, the mother being in her 40s (FitzPatrick and Boyd, 1989), might reflect some meiotic ''weakness''; equally, pure bad luck three times running is quite possible. Most de novo defects occur in the setting of an unremarkable pedigree, which is more in keeping with randomness than any substantial individual biological predisposition.

A NOTE ON THE DIAGRAMS

Following the progress of rearranged chromosomes during meiosis is not easy, so we have taken some liberties in simplifying the diagrams. Most of these diagrams depict the synapsing chromosomes at meiosis with just one chromatid; of course, the chromosome has actually replicated at this point and exists as a double chromatid entity (Figure 2–10).

NOTES

1. Cytoplasm contains the mitochondria, and transmission of mitochondrial DNA is practically entirely maternal. The mitochondrial genome has been described, somewhat whimsically, as chromosome 25, or the M chromosome. In not otherwise referring to this ''chromosome,'' we are not seeking to deny its importance or interest!

2. Since, at the level of the chromatid, there are four elements, the word *tetrad* can also be used in this setting. At the molecular level, the number of single DNA strands is eight.

3. An alternative theory of meiosis proposes that recombination precedes synapsis, and actually enables synapsis to take place (Chandley, 1993).

4. To be distinguished, in principle, from *chimerism*, which is the coexistence of more than one cell line due to the fusion of originally separate zygotes. The chimera of classical mythology was a beast with the head of a lion, the body of a goat, and the tail of a serpent.

5. The mitotic cell cycle includes interphase as well as mitosis, and we should not exclude abnormal chromosome behavior at any stage of the cycle as potentially causative of a rearrangement.

3

Deriving and Using a Risk Figure

Risk is a central concept in genetic counseling. By risk we mean the probability that a particular event will happen. Probability is conventionally measured with a number ranging from zero to 1. A probability (*P*) of zero means never, and a probability of 1 means always. For two or more mutually exclusive possible outcomes, the individual probabilities sum to 1.0 (or 100%). Thus, someone who is a heterozygote for a particular rearrangement might, in any given pregnancy, have a probability of 0.10 (10%) of having an abnormal child and a probability of 0.90 (90%) of having a normal child. We may speak in terms of risks of *re*currence or of *oc*currence: the probability that an event will happen again, or that it will happen for the first time. Risk can also be presented as *odds*: the ratio of two mutually exclusive probabilities. The odds for the preceding hypothetical heterozygote would be 9:1 in favor of a normal child.

The work *risk* has two important meanings in the English language. First, there is the scientific sense of probability that we already discussed. Second, as most people use the word, it conveys a sense of exposure to danger. Our hypothetical heterozygote runs the risk that an unfortunate outcome may occur (an abnormal child, or an abnormal result at prenatal diagnosis). In the genetic counseling clinic these meanings of risk coalesce in some ways to which the counselor needs to be sensitive. We might instead use such everyday words as *chance* or *likelihood*, which have no negative connotation, to refer to the fortunate outcome of normality. The words—*fortunate* and *unfortunate*— are also chosen deliberately: the wanted or the unwanted event will occur entirely by chance, analogous to tossing a coin, throwing a dice, or being dealt a card.

Different Types of Risk Figure

Geneticists arrive at risk figures in a number of ways (Harper, 1993), two of which have particular application to cytogenetics.

1. *Mendelian risks.* If a clear model of inheritance is known, risk figures derived by reference to that theory may be used. In practice, only Mendel's law of segregation is applied in this context. When a pair of homologous chromosomes segregate at meiosis, it is a random matter which chromosome enters the gamete that will produce the conceptus. Each has an equal chance: a probability of 0.5. As an example, the X chromosomes in the fragile X heterozygote, the normal X and the fragile X, display 1:1 segregation. This is assumed to be a *true* risk, not an estimate: it is 0.5 exactly.

2. *Empiric risks.* In the great majority of chromosomal situations, no clear theory exists from which the risk can be derived, and one must observe what happened previously in (as far as one can judge) the same situation in other families. Empiric risks thus appeal to experience, and they only *estimate* the intrinsic, true, probability. This estimate has a greater or lesser degree of precision, depending on how many data have been accumulated.

Consider, for example, the common situation of a young couple having had a child with Down syndrome. Nothing is known about nondisjunction that could provide a theoretical model on which to base a recurrence risk figure. We therefore use information obtained from surveying large numbers of other such families. It may be observed, for example, that in these families about 1 pregnancy in 100, subsequent to the index case of Down syndrome, produced another child with Down syndrome. Formally expressed, this is a segregation analysis. From this rate of 1/100 we can derive a risk figure of 1%, which we then have as the basis for advising patients. (Actually, it is not quite as straightforward as this in Down syndrome; see Chapter 16.) The more families we study, the more precise and therefore reliable the figure is (see the section below on the presentation of a risk figure).

Hook and Cross (1982) note the importance of distinguishing between the *rate* (which may be thought of as "past tense") and the *risk* (which is "future tense"). They emphasize that, while geneticists routinely extrapolate from rates in one population at one point in time, and may use these figures as risk estimates in another population and certainly at a later point in time, they should be on their guard for any evidence that a condition varies with time, geography, or ethnicity.

Doing a Segregation Analysis

Segregation analysis is essentially a simple exercise. A farmer who surveys a flock of newborn lambs and notes that 3 are black and 97 are white has done a segregation analysis. In human cytogenetic segregation analysis, the exercise involves looking at a (preferably large) number of offspring of a particular category of parent: parents who carry some particular chromosome rearrangement, or those who have had a child with a chromosomal abnormality, they themselves being karyotypically normal. The proportion of these parents' children who are abnormal is noted, and this datum serves as the point estimate of the recurrence risk.

Although segregation analysis is simple in principle, there are potential pitfalls in its application, the most important of which is *ascertainment bias*. We will deal with this problem only briefly. It is important that the counselor know of ascertainment bias and recognize whether or not it has been accounted for in the published works they consult (note, for example, Steinbach's 1986 commentary on the translocation study of Fryns et al., 1986a; and our [Sutherland et al., 1995] commentary upon the paracentric inversion review of Pettenati et al., 1995, and their [Pettenati and Rao, 1995] response). But it is not necessary to understand the complex and sophisticated mechanics of segregation analysis in detail. The reader wishing fuller instruction is referred to Murphy and Chase (1975), Emery (1986), and Stene and Stengel-Rutkowski (1988). The classic example of ascertainment bias is that of the analysis of the sex ratio in sibships of military recruits in the First World War. Adding up the numbers of brothers and sisters, there was a marked excess of males. But of course (in 1914–1918) the recruit himself had to be male. Once he was excluded from the total in each sibship the overall sex ratio was normal. Likewise, in a cytogenetic segregation analysis, the individual whose abnormality brought the family to attention—the proband—is excluded from the calculation. That person *had* to be abnormal. Furthermore, that individual's carrier parent, grandparent, and so on had to be (almost always) phenotypically normal to have been a parent. They must also be excluded from an analysis of their own sibship, if that generation is available for study. Other sibships may be included in full.

These manipulations—dropping the proband and the heterozygous directline antecedents—are the major steps to be taken to avoid the distorting effects of ascertainment bias. Another potential methodological confounder for the aficionado is *ascertainment probability*. For example, families with more affected members may be more likely to come to medical attention, which would unduly weight the data. There are means to overcome this problem.

Essential to a good analysis are good data, or at least as good as possible. Some retrospective information may be uncertain. Did a phenotypically abnormal great uncle who died as a child in 1930 have the "family aneuploidy"? (Old photos may be very helpful in this respect.) Some family skeletons may remain in cupboards unopened to the interviewer. The investigative zeal, clinical judgment, and personal qualities of the researcher are crucial in getting the right information, and getting it all.

The Derivation of a "Private" Recurrence Risk Figure

We will demonstrate some of the previously noted principles in estimating a private recurrence risk figure for the hypothetical family depicted in Figure 3–1. Six sibships are available for analysis: one in generation II, two in generation III, and three in generation IV. We determine the segregation ratio in each. It is conventional to form a table with a row for each sibship, noting the numbers of phenotypically normal (carrier, noncarrier, unkaryotyped) and phenotypically abnormal offspring. The proband (IV:4) and his heterozygous antecedents (II:1 and III:1) are excluded from their sibships. Thus, we have the following:

Parent of sibship	Affected	Phenotypically normal		
		Carrier	Noncarrier	Unkaryotyped
I:1	0	1	2	0
II:1	1	1	0	2
II:2	1	1	0	0
III:1	2	0	1	0
III:2	0	1	0	0
III:7	0	0	1	0
	4	4	4	2

(Note, in passing, I:1's heterozygosity must be inferred from his wife's and children's karyotypes. It is a subtle question whether his offspring should properly be included in the analysis, which we will not pursue here.) We see that the offspring of heterozygous parents total 14, the proband and the heterozygous antecedents having been excluded. The proportion of abnormal children is 4/14 (0.29). This, then, is a point estimate of the risk for recurrence in a future pregnancy of a heterozygote. The reader should know intuitively, and after reading the section below understand more clearly, that an estimate based on just

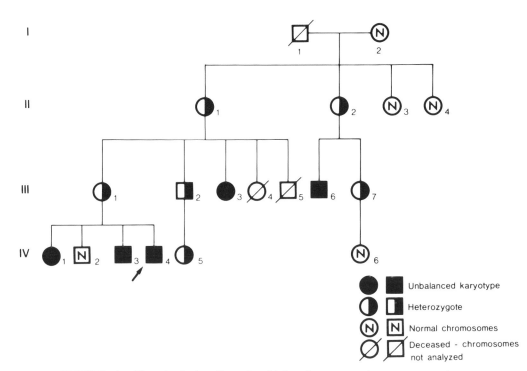

FIGURE 3–1. Hypothetical pedigree in which a chromosomal rearrangement is segregating. The proband is indicated by an arrow, as is conventional.

14 children is not going to be very precise. And what of children who died in infancy, before the family cytogenetic study had been done? Let us suppose this was the case with III:4 and 5. If there was good evidence for their having been chromosomally abnormal, a better estimate would be 6/14 (0.43).

Genetic Heterogeneity and the Use of Empiric Risk Data

It is not necessarily valid to extrapolate from one family's experience to a prediction for another. Different factors may cause an abnormality in different families. As an obvious example, it would be misleading to "lump" all Down syndrome families to determine a recurrence risk figure. "Splitting" into the different karyotypic classes of standard trisomy, familial translocations, and de novo translocations is a start. The standard trisomic category requires further splitting in terms of maternal age. In a unique case, a woman had three trisomy 21 conceptions and displayed a tendency to produce multiple cells with (differing) aneuploidies in at least skin, blood, and gonad (Fitzgerald et al., 1986). She required unique advice. And in reciprocal translocation families, uniqueness is the rule! It is generally reasonable (and often all that is feasible or possible) to apply a risk figure derived from the study of families with a similar, albeit not exactly identical, chromosomal arrangement. But occasionally a family is large enough for a "private" estimate of the recurrence risk to be made from the family itself. This estimate, if it is precise enough (see the discussion below of confidence limits and standard error), is the most valid to offer that family.

Association: Coincidental or Causal?

The counselor not infrequently encounters the problem of a chromosomal "abnormality" discovered in a phenotypically abnormal individual in whose family others—who are quite normal—are then shown to have, apparently, exactly the same rearrangement. Does a genetic risk apply then to children of the carrier, to whom the same rearranged chromosome may be transmitted? The familial paracentric inversion is a good example. In a review of 69 probands, Price et al. (1987) list the phenotypic abnormalities that led to these individuals coming to a chromosome study. There was a collection of various clinical indications, with no consistent pattern (other than that mental retardation was frequent), and several were ascertained quite by chance at prenatal diagnosis. By definition, one parent carries the same inversion; and, if the net is widened, often other relatives as well (Groupe de Cytogénéticiens Français, 1986a). In this context, and provided of course that the carrier relatives are phenotypically normal, one would reach the conclusion that the chromosome rearrangement was balanced, with no functional compromise of the genome, and that it was coincidence that led to its discovery (Romain et al., 1983a).

But when some very unusual clinical picture is associated with a paracentric inversion that is rare or previously undescribed (as most inversions are), some writers are sceptical of coincidence and propose a causal link (Urioste et al., 1994a; Fryns et al.,1994). Similarly, Wenger et al. (1995), noting the coincidence of children with an apparently balanced familial translocation, and being phenotypically abnormal, write that "the chance that two rare events in the same individual are unrelated seems unlikely to us." Here, there is a risk of deception due to "Kouska's fallacy"—Kouska was a fictional 19th-century philosopher who concluded that the combination of unlikely events that led to his parents meeting was too implausible to believe, and that therefore he himself could not exist (Lubinsky, 1986). As does Lubinsky, we must insist on the point: the proband *had* to be phenotypically abnormal, and the coexistence of a subsequently discovered different abnormal event (the karyotype) need not be seen as necessarily remarkable.

This is not to exclude the possibility of a causal link. Biological plausibility is an important criterion. It is not straightforward to explain the normality of a parent and other relatives if they carry the same abnormal chromosome. For the apparently balanced translocation, Wenger et al. (1995) offered the speculative explanation of an instability of fragile sites at or near the translocation breakpoint, while Wagstaff and Hemann (1995) provide an actual demonstration of a biological mechanism (a cryptic insertion; see p. 187). When a balanced rearrangement has a breakpoint in the region of a suspected disease locus a causal link is a reasonable proposition, the perplexing fact of a normal heterozygous parent notwithstanding, as Rizzu et al. (1995) propose in a child with Cornelia de Lange syndrome and a paracentric inv(3). It may truly be that, perhaps in no more than a very few of these apparently balanced rearrangements, a real biological mechanism exists to explain the observed karyotypic–phenotypic association. The precedent of a rigorous statistical "proof" that anticipation did not exist in myotonic dystrophy, only to fall to the real proof of molecular genetics, is an example we should not forget.

Presentation of a Risk Figure

A risk figure is a probability statement, and should be presented as such to the counselee in everyday language—for example: "there is a 50/50 chance for such and such an event"; "the risk for such and such to happen is around one chance in ten." The raw probability figure may not of itself be sufficient, and it is a test of the counselor's skill to interpret figures so as to provide empathic guidance rather than presumptuous direction. Loaded interpretative comments such as "the risk is quite high that. . . ." or " there is only a small chance that. . . ." should be used with great care. The perception of a risk figure as high or low may vary greatly according to an individual's personality and past life experiences and the way they use the language of numbers; the very act of discussing the risk may help the client see it in a less threatening light (Pearn, 1977, 1979; Kessler and Levine, 1987). A helpful perspective may be provided by noting that about 3% of all babies have a major congenital malformation or a substantial degree of mental retardation. People can come to the same risk from different positions. For example, older women having an increased age-related risk (say, 1 in 100) for a child with Down syndrome may decide against an amniocentesis if a maternal serum screening test gives a risk (say, 1 in 200) which is above the cut-off for access to amniocentesis (1 in 250) but lower than their "starting figure," whereas a younger woman with an age-related risk of, say, 1 in 500 is likely to opt for amniocentesis if she were to have the same 1 in 200 result from the screening test (Beekhuis et al., 1994).

As noted earlier, theoretical risk figures are true and empiric risk figures are estimates; the former are exact, and the latter are not. For an empiric figure we have a point estimate (e.g., 10%) and a likely range (e.g., 5–15%) of where the risk actually is. The more data that have been gathered, the more accurate the estimate and the narrower the likely range, and the more confidently, therefore, the counselor can present the figure. The likely range can be measured in different ways. The standard error, which formally measures the precision of the estimate, can be used to give a sense of the region within which the true risk can realistically be considered to lie. The 95% confidence limits define the broad range that very probably ($P = 0.95$) encompasses the true risk. Formulas to determine these parameters are set out in Appendix C.

PARENT WITH A CHROMOSOMAL ABNORMALITY

4

Autosomal Reciprocal Translocations

Reciprocal translocations are common, and every counselor can expect to see translocation families. The usual form is the simple, or two-way, reciprocal translocation: only two chromosomes, usually autosomes, are involved, with one breakpoint in each. It is this category we consider in this chapter. The special cases of translocations involving sex chromosomes, and of complex translocations, are dealt with in separate chapters.

A few translocations are associated with a high risk, as much as 20% or rarely higher, to have a malformed and mentally retarded child due to the parent transmitting an unbalanced chromosomal complement. Many translocations imply an intermediate level of risk, in the region of 5–10%. Some carriers have a low risk, 1% or less; but the woman who is a carrier, or the partner of a male carrier, may have a high miscarriage rate. Others imply, apparently, no risk to have an abnormal child, but the likelihood of miscarriage is high. Yet others, discovered fortuitously, seem to be of no reproductive significance, with carriers having no difficulties in conceiving or carrying pregnancies and having normal children. The counselor needs to distinguish these different functional categories of translocation in order to provide each family with tailor-made advice.

BIOLOGY

Simple reciprocal translocations arise when a two-way *exchange* (hence *reciprocal, rcp*) of material takes place between two nonhomologous chromosomes. The process follows the physical apposition of a segment of each chromosome, which may have been promoted by the presence in each segment of a similar DNA sequence. A break occurs in one arm of each chromosome, and the portions of chromosome material distal to the breakpoints switch positions. The portions exchanged are the *translocated segments*; the rest of the chromosome (which includes the centromere) is the *centric segment*. The rearranged chromosome is called a *derivative* (*der*) chromosome. It is identified according to

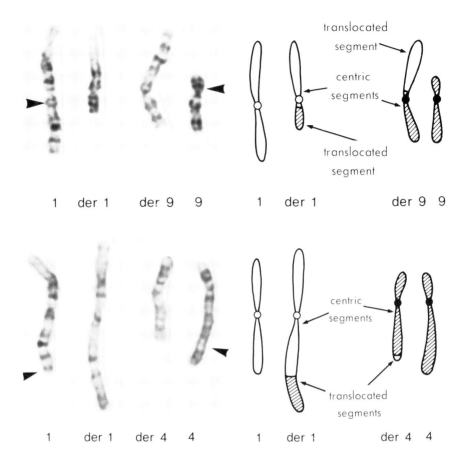

FIGURE 4–1. Reciprocal translocations demonstrating (*above*) double-segment and (*below*) single-segment exchange. Translocations are rcp(1;9)(q12;p12) and rcp(1; 4)(q44;q31.3). (Courtesy D. R. Romain and N.A. Monk.)

which centromere it possesses, as in the der(1) and der(9) depicted in Figure 4–1. When no loss or perturbation of genetic material occurs—in other words, the translocation is balanced—the phenotype of the heterozygote is normal, other things being equal. Extrapolating from prenatal and newborn studies (Van Dyke et al., 1983), about 1 person in 625 of the general population is a reciprocal translocation heterozygote. The translocation may have arisen de novo in the consultand, or may be widespread, with many carriers throughout a family and sometimes of centuries-long duration. Koskinen et al. (1993) trace a rcp(12;21) in western Finland back to a couple born in 1752!

When both translocated segments are of substantial size, we refer to this as a *double-segment*[1] exchange. The translocation shown in Figure 4–1 between a No. 1 and a No. 9, with breakpoints (arrowheads) in the proximal regions of No. 1 long arm and of No. 9 short arm, is an example of a double-segment exchange. The translocation involving breakpoints right at or actually within the centromere, with exchange of entire arms, is a particular and very rare type of double-segment exchange known as the *whole arm translocation* (Kleczkowska et al., 1986; Gravholt et al., 1994; Tümer et al, 1995). On the other hand, when one of the translocated segments is very small and comprises only the telomeric region of a chromosome arm—and thus we suppose contains no genes—this is regarded as, effectively, a *single-segment*[1] exchange. The 1;4 translocation shown in Figure 4–1, involving a substantial piece of No. 4 long arm exchanging positions with the terminal tip of a No. 1 long arm, exemplifies single-segment exchange.

The very rare category of *telomere fusion* warrants inclusion here, even though it does not, to be precise, involve a reciprocal exchange. This is the fusion at the telomere of complete, or nearly complete chromosomes, and the person has the karyotype 45,−A,−B,+t(A;B) (Rossi et al., 1993; Reeve et al., 1993).

DETAILS OF MEIOTIC BEHAVIOR

At meiosis I, the four chromosomes with segments in common come together as a quadrivalent. To match homologous segments, the four chromosomes must form a cross-shaped configuration (Figure 4–2). This is most clearly seen when the chromosomes are at the pachytene stage of meiosis I (hence, the *pachytene configuration*). As the gametocyte enters metaphase, the four components of the quadrivalent have released their points of attachment except at the tips of the chromosome arms, and a ring configuration forms. If attachment fails at one of the terminal pairings, a chain forms instead of a ring. Then, when the first meiotic cell division occurs (recall that the cell at this point is either a primary oocyte or a primary spermatocyte), the four chromosomes separate from each other, and may be distributed to the two daughter cells (may *segregate*) in a number of ways. A 2:2 segregation refers to two chromosomes going to one cell and two to the other; in 3:1 segregation three go to one cell and one to the other. The propensity for a particular segregation outcome may reflect a particular geometry of the quadrivalent, and whether it forms a ring or a chain.

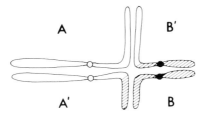

FIGURE 4–2. Pachytene configuration. The two normal (A, B) and the two translocation (A′, B′) homologs align corresponding segments of chromatin during meiosis I.

Modes of Segregation

Within these broad categories we can list the particular modes of segregation according to which chromosomes actually go where. Referring to the four chromosomes of the quadrivalent as A, B, A', and B' (see Figure 4–2) the modes of segregation are summarized as follows:

	One gametocyte with	Other gametocyte with	Segregation mode
2:2 Segregations	A & B	A' & B'	Alternate segregation
	A & B'	B & A'	Adjacent-1 segregation
	A & A'	B & B'	Adjacent-2 segregation
3:1 Segregations	A B & A'	B'	3:1 segregation with tertiary trisomy or monosomy
	A B & B'	A'	
	A' B' & A	(B)	3:1 segregation with interchange trisomy or monosomy
	A' B' & B	(A)	

In meiosis II, asymmetric segregation can happen, but this is very rare (Masuno et al., 1991). Crossing over can occur, and if it does so in the interstitial segment (between centromere and translocation breakpoint), a recombinant chromosome is formed; but almost always these gametic outcomes are either indistinguishable from other nonrecombining segregants or extremely imbalanced and very early lethal (Stene and Stengel-Rutkowski, 1982; Brandriff et al., 1986). Thus, for practical purposes, we can consider each complement to be conserved through a second meiotic division—following which, the mature gamete forms. Some of these gametes, though unbalanced, are "viable" in the sense of being "capable of giving rise to a conceptus, which would proceed through to the birth of a child." Many are not viable. The two combinations that produce interchange monosomy, (B) and (A) above, never are.

Each of these modes of segregation will now be discussed. In broad outline, the mechanics are outlined in Figure 4–3.

Alternate Segregation

In 2:2 alternate segregation, centromeres opposite each other travel to opposite poles. Note that alternate segregation is the only mode that leads to gametes with a complete genetic complement—one with a normal karyotype, the other with the reciprocal translocation in the balanced state. All other modes can be classified as "malsegregation."

Adjacent Segregation

In 2:2 adjacent segregation, adjacent centromeres travel together. There are two categories. In *adjacent-1* segregation, adjacent chromosomes with *unalike* (nonhomologous) centromeres travel to the same daughter cell (an aide-mémoire: in adjacent-*1*, the daughter cells get *one* of each centromere). Overall, *adjacent-1 is the most frequently seen mode of malsegregation* in the children of translocation heterozygotes. In *adjacent-2* segregation, which is rather un-

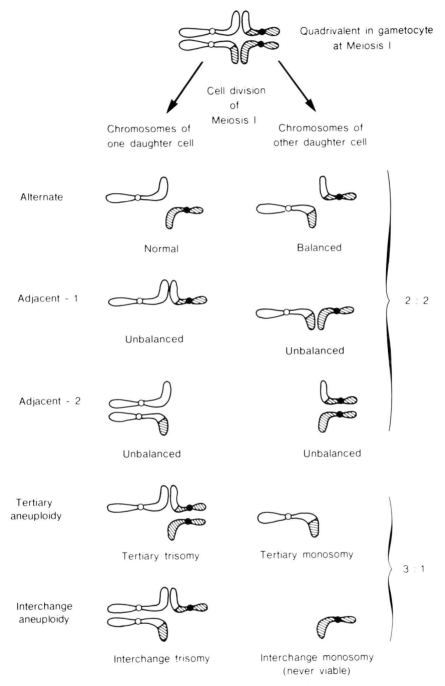

FIGURE 4–3. The categories of 2:2 and 3:1 segregation that may occur in gametogenesis in the translocation heterozygote. In the four 3:1 categories, only one of the two possible combinations in each category is depicted (both are shown in Figure 4–4).

common, adjacent chromosomes with *like* (homologous) centromeres go to the same daughter cell (another aide-mémoire: in adjacent-2, the *two* homologous centromeres go *to*gether). Thus, adjacent-2 segregation rather resembles nondisjunction.

3:1 Segregation

This is also referred to as 3:1 nondisjunction. Gametes with 24 chromosomes and 22 chromosomes are formed, and the conceptuses therefore have 47 or 45 chromosomes. Almost always, the 47-chromosome conceptus is the only viable one. Two categories exist: either the two normal chromosomes of the quadrivalent plus one of the translocation chromosomes go together (*tertiary trisomy*) or, rarely, the two translocation chromosomes and one of the normal chromosomes segregate (*interchange trisomy*). *Tertiary monosomy*, with a 45-chromosome conceptus, is extremely rare.

In theory, 16 possible chromosomal combinations could be produced in the gametes of the autosomal translocation heterozygote. Four of these we can ignore (4:0 segregants and interchange monosomies) because they are never viable. The two balanced gametes (2:2 alternate segregants) are always viable, other things being equal. Of the remaining ten possibilities, usually none or only one will be viable; occasionally two and, rarely, more than two are viable. Figure 4–4 depicts the various combinations that need to be considered (using the previously discussed 1;4 translocation as an example). In a review of 1159 rcp families, Cohen et al. (1994) found the proportions of chromosomally unbalanced offspring as follows: 71% adjacent-1, 4% adjacent-2, 22% tertiary trisomy/monosomy, and 2.5% interchange trisomy.

It is, apparently, the norm for the heterozygote to produce gametes in which many of the possible chromosomal combinations occur, albeit the proportions may differ for different translocations. Sperm karyotyping results from 27 men, heterozygous for a translocation, are summarized in Table 4–1. On average, alternate and adjacent-1 segregants are the predominant types, occurring in similar fractions (47% and 37%, respectively). Adjacent-2 at 12% and 3:1 at 5% are less frequently seen; and just one individual had a single 4:0 segregant sperm. Considerable variation occurs: some heterozygotes had no 3:1 segregants, and one had 21%; for adjacent-2, the range is 0 to 31%. It would not be surprising if a similar distribution and range of germ cell abnormalities were produced by their heterozygous sisters. Most unbalanced combinations would produce such enormous genetic imbalance that the conceptus would be lost very early in pregnancy (occult abortion), or even fail to implant. Moderate imbalances would proceed to the stage of recognizable miscarriage or to later fetal death. Those conceptuses with lesser imbalances may result in the birth of an abnormal child.

Viability is much more likely in the case of effective *single-segment* imbalance. In the unbalanced state, a partial monosomy or trisomy for the very small terminal piece is likely to contribute minimally or (if it contains no genes) not at all to the overall imbalance. This is of particular relevance in adjacent-1

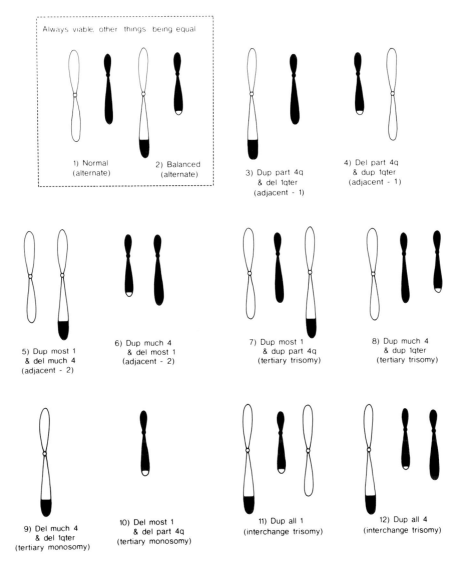

FIGURE 4–4. Segregant gametes that may be produced by the translocation het-erozygote, using the 1;4 translocation depicted in Figure 4–1 as an example (Dup = duplication, Del = deletion). The No.1 chromatin is open; No.4 chromatin is solid. Interchange monosomies and 4:0 segregants are not included.

segregation. Consider, for example, gamete (3) in Figure 4–4. The material missing from the telomeric tip of No. 1 long arm (1qter)—the telomeric cap—is so small that its loss, as far as we can tell, has insignificant phenotypic effect. For practical purposes, we can ignore this partial monosomy. So, the significant imbalance reduces to a partial 4q trisomy (trisomy 4q31.3→qter). This, as it happens, is well recognized as being a viable complement. (It is the imbalance in the children whose photograph appears in the frontispiece.) On the other hand,

Table 4—1 Chromosome segregations in sperm of 27 reciprocal translocation heterozygotes[a]

rcp	Alt	Adj-1	Adj-2	3:1	4:0
(1;2)(q32;q36)	41%	42%	6%	11%	0
(1;4)(p36.2;q31.3)[b]	46%	38%	7%	9%	0
(1;4)(p36.2;q31.3)[b]	39%	50%	8%	3%	0
(1;9)(q22;q31)	46%	38%	13%	4%	0
(1;11)(p36.3;q13.1)	33%	43%	16%	8%	0
(2;5)(p11;q15)	—	—	5%	21%	0
(2;9)(q21;p22)	43%	28%	24%	4%	0
(2;17)(q35;p13)	56%	33%	11%	0	0
(2;18)(p21;q11.2)	42%	35%	14%	8%	2%
(3;8)(p13;p21)	34%	44%	21%	1%	0
(3;15)(q26.2;q26.1)	48%	36%	12%	2%	0
(3;16)(p23;q24)	37%	41%	16%	5%	0
(4;6)(q28;p23)	46%	52%	2%	½%	0
(4;17)(q21.3;q23.2)	57%	35%	7%	2%	0
(5;7)(q13;p15.1)	40%	26%	17%	17%	0
(5;13)(q11;q33)	77%	21%	2%	0	0
(5;18)(p15;q21)	81%	16%	0	3%	0
(6;7)(q27;q22.1)	51%	49%	0	0	0
(6;14)(p24;q22)	68%	32%	0	0	0
(7;14)(q21;q13)	53%	32%	16%	0	0
(8;15)(p22;q21)	37%	38%	21%	4%	0
(9;18)(p12;q12.1)	34%	63%	0	2%	0
(10;12)(q26.1;p13.3)	61%	26%	7%	6%	0
(11;17)(p11.2;q12.3)	39%	32%	27%	3%	0
(11;22)(q23;q11)	23%	39%	23%	15%	0
(12;20)(q24.3;q11)	47%	42%	10%	2%	0
(16;19)(q11.1;q13.3)	40%	28%	31%	1%	0
Average fractions	47%	37%	12%	5%	~0

[a]Alt = alternate, adj-1 = adjacent-1, adj-2 = adjacent-2.

[b]Cousins

Sources: References in Estop et al. (1995).

in the *double-segment* exchange the imbalance contributed by each segment must be taken into account. Thus, adjacent-1 gametes have both a partial trisomy and a partial monosomy to a significant degree, and would produce a "phenotypic hybrid." Very frequently, the combination is nonviable.

If there is the possibility of viability for an imbalance, it is much the most common circumstance that there will be only one combination that is viable. Usually, this sole survivable imbalance will be one which endows a partial trisomy. It is infrequent that more than one of the imbalanced possibilities will be viable.

Predicting Segregant Outcomes

How can we determine, for the individual translocation carrier, which segregant outcomes, if any, might lead to the birth of an abnormal child? A useful ap-

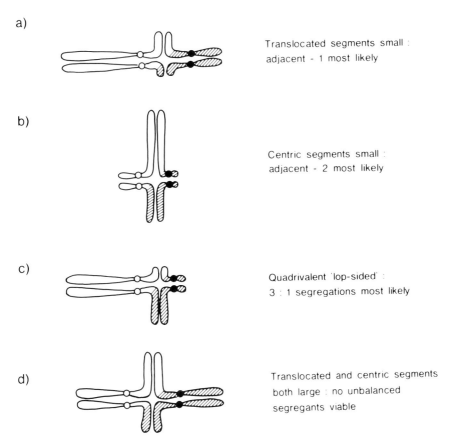

a) Translocated segments small :
adjacent - 1 most likely

b) Centric segments small :
adjacent - 2 most likely

c) Quadrivalent 'lop-sided' :
3 : 1 segregations most likely

d) Translocated and centric segments
both large : no unbalanced
segregants viable

FIGURE 4–5. Prediction of likely viable segregant outcomes by pachytene diagram drawing.

proach is to imagine how the chromosomes come to be distributed during meiosis. Following Jalbert et al. (1980, 1988), we may draw, roughly to scale, a diagram of the presumed pachytene configuration of the quadrivalent, and then deduce which modes of segregation are likely to lead to the formation of gametes, which could then produce a viable conceptus. The following (and Figure 4–5) are the ground rules:

1. We assume that alternate segregation is (*a*) frequent and (*b*) associated with phenotypic normality.
2. The least imbalanced, least monosomic of the imbalanced gametes is the one most likely to produce a viable conceptus.
3. If the *translocated* segments are small in genetic content, adjacent-1 is the most likely type of malsegregation capable of giving rise to viable abnormal offspring (Figure 4–5a).
4. If the *centric* segments are small in content, adjacent-2 is the most likely segregation (Figure 4–5b).

5. If one of the whole chromosomes of the quadrivalent is small in content, 3:1 disjunction is the most likely (Figure 4–5c). The small chromosome may be a small derivative chromosome, or a No. 13, 18, or 21.

6. If the quadrivalent has characteristics of both rules 3 and 5, or of rules 4 and 5, then both adjacent and 3:1 segregations may give rise to viable offspring.

7. If the translocated and centric segments both have large content, no mode of segregation could produce an unbalanced gamete that would lead to a viable offspring (Figure 4–5d).

Some examples to illustrate these points follow.

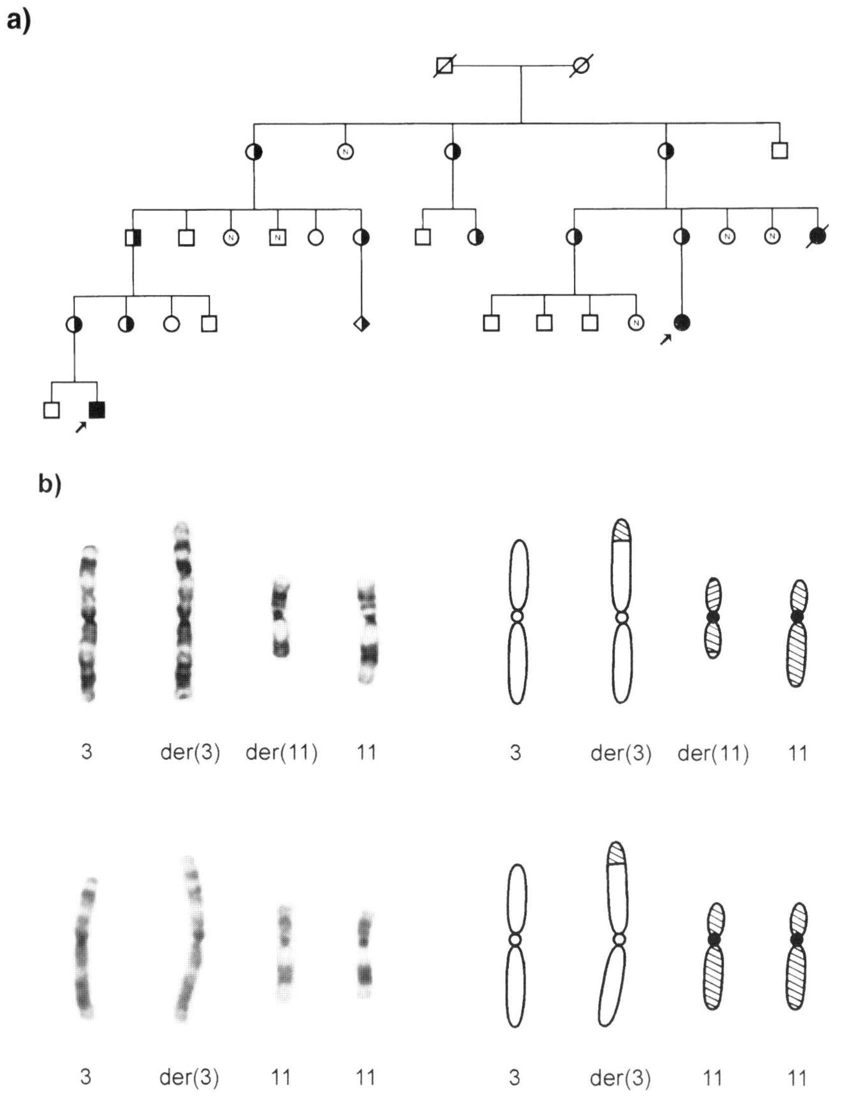

a)

b)

| 3 | der(3) | der(11) | 11 | 3 | der(3) | der(11) | 11 |

| 3 | der(3) | 11 | 11 | 3 | der(3) | 11 | 11 |

FIGURE 4–6 (legend opposite)

Adjacent-1 Segregation, Single-Segment Exchange

Many translocations involve an effectively single-segment exchange, with the translocated segment comprising a fairly small amount of chromatin (1–2% of the haploid autosomal length, HAL). This is the classical scenario within which adjacent-1 segregation occurs, and produces a phenotype capable of postnatal survival. The father with the rcp(1;4) in Figure 4–1, whose children with partial 4q trisomy are shown in the frontispiece as discussed above, is an example. Consider now the family whose pedigree is depicted in Figure 4–6a: those individuals shown as heterozygotes have the balanced translocation 46,t(3; 11)(p26;q21). A segment of chromatin consisting of almost half of the long arm of chromosome 11, and comprising 1.4% of the HAL, is translocated across to the tip of chromosome 3 short arm (Figure 4–6b). The telomeric tip of chromosome 3 short arm, which we imagine to comprise little or no phenotypically important genetic material, has moved reciprocally across to chromosome 11. The presumed pachytene configuration during gametogenesis in the heterozygote would be as drawn in Figure 4–6c. The adjacent-1 segregant gamete with −3,+der(3) (heavy arrows) produces a conceptus that has a partial 11q trisomy, as the der(3) carries the segment 11q21→qter. The loss of the 3p telomeric tip in this der(3) we presume to have no effect. No individuals are known of in this family having the other adjacent-1 combination (Figure 4–6c, light arrows): that is, the 46,−11,+der(11) karyotype, which would endow a partial 11q monosomy. Consulting Schinzel (1994), viability for the segment 11q21→qter in monosomic state is recorded in only two cases. We suppose, therefore, that it has a very high lethality in utero.

The scenario of a single survivable imbalanced form, due to a partial trisomy

c)

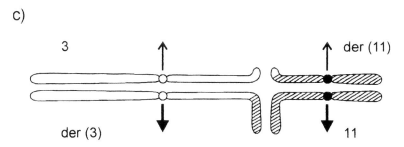

FIGURE 4–6. Adjacent-1 segregation. (a) Pedigree of a family in which there segregates a rcp(3;11)(p26;q21) having the characteristics associated with adjacent-1 malsegregation. Two independently ascertained probands have a partial 11q trisomy, and a deceased relative, who died at age 18 in an institution for the retarded, had a similar appearance from photographs, and so very probably had the same karyotype. ■● = unbalanced karyotype, ❑◑ = balanced carrier, ◙◎ = 46,N, ◈ = prenatal diagnosis, arrow = proband. (b) Partial karyotype of a translocation heterozygote (above), showing the 3;11 translocation, and a child with the unbalanced complement (below) (courtesy A. J. Watt). (c) The presumed pachytene configuration during gametogenesis in the heterozygote (No. 3 chromatin open, No. 11 chromatin crosshatched). Arrows indicate movements of chromosomes to daughter cells in adjacent-1 segregation; heavy arrows show the combination observed in this family.

from adjacent-1 segregation in a "single-segment" translocation, is the most commonly encountered circumstance in translocation families at risk for an abnormal child. (The most common scenario of all may be the family in which no unbalanced form is survivable, and the reproductive risk is confined to miscarriage, as noted below.)

Occasionally, both the partial trisomic and the partial monosomic forms are observed. A good example of this is distal 4p: both deletion and duplication for this segment are well recognized as having substantial in utero viability. Consider the translocation rcp (4;12)(p14;p13) described in a family study in Mortimer et al. (1980). The breakpoints are in distal 4p and at the very tip of 12p (12pter). The presumed pachytene configuration would be as drawn in Figure 4–5a (No. 4 chromatin open, No.12 chromatin crosshatched). With such short translocated segments (and very long centric segments), adjacent-1 segregation is the only possibility for viable imbalance. If we ignore the tiny contribution of a duplication or deletion for telomeric 12p—in other words, if we interpret this as an effective single-segment imbalance—the situation reduces to the possible adjacent-1 outcomes being a partial 4p trisomy and a partial 4p monosomy. Both of these are well-recognized entities, and apparently have substantial viability in utero. The karyotypes may be written 46,der(12)rcp(4;12)(p14;p13) and 46,der(4)rcp(4;12)(p14;p13). At least three cases of each imbalance were observed in this family.

Adjacent-1 Segregation, Double-Segment Exchange

With a double-segment translocation, an adjacent-1 imbalanced conceptus has both a partial trisomy and a partial monosomy (also called a *duplication/deficiency*). Generally, the combined effect of the two imbalances is more severe than either separately. Thus, it is infrequent that the carrier of a "double-segment" exchange can ever have a chromosomally unbalanced pregnancy proceeding through to term, or close to term. However, where both segments are small the duplication/deficiency state can be viable, and if very small, present a relatively moderate phenotype. For example, Huang et al. (1994) describe three family members with dup(14)(q32.3→qter)/del(10)(q26.1→qter) following adjacent-1 segregation from a rcp(10;14)(q26.1;q32.3), in which the dup/del for the two very small segments produced rather minor dysmorphisms and mild mental retardation; the translocation was only just discernible on high-resolution banding, and needed FISH for its clear delineation. Estop et al. (1995) report a child with an abnormal 17p, thought at first to be a de novo deletion, in whose family a balanced double-segment rcp(9;17)(q34.3;p13.3) was subsequently identified only with the use of FISH. The 17p13.3→pter translocated segment comprised 2 Mb or less, but even if it contained only one gene the translocation could still be regarded as a double-segment exchange. (It is a moot point whether some so-called single-segment exchanges might actually be in this category; but the comment in footnote 1 still stands.) A double-segment rcp(4;8)(p16.1;p23.1), in which both translocated segments are very small but nevertheless detectable on routine G-banding, is depicted in Figure 4–7. In this family, each of the

a)

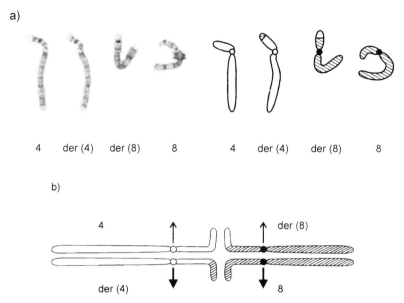

| 4 | der (4) | der (8) | 8 | | 4 | der (4) | der (8) | 8 |

b)

FIGURE 4–7. Adjacent-1 segregation, double-segment translocation with very small segments. (*a*) Parent with the translocation rcp(4;8)(p16.1;p23.1). The index case, his child, has the karyotype 46,der(4) and so has a del(4p)/dup(8p) imbalance, and an uncle has the countertype dup(4p)/del(8p) imbalance due to the 46,der(8) karyotype (not shown). (Courtesy C. E. Vaux). (*b*) The presumed pachytene configuration during gametogenesis in the heterozygote (No. 4 chromatin open, No. 8 chromatin crosshatched). Arrows indicate movements of chromosomes to daughter cells in adjacent-1 segregation. The upper combination (light arrows) would produce the dup(4p)/del(8p) imbalance, and the lower (heavy arrows) the del(4p)/dup(8p) imbalance.

adjacent-1 segregant outcomes was observed: the index case with del(4p)/dup(8p), and his uncle with dup(4p)/del(8p).

Adjacent-2 Segregation

This is an uncommon mode of segregation, limited to translocations in which the participating chromosomes both have a short arm of small genetic content; specifically, the whole short arm can be viable in the trisomic state. In fact, most cases involve an exchange between chromosome 9 and an acrocentric, or between two acrocentrics (Duckett and Roberts, 1981; Stene and Stengel-Rutkowski, 1988; Mangelschots et al., 1992; Cotton et al., 1993). The breakpoints characteristically occur in the upper long arm of one chromosome and immediately below the centromere in the long arm of the other (an acrocentric). Thus, the centric segments are small, comprising a short arm of small content and very little upper long arm.

The rcp(9;21)(q12;q11) illustrated in Figure 4–8a exemplifies the adjacent-2 scenario. At meiosis I, the form of the quadrivalent would be as drawn in Figure 4–8b. The ''least imbalanced, least monosomic'' gamete from 2:2 malsegregation is that receiving chromosome 9 and the der(9) (heavy arrows). The con-

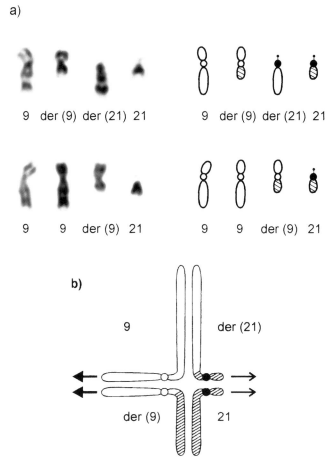

FIGURE 4–8. Adjacent-2 segregation. (*a*) Mother (*above*) has a reciprocal translo-cation rcp(9;21)(q12;q11), and her child (*below*) has the adjacent-2 karyotype 46,+der(9)rcp(9;21)(q12;q11),–21. (Courtesy C. M. Morris and P. H. Fitzgerald). (*b*) The presumed pachytene configuration during gametogenesis in the heterozygote (No. 9 chromatin open, No. 21 chromatin crosshatched). Arrows indicate movements of chromosomes to daughter cells in adjacent-2 segregation; heavy arrows show the viable combination, as observed in this family.

ceptus will have, in consequence, a duplication of 9p (and a small amount of 9q heterochromatin) and a deletion of 21p (and a miniscule amount of subcen-tromeric 21q). Although comprising a substantial piece of chromatin (1.8% of HAL), 9p is qualitatively "small" in the trisomic state. Monosomy for 21p is without effect, and the 21q loss makes little if any contribution. This combi-nation of trisomy and monosomy, together, can be viable. The countertype gam-ete with −9,+der(21) causes monosomy 9p and is not viable.

A similar picture can be seen if the acrocentric is a No. 22 (Stene and Stengel-Rutkowski, 1982). If the No. 22 long arm breakpoint is a little more distal, in q11.21–11.23, the der(9) lacks the DiGeorge critical region (p. 284), and this contributes importantly to the phenotype. Pivnick et al. (1990) and El-Fouly et al. (1991) describe children in whom the separate phenotypes due to dup(9) and deletion of the DiGeorge region could readily be distinguished (and in whom, therefore, an effective double-segment exchange is clearly demonstrated).

> The 1985 I.S.C.N.[2] cytogenetic nomenclature of adjacent-1 and adjacent-2 karyotypes can be distinguished at a glance. Both have the general form: 46,− a whole chromosome,+der. In the former, the "minus" chromosome is followed by "plus" the derivative of that same chromosome, for example, 46,−3,+der(3)t(3;11)(p26;q21) as above. In adjacent-2, the "minus" chromosome and the "plus" der are different, for example, 46,−21,+der(9)rcp(9;21)(q12;q11).

3:1 Segregation with Tertiary Trisomy

Tertiary trisomy is uncommon and may arise only when one of the derivatives is of small content. It exists in the abnormal individual as a "supernumerary" derivative chromosome, with the karyotype 47,+der. The chromosome contributing the centric segment will need to have a short arm of small genetic content; in almost all cases, complete long arms contain too much material to allow viability in a supernumerary derivative chromosome. Curiously enough, in the most common known human reciprocal translocation, practically all abnormal offspring of the heterozygote have a tertiary trisomy. This is the rcp(11;22)(q23;q11) (Figure 4–9a). The quadrivalent of this 11;22 translocation would

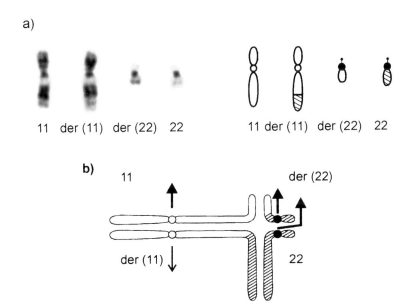

FIGURE 4–9. Tertiary trisomy. (a) The common rcp(11;22)(q23;q11). (Courtesy H. E. Dockery). (b) The presumed pachytene configuration during gametogenesis in the heterozygote (No. 11 chromatin open, No. 22 chromatin crosshatched). Arrows indicate movements of chromosomes to daughter cells in a 3:1 tertiary segregation; heavy arrows show the viable trisomic combination.

have the form outlined in Figure 4–9b. The content of the smallest chromosome, the der(22), is sufficiently small that its presence as a 47th chromosome does not impose a lethal distortion on intrauterine development, and a pregnancy could continue through to the birth of a child who would have trisomy for the segment 11q23→qter (and for the very small segment 22pter→q11). The karyotype would be written 47,+der(22)rcp(11;22)(q23;q11). Nondisjunction at meiosis II in a balanced spermatocyte is another way to arrive at the same effective partial trisomy 11q in the conceptus (Simi et al., 1992).

> This rcp(11;22) is the spectacular exception to the rule that translocations arise, in different families, at different sites. The great majority of families have a "private translocation," and some may represent the first and only case in the whole of human evolution. Apparently, few hotspots for rearrangement exist; equally apparently, 11q23 and 22q11 are remarkably hot hot-spots. One breakpoint may compromise the function of a tumor suppressor gene; there is preliminary evidence that the rcp(11;22) carrier has an increased risk for breast cancer (Lindblom et al., 1994).

At least the male heterozygote for the rcp(11;22) translocation does produce other types of unbalanced gamete (Martin, 1984), as shown on sperm chromosome study (Table 4–1), but none of these is ever viable. For No. 9 translocations, Stene and Stengel-Rutkowski (1988) point out that the risk to the female carrier for 9p trisomy is considerably less when it would arise from tertiary trisomy (1.7%) than from adjacent segregation (20%), suggesting that 3:1 disjunction in the oocyte occurs much less than 2:2 disjunction.

Note that probands in whom an extra structurally abnormal chromosome (ESAC) is discovered often are found, on parental study, to have a derivative chromosome reflecting a tertiary trisomy (Stamberg and Thomas, 1986). Winsor and van Allen (1989) describe a unique apparently harmless small ESAC due to a segregating rcp(9;15)(p24;q11.2), with three balanced 46,rcp(9;15) carriers and three 47,+der(15) individuals in the family.

3:1 Segregation with Tertiary Monosomy

If one derivative is very large, and the amount of material that is missing is "monosomically small," the 3:1 22-chromosome gamete may lead to a viable conceptus. Consider the 12;13 translocation rcp(12;13)(p13.32;q12.11) shown in Figure 4–10a. The large derivative chromosome is not far from being a composite of the two complete chromosomes. It is missing only subterminal 12p and pericentromeric No. 13. This is a "small" loss, and thus the 45,−12,−13,+der(12) conceptus is viable (Figure 4–10b). Fried et al. (1977) provide the interesting example of a child with a phenotype resembling cri du chat syndrome due to tertiary monosomy of distal 5p and pericentromeric No. 14. Courtens et al. (1994) describe an infant who died at birth with, at first sight, monosomy 21 (45,−21); but, upon review with FISH and molecular studies, a 45,−1,−21,+der(1) from a maternal translocation was appreciated. One extraordinary example is a child with 45,−16,−22,+der(16) who had monosomy for the segment 16p13→pter and had both tuberous sclerosis and polycystic kidney

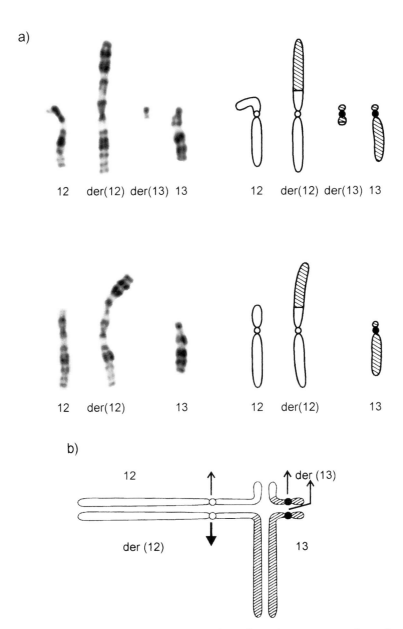

FIGURE 4–10. Tertiary monosomy. (*a*) Mother (*above*) has a reciprocal translocation between Nos. 12 and 13, 46,rcp(12;13)(p13.32;q12.11). Two children (*below*)
inherited the derivative 12, but no normal No. 12 or 13 from the mother, and have
the karyotype 45,−12,−13,+der(12). They are thus monosomic for the tip of 12p
and pericentromeric 13 (and have a near-normal phenotype). Chorionic villus sampling in a subsequent pregnancy gave a 46,XX result; an elder sister was a balanced
carrier. (Courtesy M. D. Pertile). (*b*) The presumed pachytene configuration during
gametogenesis in the heterozygote (No. 12 chromatin open, No. 13 chromatin crosshatched). Arrows indicate movements of chromosomes to daughter cells in a 3:1
tertiary segregation: heavy arrow shows the monosomic complement.

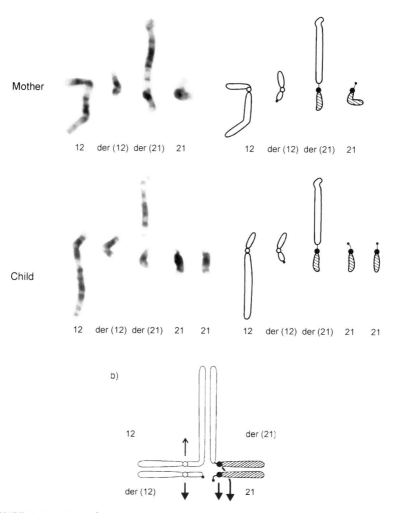

Mother

12　der (12)　der (21)　21　　　　　12　der (12)　der (21)　21

Child

12　der (12)　der (21)　21　　21　　　12　der (12)　der (21)　21　　21

b)

12　　　　　　　　　　der (21)

der (12)　　　　　　　　21

FIGURE 4–11. Interchange trisomy. (*a*) Mother (*above*) has a reciprocal translocation between Nos. 12 and 21; her child (*below*) inherited the maternal translocation
chromosomes and a "free" No. 21. The breakpoints are 12q13.1 and 21p13; an
apparent gap, comprising satellite stalk, can be discerned between the centromere
of the der(21) and its 12q component. (Courtesy R. Oertel). (*b*) The presumed pachytene configuration during gametogenesis in the heterozygote (No. 12 chromatin
open, No. 21 chromatin crosshatched). Arrows indicate movements of chromosomes
to daughter cells in 3:1 interchange segregation; heavy arrows show the trisomic
combination.

disease due to loss and disruption, respectively, of the closely linked *TSC2* and
PKD1 loci; the heterozygous 46,rcp(16;22) family members had polycystic kidney disease, due to the disruption of *PKD1* (European Polycystic Kidney Disease Consortium, 1994; Brook-Carter et al., 1994). Tertiary monosomy with a
deletion of proximal 15q can cause Prader-Willi or Angelman syndrome, ac-

cording to the parental origin of the translocation (p. 269). Tertiary monosomy is rare.

Even more rare is tertiary monosomy with a normal phenotype, due to a *telomeric fusion* translocation (Rossi et al., 1993). A practically complete chromosome, for example a No. 15 or a No. 22 from q11→qter, attaches to the telomere of a complete chromosome. The two chromosomes are fused and with all the necessary functional genetic material "present and correct"; the lost remnant contains no crucial genes. This type of translocation has been associated with infertility (Guichaoua et al., 1992). An obvious idea to explain such a fusion would be the presence of sequences in, for example, proximal 15q that closely resemble the hexameric repeats that characterize telomeric DNA; but in fact no such sequences exist. An apparent intrinsic instability of this part of 15q is reflected in its association with PWS as a "jumping translocation"—the 15q segment is attached to the terminal region of more than one chromosome in different clones of the individual, possibly as a result of somatic recombinations within ribosomal gene sequences (Reeve et al., 1993).

3:1 Segregation with Interchange Trisomy

This mode of segregation can occur only when a "trisomically viable chromosome" (i.e., 13, 18, or 21) participates in the translocation (Figure 4–11a). This chromosome (13, 18, or 21) accompanies the two translocation (interchange) elements of the quadrivalent to one daughter cell (Figure 4–11b). Interchange trisomy 21 is rare (Stene and Stengel-Rutkowski, 1988; Kotwaliwale et al., 1991; Koskinen et al., 1993) and interchange trisomies 13 and 18 extremely rare (Fryns et al., 1986b; Stene and Stengel-Rutkowski, 1988; Daniel et al., 1989; Smith et al., 1989a; Teshima et al., 1992b).

Theoretically, uniparental disomy can be an end result of interchange trisomy if one of the "trisomic" chromosomes is subsequently lost post-zygotically and if this chromosome had come from the noncarrier parent. If this chromosome is one that is subject to imprinting according to parent of origin, phenotypic abnormality

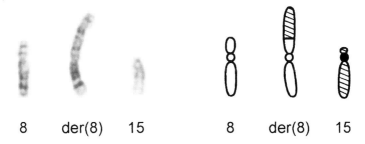

8   der(8)   15   8   der(8)   15

FIGURE 4–12. A translocation causing Angelman syndrome (AS) probably due to "corrected" interchange trisomy. The normal father has a functionally balanced translocation chromosome, 45,rcp(8;15)(p23.3;q11), as illustrated. His child with AS has apparently the same karyotype, but haplotyping with DNA markers showed that both No. 15 elements derived from the father, with no No. 15 from the mother (Smith et al., 1994). (Courtesy A. Smith.)

a)

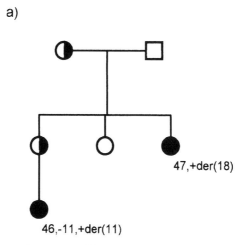

47,+der(18)

46,-11,+der(11)

FIGURE 4–13. More than one viable segregant form. (*a*) Pedigree. (*b*) Mother and one daughter have a reciprocal translocation of Nos. 11 and 18, rcp(11;18)(p15;q11) (upper). Each had one unbalanced offspring, one having 47,+der(18) due to 3:1 tertiary trisomy (middle) and the other 46,−11,+der(11) from adjacent-1 segregation (lower). The former had a complete trisomy 18p and the latter a partial 18q trisomy. (From Gardner et al., 1978; chromosome preparation courtesy C. Ho and I. Teshima.) (*c*) The presumed pachytene configuration during gametogenesis in the heterozygote (No. 11 chromatin open, No. 18 chromatin crosshatched). Heavy arrows indicate one adjacent-1 segregant movement of chromosomes, and light arrows indicate movements of chromosomes to daughter cells in a 3:1 tertiary trisomy segregation, each of which occurred in this family.

will be the consequence, notwithstanding the apparently balanced karyotype. Thus, for example, a rcp(8;15) father—such as the man with the rcp(8;15)(p22;q21) listed in Table 4–1, and 4% of whose sperm were 3:1—could have a child with Angelman syndrome. A comparable case is shown in Figure 4–12 of a man with a rcp(8;15) who had a child with UPD15 Angelman syndrome (Smith et al., 1994). Actual examples of this mechanism are extremely rare.

More than One Unbalanced Segregant Type
Sometimes a reciprocal translocation has characteristics associated with more than one type of malsegregation; so each type may be seen in the family (Niazi et al., 1978; Abeliovich et al., 1982). Consider the 11;18 translocation rcp(11;18)(p15;q11) shown in Figure 4–13. First, the translocated segments are small; 18q is known to be viable in the trisomic state, and the tip of 11p contributes a minimal/nil imbalance (i.e., this is a single-segment imbalance). Thus, one of the adjacent-1 segregants is presumed to be viable. Second, two component chromosomes of the pachytene configuration, the der(18) and No.18, are of small overall genetic content. Thus, 3:1 segregation with either tertiary trisomy or interchange trisomy is possible. In the event, the two unbalanced karyotypes in this family reflected adjacent-1 and 3:1 tertiary trisomy segregation.

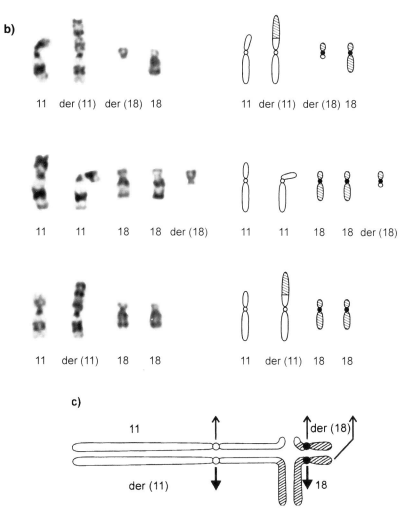

FIGURE 4–13   (Continued)

Rather more spectacular is the translocation illustrated in Figure 4–14. A mother had the karyotype 46,rcp(18;21)(q22.1;q11.2): these breakpoints are toward the end of 18q and immediately below the centromere in 21q. She had a stillborn child with tertiary monosomy, a miscarriage with adjacent-1 malsegregation (and two other unkaryotyped miscarriages), and a surviving child with tertiary trisomy. These three karyotyped pregnancy outcomes were, respectively, 45,−18,−21,+der(18); 46,−18,+der(18); and 47,+der(18). An uncle said to have had Down syndrome may have had the 46,−18,+der(18) karyotype (the der(18) includes the segment of 21 that contributes substantially to the Down syndrome phenotype), or possibly interchange trisomy with 47,+21,rcp(18;21). Some of the other possible imbalanced segregants could theoretically be viable,

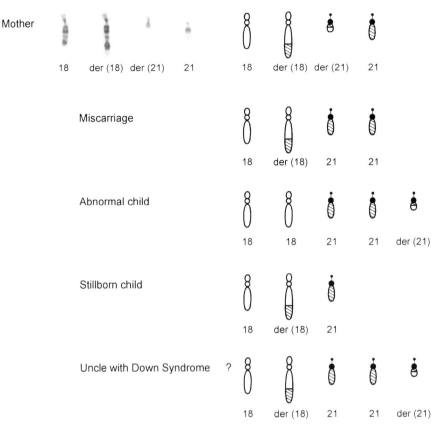

FIGURE 4–14. A translocation rcp(18;21)(q22.1;q11.2) capable of producing several viable unbalanced forms. The karyotype is illustrated of the carrier mother. She had a *miscarriage* due to adjacent-1 segregation, an *abnormal child* with a tertiary trisomy, and a *stillborn child* with a tertiary monosomy, as depicted in the cartoon karyotypes. An *uncle with Down syndrome* may have had the same adjacent-1 karyotype as in the second row, or possibly interchange trisomy 21, as depicted in the bottom row. (Courtesy M. D. Pertile).

and the reader may care to determine which ones these would be. This is due to the fact that many of these combinations have a genetically "small" imbalance. All partial trisomies and some partial monosomies for segments of chromosomes 18 and 21 can be viable as a single imbalance; and, when two different imbalances occur in combination, for example, partial trisomy 21 plus partial monosomy 18, a pregnancy may still be capable of proceeding to term, or at any rate into the third trimester.

No Unbalanced Mode Possible
Finally, for the translocation in which the quadrivalent is characterized by long translocated and long centric segments, no mode of segregation could produce

a viable unbalanced outcome. We emphasize the point that many reciprocal translocations (including whole-arm translocations; Fryns et al., 1988b) are in this category. Consider the family depicted in Figure 4–15, in which a 4;6 translocation rcp(4;6)(q25;p23) was discovered by chance at amniocentesis. The quadrivalent would have the form depicted in Figure 4–5d. It possesses none of the criteria that would allow a viable imbalance to result, by whatever mode of segregation. The translocated segments are both large (leading to double-segment imbalance); the centric segments are very large; and the content of all four chromosomes is large. It would appear that miscarriage is as far as any unbalanced conceptus could ever get. The large kindred of Madan and Kleinhout (1987) graphically illustrates this circumstance: 11 carriers had two or more miscarriages, and numerous normal children, but none had an abnormal child.

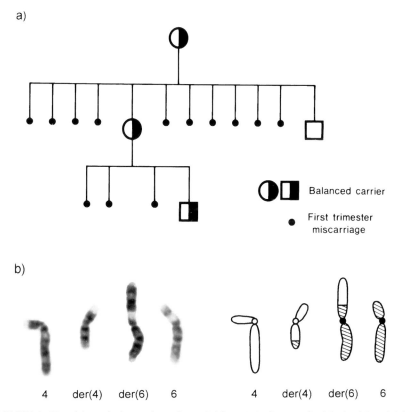

FIGURE 4–15. No unbalanced product viable. (a) Pedigree of a kindred in which mother and daughter have had multiple miscarriages, each having (b) the translocation rcp(4;6)(q25;p23) (Courtesy A. J. Watt.) The presumed pachytene configuration during gametogenesis in the heterozygote would be as in Figure 4–5d. (No. 4 chromatin open, No. 6 chromatin crosshatched) and, with large centric and translocated segments, the translocation has none of the features that enable viability of any unbalanced segregant combination.

In some such translocations identified fortuitously, for example at amniocentesis for maternal age, there may be little or no history of apparent reproductive difficulty.

Infertility

Infrequently, the mechanics of gamete formation in the translocation heterozygote are disturbed to the extent that gametogenic arrest results. The male is particularly vulnerable to this effect. This may be a consequence of failure of pairing (asynapsis or heterosynapsis) of homologous elements in the translocation chromosomes during meiosis, which promotes association of the quadrivalent with the sex chromosome vesicle, and this in turn leads to a complete spermatogenic arrest (Bourrouillou et al., 1985; Chandley et al., 1986; Luciani et al., 1987; Guichaoua et al., 1991, 1992). Translocations with breakpoints very close to the tip of a chromosome arm are more likely to lead to a chain, rather than a ring quadrivalent; and the chain configuration is associated with spermatogenic arrest (Chandley, 1988). An alternative mechanism is that the translocation compromises gametogenesis before entry into meiosis, and asynapsis or incomplete synapsis is an effect rather than a cause (Mittwoch and Mahadevaiah, 1992). Oogenesis may not be immune to the translocation obstacle (Speed, 1988; Mittwoch, 1992). Tupler et al. (1994) report two women, one with primary and the other with secondary amenorrhea, who had a balanced reciprocal translocation. Ovarian biopsy in the former, whose translocation was a de novo one, showed absence of the follicular structures in the cortex. Such cases may exemplify a translocation effect; but also, given the frequency in the population of the rcp heterozygote, it remains possible that the link is coincidental rather than causal.

Infertility may manifest as failure to maintain a pregnancy ("infecundity"), conception having been successfully achieved. We have seen a remarkable family in which, over some 10 years of marriage, the woman had innumerable very early miscarriages, about eight at 12–14 weeks, one 16 week miscarriage, and one phenotypically normal son. The husband (and the son) had the translocation 46,XY,rcp(12;20)(q15;p13). Perhaps, the quadrivalent was configured in such a way that alternate segregation was very difficult to achieve, and most sperm had an unbalanced complement. De Perdigo et al. (1991) report a possibly similar case in which they propose that heterosynapsis in the quadrivalent permitted spermatogenesis to proceed, but at the cost of producing many unbalanced gametes.

Rare Complexities

Translocations with Breakpoints at Vital Loci
The great majority of breakpoints in familial translocations between autosomes are apparently sited at points within the genome where they have no effect on its smooth running. (The same cannot necessarily be said for de novo translocations). Thus, the balanced carriers are phenotypically normal. Rarely, the point

of breakage and reunion might disrupt a gene (Brueton and Winter, 1993). In autosome translocations, examples on record include rcps having a breakpoint at 11p13 and causing aniridia (Pettenati et al., 1989); a rcp(2;20) presumably disrupting the ''Alagille critical region'' (Spinner et al., 1994); an rcp involving 7p21 in some families segregating Saethre-Chotzen syndrome (Wilkie et al., 1995); an rcp with one breakpoint at 7p13 involving the *GLI3* zinc-finger ''embryogenesis gene'' and causing Greig polysyndactyly syndrome (Vortkamp et al., 1991); an rcp(6;7)(p21.1;q11.23) disrupting the elastin gene and causing supravalvular aortic stenosis (Curran et al., 1993); and an rcp of 17q24.3–25.1 that can disrupt the *SOX9* morphogenesis gene and cause the syndrome of campomelic dysplasia with sex reversal (Tommerup et al., 1993d; Wagner et al., 1994). An important historical example is that of reciprocal translocations with one breakpoint at 17q11.2, in persons having neurofibromatosis-1, which provided an entrée to cloning the *NF-1* gene (Ledbetter et al., 1989). Similarly, the t(16;22) segregating in a family with polycystic kidney disease (noted above) enabled this gene, *PKD1,* to be isolated: the breakpoint was sited within the *PKD1* gene (European Polycystic Kidney Disease Consortium, 1994). Ambitiously, Evans et al. (1995) hope that a rcp(1;11)(q42.1;q14.3) segregating with schizophrenia in a large kindred may enable the discovery of a causative gene.

An alternative mechanism is ''position effect'': for example, a translocation with an 11p13 breakpoint can put the *PAX6* gene into a chromosomal environment which does not permit its normal expression, with consequential abnormal development of the iris (aniridia) (Fantes et al., 1995), and a translocation whose breakpoint is 50kb away from the *SOX9* locus can produce campomelic dysplasia (Wagner et al., 1994). A translocation disrupting a recessive locus would require the other chromosome to carry, coincidentally, a mutant allele for the recessive phenotype to be manifest (Alley et al., 1995). A breakpoint and a disease locus may simply be closely linked, and so the translocation and the disease cosegregate in the family (Hecht and Hecht, 1984). Constitutional translocations might convey a risk for cancer if, for example, a tumor suppressor gene is disabled, or an oncogene is separated from its controlling region. Translocations possibly implying risks for breast cancer, renal cancer, and hematologic malignancy are noted in the Genetic Counseling section.

Carrier Couple
Since rcp heterozygotes are not uncommon in the population, on rare occasions both members of a couple will, by chance, carry a translocation (Neu et al., 1988). We have seen, for example, a couple who had had several miscarriages, from 5–9 weeks' gestation. The husband's karyotype was 46,XY,rcp(7;11) (q22;q23) and the wife's 46,XX,rcp(7;22)(p13;q11.2). Presumably, their history of miscarriage reflected at least one parent transmitting, with each pregnancy, an unbalanced gamete: rather many unbalanced karyotypes, as the reader can determine, are possible! A normal child is possible if each contributes a normal or a balanced gamete to the same conceptus. It should, in theory, be reasonably likely in a given conception for the two contemporaneous gametes to have arisen from alternate segregation—as an educated guess, the chance is about 20%—

although at the time of our seeing this family only miscarriage had occurred. A child of theirs having each parental translocation would qualify as having a "complex chromosome rearrangement", and we shall follow that case in Chapter 11 (and see Figure 11–6).

GENETIC COUNSELING

The client may have these questions:

1. Is there a risk of having an abnormal child?
2. If so, what is the magnitude of the risk?
3. What would be the abnormality, and would the child survive?
4. What if the same translocation that I have is found at prenatal diagnosis?
5. What is the risk for pregnancy loss through abortion? Is pregnancy possible?
6. Is there anything else I should know?

DOES A RISK EXIST OF HAVING AN ABNORMAL CHILD?

If a family is ascertained through a liveborn aneuploid child, that very fact demonstrates viability for that particular aneuploid combination. It could happen again.

If, on the other hand, the family was ascertained by miscarriage or infertility, or fortuitously, and there is no known family history of an abnormal child, the picture is less clear. Most likely, no aneuploid combination is viable. Alternatively, a viable imbalance may be possible, but has not yet happened; or an imbalance could occasionally be viable, but usually it is not, and (so far) has led only to abortion. The approach, here, is to determine the potentially unbalanced segregant outcomes, according to the favored mode of segregation—adjacent-1, adjacent-2, or 3:1—and check if any is on record in a pregnancy that produced an abnormal child. A useful source of information is Schinzel's cytogenetic database. Where a *single-segment imbalance* is a potential outcome in a conceptus, from adjacent segregation, and if the potential imbalance comprises an aneuploidy equal to or less than one of these segments on record, viability must be assumed to be possible. If the potential imbalance comprised an aneuploidy greater than any on record, viability would be unlikely, especially if the aneuploidy is much greater. The great majority of *double-segment imbalances* from adjacent segregation due to a translocation ascertained other than by a liveborn aneuploid child would be expected to lead to lethality in utero. Some tertiary trisomies from 3:1 segregation are listed in Schinzel's database, but in most instances one has to make an educated guess, erring on the side of caution, as to whether the combination of partial trisomies from a derivative chromosome might, in sum, be viable.

Table 4—2   Broad estimates of the range of risk (%) for unbalanced offspring of translocation parent that will apply in the majority of families, according to the predicted mode(s) of segregation[a]

	Predicted segregation mode(s) and sex of heterozygous parent		
	2:2	3:1	
Ascertainment of family	Adjacent (F & M)	Ter tri/mono (F)	Ter tri/mono (M)
Liveborn aneuploid	5–30%	1–3%	1%
Other	0–5%	[0–1%]	[0–1%]

[a]Percentages are in terms of liveborn aneuploids/all liveborns. Figures in brackets are assumptions. "0–1" is probably closer to 0 than to 1. F = female, M = male, Ter tri/mono = tertiary trisomy or monosomy.

THE MAGNITUDE OF RISK

If, in a family, it is judged that there does exist a risk to have an abnormal child, a *broad* estimate of the level of risk may be derived from a consideration of four factors: the mode of ascertainment of the family; the predicted type of segregation leading to potentially viable gametes; the sex of the transmitting parent; and the assessed imbalance of potentially viable gametes. Table 4–2 outlines the ranges of risk figures that will apply to most families with respect to the first three of these factors. These percentages are expressed in terms of abnormal livebirths as a proportion of all livebirths.

A *precise* risk estimate needs to be based on the actual cytogenetic imbalance. It is scarcely possible to come up with a unifying format, given that chromatin is not uniform. Different chromosomal segments contain, of course, different genomic information. Some segments, in the trisomic state, impose a relatively mild compromise on the process of embryonic development; such as, for example, 18p and distal 4q. Other segments, although they may be of shorter length, are lethal during early pregnancy, and lead to miscarriage. Some translocations can have their own peculiar segregation characteristics, which were a priori quite unpredictable. Nonetheless, it is interesting to attempt a correlation of quantitative chromatin imbalance with risk to have a liveborn affected child. Daniel et al. (1989), Cans et al. (1993) and Cohen et al. (1994) have compared the haploid autosomal length (HAL) with viability in translocation families. Most (96%) viable imbalances comprise up to 2% monosomy, and up to 4% trisomy, with combinations of monosomy/trisomy viable only when the additive effect of x% monosomy plus y% trisomy falls within a triangular area defined by joining the 2% and 4% points on the x and y axes of a graph (see Figure 1 in Cohen et al., 1994). A few (4%) fall outside of this area, and these cases define the boundaries of a "surface of viable unbalances", reflecting the effects of qualitative differences in different segments of chromatin.

For routine practice in the genetic clinic, we suggest using the unvarnished empiric data for individual chromosome segments collected by Stengel-

Rutkowski and colleagues, as set out in their invaluable monograph (Stengel-Rutkowski et al., 1988) and discussed in a review (Stene and Stengel-Rutkowski, 1988), and to which we have already referred several times above. The figures set out in Tables 4–2 to 4–5 are summarized from their monograph; a better sense of how each figure has been derived is gained by consulting the original document. The paucity of information for some chromosomes has necessitated lumping of data for considerable lengths of a chromosome arm; the risk figures derived in this way are, naturally, composites, and indicative rather than definitive. It is prudent to err in the direction of an overestimate of risk. We assume that, in different families with (apparently) the same translocation, the genetic risks will be the same, regardless of what may have been the mode of ascertainment. And, of course, the principle always applies: if the counselee's family is large enough, do a segregation analysis to derive a "private" recurrence risk.

Adjacent-1 Segregation, Single-Segment

Specific risk figures for individual single-segment imbalances are set out in Table 4–3. A notable point is the number of risk figures which are very small: less than 1%. This most likely reflects that many imbalances are almost always lethal *in utero*, and survival through to term is exceptional. In fact, we can say that in order of frequency, there are imbalances which are (*1*) invariably lethal, (*2*) almost always lethal, (*3*) usually lethal, and—the least frequent category—(*4*) usually survivable. These risk figures are likely to be valid irrespective of the mode of ascertainment of the family or of the identity of the other chromosome contributing the telomeric tip, at least in the majority of translocations.

By way of example, imagine that the carrier aunt of the male affected case in the family shown in Figure 4–6 had sought advice about her own risk to have a baby with the same defect. The single-segment involved is 11q21→qter. As discussed above (p. 69), adjacent-1 segregation is the category that implies risk for viable imbalance in this family translocation. Consulting Table 4–3, therefore, we see that the exact segment 11q21→qter is not listed, but it comes within the compass of the segments 11qter→q13 to 11qter→q22. The best estimate of the group risk for this compass of segments is "less than 2.6%". Since the single segment in this family is at the shorter end of this compass, the upper limit of the risk estimate, namely 2.6%, is an appropriate figure to select. This is a fair reckoning of her risk (say, rounding up to 3%) to have a liveborn offspring aneuploid for 11qter→q21. The risk figure does not distinguish between a duplication or a deletion for the segment concerned, simply an aneuploidy; but since the duplication is much the more viable imbalance of the two, most if not all of the 3% figure in fact applies to the risk for the duplication.

Adjacent-1 Segregation, Double-Segment

Every double-segment translocation is likely to be a unique case (or at least no other described family is known), and risk assessment is less precise. Of course, if the family is large enough, a private segregation analysis will provide the best estimate. Otherwise, Stene and Stengel-Rutkowski (1988) recommend that one consider each segment separately. They propose the rule of thumb that the risk

Table 4—3 Specific risk figures to have a liveborn aneuploid child due to single-segment imbalance from 2:2 adjacent-1 segregation (figures are expressed as a percentage of all livebirths)[a]

			Risk	
Translocated segment that would be imbalanced			%	SD
1.	1pter	→ 1p11–34	0	
		1p35	?	
	1qter	→ q11–22	0	
		q23–32	<1.3	
		q42–43	12.2	4.7
2.	2pter	→ p11–12	0	
		p13–16	<2.5	
		p21–23	5.7	3.9
	2qter	→ q11–23	0	
		q31–32	<1.7	
		q33–36	22.9	7.1
3.	3pter	→ p11–14	0	
		p21	<2.3	
		p22–25	28.6	17.1
	3qter	→ q12–13	0	
		q21–27	<1.1	
4.	4pter	→ p11–13	7.4	5.1
		p14	15.1	4.9
		p15	29.6	8.8
	4qter	→ q11–13	?0	
		q21–34	0.8	0.8
5.	5pter	→ p11–12	3.3	2.3
		p13	7.0	2.6
		p14	29.4	11.1
	5qter	→ q13–21	?	
		q22–33	7.7	7.4
		q34	25.0	7.2
6.	6pter	→ p11–12	?	
		p21.2–24	1.3	1.3
	6qter	→ q11–16	?0	
		q21–24	20.0	17.9
		q25–26	33.3	15.7
7.	7pter	→ p11–13	4.4	3.0
		p15–21	19.1	8.6
	7qter	→ q11–21	?0	
		q22–35	<0.8	
8.	8pter	→ p11–23	9.1	3.5
	8qter	→ q11–13	2.0	2.0
		q21.2–24	11.1	6.1
9.	9pter	→ p11–13	6.4	3.6
		p21–24	16.1	4.9
	9qter	→ q11–13	0	
		q21–33	<0.8	

continued

Table 4—3 (*continued*)

Translocated segment that would be imbalanced			Risk %	SD
10.	10pter	→ p11.1	4.7	2.6
		p12–14	18.8	9.7
	10qter	→ q11–21	?0	
		q22–23	<1.4	
		q24	5.9	2.6
		q25–26	14.0	4.9
11.	11pter	→ p11–13	?0	
		p14	"Low"	
	11qter	→ q13–22	<2.6	
		q23	7.0	3.9
12.	12pter	→ p11.1	9.4	5.2
		p12	9.1	8.7
	12qter	→ q11–15	0	
		q21–24	<1.5	
13.	13qter	→ q11–33	1.6	1.1
14.	14qter	→ q11.1–31	1.0	1.0
15.	15qter	→ q11–15	0	
		q21–25	2.7	2.7
16.	16pter	→ p11.1	8.3	3.6
	16qter	→ q11.1–22	<2.6	
17.	17pter	→ p11.1–13	<2.7	
	17qter	→ q11–12	?0	
		q21–23	10.0	6.7
18.	18pter	→ p11.1–11.2	? (probably high)	
	18qter	→ q11.1–12	2.5	2.5
		q21	2.9	2.8
		q22	15.0	7.8
19.	19pter	→ p11–13.2	?0	
	19qter	→ q11–12	?0	
		q13.2–13.3	11.1	6.1
20.	20pter	→ p11.1–11.2	20.0	8.0
	20qter	→ q11.1	?0	
21.	21qter	→ q11.1–22	13.8	6.4
22.	22qter	→ q11.1–13	<2.6	

[a]One specific translocated segment is of substantial genetic content, and the other is judged to be of minimal content. For adjacent-1 segregation, the risk does not differ for the male or female heterozygote. ? = rare cases have occurred, but data too few to derive a figure. ?0 = probably no risk. 0 = apparently no risk. For segments not listed, no specific data recorded.

Source: From Stengel-Rutkowski et al. (1988).

Table 4—4   Specific risk figures for liveborn aneuploid child due to imbalance from 2:2 adjacent-2 segregation (figures are expressed as a percentage of all livebirths)

	Centric segment that would be imbalanced	Risk[a]	
		%	SD
4.	4pter → q11–13	?0	
8.	8pter → q12–13	?	
9.	9pter → q11–22	18.4	4.5
10.	10pter → q11–21	?	
12.	12pter → q11–13	?	
13.	13pter → q14–21	?	
14.	14pter → q21–22	?	
15.	15pter → q13–24	11.8	7.8
20.	20pter → q11.1	27.3	13.4
21.	21pter → q11.1–22	?	

[a]? = rare cases have occurred, but data too few to derive a figure. ?0 = probably no risk. No obvious difference exists according to sex of parent. For segments not listed, no specific data are recorded.

Source: From Stengel-Rutkowski et al. (1988).

will be *half* that of the smaller of the two risk figures. Even this may be an overestimate; in many cases, the duplication/deficiency from a double-segment imbalance will be invariably lethal in utero—a risk of 0%—notwithstanding that each segment is on record with viability in the single-segment state.

Adjacent-2 Segregation
Very few translocations are capable of producing viable adjacent-2 segregant products, and the data on specific risk levels are limited (Table 4–4). Where the potential imbalance has considerable viability, for example, trisomy 9p, trisomy 21q, the risk is likely to be substantial, and may be in the vicinity of 20%. The carrier mother in Figure 4–8 would have, from Table 4–4, an 18.4% risk for the recurrence of trisomy 9p.

3:1 Segregation, Tertiary Trisomy and Monosomy
In contrast to 2:2 segregation, the probabilities for unbalanced 3:1 outcomes differ between the sexes, with the female having the greater risk. While tertiary trisomy/monosomy is an uncommonly seen category, it is notable that the most common reciprocal translocation in the species, the 46,rcp(11;22)(q23;q11), almost always produces a viable abnormal baby only from 3:1 segregation with tertiary trisomy (Figure 4–9). The risk for this outcome is 3.7% and <0.7%, respectively, for the female and male carrier. For other translocations in this category, the risk is generally small, and is less than 2% in most cases of single-segment imbalance (Table 4–5). Nevertheless, each translocation is entitled to its individuality, and atypically higher risks are possible, as may be exemplified in the rcp(12;13) noted above and shown in Figure 4–10, in which two out of four children had a tertiary monosomy. In this case, it could be that the large translocation chromosome segregates with the normal No. 12 and 13 in the style of a Robertsonian trivalent (Figure 6–2, ''alternate''), while the tiny derivative

Table 4—5 Specific risk figures for liveborn aneuploid child due to imbalance from 3:1 single-segment segregation (figures are expressed as a percentage of all livebirths)[a]

A. Tertiary trisomy or monosomy

Segment that would be imbalanced		Risk %		SD
4.	4pter → q12–13	?		
8.	8pter → q12–13	?		
9.	9pter → q11–32	1.7 ?0	(mat) (pat)	1.7
10.	10pter → q11.1–21	?		
11.	11qter → q23[b]	3.7% <0.9%	(mat) (pat)	
12.	12pter → q11–13	?		
13.	13pter → q12–33	2.6 0	(mat) (pat)	1.8
14.	14pter → q11.1–24	2.6 <0.8	(mat) (pat)	2.6
15.	15pter → q11.1–24	<0.9		
16.	16pter → p11.1	<1.8 0	(mat) (pat)	
	16qter → q11.1–p11.1	?	(mat)	
18.	18pter → q11.1–21	<1.3 0	(mat) (pat)	
20.	20pter → q11.1	<4.4 ?0	(mat) (pat)	
21.	21pter → q11.1–22	6.9	(mat)	4.7
22.	22pter → q11.1–13	<3.5 ?	(mat) (pat)	

B. Interchange trisomy

Chromosome that would be trisomic	Risk %		SD
13	<0.2 0	(mat) (pat)	
18	<0.2 <0.3	(mat) (pat)	
21	0.5 <0.6	(mat) (pat)	0.5

[a]? = rare cases have occurred, but data too few to derive a figure. ?0 = probably no risk. 0 = apparently no risk. For segments not listed, no specific data are recorded.

[b]The common rcp(11;22)(q23;q11).

Source: From Stengel-Rutkowski et al. (1988).

segregates independently, at random. For a double-segment imbalance, the risk in most will be very small, we presume less than 0.5%; since each case is likely to be unique, an educated guess has to be made on the basis of the known phenotypes and deduced survivability for each segment separately. Stengel-Rutkowski et al. (1988) offer a detailed analysis.

3:1 Segregation, Interchange Trisomy

The risk to have a child with Patau, Edwards, or Down syndrome from an interchange trisomy is remarkably small. It may be in the vicinity of 0.5% in the female, and less than this in the male (Stengel-Rutkowski et al., 1988). Upper limits of the estimated risks are given in Table 4–5.

It is probably prudent to assume that where more than one mode of segregation can lead to a viable outcome, the overall risk will be cumulative and will be given by the sum of the individual risks. Thus, the carrier mother of the rcp(11;18) shown in Figure 4–13 would have a risk comprising three components: duplication 18q11→qter due to adjacent-1; tertiary trisomy 18pter→q11 due to 3:1; and trisomy 18 due to 3:1 interchange. From Tables 4–3 and 4–5, and choosing the closest listed segments, these risks are 2.5%, <1.3%, and <0.2, respectively, for a total of <4.0%. The lowest risk, namely zero, applies in the case of imbalances of large genetic content, and in families interpreted as being in this category, prenatal diagnosis could be seen as unnecessary (Vauhkonen et al., 1985).

> The risk for detection of abnormality at prenatal diagnosis is greater than that of having a liveborn aneuploid child. This is because there is differential survival throughout pregnancy, with spontaneous loss more likely in an abnormal than in a normal pregnancy. Very unbalanced conceptions will abort before the time of prenatal diagnosis. Daniel et al. (1989) derived an overall figure of about 25% for carriers to have an unbalanced fetal karyotype detected at amniocentesis when ascertainment was through a previous aneuploid child, and about 5% when it was through recurrent miscarriage. The likelihood of finding an unbalanced karyotype at second-trimester prenatal diagnosis peaks, at 35%, with the carrier whose risk to have an abnormal livebirth is in the "medium" range of 5 to 10% (Stene and Stengel-Rutkowski, 1988).

PHENOTYPE AND SURVIVABILITY

A major degree of dysmorphogenesis, involving several body systems, and globally disordered brain function constitute the usual picture in viable autosomal imbalance (at least those detectable by current cytogenetic technology). Many clients will come with the knowledge of the particular phenotype of at least one of the viable segregant outcomes—the proband in their own family. The same imbalance in a future pregnancy would be expected to lead to a similar physical and mental phenotype. Survivability is less predictable because, for many conditions, there is a fine line between relative robustness and a fragile hold on existence, intrapartum and postnatally. Whether or not there is a heart defect (a frequent malformation in many chromosomal disorders; Epstein, 1986; Pierpont et al., 1987) may be a major factor in this. As for the phenotype of potentially survivable outcomes other than those already exemplified in the family, reference to the chromosomal catalogs (Schinzel, de Grouchy and Turleau) and to the journal literature provides a guide. An interesting question, currently being addressed, is whether partial aneuploidies due to familial reciprocal translocations might express different phenotypes according to the sex of the transmitting parent (Schinzel, 1993a).

THE BALANCED TRANSLOCATION IN THE FETUS

For many years, the conventional wisdom has been that if the same (balanced) karyotype found in the carrier parent is detected at prenatal diagnosis, there is no increased risk for phenotypic abnormality in the child. But some have doubted this, notably Fryns et al. (1986a) in Leuven. These workers had claimed from their own material an apparent excess (17%) of mental and/or physical defects in these translocation children and proposed a causal link. Others remained sceptical and imputed ascertainment bias as the confounding factor (Steinbach, 1986). Upon reevaluating and extending their data (Fryns et al., 1992) the effect remained, albeit at a smaller level (6.4%, which would include the background risk); this figure remains to be confirmed by others. Theoretical mechanisms whereby a ''balanced'' rearrangement could have an effect include cryptic unbalanced defect beyond the resolution of routine cytogenetics, uniparental disomy, and unmasking a recessive allele on the normal homolog.

Wagstaff and Hemann (1995) provide a disconcerting example of a cryptic unbalanced defect: an apparently balanced reciprocal translocation which turned out to be a complex chromosome rearrangement with a tiny segment from the breakpoint of one of the translocation chromosomes inserted into a third chromosome (p. 187 and Figure 11–7). In families in which the balanced translocation has been transmitted to numerous phenotypically normal individuals such a scenario is unlikely, since consistent cosegregation of the ''cryptic chromosome'' to give an overall balanced complement in all these persons would be improbable. Where the translocation is of more recent origin, perhaps de novo in the parent, the possibility may be more real.

A separate concern relates to uniparental disomy (UPD). An apparently balanced reciprocal translocation transmitted from a carrier parent may be structurally balanced but functionally imbalanced. What looks like alternate segregation in the fetus could actually have been 3:1 interchange trisomy, with a postconceptual ''correcting'' loss of the homolog in question—but this homolog had been the one contributed by the noncarrier 46,N parent. If this is a chromosome subject to imprinting (p. 287), phenotypic defect may result (Nicholls et al., 1989; Temple et al., 1991). It is becoming apparent that such a scenario is an uncommon event. James et al. (1994) studied 21 individuals with an inherited balanced reciprocal translocation and having various phenotypic (mostly functional neurological) abnormalities, and none had UPD.

If an important additional risk due to one or other of the above scenarios really does exist, it is surely small, perhaps no more than "a percent or so" that a child with the "balanced" parental karyotype might have a defect of mostly unpredictable severity and extent. In due course, molecular and FISH studies along the lines of Wagstaff and Hemann's (1995) approach may become practicable investigations that confirm that a simple, apparently balanced reciprocal translocation truly is balanced, at any rate in families with a phenotypically abnormal individual having the family "balanced" translocation; and in the case of imprintable chromosomes, confirmation of biparental inheritance at prenatal diagnosis may become an optional additional test. In the meantime, it remains true that in the great majority the balanced translocation really is balanced, structurally and functionally, and will have, of itself, no detrimental effect. Thus, in practical terms, it would be appropriate to continue a pregnancy when the fetal karyotype is the same as that of the carrier parent, and with considerable (if not absolute) confidence in the likelihood of a normal outcome.

PREGNANCY LOSS AND INFERTILITY

Miscarriage

Conceptuses with large imbalances will abort. Against the background population risk of 15% for a recognized pregnancy to miscarry, the risk for the translocation carrier is rather greater, and is in the range of 20 to 30% (Stengel-Rutkowski et al., 1988). An increasing viability of gametes implies a correspondingly diminishing likelihood of pregnancy loss by miscarriage. In practical terms, patients can be encouraged that miscarriage, in this setting, is the natural elimination of a severe abnormality, which provides the opportunity to make a fresh, and hopefully, a more fortunate, start. Optimism has to be muted, however, in the setting of a family history of many miscarriages, which may indicate a propensity for the production of unbalanced gametes.

Infertility
Infrequently, some male translocation carriers are infertile with a spermatogenic arrest, as discussed above. There is little (if any) increased incidence of infertility in the female: oogenesis is a more robust process in the setting of an abnormal synapsis.

OTHER ISSUES

Associated Mendelian Condition

Rare translocations are associated with a Mendelian disorder due either to the breakpoint disrupting or influencing a locus or to a coincidental linkage of a mutation near the breakpoint. We noted some examples in the Biology section earlier. In such families, over and above any risk associated with unbalanced segregants, one should discuss the risk of transmitting the abnormality peculiar to that chromosome.

Cancer Risk

In three translocations there is some evidence to suggest that the rearrangement may disrupt a tumor suppressor gene and comprise a ''first hit'' in a cascade of events leading to the cellular phenotype of cancer. These are the common rcp(11q;22q) which may increase the risk for breast cancer; a t(3;8) possibly predisposing to renal cancer; and a t(3;6) possibly predisposing to hematologic malignancy (Cohen et al., 1979; Markkanen et al., 1987; Lindblom et al., 1994). According to the strength of these proposed associations, heterozygotes should receive appropriate counseling, and entry into a cancer surveillance program may well be appropriate.

Interchromosomal Effect

There was originally concern that a reciprocal translocation heterozygote might be prone to produce gametes aneuploid for a chromosome not involved in the translocation, specifically, in this context, chromosome 13, 18, 21, or X. Warburton (1985) reviewed the associations of reciprocal translocations and trisomy 21 from unbiased (amniocentesis) data and found no evidence to support the contention. More directly, numerous sperm karyotyping studies have shown no excess of abnormalities unrelated to the translocation (Martin and Rademaker, 1990). Jacobs' (1979) assessment thus remains valid: ''there is no indication that parents with a structural abnormality are at an increased risk of producing a child with a chromosomal abnormality independent of the parental rearrangement . . . [and] their recurrence risk for such an event is the same as the incidence rate in the population.''

NOTES

1. There is scope for confusion in the use of these terms: of course, all reciprocal exchanges, by definition, involve two segments. A true single-segment exchange—that is, a one-way translocation—is generally considered not to exist, in that a segment of chromosome cannot attach to an intact telomere, although there are rare exceptions to this rule (A. O. Martin et al., 1986a; Rossi et al., 1993). The distinction begins to break down when a translocated segment is very small but could still contain genes, such as the ≤2 Mb 17p13.3→pter segment in Estop et al. (1995) discussed on p. 70. Be this as it may, the terms double- and single-segment exchange, used carefully, serve a practical purpose.

2. The 1995 I.S.C.N. changes these rules. The ''minus'' chromosome in adjacent-1 is now no longer indicated, for example, 46,der(3)t(3;11)(p26;q21) and the ''−3'' is taken as read. Adjacent-2 nomenclature is distinguished by the inclusion of the ''minus'' chromosome, for example, 46,+der(9)t(9;21)(q12;q11),−21, although note in this example the new custom of tail-end placing of the ''−21'', reflecting its numerical rank. Sometimes the old nomenclature, and sometimes the new, are used in this book. See also Appendix B.

5

Sex Chromosome Translocations

Translocations between a sex chromosome and an autosome, and exceptionally between two sex chromosomes, need to be considered separately from translocations between autosomes. The sex chromosomes have unique qualities that have an important influence on the nature of sex chromosome–autosome translocations. The X is capable of undergoing genetic inactivation, and it appears often to be vulnerable to the presence of a breakpoint. The Y chromosome is composed of chromatin which is, in large part, permanently inert.

In this chapter, we consider translocations involving carriers who are phenotypically normal, or nearly so, and seek advice about the outlook for their own procreation.

BIOLOGY

The X Chromosome and the X-Autosome Translocation

The normal female has two X chromosomes, yet the possession of only a single X is sufficient to produce normality in the 46,XY male. Are the sexes really so genetically different? Does the female really need a second X? The answer is a qualified no. The second X is largely surplus and is subject to genetic inactivation very early in the life of the female. At around the second week following conception one of the X chromosomes in every cell of the female conceptus is randomly genetically inactivated—a process called *lyonization*. In all descendant progeny cells, the same X chromosomes remain inactive and active, respectively. This dosage compensation allows for a functional monosomy of most of the X chromosome. Inactivation is initiated at an X inactivation center (XIC) in Xq13 and spreads in both directions along the chromosome (Figure 5–1). Within the XIC is a gene *XIST* which is *cis*-acting (that is, it can influence only the chromosome it is actually on) and is transcribed only from the inactive X. This transcript is not translated into protein, but functions as an RNA molecule. *XIST*

95

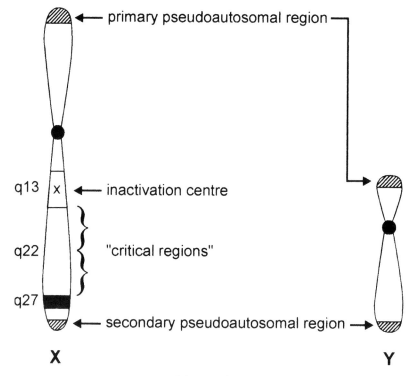

FIGURE 5–1.   Important regions of the sex chromosomes.

(*X* [*i*nactive] *s*pecific *t*ranscript) must be present for X-inactivation to happen, but it is not necessary for its maintenance once it has occurred (Brown and Willard, 1994); epigenetic changes, such as methylation of CpG islands, are thought to have a role in maintaining the inactivated state (Disteche, 1995). The inactive X replicates late during the cell cycle; the active X replicates early, along with the autosomes.

But for some purposes a second X chromosome is crucial. Not all genes on the X chromosome are inactivated and thus some loci are, in the normal female, functionally disomic. There is a block to the spread of inactivation into the primary pseudoautosomal segment, which comprises the terminal 2.6 megabases of Xp in band p22.3 (Figure 5–1); this segment has a homologous region on distal Yp. There is a secondary pseudoautosomal region which extends over 320 kb within distal Xq, having homology with distal Yq (Freije et al., 1992; Kvaløy et al., 1994). An obligate recombination event occurs in the primary pseudoautosomal regions of the X and the Y chromosome at male meiosis; recombination between the secondary regions, if it occurs, is infrequent. Certain other X-borne loci other than in the pseudoautosomal regions (some of which have homologs on the Y) are not subject to inactivation, and disomic expression in the female (and, for some, in the male) is normal (Disteche, 1995).

Patterns of Inactivation in the Balanced Translocation Carrier

The balanced X-autosome translocation carrier has two translocation chromosomes, with the X segment in one containing the XIC and the X segment in the other lacking the XIC. The latter segment, having no physical connection to the XIC on the other derivative chromosome, is beyond its influence, and is always active. The only way, then, for the karyotypically balanced female X-autosome heterozygote to achieve a functionally balanced genome is to "use," as her active X complement, the two parts of the X in the two translocation chromosomes: together, they add up to an equivalent whole, and functioning, X chromosome. The other, intact, X chromosome is inactive (Figure 5–2, upper). Probably the mechanism to achieve this is as follows. Inactivation is initiated at random in each cell, at either of the XICs. Some cells will be functionally balanced, with the intact X inactive, as described above, while others, in which the intact X is active, will have a functional X disomy. Cell selection then eliminates the functionally disomic X lines. This mechanism is successful in

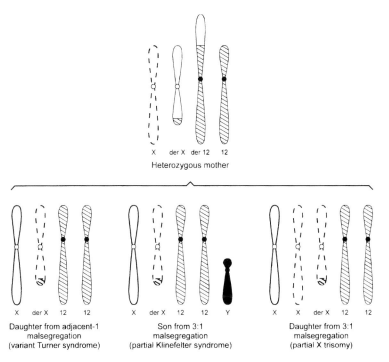

X   der X   der 12   12

Heterozygous mother

X   der X   12   12

Daughter from adjacent-1
malsegregation
(variant Turner syndrome)

X   der X   12   12   Y

Son from 3:1
malsegregation
(partial Klinefelter syndrome)

X   X   der X   12   12

Daughter from 3:1
malsegregation
(partial X trisomy)

FIGURE 5–2.   Mother with balanced X;12 translocation, showing patterns of inactivation in herself and in her two chromosomally unbalanced children with partial Turner and partial Klinefelter syndrome, respectively. It is depicted as an effectively single-segment exchange, with the autosomal breakpoint at the telomeric tip of 12p. Broken outline indicates inactivated chromosome. The phenotype of a theoretical third child with a partial X trisomy (*bottom right*) might be predicted to be close to normal. These three segregations are represented in *b, d,* and *d* in Figure 5–4.

about three quarters of heterozygotes; and aside from a possible gonadal effect (see below) such individuals are phenotypically normal.

In one quarter of structurally balanced female X-autosome heterozygotes, however, the mechanism fails and some functionally disomic cells survive, come to be a constitutional part of the soma, and cause phenotypic abnormality. Only cells with small disomies can survive. Thus, we more commonly observe, in these females, translocation breakpoints in distal Xp or distal Xq (Xp22 and Xq28), which would impart disomy for only a very small segment of either distal X short arm or distal X long arm (Schmidt and Du Sart, 1992; Du Sart et al., 1992). There may also be a contribution to phenotypic abnormality from functional partial monosomy of the autosomal segment on the translocation product which has the XIC, due to spreading of inactivation into the autosomal chromatin.

Inactivation status has been assessed by replication-banding, enabling distinction of the early and the late replicating X chromosomes. Only a small number of cells, a hundred or so, can realistically be studied by this technique, and only from the tissue represented by the sample taken (usually blood). More recently, molecular means to examine X-activation status (the use of methylation sensitive restriction nucleases) have enabled a more powerful approach. A complete concordance of translocation X/active and normal X/inactive in the representative tissue analyzed would indicate that the same 100:0 proportion applied elsewhere in the soma—at least in the phenotypically normal heterozygote. Since it is impossible ever to test the entire soma (and in particular the brain) it would have to remain an open question, in a phenotypically abnormal but structurally balanced X-autosome heterozygote, whether a 100:0 ratio in some peripheral tissue(s) truly reflected the activation status in every tissue. Abnormal individuals showing incomplete concordance of inactivation status may have quite different ratios in different tissues: say, 80:20 in blood and 30:70 in skin (Schmidt and Du Sart, 1992).

Patterns of Inactivation in the Unbalanced Offspring

In the karyotypically unbalanced child of an X-autosome heterozygote, the effects of chromosomal imbalance may be mitigated by selective inactivation of the abnormal X—note that this is the reverse of the case in the balanced carrier (Figure 5–2, lower). If the derivative X contains a significant amount of autosomal material, inactivation spreading into the autosomal chromatin may convert this structural autosomal trisomy into a functional disomy (e.g., Leisti et al., 1975; Pallister and Opitz, 1978; Morichon-Delvallez et al., 1982; Williams and Dear, 1987; Schanz and Steinbach, 1989). Petit et al. (1994) describe the case of a normal grandmother with a balanced t(X;4)(p22.1;p14) who had a 46,X,der(X) daughter in whom the additional 4p material on the X-4 translocation was inactivated in all cells studied (except for the most distal band, 4p16). Her only significant problems were social and personality difficulties; the physical phenotype was unremarkable. (Most extraordinarily, this woman herself had a daughter with the same unbalanced karyotype, the same inactivation pat-

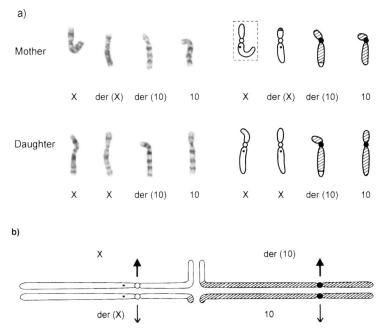

FIGURE 5–3. Functional X disomy. (*a*) Mother with balanced X;10 translocation (*above*), and her daughter with a 46,XX,-10,+der(10) karyotype from adjacent-1 segregation (*below*). The translocation is (X;10)(p22.31;q26.3). Dashed outline on cartoon karyotype indicates preferentially inactivated chromosome; dot indicates X inactivation center. The der(10) contains Xp material in the translocated segment, which cannot be inactivated, and so the daughter has functional X disomy. Since the 10q breakpoint is in the terminal band we may regard this as an effectively single-segment exchange, with the phenotype of severe mental deficit and minor dysmorphism due entirely to disomy for the small Xp22.31→pter segment (Courtesy A. Ma and H. R. Slater). (*b*) The presumed pachytene configuration during gametogenesis in the mother (X chromatin open, No. 10 chromatin crosshatched, dot indicates X inactivation center). Arrows indicate movements of chromosomes to daughter cells in adjacent-1 segregation; heavy arrows show the combination observed in this family. This is essentially the segregation *a* in Figure 5–4, but with an Xp breakpoint.

tern, and phenotypic abnormalities essentially confined to personality.) The extent of spread of inactivation is variable and unpredictable (Summitt et al., 1978; Carpenter et al., 1980; Keitges and Palmer, 1986; Ponzio et al., 1987; Romain et al., 1988). Figure 5–5 shows an example of incomplete spread of inactivation into the autosomal segment.

On the other hand, if the X-originating translocated segment in the derivative autosome does not contain the XIC, it cannot be inactivated, and there will be, in addition to the autosomal monosomy, a functional partial X disomy (Sivak et al., 1994). Figure 5–3 demonstrates a functional disomy for a part of Xp (Xp22.31→pter) in an unbalanced daughter; in this instance, since the autosomal breakpoint is at the telomere, we assume there to be little or no effect from a 10q monosomy. Gustashaw et al. (1994) describe a similar case in which they could be sure the partial functional X disomy was the sole cause of the abnormal phenotype, since the autosomal breakpoint was in 13p and loss of one acrocentric short arm is, of itself, without phenotypic consequence.

The der(X) may contain no autosomal material (other than a telomeric tip) and thus comprise, essentially, a deleted Xp or Xq chromosome. In this case, inactivation will proceed as in any individual with 46,X,del(X), with preferential inactivation of the deleted X. Leichtman et al. (1978) provide an example in a three-generation family with seven persons having an Xp deletion Turner syndrome variant on the basis of a segregating rcp(X;1).

MEIOSIS

Meiosis proceeds differently in the female and the male. In the female, a quadrivalent presumably forms, just as in the two-way translocation between autosomes. Given the greater survivability of X imbalances, and the lessened effect of autosomal imbalance resulting from spreading inactivation, a greater number of gametes may be viable than from the autosome–autosome translocation. The "rules" of segregation may not apply; for example, a viable adjacent-2 malsegregation can occur with a derivative chromosome having a large centric segment. The coexistence of tertiary monosomy and adjacent-2 in the family described in Figure 5–7, two otherwise uncommon segregations, reflects the unique characteristics of the X-autosome translocation. In the male, it may be that a trivalent forms involving the translocation chromosomes and the intact autosome, or perhaps a quadrivalent which includes the Y. Disturbance of the sex vesicle formation presumably occurs, and this, presumably, is why the male with an X-autosome translocation is almost invariably infertile (Schmidt and Du Sart, 1992).

Figure 5–4 sets out certain segregant outcomes that may be viable in gametes produced by the female heterozygote in the three categories of single-segment translocation with the X, or with the autosomal segment involved, and in the double-segment translocation, as discussed below. For simplicity, the X breakpoints are depicted only in the long arm, but of course short arm breakpoints occur.

Categories of Translocation and Modes of Segregation

Single-Segment Exchange

If one of the translocation breakpoints is at the telomeric tip of either the X or the autosome, and thus only one of the translocated segments comprises an important amount of chromatin, this is an effective "single-segment exchange" (and see p. 61). The first column in Figure 5–4, segregations *a-d*, depicts the general form of a translocation in which the single important exchanged segment comprises *X* chromatin. A particular example is shown in Figure 5–2, in which the derivative X chromosome is deleted for a large segment of Xq, and has only the telomeric tip of 12p in exchange. A child receiving this abnormal Xq- in

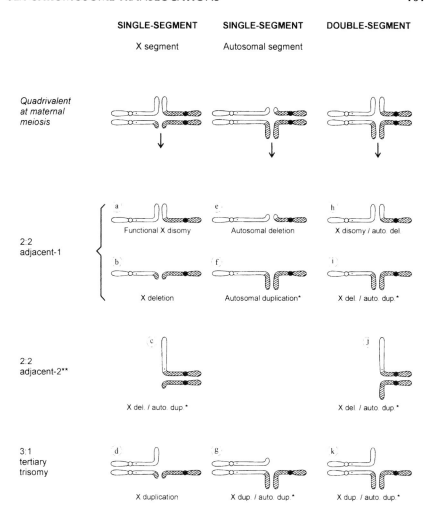

FIGURE 5–4. Major categories of malsegregation in the X-autosome female carrier. Crosshatched = autosomal chromatin, open = X chromatin, dot = X inactivation center. "Single-segment" and "double-segment" are defined in the text. 3:1 interchange malsegregations not shown. X exchanges can occur in either Xp or Xq; only Xq exchanges shown here. Circled letters provide reference points for text comments.

*Effect of autosomal imbalance in female offspring may be lessened by spreading of inactivation into the autosomal segment.

**Only one type of adjacent-2 segregant is shown, the −X,+der(A) combination, which is seen only when the X translocated segment comprises almost all of Xq and thus includes the XIC.

place of a normal X, or as an additional chromosome, could present with a partial form of a sex chromosome aneuploidy syndrome. Thus a daughter with 46,X,−X,+der(X) from adjacent-1 malsegregation (*b* in Figure 5–4) may have a variant form of Turner syndrome. From tertiary trisomy (*d* in Figure 5–4), a son with 47,XY,+der(X) could have incomplete Klinefelter syndrome; and a 47,XX,+der(X) daughter might show the 47,XXX phenotype to a diminished degree. Conceptions with $46,-12,+$der(12) from adjacent-1 segregation (*a* in Figure 5–4) would be functionally disomic for a large, and unsurvivable, amount of Xq, and would abort. However, if the translocated X segment is small, the functionally disomic X state may be viable. This is shown in Figure 5–3, in which the phenotypically abnormal daughter has a $46,-10,+$der(10) karyotype and is functionally disomic for the small amount of Xp22.31→pter.

The single segment may be of *autosomal* origin, with only the telomeric tip of Xp or Xq translocated in exchange (middle column, Figure 5–4, segregations *e–g*). The imbalanced conceptions from 2:2 malsegregation would be partially monosomic or partially trisomic for the autosomal segment: $46,-A,+$der(A) and $46,-X,+$der(X) respectively (segregations *e* and *f* in Figure 5–4). The partial trisomic state may, in the $46,X,-X,+$der(X) female, have an attenuated phenotype due to spreading of inactivation from the XIC of the der(X) into the autosomal segment. The $46,Y,-X,+$der(X) male conceptus, in which no X inactivation occurs, would show the undiluted effect of the partial autosomal trisomy. The partially monosomic state, $46,-A,+$der(A), would be no different than if the other chromosome participating in the translocation had been an autosome, instead of an X.

Double Segment Exchange

In a double-segment exchange with *adjacent-1* segregation (right column, Figure 5–4, segregations *h–i*), there may be, in the unbalanced conceptus, effects of a combined X functional disomy and autosomal monosomy, or of X monosomy (or nullisomy) and autosomal trisomy. These effects may, in the $46,X,-X,+$der(X) female (adjacent-1 segregation *i*), be considerably modified by spreading of inactivation. Consider the rcp(X;16) illustrated in Figure 5–5. The $46,-X,+$der(X) daughter has both a monosomy for most of Xp, giving a Turner-like phenotype, and a structural trisomy for most of 16p. Following spread of inactivation in the der(X) into its autosomal segment in a fraction of cells, the 16p trisomy has been converted, in these cells, into a functional 16p disomy. In 76% of cells, however (and in the cell illustrated), the inactivation has not spread into the 16p segment. Thus she has, effectively, a mosaic 16p trisomy/disomy. This same combination with a Y replacing the X as the intact sex chromosome, $46,Y,-X,+$der(X), with nullisomy Xp/trisomy 16p, would be lethal in utero. The other adjacent-1 conceptions with $46,XX,-16,+$der(16) and $46,XY,-16,+$der(16) (light arrows, Figure 5–5b) would not be similarly "correctable" and would have a very large functional imbalance, with monosomy 16p/functional disomy Xp, and would presumably abort spontaneously early in pregnancy.

Adjacent-2 segregation in most translocations produces trisomy for much of one chromosome along with monosomy for much of the other which is not, in the usual autosome-autosome translocation, remotely viable (e.g., segregation 5 in Figure 4–4). But such an enormous degree of structural imbalance can be accommodated in some X-autosome translocations, in a female conceptus. Firstly, consider the case of the intact autosome and the derivative autosome being transmitted together: $46,X,-X,+$der(A). Provided the X segment includes the

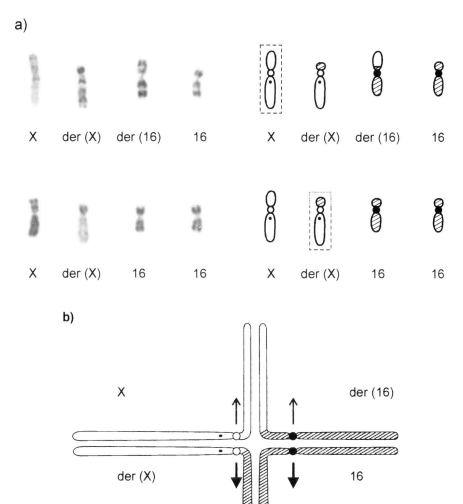

a)

X   der (X)   der (16)   16   X   der (X)   der (16)   16

X   der (X)   16   16   X   der (X)   16   16

b)

X   der (16)

der (X)   16

FIGURE 5–5. Spread of inactivation into autosomal segment. (*a*) Mother with balanced X;16 translocation (*above*), and her daughter with a 46,X,-X,+der(X) karyotype from adjacent-1 segregation (*below*). The translocation is (X;16)(p11;p12). Replication-banding shows active (darker-staining) and inactive (lighter-staining) chromosome segments. The normal X is inactivated in all cells analysed in the mother (dashed outline on cartoon karyotype; dot indicates X inactivation center). The daughter's abnormal X lacks Xp and contains distal 16p material. This chromosome is preferentially inactivated (dashed outline), but in 76% of cells analyzed (lymphocytes) the inactivation has not continued through the translocated 16p segment (dotted outline). The phenotype is the combined result of the Xp monosomy and a "partial" 16p trisomy. The child is short and has a developmental age of about 2$\frac{1}{2}$ at a chronological age of 4 years. (Courtesy C. E. Vaux). One other daughter had the same balanced translocation as the mother, and showed consistent inactivation of the normal X chromosome in blood lymphocytes, but suffered intellectual deficit. (*b*) The presumed pachytene configuration during gametogenesis in the mother (X chromatin open, No. 16 chromatin crosshatched, dot indicates X inactivation center). Arrows indicate movements of chromosomes to daughter cells in adjacent-1 segregation; heavy arrows show the combination observed in this family. This is essentially the segregation *i* in Figure 5–4, but with an Xp breakpoint.

XIC (segregation j in Figure 5–4), inactivation can spread from the XIC in both directions and into the autosomal segment, counteracting the effect of the autosomal duplication, at least partially. The concomitant partial X monosomy is, of itself, a viable state. The child would be expected to display a partial Turner phenotype, upon which the effect of a variably inactivated partial autosomal trisomy would be added. In the case of Leisti et al. (1975), the mother carried a rcp(X;9)(q11;q32) and her daughter's karyotype was 46,X,−X,+der(9). Inactivation spread through much of the autosomal segment, which very substantially, although not entirely, neutralized the effect of the partial trisomy 9: she had a Turner phenotype with superadded microcephaly and mental defect. The case in Williams and Dear (1987) is similar, with a retarded and dysmorphic child having the karyotype 46,X,−X,+der(10)t(X;10)(q11; q25)mat, but inactivation into the autosomal segment did not extend past the centromere of the der(10). This left the child with an effective duplication of 10p, along with the X deletion (Figure 5–6). An adjacent-2 male conception in this setting, being nullisomic for a large part of X, would be lethal in utero.

Secondly, viability is also possible in one rare circumstance of an intact X and the der(X) being transmitted together, with the adjacent-2 karyotype 46,XX,−A,+der(X). The der(X) must contain an XIC; its autosomal segment must comprise a very substantial amount of the chromatin of that autosome; and there must be little or no spread of inactivation beyond the X segment of the translocation chromosome into the autosomal segment. In this way, the autosomal component can maintain sufficient genetic activity to produce a viable phenoype. Only autosomes with "genetically small" short arms, such as chromosome No. 22, could enable these criteria to be met. An example from a maternal rcp(X;22)(p21.3;q11.21) is noted in the legend to Figure 5–7 (this scenario is not included in Figure 5–4).

These same criteria may apply to viable *tertiary monosomy* from 3:1 segregation of an X-autosome translocation, and the rcp(X;22) in Figure 5–7 again provides an example. The der(X) comprises most of an X and all, or almost all, of 22q. In the index case having the tertiary monosomy state 45,X,−X,−22,+der(X), the der(X) chromosome is preferentially inactivated but inactivation has not (on blood lymphocytes) spread through to the 22q component of the der(X) and a functional 22 disomy is maintained, or nearly so. Thus, the important structural imbalance may be limited to the Xp21.3-pter deletion (loss of 22p being without effect), and a Turner-like phenotype might be predicted. It remains open that inactivation elsewhere in the soma could differ from the pattern observed on peripheral blood, with a degree of functional 22q monosomy in some tissues.

From each of the categories of single and double segment exchange, *3:1 interchange trisomy* could theoretically produce Klinefelter syndrome or "XXX syndrome," and *interchange monosomy* could produce 45,X Turner syndrome (not shown in Figure 5–4). We are aware of only one such outcome, an infertile woman with 47,XX,−12,+der(X),+der(12) from a 46,X,rcp(X;12)(q22;p12) mother (Madan et al., 1981).

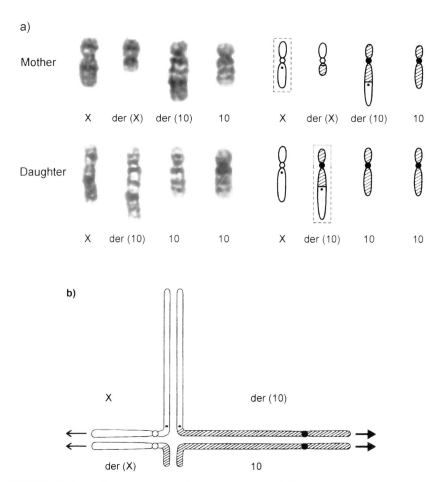

FIGURE 5–6. Adjacent-2 segregation. (*a*) Mother with balanced X;10 translocation (*above*), and her daughter with a 46,X,−X,+der(10) karyotype (*below*), on G-banding. The translocation is (X;10)(q11;q25). Replication-banding showed the normal X to be inactivated in all 30 lymphocytes analysed in the mother (dashed outline on cartoon karyotype; dot indicates X inactivation center). The daughter's der(10) was preferentially inactivated (dashed outline) in 50/50 cells, but the inactivation did not continue through to the 10p segment (dotted outline). The phenotype is the combined result of the 10p duplication and Xp monosomy. From Williams and Dear (1987), with the permission of the British Medical Association, courtesy J. Williams. (*b*) The presumed pachytene configuration during gametogenesis in the mother (X chromatin open, No. 10 chromatin crosshatched, dot indicates X inactivation center). Arrows indicate movements of chromosomes to daughter cells in adjacent-2 segregation; heavy arrows show the combination observed in this family. This is segregation *j* in Figure 5–4.

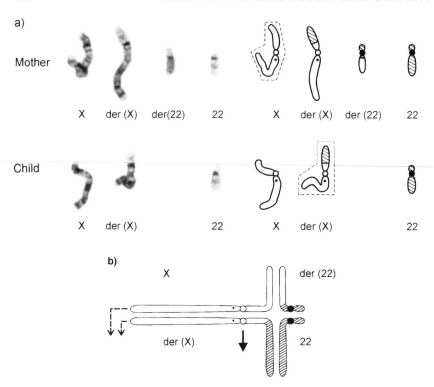

FIGURE 5–7. 3:1 tertiary monosomy segregation. (*a*) Mother with balanced (X;22)(p21.3;q11.21) translocation (*above*), and her newborn daughter with minor physical anomalies having a 45,X,−X,−22,+der(X) karyotype (*below*), on G-banding. The der(X) was positive for the probe sc11.1, which recognizes a sequence in the DiGeorge critical region. On replication-banding, the normal X is inactivated in all cells analysed in the mother (dashed outline on cartoon karyotype; dot indicates X inactivation center). The daughter's der(X) chromosome is preferentially inactivated (dashed outline), and showed, in 50/50 cells, no inactivation going through to its 22 component (dotted outline). The presumed genetic imbalance is thus a partial Xp monosomy in all tissues; whether inactivation may have spread into 22 chromatin in some tissues, causing a "mosaic" functional partial 22q monosomy, remains an open question (the child did not display a DiGeorge phenotype). The maternal grandmother is also a carrier, and the mother's sister with a mild intellectual deficiency had the adjacent-2 karyotype 46,XX,+der(X),−22. (Courtesy T. Burgess.) (*b*) The presumed pachytene configuration during gametogenesis in the mother (X chromatin open, No. 22 chromatin crosshatched, dot indicates X inactivation center). Heavy arrow indicates movement of the der(X) chromosome to one daughter cell in 3:1 segregation to give the monosomic combination, and dashed arrows show the movement of chromosomes in the adjacent-2 combination, these being the two malsegregations observed in the family. Neither is represented in Figure 5–4.

The X "Critical Regions"

The location of breakpoints in the X chromosome involved in an X-autosome translocation, unlike those in autosomal translocations, may affect gonadal function. A breakage and reunion within two "critical regions" often leads to

Table 5—1   Occurrence of gonadal dysgenesis (primary and secondary) in t(X;A) women according to X-chromosome breakpoint

Breakpoint	Gonadal dysgenesis	Normal gonadal function
Xpter–q12	5	37
q13	4	8
q13–q22	20	1
q22	11	6
q22–q25	7	1
q26	3	5
q27–qter	1	9

Source: From Therman et al. (1990).

gonadal dysgenesis. These regions are regarded as being Xq13–q22 and Xq22–q27, separated by a narrow region within Xq22 which is not critical (Therman et al., 1990) (Figure 5–1). Breakpoints within these regions carry an increased risk for primary or secondary ovarian failure (Table 5–1). Premature ovarian failure (defined as secondary amenorrhea before age 40) is particularly associated with breaks in Xq26.1–q27 and Xq13.3–q21.1, and there may be gene clusters in these regions that determine ovarian activity (Powell et al., 1994). However, as Table 5–1 shows, no particular breakpoint is certain to cause gonadal dysgenesis, nor certain to allow normal gonadal function.

Origin of the X-autosome Translocation

All de novo X-autosomal translocations so far studied have been of paternal origin, which may reflect the availability in male meiosis of the largely unpaired X to exchange with other chromosomes (Powell et al., 1994). Giacalone and Francke (1992) did a molecular dissection on a de novo rcp(X;4)(p21.2;q31.22) in a girl with Duchenne muscular dystrophy, and proposed a format whereby two GAAT sequences 5kb apart in Xp, and one GAAT in 4q, came together during meiosis in spermatogenesis, deleted the 5kb length in Xp (which comprised a small part of the dystrophin gene), and reformed as a der(X) and a der(4). Once a balanced translocation is established in a family, male infertility dictates that transmission thereafter will be matrilineal.

> Certain breakpoints are on record as being associated with particular X-linked Mendelian disorders (Table 2 in Schlessinger et al., 1993). These are seen in females with de novo X-autosome translocations in which the actual locus has been disrupted. With preferential inactivation of the normal X there is no functional copy of the normal allele. A notable example of this is the female Xp21–autosome translocation heterozygote who has Duchenne/Becker muscular dystrophy (Bodrug et al., 1990) (Figure 5–8). We comment upon the de novo X-autosome translocation identified at prenatal diagnosis on p. 366.

The Y Chromosome and Y-Autosome Translocations

The particular raison d'être of the Y chromosome is to bring about male development. The testis-determining gene, *SRY* (see p. 294), lies in the euchro-

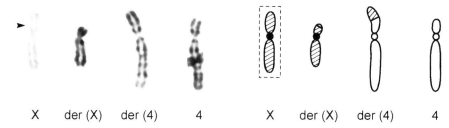

X   der (X)   der (4)   4   X   der (X)   der (4)   4

FIGURE 5–8. A de novo X-autosome translocation 46,X,rcp(X;4)(p21;p16) in which the dystrophin locus at the Xp21 breakpoint is presumed to be disrupted in a 7-year-old girl. The approximate position of the dystrophin locus is indicated (arrowhead) on the intact X. The intact X is preferentially inactivated, as shown here with replication-banding and indicated in dashed outline on the cartoon karyotype, and in consequence very little dystrophin is produced, and the girl has a Becker-like muscular dystrophy. (Courtesy J. A. Sullivan).

matic region on the short arm, just 5 kb proximal to the pseudoautosomal boundary (Sinclair et al., 1990). As noted above, the primary pseudoautosomal regions of the Y and X short arm contain homologous loci, and certain other loci elsewhere in the Y have homologs on the X (Disteche, 1995). Postulated Y-specific genes for height and spermatogenesis have yet to be identified; the gene *DAZ* (deleted in azoospermia) is a candidate for the latter (Reijo et al., 1995). About half the Y—the amount is variable—comprises the genetically inert heterochromatic region of the long arm (Yq11→qter), which contains highly repetitive DNA sequences.

Y-autosome translocations fall into two major Yq-breakpoint categories (Smith et al., 1979; Sheehy et al., 1987), and two rare Yp-breakpoint forms, as follows.

Acrocentric Short-Arm and Y-Long-Arm Translocation

The autosome in the Y-autosome translocation is an acrocentric (Figure 5–9a), with the breakpoint on its short arm, while the Y breakpoint is in the Yqh heterochromatin. In about half of the translocations, the acrocentric is a No.15 and next most commonly a No. 22 (Cohen et al., 1981). Thus, there is no loss or gain of euchromatin; the result is that one acrocentric carries some phenotypically irrelevant Y heterochromatin (Yqh), looking rather like (and sometimes mistaken for) a very long short arm (Neumann et al., 1992). The majority are clinically innocuous; perhaps they all are, and reports of clinical abnormality simply reflect chance associations. This type is usually familial, males and females being equally involved; fertility is unaffected (Chandley, 1988). Phenotypic normality for the t(Yq22p) has been reported in the homozygous state (Leschot et al., 1986).

Nonacrocentric Short-Arm and Y-Long-Arm Translocation

These are apparently balanced Y-autosome translocations in which the autosomal breakpoint is elsewhere than at an acrocentric short arm (Figure 5–9b). This

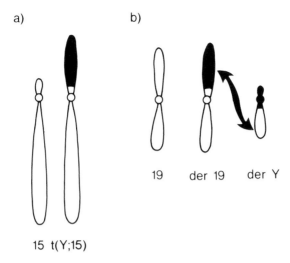

15 t(Y;15)

19   der 19   der Y

FIGURE 5–9. (*a*) The Y-autosome translocation involving an acrocentric autosome, with the breakpoint in the acrocentric short arm. The karyotype is unbalanced, but the phenotype is normal. (*b*) The Y-autosome translocation with the autosomal break-point elsewhere than an acrocentric short arm. The karyotype is apparently balanced, but the phenotype is abnormal. White = autosome, black = Y chromosome.

is a rare condition, classically occurring as a de novo event (Moreau et al., 1987), although familial cases have been recorded (Teyssier et al., 1993). The phenotype is usually abnormal, with azoospermia/hypogonadism a very frequent feature (Chandley, 1988) and mental retardation and physical malformation common. Most, but not all, are male. The infertility may be a result of abnormal sex vesicle (X–Y association) formation disrupting meiosis and causing sper-matogenic arrest (Maraschio et al., 1994); other phenotypic abnormalities may reflect a disruptive effect at the breakpoints (Erickson et al., 1995) or a deletion of autosomal material distal to the breakpoint.

Rare Forms with Y-Short-Arm Translocation

(*1*) In the Yp-autosome translocation, the testis-determining region of the Y is translocated to an autosome, usually an acrocentric (Farah et al., 1994). The individual, phenotypically male, has 45 chromosomes, including the Y+autosome fusion product. Those few who are phenotypically normal and fertile provide a fascinating example of a sex-determining mechanism seen in some other species (Callen et al., 1987). The translocated Y segment may be beyond the level of cytogenetic resolution, and the karyotype appears as 45,X (Abbas et al., 1990). (*2*) A handful of cases of Prader-Willi syndrome (PWS) have been due to a fusion between a Y and a No. 15, with breakpoints in Yp and at 15q12–13 (Vickers et al., 1994), with the karyotype 45,X,−Y, der(15)t(Y;15). These individuals do not reproduce, and we leave further com-ment on this category to the section on PWS (p. 269).

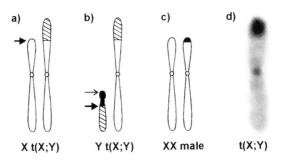

FIGURE 5–10. Three ways in which X-Y translocations are seen. (*a*) with a normal X (in a female); (*b*) with a normal Y (in a male); and (*c*) in a "46,XX male". White indicates X chromosome, black indicates Y euchromatin, crosshatching indicates Yq heterochromatin. In the classical t(X;Y) as in (*a*) and (*b*), and a C-banded example of which is shown in (*d*), the breakpoints occur at Xp22.3 and Yq11 (heavy arrows). (Courtesy M. D. Pertile). In the "46,XX male" with t(X;Y), the Y breakpoint is in Yp, proximal to the *SRY* gene (light arrow).

The X–Y Translocation

The Classical X–Y Translocation

Three different forms of this very rare translocation exist. The classical form (Bernstein, 1985; Ballabio and Andria, 1992) has breakpoints in the distal X short arm (Xp22.3) and in the proximal Y long arm (Yq11). This translocation is readily recognized cytogenetically, and the important genotypic defect is deletion of the distal segment of X short arm with loss of the pseudoautosomal region and a variable amount of X-chromatin proximal to the pseudoautosomal boundary. Thus, the person who is 46,X,t(X;Y)—usually a female—has a partial monosomy for this very small segment; and the 46,Y,t(X;Y) individual—always a male—is partially nullisomic (Figure 5–10). The female heterozygote is characteristically short (height is generally 150 cm or under), fertile, and of normal intelligence. With a more distal breakpoint, close to the actual pseudoautosomal boundary, stature may be normal (Gabriel-Robez et al., 1990). One de novo t(X; Y) girl whose abnormal chromosome was genetically active in 91% of blood cells had hypoplastic internal genitalia and polycystic ovaries (Kuznetzova et al., 1994). The male hemizygote is characteristically mentally impaired, and if the breakpoint is more proximal may manifest Mendelian diseases whose loci are in the region, such as steroid sulfatase deficiency, anhydrotic ectodermal dysplasia, chondrodysplasia punctata, and Kallmann syndrome (Figure 12–4) (Allderdice et al., 1983a; Franco et al., 1991; van Maldergem et al., 1991; Wulfsberg et al., 1992). In the male with a more distal breakpoint intelligence can be intact (although psychological disturbance may be associated); infertility is likely, and may indeed be invariable, due to spermatogenic arrest (Gabriel-Robez et al., 1990).

The majority of cases are familial. Presumably, the X–Y chromosome arose following a reciprocal exchange between the X and Y during spermatogenesis in the individual fathering the originating (female) translocation carrier in the family. This event is facilitated by the apposition of X and Y segments having a high degree of homology; for example, a cross-over between the Kallmann locus on the X chromosome and a Kallmann-like nonfunctional pseudogene on the Y chromosome long arm (Guioli et al., 1992). In the female, the pattern of X-inactivation tends toward inactivation of the t(X;Y) but is variable and unpredictable (Gabriel-Robez et al., 1990). In the case of Kuznetzova et al. (1994) noted above, predominant (91%) activation of the t(X;Y) was associated with gonadal dysgenesis.

> Some cytogenetically apparently identical X–Y translocations are associated with the microphthalmia and linear skin defect (MLS) syndrome in the 46,X,t(X;Y) female (Al-Gazali et al., 1990; Temple et al., 1990). The phenotype may result from the effect of disruption of an ''Aicardi–Goltz gene'' on the t(X;Y) chromosome in parts of the soma in which the normal X chromosome is inactivated, with nonexpression at this locus in these tissues, but this remains to be proven (Lindsay et al., 1994; Ballabio, 1995).

The Cryptic Xp–Yp Translocation

The second form of the X–Y translocation is usually not visible (or barely visible) to the cytogeneticist without the use of FISH using Yp sequences as probe. Again, the X breakpoint is within Xp22.3; but the Y breakpoint is in the short arm, proximal to the testis determining gene (*SRY*). The genotypic consequences are loss of the distal region of the X chromosome, and more importantly, the transfer of the *SRY* gene onto an almost intact X chromosome. Thus, the person is male. The karyotype would initially appear to the cytogeneticist as 46,XX or 45,X. This translocation accounts for about 80% of XX males, and some 45,X males. It arises from an abnormal X–Y recombination during paternal meiosis (Weil et al., 1994), and is always sporadic. Such males are invariably infertile.

"46,XYq−" with Cryptic Xq–Yq Interchange

A third category is the X–Y translocation arising de novo from an exchange in paternal spermatogenesis between Yq and distal Xq, producing an apparent Yq− chromosome which actually contains a very small segment of distal Xq. The functional distal Xq disomy produces a severe phenotype (Lahn et al., 1994).

GENETIC COUNSELING

The X-Autosome Translocation

Fertility is affected in the X-autosome heterozygote and hemizygote. Approximately half of the female carriers, and practically all males, are likely to be infertile (Mattei et al., 1982; Kleczkowska et al., 1985; Chandley, 1988; Therman et al., 1990; Schmidt and Du Sart, 1992). If fertile, the female heterozygote has a substantial risk for having abnormal offspring due to the transmission of an unbalanced chromosomal constitution. At one end of the scale, the abnormality might be rather mild (e.g., partial Klinefelter syndrome, partial X trisomy). At the other end, it could be severe (e.g., partial X disomy or autosomal aneuploidy, not modified by inactivation). The counselor should determine the theoretical gametic combinations from the particular category of translocation, with reference to the examples described in the Biology section. Adjacent-1 and 3:1 tertiary trisomy are the major malsegregation modes to be considered. Figure 5–4 provides a guide but each translocation needs to be assessed on its own merits. The following general comments apply to each of the three categories noted in Figure 5–4:

1. A single-segment translocation with an X segment of large size would imply a risk for partial Turner, partial Klinefelter, and partial XXX syndromes (Figure 5–2; Figure 5–4, left column). A single-segment translocation with an X segment of small size would imply a risk not only for these three partial sex chromosome aneuploidies, but also for functional disomy for a small distal Xp or Xq segment, which would have a severe outcome (e.g., Figure 5–3).

2. A single-segment translocation with an autosomal translocated segment of "viable size" (Figure 5–4, middle column) implies a risk for partial autosomal trisomy or monosomy from adjacent-1 segregations; in the female conceptus, the trisomy may be modified by spreading of inactivation, but this is unpredictable. Selective inactivation of the der(X) may enable viability of 47,+der(X) tertiary trisomy; no useful prediction of the degree of phenotypic defect in this setting is presently possible.

3. Any 2:2 unbalanced segregant from a double-segment translocation (Figure 5–4, right column) has a combined duplication/deficiency, and spontaneous abortion is probable. But spreading of inactivation in a female conception may attenuate a partial autosomal trisomy and allow for survival, albeit with phenotypic defect. As in the previous category, the tertiary trisomic 47,+der(X) may be viable.

The Level of Risk

The risk for most female heterozygotes, who are fertile, will be "substantial." An otherwise nonviable unbalanced conception may survive because inactivation tempers the imbalance and some conceptions with the structurally balanced complement may be functionally unbalanced due to aberrant inactivation patterns. The risks to have a liveborn child with a structural and/or functional aneuploidy may be in the range of 20 to 40%. As we discuss above, the components making up the total risk may include very mild abnormality through severe mental and physical defect. Only with the 46,XX and 46,XY karyotype can one be confident of normality, other things being equal.

The Balanced X-Autosome Detected Prenatally

A balanced X-autosome karyotype identified at prenatal diagnosis, the fetus being *female*, is not necessarily associated with the same phenotype as that of the mother. A normal mother would have, presumably, a "perfect" 100:0 concordance of activation status, with respect to the translocation X and the intact X (see above). But the protective mechanism could fail in a daughter of hers, and some tissues could express a functional partial X disomy, with consequential phenotypic defect. The distribution of cases in the review of Schmidt and Du Sart (1992) suggests a risk of about 25%, although ascertainment bias may have somewhat exaggerated this figure. The risk in a liveborn child is less when the X breakpoint is proximal to Xp22 or Xq28, since if there had indeed been a functional imbalance it may not have allowed intrauterine survival, as discussed above in the Biology section. It remains to be shown whether X-inactivation studies at amniocentesis would be predictive of phenotype. Too little information exists concerning the phenotype of the *male* "hemizygote" born to a female X-autosome heterozygote for any firm advice to be offered. Normality has been recorded in this setting (Buckton et al., 1981; Kleczkowska et al., 1985), but so has major genital defect (Callen and Sutherland, 1986). Fetal ultrasonography may be useful. Otherwise normal male carriers would almost certainly be infertile.

Y-Autosome Translocations

The Yqh-Acrocentric Translocation

These can be regarded as no more than interesting variant chromosomes, and of no clinical significance.

The Apparently Balanced Y-Autosome Translocation

Most Y-autosome carriers are either mentally retarded or infertile. For those who are fertile, risk data are too few to form a secure base for genetic counseling. From first principles, unbalanced forms would be possible, and it may be appropriate to raise the option of prenatal diagnosis. The same balanced Y-autosome translocation can behave differently in different male members of a family in terms of fertility (Teyssier et al., 1993).

The Yp-Acrocentric Translocation

The very rare fertile carrier of a translocation between the euchromatic region of Yp and an acrocentric would be expected to have normal sons and daughters in equal proportion. Theoretical concern about an increased risk for an XXY or 45,X offspring might be seen as grounds for prenatal diagnosis.

The Classical X–Y Translocation

The female with an X–Y translocation is usually fertile and of normal intelligence. She has a 50% risk for having a child, whether a son or daughter, who would have the translocation. An X–Y translocation son may be abnormal according to the extent of distal Xp nullisomy (Wulfsberg et al., 1992). If the mother is short, an X–Y translocation daughter would also be short. As with Turner syndrome, growth hormone treatment may be appropriate for such a child. She would probably be fertile. A child receiving her normal X would be 46,XX or 46,XY.

The male X–Y translocation carrier is characteristically, and perhaps invariably, infertile.

6

Robertsonian Translocations

The American insect cytogeneticist W. R. B. Robertson first described translocations of chromosomes resulting from the fusion of two acrocentrics in his study of insect speciation in 1916. This type of translocation is named Robertsonian (abbreviation *rob*) in his honor. There are five human acrocentric autosomes—Nos. 13, 14, 15, 21, and 22 (the 13, 14, and 15 are the D group chromosomes, and the 21 and 22 comprise the G group). All are capable of participating in Robertsonian translocations. The composite chromosome thus produced includes the complete long arm chromatin of the two fusing chromosomes, although it lacks at least some of the short arm chromatin. These translocations are among the most common balanced structural rearrangements seen in the general population with a frequency in newborn surveys of about 1 in 1,000 (Blouin et al., 1994). Historically, the most important Robertsonian translocations are the D;21 and G;21, which are the basis of familial translocation Down syndrome. In recent years, the role of uniparental disomy has come to be recognized; in the Robertsonian context, this is of relevance with the two imprintable acrocentric chromosomes, Nos. 14 and 15.

In this chapter we consider the case of the phenotypically normal person who carries, in balanced form, a Robertsonian translocation. We generally use a short cytogenetic description for the carrier state, for example, 45,XX,rob(14q21q) or simply rob(14q21q). The correct 1995 I.C.S.N. designation for a centric fusion Robertsonian translocation would be 45,XX,rob[or der](14;21)(q10;q10).

BIOLOGY

The great majority of balanced Robertsonian translocations involve two different chromosomes (a *nonhomologous* translocation); those involving the fusion of homologs (*homologous* translocation) are very rare. Nonhomologous translocations can be transmitted through many generations, whereas the homologous

Table 6—1   The frequency of Robertsonian translocations (relative frequencies in literature review [most cases biased ascertainment], and in studies in which ascertainment was unbiased)

Translocation		Literature review	Unbiased ascertainment
	13;13	3%	2%
	14;14	½%	(0)
	15;15	2%	(0)
D;D	13;14	33%	74%
	13;15	2%	2%
	14;15	2%	5%
	13;21	2%	1%
	13;22	1%	2%
	14;21	30%	8%
D;G	14;22	1%	2%
	15;21	3%	½%
	15;22	½%	1%
	21;21*	17%	3%
G;G	22;22	1%	(0)
	21;22	2%	½%

ªMost are i(21q) Down syndrome; the figure for true rob(21q21q) is probably near ½%.

Source: From Hook and Cross (1987b) and Therman et al. (1989).

translocation is almost always seen as a de novo event in the consultand. As Table 6–1 attests, the rob(13q14q) and the rob(14q21q) are predominant. If we exclude the ''rob(21;21)'', most of which are actually isochromosomes for 21q (Robinson et al., 1994), the rob(13q14q) accounts for around 75% of all Robertsonian translocations in unbiased studies. Balanced carriers for any of the five homologous translocations seem to be of about equal rarity.

There are three possible mechanisms of formation of the *nonhomologous* translocation: fusion at the centromere (centric fusion), union following breakage in one short arm and one long arm (essentially, a whole-arm reciprocal translocation), and union following breakages in both short arms (Guichaoua et al., 1986) (Figure 6–1). The former two produce a translocation chromosome with one centromere (monocentric), and the latter results in a chromosome with two centromeres (dicentric). The predominant rob(13q14q) and rob(14q21q) translocations are, in fact, always dicentric (Earle et al., 1992a; Han et al., 1994a). In some dicentric chromosomes, one centromere is ''suppressed,'' and the chromosomes appear monocentric. This heterogeneity of formation is not of any clinical significance that can presently be discerned. In the reciprocal type, the other product may rarely survive as a stable small bisatellited ''extra structurally abnormal chromosome'' (Schmutz and Pinno, 1986). The propensity to recombine may be the consequence of an attraction between similar sequences shared by acrocentric chromosomes (Choo et al., 1988). The predominance of the rob(13q14q) and the rob(14q21q) may be due to homologous but inverted segments in these pairs of chromosomes that encourage cross-over (Therman et al., 1989). The specific case of the rob(14q21q) in de novo translocation Down

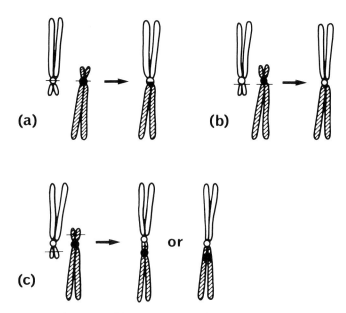

FIGURE 6–1. Mechanisms of formation of Robertsonian translocations. Centric fusion, giving a monocentric chromosome (*a*); breakage in one short arm and one long arm, giving a monocentric (*b*); and breakage in both short arms, giving a dicentric or, after suppression of one centromere, a monocentric (*c*).

syndrome most likely reflects translocation of one No. 21 chromatid to a No. 14 at maternal meiosis, and in general the de novo rob is of predominantly maternal origin (Petersen et al., 1991; Shaffer et al., 1992). Just as a Robertsonian can form de novo from the fusion of chromosomes, so can it (very rarely) revert to two separate chromosomes by a "back-mutational" fission (Fryns et al., 1979; Pflueger et al., 1991).

The *homologous* Robertsonian translocation is most likely to have formed not during meiosis, but after conception, and probably in one of the very first cell divisions (Robinson et al., 1993a, 1994; Blouin et al., 1994). The paternal and the maternal homologs fuse to form the translocation, in which, therefore, the two arms are heterozygous. Some homologous Robertsonian translocations are actually isochromosomes arising from the one homolog, and these can form at meiosis II or at a very early postzygotic stage. The formation of the isochromosome is discussed on p. 265.

Nucleolar Organizing Regions (NORs) and the Robertsonian Translocation

The NORs are located on the short arms of the acrocentric chromosomes and comprise multiple copies of genes coding for ribosomal RNA. When a Robertsonian translocation forms, the NORs of two of the fusing chromosomes are lost, at least with the rob(13q14q) and rob (14q21q). Thus, an individual with a Robertsonian translocation has eight NORs instead of the usual ten. Not all

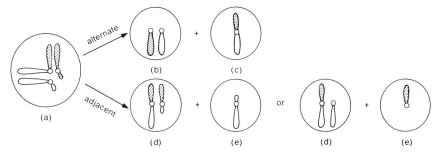

FIGURE 6–2.   Meiotic behavior of the Robertsonian translocation. Trivalent at synapsis (*a*); normal (*b*) carrier (*c*) gametes from alternate segregation; and disomic (*d*) and nullisomic *(e)* gametes from adjacent segregation.

NORs are active: as judged by silver (Ag-NOR) staining, most individuals have four to seven per cell that are active (Varley, 1977). Presumably, a minimum number are necessary for normal cellular function.

The Nonhomologous Robertsonian Translocation

MEIOSIS

This Robertsonian translocation chromosome comprises the long arm elements of two different acrocentric chromosomes. At meiosis in the heterozygote, the translocation chromosome and the two normal acrocentric homologs synapse as a trivalent. Following 2:1 segregation, six types of gamete are produced. Alternate segregation leads to the production of normal and balanced gametes; and adjacent segregation produces two types of disomic and two types of nullisomic gamete (Figure 6–2). In obvious contrast to what happens with the reciprocal translocation, the chromosomally abnormal conceptuses essentially have complete aneuploidy. Only unbalanced conceptuses that are effectively trisomic for chromosome 13 or 21 can survive well into or right through pregnancy (whether to fetal death, stillbirth, or livebirth). Fetal trisomies 14, 15, and 22 are expected to end in miscarriage in the first trimester.

Alternate segregation is, apparently, favored. Translocation Down syndrome and translocation trisomy 13 are scarcely ever seen in the offspring of the male heterozygote (Abe et al., 1975; Boué and Gallano, 1984; Mori et al., 1985; Daniel et al., 1989; Pellestor, 1990). The characteristic *cis*-configuration of the trivalent at meiosis, with the two intact chromosomes lined up together opposite the matching q arm components of the translocation, is the probable reason that symmetric segregation usually occurs, with only small numbers of disomic sperm produced from asymmetric segregation (Table 6–2) (Syme and Martin, 1992). Likewise for the female rob(13q14q), translocation trisomy 13 is a rare observation (Table 6–3). In marked contrast, for the female rob(Dq21q) and rob(21q22q) carrier the risk for a translocation Down syndrome child is sub-

Table 6—2 Frequency of "viable" disomic sperm produced by six Robertsonian heterozygotes

Case	Disomic karyotypes	% sperm with this karyotype	Potential phenotype in child
rob(13q14q)	23,−14,+rob(13q14q)	2.5%	Translocation trisomy 13
	23,−13,+rob(13q14q)	2.5%	UPD 14(pat) syndrome[a]
rob(13q14q)	23,−14,+rob(13q14q)	10%	Translocation trisomy 13
	23,−13,+rob(13q14q)	4%	UPD 14 (pat) syndrome[a]
rob(13q15q)[b]	23,−15,+rob(13q15q)	0	(Translocation trisomy 13)
	23,−13,+rob(13q15q)	0	(Angelman syndrome[a])
rob(14q21q)	23,−14,+rob(14q21q)	4%	Translocation Down syndrome
	23,−21,+rob(14q21q)	4%	UPD 14 (pat) syndrome[a]
rob(15q22q)	23,−15,+rob(15q22q)	6%	None[c]
	23,−22,+rob(15q22q)	1%	Angelman syndrome[a]
rob(21q22q)	23,−21,+rob(21q22q)	2%	None[c]

[a]Following "correction" by loss of homolog from mother; only one recorded case of this known for UPD 14(pat) (see text)

[b]Had fathered a child with translocation trisomy 13.

[c]Trisomy 22 is practically certain to miscarry.

Source: From Balkan and Martin (1983), Pellestor et al. (1987), Martin (1988b), Pellestor (1990), Martin et al. (1992), and Syme and Martin (1992).

stantial. It may be that with these two 21-translocations in the female the frequency of adjacent segregation is not greatly less than alternate, with subsequent selective loss of some trisomic conceptuses. In the sperm studies noted in Table 6–2, the numbers of normal and balanced sperm have been, as theoretically expected, approximately equal; an excess of the balanced state observed at prenatal diagnosis in the rob(13q14q) heterozygote, whether male or female, likely reflects ascertainment bias (Table 6–3).

Postzygotic "Correction" and Uniparental Disomy

An initial translocation trisomy may be "corrected" by mitotic loss of one of the free homologs and lead to uniparental disomy (UPD) in the embryo. For example, a presumed mechanism whereby UPD 15 could arise from a rob(13q;15q) parent is outlined in Figure 6–3. Essentially, adjacent segregation produces a trisomic 15 conception, and then loss of the No. 15 contributed from the other parent, at an early postzygotic stage, "corrects" the karyotype. UPD has no abnormal effect if the chromosome is not subject to imprinting; chromosomes 13, 21, and 22 are in this category. If there is UPD for an imprintable chromosome—in this context, chromosome No. 14 or No. 15—a UPD syndrome would result. For UPD 15, the syndromes are Prader-Willi syndrome (PWS) or Angelman syndrome (AS). A mother with, for example, 45,XX,rob(13q15q) could have a 45,rob(13q15q) child with PWS; and a father with, say, 45,XY,rob(14q15q), could have a 45,rob(14q15q) AS child (Smith et

Table 6—3 Frequency of unbalanced complements detected at prenatal diagnosis by amniocentesis in the Robertsonian translocation heterozygote

| | | | | Results | | |
| | | | | | Unbalanced | |
Translocation	Parent	Number studied	Normal (%)	Balanced (%)	(n)	(%)
rob(13q14q)	Mother	293	37	63	1	0.3
	Father	141	27	71	2	1.4
rob(13q15q)	Mother	9	11	89	0	—
	Father	7	14	86	0	—
rob(13q21q)	Mother	12	33	50	2	17
	Father	9	44	56	0	—
rob(13q22q)	Mother	2	—	—	0	—
	Father	5	—	—	0	—
rob(14q15q)	Mother	6	—	—	0	—
	Father	2	—	—	0	—
rob(14q21q)	Mother	208	35	50	31	15
	Father	74	45	54	1	1.4
rob(14q22q)	Mother	2	—	—	0	—
	Father	6	—	—	0	—
rob(15q21q)	Mother	9	44	56	0	—
	Father	6	33	67	0	—
rob(15q22q)	Mother	5	—	—	0	—
	Father	2	—	—	0	—
rob(21q22q)	Mother	30	43	43	4	13
	Father	3	—	—	0	—

Source: From Boué and Gallano (1984) and Daniel et al. (1989).

al., 1993; Nicholls et al., 1989). The phenotypic consequences of a parent-of-origin effect due to UPD could be exacerbated by a coexisting residual low-grade fetal disomy/trisomy mosaicism and by placental dysfunction due to trisomy of the placenta (if the ''correction'' from trisomy to disomy occurs during formation of the cell line that gives rise to the embryo) (Papenhausen et al., 1995).

With respect to the rob(13q14q), Healey et al. (1994) describe a mother and her abnormal child with UPD 14(mat) each having the karyotype 45,rob(13q14q) and review three other cases. A unique case is that of Wang et al. (1991) who describe an abnormal child with UPD 14(pat) having the karyotype 45,rob(13q14q), whose father was 45,rob(13q14q) and whose mother carried a balanced rcp(1;14). We presume the union of an adjacent-1 disomic 14 sperm and a 3:1 interchange nullisomic 14 ovum (an actual example of gametic complementation, not postzygotic correction). UPD 14 due to familial rob(13q14q) seems a rare occurrence, as an obvious excess of children with abnormal phenotypes in families segregating this common translocation has not been observed, and most of the very few recognized cases of UPD 14 with a

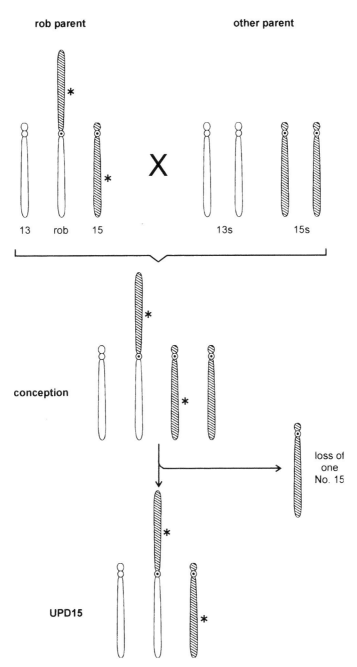

rob parent   **other parent**

13   rob   15   13s   15s

conception

loss of
one
No. 15

UPD15

FIGURE 6–3. Uniparental disomy 15 from a rob(13q15q) parent. The heterozygous parent produces a gamete with the translocation, and with a free No. 15, and the conception has trisomy 15. Subsequently, the No. 15 from the other parent is lost. (No. 13 elements white, No. 15 elements crosshatched. The two No. 15 elements from the carrier parent are asterisked.)

rob(13q14q) have been de novo aberrations. But now that UPD 14 phenotypes, maternal and paternal, have been proposed, it would not be surprising if review of some rob(13q14q) families, and of families with other Robertsonians involving a No. 14, yields some previously unsuspected cases.

Association with Infertility

Infertility includes the inability to achieve conception and the inability to sustain a pregnancy through to livebirth (the latter also called "infecundity"). An intriguing observation is that an approximately sevenfold excess of Robertsonian heterozygotes is found among couples who are infertile (Tharapel et al., 1985). Yet cytogenetic study of the abortus may show the balanced translocation complement, rather than an unbalanced form. One suggestion is that an insufficient number of actively functional NORs may cause the pregnancy to abort (Gosden et al., 1978). A rob(D;D) associated with spontaneous abortion is usually carried by the mother. Perhaps the female has a greater propensity to produce adjacent segregants than the male, and these also contribute to the miscarriage excess.

A tenfold excess of Robertsonian heterozygosity is found in men presenting with infertility due to oligospermia (Chandley, 1988; Guichaoua et al., 1990; De Braekeleer and Rao, 1991). The association is most marked in severe oligospermia (sperm count $<10^6$/ml). A case has been made that, in this setting, synapsis is incomplete in the trivalent, and the heterochromatic regions of the short arms remain unpaired; these "exposed" regions then interfere with pairing in the X–bivalent, so that spermatogenesis is blocked from further progression (Luciani et al., 1987; Johannisson et al., 1987). Guichaoua et al. (1990) have directly observed the asynapsed short arms of the trivalent associating with the X–Y bivalent in testicular tissue from a oligospermic man heterozygous for a rob(14q22q), and Navarro et al. (1991) have similarly studied a rob(13q14q) man. Mice with several Robertsonian translocations show spermatogenic arrest if the translocations form a chain and associate with the sex chromosomes (Johannisson and Winking, 1994). Another suggestion is that, with a monocentric translocation, deletion of a normal "spermatogenesis allele" at proximal 14q causes hemizygosity of a recessive gene on the normal No. 14 (Therman et al., 1989). This scenario does accommodate the observation that male relatives with the same translocation can be fertile. The high frequency of male infertility in the general population (Skakkebæk et al., 1994) precludes straightforward interpretation in the individual infertile man with 45,XY,rob(13q14q).

Rare Complexities

Can a Robertsonian translocation set the stage for a further structural rearrangement? A case such as that of Bonthron et al. (1993) of a rob(14q21q) carrier whose apparently balanced rob(14q21q) phenotypically abnormal child actually had a "molecular deletion" at 14q32 we rather presume was a rare coincidental event. A causal link between the No. 14 existing as a translocation and its undergoing an interstitial deletion cannot entirely be excluded, but it is difficult to imagine a genetic mechanism.

An interesting curiosity is the extremely rare case of a union between Robertsonian heterozygotes (Rockman-Greenberg et al., 1982; Martinez-Castro et al., 1984; Eklund et al., 1988). For example, Martinez-Castro et al. (1984) describe three phenotypically normal siblings who have a diploid number of 44, with their No. 13s and their No. 14s existing as a pair of (13q14q) Robertsonian translocations. The reader may care to construct a theoretical balanced karyotype with 2n = 41 and five Robertsonian translocation chromosomes.

The Homologous Robertsonian Translocation (or Acrocentric-derived Isochromosome)

This Robertsonian translocation chromosome comprises the long arm elements of two acrocentric chromosomes which are the same. If the rearrangement is actually an isochromosome due to the nonseparation of long arm sister chromatids, each long arm is an exact copy of the other. Only two segregant outcomes are possible at meiosis in this 45,rob heterozygote. Either the gamete will receive the translocation chromosome, and be effectively disomic, or it will not, and be nullisomic. Essentially, this is 1:0 segregation (or "1+1":0 segregation). No balanced gamete is possible. Thus, if the other gamete is normal, only trisomic or monosomic conceptions are possible. Occasionally, conceptuses with translocation trisomy 13 are viable, and translocation trisomy 21 not infrequently survives to term. Any of the other unbalanced possibilities (trisomies 14, 15, and 22, and any of the monosomies) are never (or virtually never) viable, *except* in the event that a postzygotic "correction" takes place. If, say, in the case of an unbalanced 46,−22,+rob(22q22q) conception, the free No. 22 were lost at a very early mitosis, genetic balance in this cell line would be restored, with a 45,−22,−22,rob(22q22q) karyotype. Provided the unbalanced cell line contributed negligibly or not at all to the embryo, and provided there were no effect due to uniparental disomy (and in the case of No. 22, there is not), the child would be normal. This scenario has been inferred in only a handful of families worldwide (Stallard et al., 1995).

> An individual mosaic for a homologous Robertsonian translocation, or for a "Robertsonian isochromosome," could produce either chromosomally normal children or conceptions/children with trisomy/monosomy. Bartsch et al. (1993) note some recorded cases of parental mosaicism for 47,+i(21q) and describe their own unique case of a woman with 47,+i(21p)/47,+i(21q)—some hundreds of cells from blood, gonad, marrow, skin were 47,+i(21p), and one single blood cell was 47,+i(21q)—who had two children with Down syndrome due to the karyotype 46,−21,+i(21q). In her case, clearly, the isochromosomes arose as a postzygotic event, with classic centromere misdivision during a mitotic cycle in a 47,+21 preembryo the probable mechanism; the 47,+i(21p) line came to be the predominant in most tissues, but the i(21q) line had at least some representation in gonad and blood.

GENETIC COUNSELING

The Nonhomologous Translocation Carrier

Infertility and Miscarriage

The Robertsonian translocation involving nonhomologs is occasionally associated with repeated spontaneous abortion and male infertility. It is unclear whether these associations are causal or fortuitous (see above, Biology). We can theorize that in some miscarrying couples, a number of nonviable adjacent segregants may have been produced; and in some infertile males, the translocation may disrupt spermatogenesis. Cytogenetic analysis of products of conception, and of testicular biopsy, respectively, may cast some light. It remains possible that some other cause underlies the problem.

RISKS TO HAVE ABNORMAL OFFSPRING FROM INDIVIDUAL TRANSLOCATIONS

Figures for risks of detection of an unbalanced form at prenatal diagnosis are set out in Table 6–3, taken from data in European and North American collaborative studies (Ferguson-Smith, 1983; Daniel et al., 1989). Detailed comments on each translocation follow.

The More Common Translocations

rob(13q14q)

The rob(13q14q) is by far the most common Robertsonian translocation (Figure 6–4). Indeed, it is the most common single rearrangement in the human race. As noted above, in literature studies this "uninteresting" translocation accounts for only 40% of all published cases, but in unbiased surveys its true proportion of all Robertsonians is about 75%. Since 1 in 1000 persons is a rob heterozygote, the prevalence of the rob(13q14q) carrier is 0.075%, or about 1 person in 1,300. Two unfortunate outcomes are possible from the pregnancy of the heterozygote. *Firstly*, translocation trisomy 13 can result from adjacent-1 segregation, with a typical Patau syndrome phenotype. The risk for this is small. Almost all instances are index cases in families, not secondary cases. In a European collaborative study, none of 230 prenatal diagnoses had an unbalanced karyotype (Boué and Gallano, 1984), suggesting a risk of less than 0.4%. An incidence in Daniel et al.'s (1989) North American data of 3/204 may have been influenced by ascertainment bias. *Secondly*, there is the risk of having a child with UPD (uniparental disomy) 14, which seems likely to be very small. The counselor will need to consult current sources for the best information on the UPD 14 risk, such as it may be (and see below).

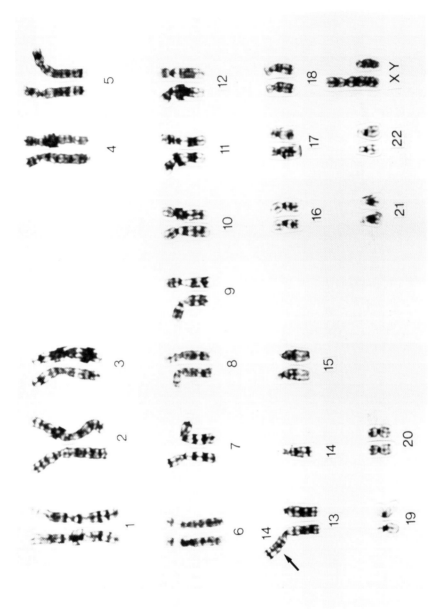

FIGURE 6–4. The balanced rob(13q14q) in a phenotypically normal male.

rob(14q21q)

The rob(14q21q) is the most important Robertsonian translocation in terms of its frequency and genetic risk. Most familial translocation Down syndrome is due to the rob(14q21q) (Figure 6–5). Adjacent segregation may lead to the conception of translocation trisomy 21 (Figure 6–6). At amniocentesis, the female heterozygote has a risk for translocation trisomy 21 of about 15% (Ferguson-Smith, 1983; Boué and Gallano, 1984; Stene and Stengel-Rutkowski, 1988; Daniel et al., 1989). The risk to the female carrier of having a liveborn child with translocation Down syndrome is a little less (around 10%): this likely reflects the loss, through spontaneous abortion, of a fraction of Down syndrome fetuses after the time during gestation when prenatal diagnosis is done (see also p. 328). We comment below about the presumed very small risk for UPD 14, and the uncertainty, as yet, whether prenatal diagnosis is justified.

The risk for the male heterozygote is very different. Very few examples of Down syndrome due to paternal transmission of a rob are known; a risk figure of 0.5% or less may be appropriate to offer. The risk for UPD 14 we suspect would be at least as small, and probably smaller, than for the female, but we presently have no data to buttress this suspicion.

The Rare Translocations

rob(13q15q)

Few data are available concerning genetic risks to the carrier (Mori et al., 1985; Daniel et al., 1989). We would expect these individuals are no more likely to produce adjacent segregants than the rob(13q14q) carrier, and a similar risk of 0.5% or less for translocation trisomy 13 may therefore apply. The risk for UPD 15 is not known (and see below). Five cases of UPD 15(mat) from a rob(13; 15) are on record (Smith et al., 1993); we know of no case of UPD 15(pat) in this setting.

rob(13q21q)

In Boué and Gallano's (1984) study, the risk for translocation Down syndrome, in terms of the likelihood of detection at amniocentesis, was 10% for the female, and in Daniel et al.'s (1989) study, the figure was 17%. This 10–17% range suggests there is no real difference from the 15% that applies to the common rob(14q21q). The risk for the male heterozygote is low, and probably similar to the 0.5% or less proposed for the male rob(14q21q) carrier. A 0.5% or less risk for translocation trisomy 13 may apply, for either sex. UPD is not a concern.

rob(13q22q)

We presume the risk for translocation trisomy 13 would be ''small'' and perhaps similar to that for the rob(13q14q). In Boué and Gallano's (1984) study of 262 Robertsonian prenatal diagnoses not involving chromosome 21, there were only three rob(13q22q) cases, and in fact one of these showed trisomy 13; no unbalanced karyotypes were diagnosed in Daniel et al.'s (1989) seven cases. UPD is not an issue.

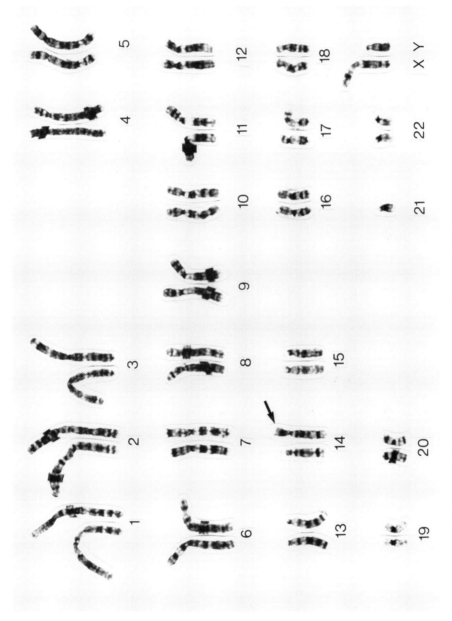

FIGURE 6–5. The balanced rob(14q21q) in a phenotypically normal male.

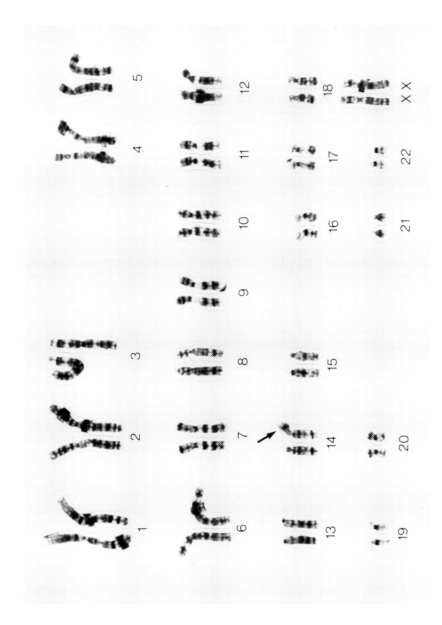

FIGURE 6–6. The unbalanced rob(14q21q) in a girl with translocation Down syndrome.

rob(14q15q)

Adjacent segregants (translocation trisomy 14, translocation trisomy 15) are invariably lethal in utero. UPD 14 or UPD 15 are possible outcomes, although the only proven case on record is a child with UPD 15(mat) (Smith et al., 1993). An abnormal 45,rob(14q15q) daughter of a 45,rob(14q15q) father described in Monteleone et al. (1978) has a phenotype rather reminiscent of *maternal* UPD 14, as set out below; the case in this individual remains open.

rob(14q22q) and rob (15q22q)

The potentially trisomic states from these translocations (trisomy 14, 15, or 22) would all be anticipated to abort spontaneously. Neu et al. (1975) record the segregation of a rob(14q22q) chromosome in a large family, in which some carriers had an increased miscarriage rate. We comment below on UPD.

rob(15q21q)

From Boué and Gallano's (1984) small series of nine carrier mothers, one (11%) had translocation trisomy 21 detected at amniocentesis; and in Daniel et al.'s (1989) data, the fraction was 0/9. These figures derive from too small a body of data to be sure, as yet, that the risk is truly different from the more solidly based 15% which applies to the rob(14q21q) female carrier. Again, we suppose a low risk (less than 0.5%) for the male carrier in terms of Down syndrome. The possibility of UPD is noted below.

rob(21q22q)

For a rob(21q22q) carrier parent, the risks for detection of translocation trisomy 21 are about the same as for the rob(14q21q), according to the sex of the parent (see above) (Boué and Gallano, 1984). UPD need not be a concern.

Uniparental Disomy

UPD is a recently recognized cause of concern with the Robertsonian translocation; or to be precise, those translocations involving a No. 14 or a No. 15. The four syndromes that can arise are UPD 14(mat), UPD 14(pat), UPD 15(mat), and UPD 15(pat). (UPD 13, 21, and 22, maternal and paternal, have no phenotypic effect.) UPD 15(mat) and UPD 15(pat) are better known as Prader-Willi and Angelman syndrome, respectively. UPD 14(mat) can be associated with growth retardation with a relative macrocephaly, mild developmental delay, and a mildly dysmorphic facies (Healey et al., 1994), but a milder phenotype with normal intellect has been recorded (Temple et al., 1991). Indeed, Papenhausen et al. (1995) describe a completely normal phenotype in a woman with UPD 14(mat) with a 45,rob(14q14q) karyotype who had presented with a history of multiple miscarriages, casting some doubt on the role of this particular UPD in producing a pathogenic effect. UPD 14(pat), from two recorded cases (Wang et al., 1991; Papenhausen et al., 1995), may produce a severe intellectual defect and dysmorphism. UPD in the context of a familial Robertsonian translocation seems likely to be an infrequent, perhaps rare, occurrence. James et al.

(1994) made a specific search in a group of 14 phenotypically abnormal balanced rob carriers, in most of whom the translocation was inherited, and identified only one case of UPD.

Wang et al. (1991) raise the question "whether we should consider any changes in counseling when prenatal diagnostic studies find that a fetus has inherited a balanced translocation from one of the parents". We are not yet sure how to answer this question. We do not have an accurate idea of the risk to the male or female heterozygous for any of a rob(13q14q), rob(13q15q), rob(14q15q), rob(14q21q), rob(14q22q), rob (15q21q), or rob(15q22q) for having a child with UPD. An educated guess that the risk for UPD is at the low end of the range 0.1 to 0.5%, at least for the common rob(13q14q) and rob(14q21q), may turn out to be correct, but we can make no firm statement at this time. We cannot yet say if it would be warranted routinely to offer chromosomal prenatal diagnosis and then to proceed to parent-of-origin studies to check for UPD (in centers where the facility for this is available) if the balanced 45,rob karyotype is shown in the fetus; this course of action at least warrants consideration. Counselors will need to consult the most recent literature to keep abreast. With so little data to go on for the more rare translocations which include a No. 14 or No. 15 as a component chromosome, a different (perhaps greater) propensity for UPD cannot be excluded, and a more circumspect attitude may be called for. There is an impression that a greater level of concern applies to the mother carrying a rob with a No. 15, and a firmer case may exist for UPD analysis in this setting. Maternal and paternal UPD 13, 21, and 22 are, apparently, without phenotypic effect, and need not be a cause for concern. We have referred above to the challenging observation of Papenhausen et al. (1995) of phenotypic normality in one case of UPD 14 (mat).

Interchromosomal Effect

The concept of an "interchromosomal effect" has been invoked in the setting of the balanced Robertsonian heterozygote. Can a translocation somehow influence the distribution of another chromosome not involved in the rearrangement, with the production of a gamete aneuploid for a chromosome not involved in the translocation? Anecdotal reports of Down syndrome children born to rob carriers (e.g., Farag et al., 1987) suggested this possibility. However, formal segregation studies in large numbers of families with a rob(13q14q) or with trisomy 21 show no excess of trisomic offspring or of parental Robertsonian translocations, respectively (Harris et al., 1979; Lindenbaum et al., 1985). Therman et al. (1989) ascertained no Robertsonian translocation through a trisomic child other than one which included the trisomic chromosome. Sperm karyotypes of male heterozygotes show no excess of disomy for other chromosomes (Pellestor, 1990; Syme and Martin, 1992). These pieces of evidence amass a rather strong case that the Robertsonian translocation influences the segregation of no chromosomes other than those of which it is comprised.

The Homologous Robertsonian Translocation Carrier

We refer to these rearrangements as "rob" recognizing, as discussed above, that some such cases could actually involve an acrocentric-derived isochromosome.

Practically all conceptions of the heterozygote result in either trisomy or monosomy. Monosomy results in occult abortion. Trisomy 14 and 15 always, and trisomy 22 virtually always, miscarry. Most trisomic 13 pregnancies miscarry, although some endure until the third trimester; while many trisomic 21 pregnancies will proceed through to the birth of a child with Down syndrome. No normal child could be produced. Appropriate advice for these carriers is to consider sterilization. Alternatively, the use of donor sperm/ova allows some couples to have a normal child.

> The only exception to the bald statement that a normal child is impossible would be in the event of a post zygotic "correction" with loss of the free homolog from the noncarrier parent (Stallard et al., 1995). If this occurred in the blastocyst, in the cell destined to give rise to the inner cell mass and hence the embryo, the child would then have the same balanced Robertsonian translocation as the parent. Alternatively, if the other parent contributes a nullisomic gamete, a disomic conceptus would result. In either case, there would be UPD. Although each of these mechanisms could—in the case of the rob(13q13q), rob(21q21q), and rob(22q22q)—lead to the birth of a normal child, they are highly unlikely to happen, and are scarcely outcomes that can realistically be offered in genetic counseling. We suppose that most couples hoping to have a normal child from these two mechanisms would, in fact, most likely produce no more than a long series of miscarriages. The rob(15q15q) carrier, at least, could never have a normal child, even if "correction" occurred, since the UPD leads to an abnormal phenotype: a unique example of an absolutely 100% genetic risk.

Specific comments relating to the risk for abnormal offspring in each type of rob follow.

rob(13q13q)

The carrier parent can produce only monosomic or trisomic 13 conceptions, and these would either miscarry or, in the case of trisomy, produce a very abnormal child. The sole recorded exception to this statement is given in Stallard et al. (1995), of a normal mother and daughter with uniparental isodisomy 13, in whom the translocation may actually have been an isochromosome 13q. The unique case in Almeida et al. (1983) of a ring 13 son from a 13;13 translocation mother is of academic interest.

rob(14q14q), rob(15q15q)

Trisomies and monosomies for chromosomes 14 and 15 are not viable, and thus all pregnancies of these heterozygotes would be expected to terminate in occult abortion or miscarriage. Even if "correcting" UPD did happen, the child would be abnormal, with UPD 14(mat)* or UPD 14(pat), or Prader-Willi or Angelman syndrome, according to the translocation, and the sex of the transmitting parent. Thus it is, in theory and in reality, impossible to have a normal child from any gamete of the heterozygote (barring a back-mutational fission of the translocation, which has never been seen in this context. For the record, Neri et al. (1983) report one category of presumed structural change in a rob(15q15q), a r(15) son of a rob(15q15q) mother).

rob(21q21q)
Although the rob(21q21q) is extremely rare, every counselor knows about this famous translocation. It is a classic example of a genetic risk of (practically) 100%. All pregnancies continuing to term can be expected to produce a child with Down syndrome. Sudha and Gopinath (1990), for example, report a couple who had 13 pregnancies, with 4 children proven or presumed to have had DS, and 9 miscarriages. The mother was 45,rob(21q21q). These carriers can never have a normal child (except in the theoretical circumstance of post zygotic correction as discussed above).

rob(22q22q)
All conceptions would be monosomic or trisomic 22, other things being equal. For example, one carrier woman had 24 miscarriages, but no normal child (Farah et al., 1975). Three cases are recorded of postzygotic correction, as discussed above, with the birth of a normal child. This is not a realistic hope to offer in the individual case.

---

* But note the observation of phenotypic normality in one case; see Papenhausen et al. (1995) as discussed above.

7

Centromere Fissions

Centromere fission results when a metacentric or submetacentric chromosome splits at the centromere, giving rise to two stable telocentric products. In a sense, this is the reverse of what happens in the Robertsonian fusion. The heterozygote, a phenotypically normal individual, thus has 47 chromosomes. Centromere (or centric) fission is the rarest of all chromosome rearrangements: we know of only eight families on record (Del Porto et al., 1984; Elakis et al., 1993; Bogart et al., 1995). Just five chromosomes—4, 7, 9, 10, and 21—have been involved.

BIOLOGY

A nonacrocentric chromosome undergoes a horizontal splitting at the centromere (Figure 7–1). Two new telocentric chromosomes result. One comprises the short arm of the original and the other its long arm. The heterozygous person (47, cen fis) may have a balanced complement of genetic material and thus be phenotypically normal. The process of fission itself, however, may lead to genetic imbalance (Rivera and Cantú, 1986)

At meiosis in the heterozygote, the centric fission products presumably form a trivalent with the intact homolog; 2:1 segregation, essentially as in the Robertsonian carrier, then follows. Alternate segregation produces normal and balanced centric fission gametes, while adjacent segregation leads to gametes disomic or nullisomic for either of the fission products (Figure 7–2). Monosomy would probably be associated with occult abortion and trisomy with miscarriage or, in exceptional cases, with the live birth of an abnormal child. Thus far, only trisomies for 4p and 9p are on record.

The paucity of data does not allow for a good assessment of the genetic risk run by the centric fission carrier. Dallapiccola et al. (1976) reported a chromosome 4 centric fission (Figure 7–3) in a woman who had had two children with trisomy 4p and one normal child. Fryns et al. (1980) describe a man and his

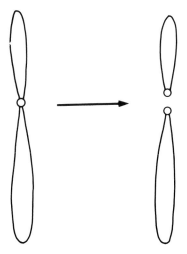

FIGURE 7–1. The process of centric fission. Two whole arm products are generated.

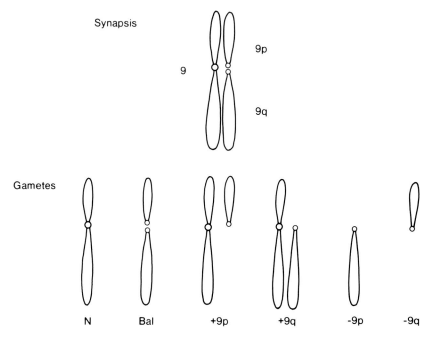

FIGURE 7–2. The six possible gametes arising from 2:1 segregation in a 47,cen fis(9) heterozygote. The first three could give rise to a viable conceptus.

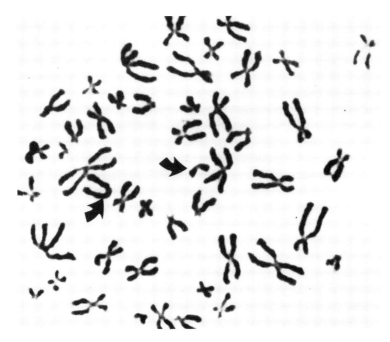

FIGURE 7–3. Metaphase from a woman with a centric fission of chromosome 4. The 4p and 4q chromosomes are arrowed. (Reproduced from Dallapiccola et al., 1976, with the permission of Springer-Verlag.)

normal daughter having a centric fission of chromosome 10. Elakis et al. (1993) record centric fission of chromosome 10 in a normal woman and her phenotypically abnormal fetus; the fetal defect was presumed to be coincidental. Recurrent abortion in the family of Janke (1982) may well have been a result of asymmetric segregation of a chromosome 7 centric fission. Bogart et al. (1995) record a de novo fis(21) in a normal child, identified at routine amniocentesis. Whether this might imply a genetic risk in the next generation, with the possibility of asymmetric segregation of the 21q elements and a child with Down syndrome, is at this point speculative.

GENETIC COUNSELING

The centric fission heterozygote has a significant risk of having a phenotypically abnormal child in those cases in which a whole arm aneuploidy is viable. The 4p and 9p trisomies are the only examples known so far. It is most unlikely that any combination other than the short arm trisomy could be viable. Five to 25% is an educated guess of the likely risk range. Prenatal testing is certainly advisable. Of the phenotypically normal offspring of the heterozygote, half would be expected to have the centric fission and half to have normal chromosomes.

For the heterozygote in whom neither whole arm imbalance is viable—an obvious example would be a 47,fis(1)—no risk for a liveborn abnormal child exists.

8

Inversions

Inversions (inv) are intrachromosomal structural rearrangements. Much the most common is the *simple* (or single) inversion. If the inversion coexists with another rearrangement in the same chromosome it is a *complex* inversion. The simple inversion comprises a two-break event involving just one chromosome. The intercalary segment rotates 180°, reinserts, and the breaks unite (Figure 8–1). The rearranged chromosome consists of a central *inverted* segment and flanking *distal* or *noninverted* segments. If the inverted segment includes the centromere, the inversion is *pericentric*; if it does not, it is *paracentric*. Figure 8–2 depicts two different pericentric inversions of chromosome 3. Note that the pericentric inversion has one break in the short arm and one in the long arm, whereas in the paracentric both breaks occur in the same arm. Thus, when reading cytogenetic nomenclature, one can tell which is which: for example, 46,XX,inv(3)(p25q21) is pericentric and 46,XY,inv(11)(q21q23) is paracentric.

The heterozygote is, other things being equal, a phenotypically normal person. The reorientation of a sequence of genetic material apparently does not influence its function, and breakage and reunion at most sites do not perturb the smooth running of the genome. Some inversions of the X may be an exception to this rule: a breakpoint involving the X long arm within the "critical region" can cause gonadal insufficiency. Some pericentric breakpoints occur at preferential sites, including 2p13, 2q21, 5q13, 5q31, 6q21, 10q22, and 12q13 (Kleczkowska et al., 1987), and certain paracentric breakpoints are likewise overrepresented (Price et al., 1987; Hales et al., 1993; Estop et al., 1994). In the event that a breakpoint occurs within a gene the inversion could be directly pathogenetic. Rare examples include a pericentric inv(16)(p13.3q13) disrupting the Rubinstein-Taybi syndrome locus, an inv(17)(q12q25) disrupting *SOX9* and causing campomelic syndrome, and an inv(X)(p11.4q22) compromising the Norrie syn-

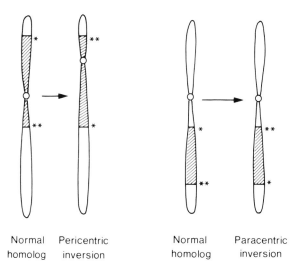

Normal   Pericentric   Normal   Paracentric
homolog   inversion   homolog   inversion

FIGURE 8–1.   The structure of the pericentric (*left*) and paracentric (*right*) inversions. The inverted segment is crosshatched.

drome gene (Lacombe et al., 1992; Maraia et al., 1991; Pettenati et al., 1993). A paracentric inv(2)(q35q27.3) provided, in fact, the entrée to the mapping of the Waardenburg syndrome locus to 2q35 (Ishikiriyama et al., 1989). The inv(2), inv(16), and inv(17) were de novo rearrangements; the inv(X) had been transmitted through four generations.

"Inversions" having a breakpoint within the heterochromatic regions of chromosomes 1, 9, 16, and Y are frequently seen, and are to be thought of as variants, not abnormal chromosomes (see Chapter 15). The most common inversion in humans not involving centromeric heterochromatin is the inv(2)(p11q13). Homozygosity for this inv(2) appears to be without deleterious effect (Gelman-Kohan et al., 1993). Other inversion variants include the following: inv(3)(p11q11) and inv(3)(p11q12), inv(3)(p13q12), inv(5)(p13q13), and inv(10)(p11.2q21.2).

Excluding these variant forms, inversions are a fairly uncommon rearrangement. Estimates of frequency range from about 0.12–0.7‰ (pericentric) and about 0.1–0.5‰ (paracentric) of individuals (Van Dyke et al., 1983; Kleczkowska et al., 1987; Worsham et al., 1989; De Braekeleer and Dao, 1991; Pettenati et al., 1995).

The Pericentric Inversion

BIOLOGY

The Autosomal Pericentric Inversion

MEIOSIS

The inversion heterozygote may produce chromosomally unbalanced gametes. The chromosomal imbalance is a result of the formation of a recombinant (rec)[1]chromosome. This is *aneusomie de recombinaison*—aneusomy due to recombination. Recombination occurs if there is, within the inverted segment, a cross-over between the inversion chromosome and the normal homolog.

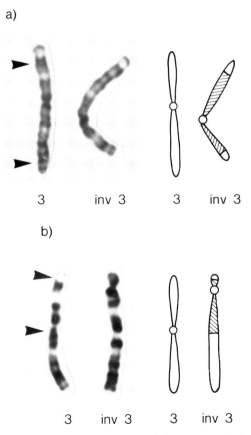

a)

3   inv 3   3   inv 3

b)

3   inv 3   3   inv 3

FIGURE 8–2. Two pericentric inversions of chromosome 3. Both of the noninverted segments are small in one (a) and one is large in the other (b). (Courtesy N. A. Monk and L. M. Columbano-Green.)

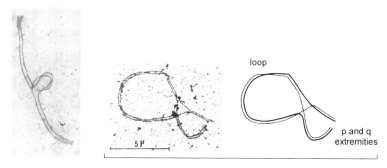

FIGURE 8–3. Inversion loop in meiosis, direct observation. *Left,* inversion loop in a mouse study. (Courtesy Y. Rumpler.) *Right,* spermatocyte study of a man with inv(6)(p22q22.2) (From De Perdigo et al., 1989, courtesy Y. Rumpler and with the permission of Springer-Verlag.)

Synapsis and Recombination

Classically, crossing-over follows the reversed loop model (Figures 8–3 and 8–4). This configuration of the bivalent allows optimal alignment and pairing of matching segments of the inversion chromosome and its normal homolog (homosynapsis). One cross-over within the inversion loop, between a chromatid of the normal homolog and a chromatid of the inversion chromosome, leads to the production of two complementary recombinant chromosomes. One of these has a duplication of the distal segment of the short arm and a deletion of the distal segment of the long arm (chromosome c-c' in Figure 8–4); and the other chromosome (d-d' in Figure 8–4) has the opposite. Thus, the conceptuses that result would have *either* a partial trisomy for one distal segment and a partial monosomy for the other *or* vice versa. Almost always, only one of these—the least monosomic—is ever viable. Consider the recombinant 7 due to a paternal inversion illustrated in Figure 8–5. There is a duplication for the substantial segment 7p14.2→pter and a deletion for only the tiny segment comprising the distalmost sub-band of 7q (7q36.3→qter). The countertype form, having a monosomy for 7p14.2→pter (and trisomy 7q36.3→qter) would, we suppose, cause a miscarriage.

The cytogenetic nomenclature to describe the recombinant karyotype is straightforward. In the above case, for example, we have

> Parent: 46,XY,inv(7)(p14.2q36.3)

> Recombinant offspring (c-c'):   46,XY,rec(7)dup(7p)inv(7)(p14.2q36.3)

It is not necessary to put "dup(7p)*del(7q)*"—the complementary deletion is taken as read. More fully, the nomenclature is

> 46,XY,rec(7)dup(7p)inv(7)(pter→p14.2::q36.3→p14.2::q36.3→qter)pat.

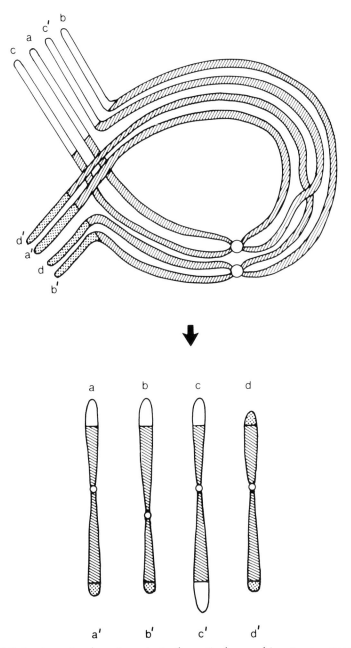

FIGURE 8–4. Inversion loop in meiosis, theoretical recombinant outcomes (based on the inv(3) shown in Figure 8–2a). Both sister chromatids are shown. The inversion (centromeric) segment is crosshatched, the long arm noninverted segment is stippled, and the short arm noninverted segment is open. The four possible gametic outcomes following one cross-over within the inversion loop are depicted. Chromosomes a–a' and b–b' are the intact homolog and the inversion, respectively; chromosomes c–c' and d–d' are the dup p and dup q recombinant chromosomes.

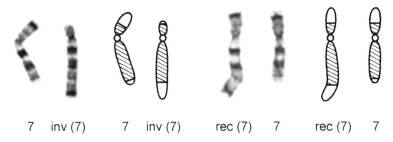

7   inv (7)   7   inv (7)   rec (7)   7   rec (7)   7

FIGURE 8–5. Inversion 7 in father (*left*) of an abnormal child with a recombinant 7 (*right*). The recombinant chromosome has a duplication of just over half of 7p and a minuscule deletion involving the distalmost sub-band of 7q. The child has a triple amount of the segment p14.2→pter. The karyotypes are 46,inv(7)(p14.2q36.3) and 46,rec(7)dup(7p)inv(7)(p14.2q36.3)pat. (Courtesy S. M. White.)

This complex twisting of the chromosomes to form a loop may only occasionally take place. In an inversion with a short inverted segment (Figure 8–6a), a partial pairing may occur. Both distal segments, or sometimes just one, align in homosynapsis. The inverted segment and the corresponding part of the normal homolog either ''balloon out'' (asynapsis of the inversion segment) or lie adjacent but unmatched (heterosynapsis) (Gabriel-Robez and Rumpler, 1994). Thus, no crossing-over can occur within the inverted segment, and recombinant products do not form. Conversely, some inversions with long inverted and very short distal segments may undergo synapsis of the inverted segment only, with the distal segments at each end remaining unpaired (Figure 8–6b). Recombination can occur in this setting. The quality of the chromatin may of itself have an influence. Complete homosynapsis with formation of a loop may require that both breakpoints are in G-light bands; heterosynapsis is associated with one or both breakpoints being in a G-dark band (De Perdigo et el., 1989; Ashley, 1990).

Sperm studies in inversion heterozygotes give an indication of the frequency with which recombination happens, at least in male gametogenesis (Martin, 1988a). We can separate these into those with a long inversion segment and those in which it is short (in terms of haploid autosomal length, HAL). In three longer inversions, inv(3)(p25q21), inv(7)(p13q36), and inv(8)(p23q22), the proportions of recombinant chromosomes were respectively 31%, 25%, and 11%, while no recombinants were seen in two with shorter inversion segments, inv(20)(p13q11.2) and inv(1)(p31q12) (Martin, 1991, 1993; Jenderny et al., 1992; Navarro et al., 1993; Martin et al., 1994b). In one very short ''normal variant'' pericentric chromosome 3 inversion, inv(3)(p11q11), no recombinant chromosomes were seen (Balkan et al., 1983). Thus, from first principles, and from observing outcomes in these few gametes, we suppose that the longer the inverted segment, the more likely it is that recombination will occur. Theoretically, a ''correcting'' second cross-over might take place in a very long inversion segment, but this is not a concept we can usefully apply to risk estimation.

Segment Content and Viability

While a long inversion segment can set the stage for recombination, what determines the viability of the recombinant conceptus is the *functional content* of the *non*inverted (distal) segments. We speak of a "genetically small" content if the combined effect of a duplication and deletion does not cause lethality during pregnancy but allows development to proceed to the stage of livebirth. Thus, only those heterozygotes who have inversions with genetically small distal segments will ever have a chromosomally unbalanced phenotypically abnormal liveborn child. The inversions shown in Figures 8–2a and 8–5 illustrate this case. Inversion heterozygotes in whom one or both distal segments are genetically large (e.g., Figure 8–2b) cannot have an abnormal recombinant child, although they may have an increased risk for miscarriage. Any recombinants produced in such a person would impart a degree of imbalance that would be lethal in utero.

Genetic content corresponds fairly well to chromosome length. In inversion families in which recombinant children have been born, the distal segments together comprise, on average, only 35% of the total chromosome length, whereas in families having no known recombinant offspring, the figure is 62% (Kaiser, 1988). Nevertheless, if the distal segments comprise "genetically small" material, a larger fraction would not necessarily exclude a reproductive risk. Consider the inv(13)(p11q14) and inv(13)(p12q13), in which the distal segments comprise as much as 75% of the chromosome length (Kaiser, 1988). Although the imbalance in the recombinant is large in terms of haploid autosomal length, the result in the dup(q) form is, in effect, a partial trisomy 13 (the partial monosomy for 13p

a)   b)

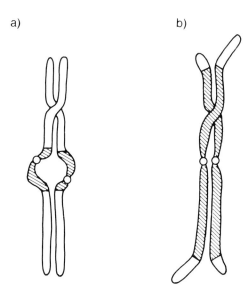

FIGURE 8–6. Alternative models for meiotic pairing, in which only a partial synapsis is achieved. Synapsis of (a) both distal segments; (b) the inverted segment.

being without phenotypic influence). This is, of course, sufficiently genetically small to allow intrauterine and postnatal survival. Similarly, an inversion in chromosome 18 can have distal segments which may be long relative to a short inversion segment, but they are still small genetically, and the dup+del combination can be viable (Schmutz and Pinno, 1986; Ayukawa et al., 1994).

As noted above, almost always only one recombinant form is ever viable. This is rather impressively illustrated in Allderdice et al. (1975) in a kindred with the well-known inv(3)(p25q21). Numerous cases of known and suspected dup(3q) children have been born, but none with the countertype del(3q). There is not even an increase in the miscarriage rate, suggesting that the del(3q) is lethal very early in pregnancy and causes "occult abortion". Viability with both recombinant forms from the same inversion, the dup/del and the reciprocal del/dup, is very rarely seen. Kaiser (1984) records this only in the case of inv(5)(p13q35), inv(13)(p11q22), and inv(18)(p11q21), and Hirsch and Baldinger (1993) add an inv(4)(p15.32q35). These four instances have this quality in common: the noninverted segments are not only short, but remarkably small in terms of genetic content.

It is instructive to consider the inv(4)(p15.32q35) in Hirsch and Baldinger (1993). The four separate segmental imbalances are all well known individually to be viable. Distal 4p- is, of course, the basis of the Wolf-Hirschhorn syndrome; distal 4p trisomy has syndromic, if not eponymic, status; distal 4q produces only a relatively mild trisomic phenotype (see the frontispiece figure); and distal 4q deletion, at 4% of the length of chromosome 4 and thus 0.25% of the haploid autosomal length, imposes only a small partial monosomy. So, the respective imbalances in the combined states—the del(4p)+dup(4q) and the dup(4p)+del(4q)—remain sufficiently small to be viable, at least much of the time. The index case, with the former imbalance, is a severely retarded child with a Wolf-Hirschhorn phenotype; and an aunt, having the latter combination, had rather minor dysmorphism and mental retardation. The inverted segment is very long: 87% of the total length of No. 4. Therefore, a cross-over within the inverted segment is, we assume, very likely to take place. Surely, the genetic risks to heterozygotes for this inv(4) would be high. An even higher risk might apply to the inv(13)(p11q22) described in Williamson et al. (1980) in a family with several documented, suspected, or possible recombinant abnormal offspring: here, the contribution of 13p imbalance to the two recombinant states— the del(13p)+dup(13q) and the dup(13p)+del(13q)—has no phenotypic effect, and the effective "single-segment" imbalances of dup(13)(q22→qter) and del(13)(q22→qter) are well known to be viable. Applying the principles of "private segregation analysis" set out in Chapter 3, the risk for a recombinant form in this family is 50%. We emphasize again the point that, while the length of the inverted segment may influence the likelihood of recombination happening, it is actually the combined genetic content of the distal segments that is the direct determinant of viability of the recombinant form.

Inversions with very small distal segments may stretch the limits of cytogenetic detection. Biesecker et al. (1995) describe an inv(22) with the long arm breakpoint in subtelomeric 22q, with the terminal 23-30 centimorgans of 22q now attached to 22p, which required molecular analysis with microsatellite markers and then FISH with a distal 22q cosmid probe for its identification. Due to the relative lack of G-band landmarks in 22q, and the normal variation that occurs with 22p, the defect was not recognized on a 450-band cytogenetic study. The mother carrying this inversion would have had, presumably, a risk approaching 50% to have a further abnormal recombinant child. It remains to be discovered what fraction of "cytogenetically normal" retarded and malformed children actually have cryptic rearrangements such as this family exemplifies; it is interesting that in their study, which was specifically set up to address this question, this case was only the ninth to be enrolled.

Pericentric Inversions Are Frequently Innocuous

Many pericentric inversions are not associated with any discernible reproductive problems. The families of Voiculescu et al. (1986) and Rivas et al. (1987) are not atypical—an inversion chromosome transmitted through several generations, with numerous carriers identified, and no difference between the offspring of carriers and those of noncarriers in the incidences of abortion and neonatal death.

Rare Complexities

Uncommonly, the inversion heterozygote can be infertile (Groupe de Cytogénéticiens Français, 1986b; De Braekeleer and Dao, 1991). Abnormal synapsis of the chromosome pair can affect cellular mechanics at meiosis in the male, more likely if the inversion involves a larger chromosome, arresting spermatogenesis and causing sterility (Gabriel-Robez and Rumpler, 1994). Meschede et al. (1994), for example, describe azoospermic brothers, one with histologically documented arrest at the level of the primary spermatocyte, each heterozygous for an inv(1)(p34q23) inherited from their mother.

An inversion may, rarely, set the stage for the formation of a different type of rearrangement. Navarro et al. (1993) identified 2 sperm out of 140 examined from an inv(7)(p13q36) carrier to have an "inversion within inversion." A submicroscopic alteration could occur in parent–child transmission, with a locus or small number of loci disrupted or removed; unequal cross-over within the inversion loop is a possible mechanism. A remarkable example is a familial inv(15)(p11q13) which, when transmitted from mother to child, underwent loss of the region that contains the putative Angelman syndrome (AS) locus (Webb et al., 1992). The loss was not detectable cytogenetically—the child appeared to have the same inversion that his mother and grandfather carried—but was revealed on molecular analysis. The child had AS. Kähkönen et al. (1990) likewise describe a child with Prader-Willi syndrome and a 15q11 deletion whose father and grandmother were 46,inv(15)(p11q12). More speculatively, Urioste et al. (1994a), for example, suggest this type of mechanism in a child with a short rib/polydactyly syndrome, mother and child having the same apparently balanced inv(4)(p16q13.2). It remains entirely possible that associations like this are fortuitous (p. 53).

Some inversions have been discovered in the setting of a child with an aneuploidy such as trisomy 21, and "interchromosomal effect" has been invoked (Groupe de Cytogénéticiens Français, 1986b). More likely, these associations are fortuitous: sperm studies endorse this inference (Martin, 1993). It is intriguing to note that one case of cystic fibrosis due to maternal uniparental isodisomy 7 occurred in the setting of a maternal pericentric inversion variant for chromosome 7. This link seems more likely coincidental than causal (Voss et al., 1989). In one instance, "intrachromosomal effect" in an inv(21) caused trisomic and monosomic 21 conceptions (Gabriel-Robez and Rumpler, 1994).

Collectors of remarkable cases will find fascinating the report of Allderdice et al. (1991). They studied a kindred (mentioned also above) with a segregating inv(3)(p25q21) which originated from a couple marrying in 1817 and which was quite widely spread over the maritime provinces of Canada and other parts of eastern Canada and the northeastern United States. In the course of the study, a normal man was found to have two recombinant 3 chromosomes: one with a dup(q)+del(p) and the other with a complementary dup(p)+del(q), such that his karyotype was balanced. Probably, both of his parents were inv(3)(p25q21) heterozygotes; one produced one recombinant gamete and the other the other. Theoretically, he could produce a sperm with a "correcting" recombination that would make a balanced inversion or a normal chromosome; in fact he was infertile.

The Pericentric Inversion X

Pericentric inversions of the X are rare indeed (Duckett and Young, 1988; Therman et al., 1990; Schorderet et al., 1991). The X inversion forms in the same way as an autosomal inversion, but the implications are different. This is because (1) breakpoints in certain parts of the X (its critical region) may have an influence on the phenotype of the female; (2) X chromosomal imbalance in the 46,X,rec(X) female may be mitigated by selective inactivation of the abnormal X; and (3) the 46,Y,rec(X) conceptus will have a partial X nullisomy and functional X disomy. The inv(X) can be transmitted both by the males and females. Baumann et al. (1984) and Schorderet et al. (1991), for example, describe families with an inv(X) transmitted through four generations, with all carriers—female heterozygotes and male "hemizygotes"—being phenotypically normal.

Let us look at the differing situations for the female and male inv(X) carrier. Outwardly, the *female* heterozygote appears normal. The concept of "position effect" is of practical importance in the context of X rearrangement. If the long arm breakpoint lies within the segment Xq13→q22 or Xq22→q26, gonadal dysfunction may occur (Therman et al., 1990). There may be primary amenorrhea; or, after a fertile period in early adulthood, the menopause comes prematurely.

Meiosis would be expected to proceed according to one of the preceding scenarios (see Figures 8–4 and 8–6), with recombination within the inverted segment a possibility. While there is little practical experience to go on, we presume that an ovum with a normal X or the intact inv(X) would produce a normal child. If, in that family, the balanced inversion is associated with normal gonadal function in the female, a daughter would be expected to have, likewise, normal puberty, fertility, and menopause at the usual time. This family information may not be accessible (or may not exist). In the family of Soler et al. (1981), for example, a hemizygous father had three sons and three daughters—each daughter, of course, an obligate heterozygote. He, apparently, had no gonadal deficiency, but his two older daughters had menopause at 37 and 34 (the youngest was only 30). There was no family history recorded antecedent to him.

An ovum carrying a recombinant X would have two very different results, depending on whether it is fertilized by an X- or a Y-bearing sperm, as follows.

1. The 46,X,rec(X) conceptus. Where one or both of the noninverted segments are small the duplication/deficiency associated with a recombinant X would have a mild or even imperceptible effect on the phenotype. Consider the case presented by Buckton et al. (1981) (Figure 8–7). One of the breakpoints is at the tip of the short arm, and the other is in proximal Xq. The recombinant chromosome (characteristically the inactive X) with a deficiency of the tip of Xp and a duplication of distal Xq (Figure 8–7, lower right) was, in this family, associated only with shortness of stature. The partial Xq trisomy, apparently, made no discernible contribution to the phenotype. A 26-year-old mother with the rec(X) herself had a rec(X) daughter: unarguable evidence that oogenesis had not (at least until age 26) been compromised. Where the partial monosomy involves larger segments, and particularly of the short arm, a Turner-like phenotype with the risk of ovarian deficiency eventuates.

2. The 46,Y,rec(X) conceptus. There will be a *nulli*somy for the deficient X segment. If this segment constitutes any but the tiniest length of chromatin, the conceptus would not be viable. Nullisomy for a tiny telomeric segment may be viable, but with major dysmorphogenesis. Further, the concomitant disomy X is functional, not being subject to inactivation, and therefore of itself produces a major deleterious effect (Groupe de Cytogénéticiens Français, 1986b).

In the *male* inv(X) hemizygote, the rearrangement apparently has no effect on phenotype or on reproduction. Meiosis proceeds unperturbed (of course, there can be no recombination within the inverted segment). All his daughters will be heterozygotes. Many will have normal gonadal function, although a family history of premature ovarian failure might predict the same problem (see also above). Sons receive his normal Y, and their mother's X chromosome.

The Pericentric Inversion Y

A pericentric inversion of the Y, inv(Y)(p11q13), is not uncommon in the general population (Verma et al., 1982; Tóth et al., 1984). It has no phenotypic effect and implies no risk for having an abnormal child. It may be regarded as a normal variant. Meiosis proceeds as it would in the 46,XY male.

GENETIC COUNSELING

The Autosomal Pericentric Inversion

Variant Forms

The not uncommon inv(2)(p11q13) is probably quite innocuous (MacDonald and Cox, 1985; Groupe de Cytogénéticiens Français 1986b; Daniel et al., 1989);

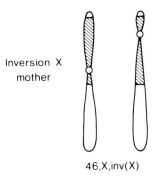

Inversion X
mother

46,X,inv(X)

female recombinant conceptuses

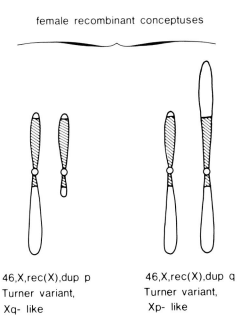

46,X,rec(X),dup p   46,X,rec(X),dup q
Turner variant,   Turner variant,
Xq- like   Xp- like

FIGURE 8–7. Possible reproductive outcomes following recombination within the inverted segment of an X inversion (from the case in Buckton et al., 1981). The normal X on the left has been contributed by the father. Male recombinant conceptuses are not shown: the combination of X nullisomy and functional X disomy in the 46,Y,rec(X) conceptus is almost always lethal in utero.

a proposed twofold risk for miscarriage (Djalali et al., 1986) has yet to be tested prospectively. No genetic risks are known to be associated with the other inversion variants noted in the Biology section—''inversions'' of 1, 9, 16, and Y heterochromatin, inv(3)(p11–13q11–12), inv(5)(p13q13), inv(10)(p11.2q21.2). We exclude these inversion variants from the discussion below.

Table 8—1   Autosomal pericentric inversions from the literature associated with the birth of a recombinant offspring, listed in "numerical" order, and at the level of band (i.e., not sub-band) precision

Chromosome	Inversions		
2	p25q34		
3	p23q25	p25q13	p25q21[a]
	p25q23	p25q25	p26q26[a]
4	p12q33	p13q35	p14q25
	p14q35	p15q35[a]	
5	p13q13	p13q33	p13q35
	p14q35	p14qter	
6	p21q27	p23q23	p25q22
	p25q25		
7	p15.1q36	p22q32	
8	p23.1q22.1[a]		
9	p21q31	p22q32	
10	p11q25	p11q26[a]	p13q26
	p15q24[a]	p15.1q25.2	
11	p11q25		
13	p1q13	p1q14	p1q21
	p1q22[a]	p1q31	
14	p1q23	p1q24	
15	p1q22		
17	p11q25	p13q25	
18	p11q11	p11q12	p11q21[a]
	p11q22		
20	p11q13		
21	p1q21[a]	p1q22	
22	p1q12		

[a]Reported in more than one family.

RISKS OF HAVING AN ABNORMAL CHILD

Ascertainment via Recombinant Child

Identification of a family through a recombinant individual proves the viability of at least one of the two recombinant chromosomes. Table 8–1 lists inversions for which a carrier is known to have had a recombinant child. There have been various empiric estimates of the *overall* level of risk to the heterozygote in families ascertained through an abnormal child. From a number of studies, a consensus range for the usual risk to have a liveborn abnormal child due to recombination is 5–10% (Sherman et al.,1986; Stene, 1986; Groupe de Cyto-généticiens Français, 1986b; Daniel et al., 1988). As a general rule, the longer the inversion segment—and, consequently, the shorter the distal segments—the greater the risk to produce a viable recombinant gamete. Very long inversions, such as that in Roberts et al. (1989), an inv(10) which comprised 80% of the whole chromosome, would imply the highest risks: in this particular case, two out of the carrier father's three children were recombinant. For the majority of families, there is probably no risk difference depending on sex of heterozygote (Kaiser, 1984; Stene, 1986); but in some families, the female heterozygote may run a greater genetic risk (Sutherland et al., 1976; Pai et al., 1987).

Daniel et al. (1989) pooled American, Canadian, and European data to derive risks for an unbalanced karyotype at amniocentesis and derived (from rather small data) a figure of 10–15% for inversions with small distal segments in a family in which a previous affected child had been born.

Each individual inversion carries its own *individual* risk. This may be arrived at by analyzing the client's family, studying the literature, and assessing the degrees of imbalance potentially arising in the recombinant conceptuses. A specific figure has been derived for one relatively common inversion, the inv(8)(p23q22): the risk for liveborn recombinant offspring, for both maternal and paternal transmission, is 6% (Smith et al., 1987). With inversions of 18, with breakpoints at p11 and at q11, q12, or q21, a "group risk" of 8% applies (Ayukawa et al., 1994). In due course, figures may be determined for other inversions seen in more than one family, such as the inv(3)(p25q21), inv(4)(p14q35), inv(10)(p11q25), and inv(13)(p13q21). The existence of several affected individuals enables a clear picture of the range of phenotype to be put together (Sujansky et al., 1993).

No Family History of Recombinant Form

For families identified by means other than through the birth of an abnormal child (e.g., discovered fortuitously at prenatal diagnosis), the *overall* risk is—for what this figure is worth—around 1%. The *individual* risk, which is what really matters, depends on the actual inversion. Is the inversion chromosome on record (Table 8–1) as being associated with viable imbalance? Or, does the inversion segment include and extend beyond the inversion segment of one of these recorded case? In this circumstance, a significant risk surely does apply (see above). Is the inversion segment much shorter in length than any of those listed in Table 1? Here, the risk may be as low as zero. The level of risk can be assessed from a study of the counselee's family, noting the reproductive histories of other heterozygotes, and from a consideration of the degrees of potential imbalance in a conceptus. As a rule, any chromosome with a short (less than one-third) inversion segment is most unlikely ever to lead to a viable recombinant product (Kaiser, 1988).

Nevertheless, one should determine the composition of the theoretically possible recombinant gametes and gauge whether the resulting partial trisomy and partial monosomy might be viable. This applies in particular to inversions of chromosomes 13, 18, and 21, since partial trisomies and partial monosomies of these chromosomes are well recognized as viable. If, in any inversion chromosome, one breakpoint is very close to the telomere, one recombinant form will impose very little partial monosomy. The contribution of the duplication can then be assessed on its own, and reference to the viability of this segment in other cytogenetic contexts (translocation, de novo rearrangement) will likely provide a valid comparison. For example, had the father in Figure 8–5 been identified before he had had children, we could have deduced that the rec(7)dup(7p) genotype might survive to term, knowing that the databases of Stene and Stengel-Rutkowski (1988) and Schinzel (1994) record a viable phenotype for trisomy 7p14→pter.

General Comments

Whether inversion heterozygotes have a risk for having children with other categories of chromosome abnormality is unclear. Do carriers of inversions of 13, 18 and 21 run an increased risk for trisomy of the respective chromosome? If they do, the rarity of cases indicates the risk must be very small. A suggested interchromosomal effect, for an inversion of any chromosome that would impart an increased risk for, in particular, trisomy 21 remains to be confirmed (Groupe de Cytogénéticiens Français, 1986b; Kleczkowska et al., 1987). The possibility of deletion within the inversion loop, or at its boundaries, is exemplified by the Angelman case of Webb et al. (1992); but, for most inversions at least, the risk for this we suppose to be very small, and bordering upon ''negligible.'' Except in a very few special cases, it would not be feasible to attempt to detect such deletions in routine practice.

Prenatal diagnosis should be offered to the following individuals:

1. Any heterozygote in whose family a recombinant child has been born.
2. A heterozygote for any of the inversions listed in Table 8–1.
3. A heterozygote for an inversion involving a segment longer than, but including, a region listed in Table 8–1.
4. Any other heterozygote for whom the theoretical recombinant product(s) might be viable. Many inversions of chromosomes 13, 18, and 21 will fall into this category.
5. Molecular analysis to exclude deletion in the Prader-Willi/Angelman region of 15q11–13 may be appropriate in an inversion having a breakpoint within or adjacent to this segment (and see p. 269). Where there is a breakpoint in distal 11p, ultrasonography to exclude a Beckwith phenotype may be advisable (and see p. 290).

Of the phenotypically normal offspring, approximately half will have normal chromosomes and half will be inversion heterozygotes (Groupe de Cytogénéticiens Français, 1986b).

The Inversion X

The *female* heterozygote could have a premature menopause if the long arm breakpoint is in the critical region and if there is a family history of early ovarian failure; and a piece of practical advice would be to have children sooner rather than later. She has a risk, perhaps in the range of 10–20%, of producing an abnormal daughter with a recombinant X. The abnormality is likely to be either mild (partial Turner syndrome variant with primary amenorrhea) or very mild (a period of fertility, but with premature menopause), depending on the degree of partial X monosomy associated with the recombinant chromosome. For the most part, no risk exists for having an abnormal son because recombinant male conceptuses, having partial X nullisomy and disomy, would be nonviable. Only when the breakpoints are very close to the telomere is male viability possible (e.g., Groupe de Cytogénéticiens Français, 1986b). Such a child would have major physical abnormalities and mental retardation, probably severe.

All daughters of the *male* heterozygote would be inv(X) heterozygotes. Other things being equal, they will be phenotypically normal. If the long arm breakpoint is in the "critical region" and if heterozygous female relatives have had ovarian deficiency (e.g., primary amenorrhea, premature menopause), they may develop the same problem. All sons would have a 46,XY karyotype.

The Inversion Y

All the sons of the inv(Y) carrier are, themselves, inv(Y) carriers. They are all normal and, other things being equal, have normal gonadal function. All the daughters would be 46,XX.

The Paracentric Inversion

BIOLOGY

MEIOSIS

Classical theory has it that the heterozygote for an autosomal paracentric inversion cannot produce a viable unbalanced progeny. If a recombinant gamete is formed following a cross-over in the inverted segment, the chromosome would be either acentric (lacking a centromere) or dicentric (Figure 8–8). An acentric chromosome is never viable, since it lacks a point of attachment to the spindle fibers. The dicentric is generally considered a lethal impediment, being attached to spindle fibers pulling in opposite directions, with the chromosome thus suspended between the daughter nuclei at telophase and excluded from either cell (although rare stable dicentric chromosomes, other than a Robertsonian, have been observed in phenotypically normal persons; Wang and Li, 1993; Wandall, 1994). Alternatively, if the dicentric were to be included in the nucleus of a gamete, McClintock's classical breakage-fusion-bridge cycle might impose an eventually insuperable obsta-

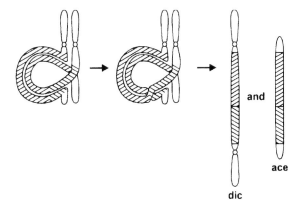

FIGURE 8–8. Theoretical recombinant products from classical cross-over in paracentric inversion. One is acentric (ace) and the other dicentric (dic).

cle to continuing cell division as the chromosome is tugged in two directions by its two centromeres in succeeding mitoses after formation of the zygote.

Recombination with Viable Products

Classical theory remains valid in essence, some exceptions notwithstanding. The abnormal process of ''U-loop recombination'' (Feldman et al, 1993; Mitchell et al., 1994) is a mutational event, not a predictable consequence of a ''normal'' meiotic process (albeit in a chromosome that is abnormal). The cross-over within the inversion loop, instead of continuing on in the same direction along the chromatid, reverses upon itself. The mechanism is illustrated in Figure 8–9. According to this construction, the resulting recombinant chromosomes would have either a duplication of that part of the inversion loop proximal to the cross-over, and a deletion of that part distal to it, or vice versa. A cross-over (or, rather, chromatid breakage with abnormal reunion) at one of the entry points to the loop would produce a duplication alone or a deletion alone. Feldman et al. (1993) review the inversion duplication (inv dup) chromosome, and notably, of the six familial cases on record, five may have been due to presumed U-type recombination from a maternal paracentric inversion. Chia et al. (1992) describe a similar case, a man with 46,inv(18)(q12.1q23) who had a child with a duplication/deletion 18q syndrome due to a presumed rec(18)(pter→q21.3::q21.3→q12.1::q23→qter) chromosome, as shown in Figure 8–9. In their exhaustive review, Pettenati et al. (1995) collected about a dozen similar cases. These cases represented offspring in 3.8% of their series of 446 paracentric inversions; but since *all* of these offspring were probands, and some we actually doubt were truly paracentric recombinants, we presume the actual reproductive risk due to U-loop recombination would be a much smaller figure (Sutherland et al., 1995). The last word on this issue has yet to be spoken (Pettenati and Rao, 1995).

Classical theory needs to accommodate the phenomenon of centromere suppression which, extremely rarely, can allow the recombinant to function stably

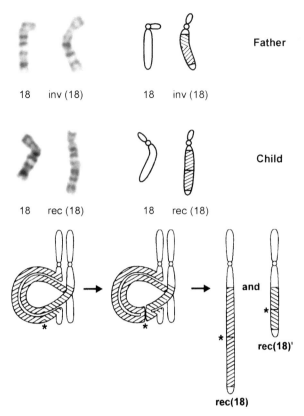

FIGURE 8–9. *Above,* father has paracentric inversion of 18q, inv(18)(q12.1q23). The inverted segment is shown crosshatched (crosshatching changes slope at q21.3). Child has duplication of the segment q12.1→21.3 on the recombinant chromosome (shown crosshatched) and deletion q21.3→q23. (Courtesy N. L. Chia and L. R. Bousfield.) *Below,* proposed mechanism of U-loop exchange depicted; asterisk indicates point of U-loop. The position of the point of exchange within the inversion loop (in this case, q21.3) determines the nature of the imbalance. There is duplication of chromatin proximal to the cross-over point (q12.1→q21.3), and deletion of distal chromatin (q21.3→q23), as in the child's rec(18); and vice versa in the complementary product, rec(18)′. (An alternative interpretation is that the father's rearrangement is a within-arm insertion of 18q, rather than an inversion, in which case the karyotype of the child would have been derived from recombination in the inserted segment.)

as, in effect, a monocentric. The chromosome attaches to the spindle fiber of only one daughter nucleus. "Extremely rarely" could, at this writing, be defined as two recorded cases from an autosomal paracentric inversion. Mules and Stamberg (1984) describe an infant dying as a neonate with a rec(14) whose mother had an inv(14)(q24.2q32.3), and Worsham et al. (1989) studied in considerable detail a child with a rec(9) from a maternal inv(9)(q22.1q34.3). These two cases share the features of a large inversion involving almost all of a long arm, and the short arms (14p and 9p respectively) being genetically "small": in other words, the dup p+q/del q combination did not impose a lethal imbalance. Only in this setting, and if the dicentric chromosome were stable, could recombination lead to the birth of an abnormal child.

> A mechanism reminiscent of paracentric inversion recombination may be the cause of some isochromosome Xq Turner syndrome (H. F. Willard). Two zinc-finger genes (ZXDA and ZXDB) in proximal Xp, just above the centromere, have about 98% homology, and transcribe in opposite directions. In X-to-X synapsis in some meioses, a small inversion loop in proximal Xp can enable ZXDA (the more centromeric locus) in one Xp to match up with ZXDB on the other Xp, and vice versa. Then, a cross-over between the two ZXD loci generates an isodicentric chromosome Xqter→cen→ZXDA::ZXDA→cen→Xqter.

A minuscule number of cases of other sorts of viable recombinant offspring are known (Worsham et al., 1989). A dicentric recombinant chromosome, pulled in two directions, may rupture and yield a deletion. The abnormal synapsis may set the stage for some other type of rearrangement to form, such as excision of an inversion loop and unequal crossing-over at the base of an inversion loop. Phelan et al. (1993) report the unique case of father with an inv(9)(p13p24) having a child with a rec(9) containing a tandem duplication, which they propose came from breakage and reunion between *sister* chromatids within the inversion loop.

Some inversion carriers have been ascertained through their having had many miscarriages. In most of these, surely, the discovery was fortuitous. In a very few, theoretical dicentric recombinant products might convey a genetic imbalance that could allow at least some weeks of in utero growth before miscarrying (Bocian et al., 1990; Bell et al., 1991). The nine miscarriages suffered by the carrier grandmother in the family in Worsham et al. (1989) we might more readily imagine to have been due (some of them at any rate) to recombinant gametes, the dicentric state having been proven in her index grandchild.

X Chromosome

If a paracentric inv(X) is associated elsewhere in the family with normality, no defect would be anticipated in future heterozygotes or hemizygotes (Neu et al., 1988). Breakpoints in the critical region in Xq might compromise ovarian integrity: for example, Dar et al. (1988) describe a woman with a de novo inv(X)(q13q24) who had ovarian dysgenesis with primary amenorrhea and no spontaneous pubertal development, and Dahoun (1990) reports a similar case, in which the somatotype was that of Turner syndrome, with an Xp inversion (p11.2p22.1).

Paracentric Inversions Are Usually Innocuous

The above compendium notwithstanding, the observed facts attest to the general innocuousness of the autosomal paracentric inversion: concerning either the heterozygous state per se, or a risk for chromosomally unbalanced offspring. Price et al. (1987) review 104 cases of autosomal paracentric heterozygosity. While most of these had an abnormal phenotype, this was, of course, the reason they had the chromosome test done in the first place: by definition, they had to be abnormal. No clear consistent pattern amongst phenotypes of presenting cases is apparent. In their major review, Pettenati et al. (1995) could be confident about a causal association with a specific phenotype only in the paracentric inv(X), and not with any autosomal inversion. Heterozygotes whose ascertainment was unbiased show no discernibly increased incidence of phenotypic abnormality (Madan et al., 1984; Callen et al., 1985). Fryns et al. (1986c, 1994) propose that the balanced state may of itself cause abnormality in the child, even though the parent is normal; it could be that most and possibly all of the associations they observed were coincidental and accounted for by biased ascertainment. Nevertheless, the possibility of locus disruption does exist, as rare de novo cases exemplify (Ishikiriyama et al., 1989; Maraia et al., 1991), and, as with the reciprocal translocation, cryptic defects may, rarely, belie an apparently simple and balanced karyotype. The intriguing observation of Cornelia de Lange syndrome (CDLS) in a child with a maternally inherited balanced paracentric inv(3q), in which the 3q27 breakpoint is in the vicinity of a postulated CDLS locus, awaits clarification (Rizzu et al., 1995).

The Groupe de Cytogénéticiens Français (1986a) note that the reproductive fitness of heterozygotes in 32 French families was normal. One quite commonly seen inversion studied in a number of families in several parts of the world is the inv(11)(q21q23). No abnormalities directly attributable to this inversion have ever been documented (Madan et al., 1990; Chodirker et al., 1992). It may be founder effect, or recurring mutation, that is the basis for its frequency. In the one sperm study on a paracentric inversion heterozygote, having the relatively common inv(7)(q11q22), Martin (1986) found no recombinants. The smallness of the inversion segment may have been a factor militating against formation of a synaptic loop. (It is not without interest to note that a similar inversion is the norm in the gorilla No. 7, so this human form could perhaps be thought of as a "back mutation" to that of the ancestral primate.)

Rare Complexities

Watt et al. (1986) raise the possibility that the paracentric inversion might have an "interchromosomal effect." They note an apparently high level of reported associations, within families, of an inversion plus some other chromosomal defect. We suspect this is artefactual; as these authors note, ascertainment and publication biases are potential confounders in this setting. Pettenati et al. (1995) reached a similar conclusion.

> Mendelian loci can be vulnerable when chromosomal rearrangement happens, due either to direct disruption, or to "position effect". A probable example—and one that does imply a high recurrence risk—is exemplified by the family reported in Norman et al. (1992). A mother had one child with Beckwith syndrome and a presumably affected fetus, all three carrying an apparently balanced inv(11)(p11.2p15.5). The Beckwith locus is normally subject to maternal imprinting. Speculatively, the inversion influenced the Beckwith locus such that imprint-

ing failed in the transmitted chromosome, and biallelic expression at the locus led to the abnormal phenotypes (Weksberg et al., 1993b). Another case is the inv(15)(q11q13) family in Clayton-Smith et al. (1993), in which cousins had Angelman syndrome and Prader-Willi syndrome.

TECHNICAL COMMENT

Paracentric inversions can be technically difficult to detect. Gross chromosome morphology is not altered, and unless major landmark bands are shifted, the rearrangement may go unnoticed. Only with the use of good quality, high-resolution banding are paracentric inversions likely to be detected regularly. These cytogenetic difficulties may be why relatively few cases of this type of inversion have been published. Also, for technical reasons, reported cases of recombination in the literature should be regarded with caution; some "inversions" are likely actually to be intrachromosomal insertions ("paracentric shifts"). The cytogenetic distinction can be difficult to make (Callen et al., 1985; Groupe de Cytogénéticiens Français, 1986a; Webb et al., 1988). We have seen a family in which the index case seemed to have an unbalanced translocation at distal 4p, but the normal mother and grandfather had the same anomaly which could then be reinterpreted as a one-band paracentric inversion, inv(4)(p15.3p16.3) (Smith et al., 1992).

GENETIC COUNSELING

On practical grounds, the reassuring point to note is that practically all paracentric inversion heterozygotes identified have been discovered fortuitously, and not through the birth of a child with an abnormality attributable to the parental inversion (Madan et al., 1984, 1990; Groupe de Cytogénéticiens Français, 1986a). Apparently, the genetic risks to offspring are extremely small. In the U.S. collaborative study described in Daniel et al. (1988), there were no unbalanced karyotypes in 30 prenatal diagnoses. We remain unconvinced that paracentric inversions have any interchromosomal effect (Madan, 1988). It remains possible, but is yet to be proven, that any risk exists due to submicroscopic molecular damage occurring during gametogenesis in a paracentric inversion chromosome.

A tiny handful of abnormal offspring (noted above) refute a complete harmlessness in the parental paracentric inversion: whether due to classic recombination with a dicentric chromosome, to the generation by U-loop "recombination" of an inverted duplication (inv dup) chromosome, or to the rupture of a recombinant which produces a viable monocentric product. Whether this would warrant prenatal diagnosis, when a parent is a carrier, is a matter for debate. Even where a classic or U-loop recombinant might on theoretical grounds be viable, the risk of it occurring, while its exact magnitude is unknown, is surely "very small." An educated guess that it lies in the range of 0.1 to 0.5% may turn out to be correct, or perhaps an overestimate. We suggest that an offer of amniocentesis be discretionary in the case of a fortuitously discovered inversion, and would regard it as not inappropriate if the offer were declined. A firmer stance may be appropriate if there has been a previous history of an apparently associated reproductive abnormality. For those who did proceed, we would expect practically every prenatal diagnostic test to reveal a normal karyotype or the same balanced inversion; and, if so, we would anticipate the child to be normal, other things being equal.

In the particular case of inversions having breakpoints in distal 11p and proximal 15q, a case could possibly be made for prenatal diagnosis concerning, respectively, ultrasonographic assessment for Beckwith syndrome stigmata, and molecular analysis of the Prader-Willi/Angelman region.

NOTE

1. Note that this is one of the few occasions on which this abbreviation is used. This emphasizes the unusual point that, in the situation of an inversion, the abnormal unbalanced chromosome transmitted from parent to child is a *new* arrangement. Contrast this with the relatively common situation of the derivative chromosome, which is transmitted intact from a reciprocal translocation heterozygote.

9

Insertions

Insertions are a type of translocation: sometimes the expression ''insertional translocation'' is used. Three breaks are required. The first two breaks release an interstitial segment of chromosome, which is then inserted into the gap created by the third break. In the *inter*chromosomal insertion, a segment from one chromosome is inserted interstitially into another chromosome; there is no reciprocal exchange. In the *intra*chromosomal insertion, a segment is inserted into another part of the same chromosome. The segment may be inserted ''right way around''—that is, with the same orientation to the centromere as before; this is a *direct* insertion (dir ins). Or it may be reversed—an *inverted* insertion (inv ins). With a very small segment, its orientation toward the centromere may not be distinguishable. In the phenotypically normal heterozygote, the rearrangement is assumed to be balanced. A single recorded case documents a four-break rearrangement with a reciprocal exchange of interstitial segments (Wang et al., 1994).

The Interchromosomal Insertion

BIOLOGY

The format of the rearrangement is depicted in Figure 9–1. The recipient chromosome now carries the insertional segment, and the donor chromosome lacks it. In theory, two categories of meiotic behavior are possible.

MEIOSIS

1. Independent Synapsing of Homologous Pairs

Meiosis could proceed in the usual fashion, with homologs pairing independently as bivalents. In essence, we can suppose that the insertional segment is

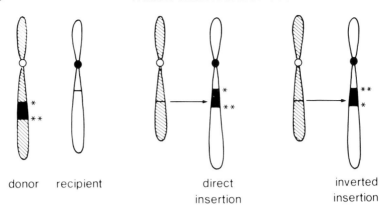

donor   recipient   direct   inverted
                                insertion   insertion

FIGURE 9–1. The formation of an interchromosomal insertion. The *direct* insertion has the same orientation to the centromere; the *inverted* insertion has the opposite orientation.

disregarded and that the homologs synapse, with segments matching for as much of their length as they are able. The insertional segment could be thrown into a loop[1] to accommodate this (Figure 9–2). (Some crossing over will presumably occur between synapsed regions, but this would not alter segregation outcomes.) Alternatively, homologs may pair along their full lengths, which would bring some nonmatching segments ''incorrectly'' alongside each other (''heterosynapsis''). Then, with normal segregation of the two bivalents, independently of each other, two alternative pairs of gametes are possible. Thus, overall, gametes of four possible segregant types, in the ratio 1:1:1:1, would arise—two with a correct amount of genetic material, and two not. The former two combinations would give rise to 46,N and the balanced insertion carrier. The two unbalanced combinations would produce one conceptus with a partial trisomy (duplication) and the other with a partial monosomy (deletion) for the insertional segment (Figure 9–2). Note that the imbalances will be pure trisomy or pure monosomy (not mixed trisomy/monosomy as in reciprocal translocations and inversions). It makes no difference whether the insertion is direct or inverted.

The viability of the conceptuses—in other words, the risk to the heterozygote of having an abnormal child—depends on the degree of the aneuploid states. Consider the example illustrated in Figure 9–3. A small segment from the middle of chromosome 8 long arm (8q21.2→22) has been removed and is inserted within the No. 10 long arm. This segment comprises about 0.4% of HAL (haploid autosomal length). The heterozygote for this rearrangement could produce two types of unbalanced conceptus: one with a duplication of the segment 8q21.2→22 and one with this segment deleted. Figure 9–2 depicts these combinations (shaded chromosome is No. 8, clear chromosome is No. 10, black segment is 8q21.2→22). In this family (Figure 9–4), only the duplication was observed. These individuals had mild to moderate mental retardation and minor physical anomalies (Bowen et al., 1983). A segregation analysis of the family was done, and the segregation ratio was close to 1:1:1:0 for normal:balanced:

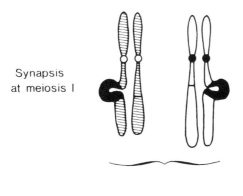

Synapsis
at meiosis I

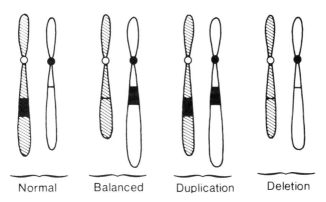

Normal   Balanced   Duplication   Deletion

FIGURE 9–2. Gamete production following independent pairing of the two sets of homologs—based on the ins(10;8) in Figure 9–3.

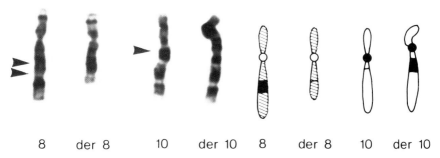

8   der 8   10   der 10   8   der 8   10   der 10

FIGURE 9–3. An insertion from chromosome No. 8 to No. 10, ins(10;8) (q21;q21.2q22). The breakpoints are arrowed. (From Bowen et al., 1983, with the permission of A. R. Liss, Inc.) Note that, according to the I.S.C.N., the recipient chromosome is listed first, and the donor chromosome second.

161

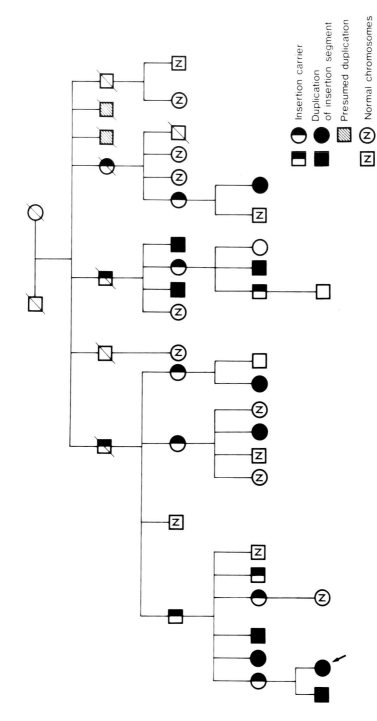

FIGURE 9–4. The pedigree of the family in which the insertion illustrated in Figure 9–3 was segregating.

Insertion carrier

Duplication of insertion segment

Presumed duplication

Normal chromosomes

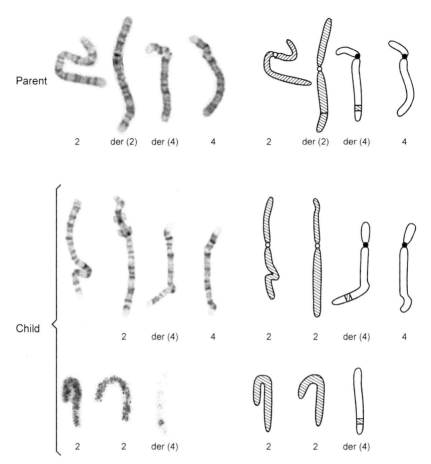

| 2 | der (2) | der (4) | 4 |
| 2 | der (2) | der (4) | 4 |

| 2 | der (4) | 4 |
| 2 | 2 | der (4) | 4 |

| 2 | 2 | der (4) |
| 2 | 2 | der (4) |

FIGURE 9–5. A very small insertion, needing FISH to be seen clearly. The karyotype of the carrier parent (*upper*) is 46,inv ins(4;2)(q32;q34q33.1). The child is duplicated for the segment 2q33.1→q34, but this is difficult to appreciate on the G-banded karyotype (*middle*). FISH using chromosome in situ suppression (CISS) with a chromosome 2 specific paint (*lower*) shows clearly the small insertion segment from No. 2 present in the der(4). (Courtesy M. Curtis.)

partial trisomy:partial monosomy. This implies a normal viability for the partially trisomic conceptus and complete nonviability for the partially monosomic state. Thus, in this family, the risk for having an aneuploid child is $1/1+1+1+0$, or 33%. This assessment is an example of a ''private'' segregation analysis (see Chapter 3).

An insertion of a very small segment may be difficult to detect. Consider the insertion in Figure 9–5, in which two small sub-bands from 2q (2q33.2 and 33.3) and adjoining parts of q33.1 and q34 are inserted into No. 4. This is only about 0.3% of HAL. This rearrangement was at the limit of detection of high-resolution G-banding and required FISH for its clear recognition. In this family, three of five children had a duplication of the insertion, inheriting from the carrier parent the normal No. 2 along with the derivative No. 4 containing the insertional segment (2q33.1→34). The children with this very short duplication had a clinical picture of poor speech development, distractable and aggressive behavior, and subtle facial dysmorphism.

2. Formation of a Quadrivalent

Probably only in exceptional cases, with large insertional segments (Walker and Bocian, 1987), a quadrivalent forms, enabling recombination within the insertional segments. Thus, recombinant chromosomes could form. With the *direct* insertion, these would be monocentric, and therefore functional. *Inverted* insertions, on the other hand, would be associated with dicentric or acentric recombinant chromosomes, with the resulting gametes predicted to be nonviable.

Consider the case of the large *direct* insertion depicted in Figures 9–6 and 9–7. Much of the material within the chromosome 5 long arm (q11→22) has been removed and inserted within the distal long arm of chromosome 1. A pachytene configuration at meiosis I such as that depicted would allow for complete synapsis of homologous segments. If no cross-over occurred in the insertional loop (and assuming 2:2 disjunction with symmetric segregation of centromeres) the same four outcomes noted in the preceding section would eventuate. The gametic combination [a,c] would produce a del(5q11→22), and the combination [b,d] would produce a duplication for this segment. But if a cross-over did occur, two recombinant chromosomes would be formed, and now three further unbalanced outcomes from symmetric 2:2 disjunction would be possible: gametes [b',d'], [b',c] and [a,d'] in Figure 9–6. The duplication/deletion combinations, [b',c], and [a,d'], are judged to be nonviable, although they might cause miscarriage. The ''least imbalanced, least monosomic'' combination is the ''dup ins'' [b',d'], which leads to a partial trisomy for the insertional segment, 5q11→22. This was, in fact, the karyotype of the proposita in this family (Figure 9–7). Actually, this karyotype endows the same genetic imbalance as would the nonrecombinant [b,d] gamete; so in practical terms, it made no difference that this recombination did happen.

Although the range of abnormality may thus be greater in the case of the heterozygote for a large direct insertion because of the additional risks for gametes having recombinant chromosomes, the outlook is not so discouraging in practice. Often the extent of imbalance associated with a recombinant chromosome is so substantial that nonviability is very likely. In other words, these abnormal pregnancies are lost at an early stage, and do not produce an abnormal child. Each family needs to be assessed individually. The counselor may find it useful to follow the format outlined in Figure 9–6 in making this assessment, in terms of what combinations of imbalanced segments might arise.

As for the *inverted* insertion, if a quadrivalent did form and recombination occurred, an acentric or a dicentric chromosome would result. Such a chromosome, in addition to being genetically unbalanced, would be unstable and com-

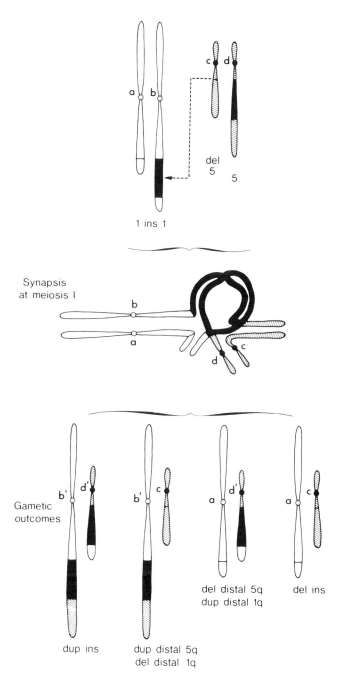

FIGURE 9–6. Gamete production following formation of a quadrivalent in the interchromosomal insertion, with a single cross-over having occurred in the insertion loop (from the case of Jalbert et al., 1975). Only one of each sister chromatid is shown. Recombinant chromosomes noted as b′ and d′.

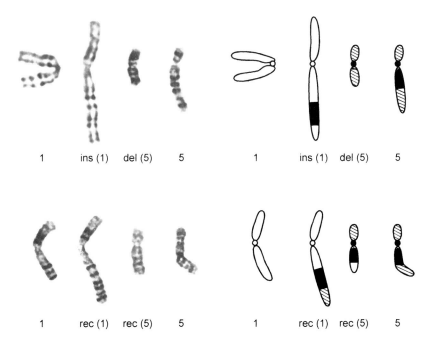

FIGURE 9–7. Interchromosomal insertion with recombinant chromosomes in phenotypically abnormal offspring. Partial karyotypes of 46,ins(1;5)(q32;q11q22) carrier parent (*above*) and her recombinant child with 46,rec(1)rec(5)dup(5q)ins(1;5)(q32; q11q22) (*below*). The latter is the [b',d'] combination in Figure 9–5. The child is trisomic for the segment 5q11→q22. Cartoon karyotype: white = chromosome 1, black = 5q11→q22, crosshatched = remainder of 5. (From Jalbert et al., 1975, courtesy P. Jalbert, and with the permission of the British Medical Association.)

promise the progress of further cell cycles. Thus, the conceptus would be nonviable very early postconception.

Gametogenesis Studies

Gametic analysis has been reported in two insertion heterozygotes. Goldman and Hultén (1992) examined testicular material from an ins(6;7) heterozygote and demonstrated independent synapsis of the No. 6 and No. 7 homologous pairs at diakinesis with the two bivalents occupying quite separate parts of the nucleus. This is a direct demonstration that the segregation scenario set out in Figure 9–2 does happen. Testicular tissue and sperm from one ins(3;10) carrier was studied in a three-country (England, Germany, and Canada) collaboration (Goldman et al., 1992). A very small segment of No. 10 (p13→p14) was inserted into No. 3 at q13.2. In meiosis I, the pairing chromosomes did not "loop out" the nonhomologous segments; but in fact the normal No. 3 appeared to pair fully with the der(3), and likewise the No. 10 and the der(10). This may be heterosynapsis. Sperm karyotyping showed, as expected from the theoretical considerations noted above, similar proportions of gametes with normal, balanced, duplication, and deletion chromosomes: the actual figures were 22%,

32%, 24%, and 22%, respectively. No recombinant forms were seen. Possibly, small insertions may, as a rule, show similar meiotic behavior, with absence of looping out and no quadrivalent formation.

GENETIC COUNSELING

Insertions are among rearrangements implying the highest reproductive risk. Families like the one in Abuelo et al. (1988), presenting through multiple miscarriage, are exceptional; usually, families come to attention through having had an abnormal child. Pooled data from a number of insertion families (see the bibliography in Walker and Bocian, 1987; van de Vooren et al., 1984) indicate an average risk of having an abnormal child of 32%. It may reach 50%. The risk is greater in the small-segment insertion, and smaller in the large-segment. Offering prenatal testing should certainly be the rule. Of the phenotypically normal offspring, approximately half will have normal chromosomes and half will be insertion heterozygotes. A more detailed discussion follows.

For the *short* insertion (say, <1% of HAL), the segregation ratio at conception would be expected to be 1:1:1:1 for normal:balanced:duplication:deletion (meiosis proceeding as described in the first subsection under Biology). If the insertional segment is not only short but also genetically "small," both trisomically and monosomically, the maximum risk of having a liveborn aneuploid child would approach 50% $(1+1/1+1+1+1)$. The segment 18q11→21 (HAL = 0.8%), for example, meets these criteria, as seen in the insertion family presented in Chudley et al. (1974). Carriers for this insertion had the four karyotypic classes of offspring—insertion heterozygotes, karyotypically normal individuals, individuals with a duplication for a small segment of 18q, and individuals with the same segment deleted—in approximately equal numbers. If viability is reduced or impossible for the trisomic or monosomic conceptuses, the risk would be correspondingly less. Trisomic lethality presumably increases with an increasing fraction of HAL, with monosomic imbalances being more lethal.

It may not be possible to make a clear judgment, based on the literature, about the qualitative content of the imbalance, because the insertion involves an *interstitial* segment of chromosome, whereas the chief part of data on record relates to *distal* segments. Nevertheless, Schinzel's cytogenetic database should certainly be consulted; some more distal insertional segments may well be bounded within terminal duplications and deletions that have been described. An insertion segment of this sort would, presumably, be at least as viable as these duplications/deletions; the phenotype it would produce might be similar or, since the extent of the insertion segment would be less, it could be somewhat less severe. Of course, any unbalanced child in the counselee's family will provide proof of viability, and an illustration of that particular phenotype. A study of the wider family may provide a guide to the recurrence risk—a "private" segregation analysis, as illustrated above in the Biology section. But in any case, the starting point with a counselee having a short insertion is that the risk for an abnormal child is high, by which we mean in the range of 10 to 50%.

For the direct insertion involving a *longer* segment (say, 2% of HAL), there is theoretically an additional risk for the formation of recombinant duplication and deletion chromosomes. (An insertion loop may form, as described earlier in the section on Formation of a Quadrivalent.) But in fact the deletion for a long segment (whether the result of a nonrecombinant or recombinant chromosome) would almost always impose a nonviable degree of partial monosomy. The dup/del combinations (see Figure 9–6) are even more unbalanced, leading to spontaneous abortion. Thus, only the duplication (whether nonrecombinant or recombinant) is likely to allow for viability. In the great majority of cases, therefore, the segregation ratio for pregnancies going to term is 1:1:x:0 for normal:balanced:partial trisomy:other imbalances, where x is less than 1, and probably very much less than 1. As an educated guess, the risk for an abnormal child is likely to be in the range of 0 to 5%. In the family of Jalbert et al. (1975) discussed above, the insertional segment (5q11→q22) comprised 2.2% of HAL, and this duplication did allow survival, although the child was dysmorphic and severely mentally retarded. This case is the sole example of dup (5q11→q22) in Schinzel's database. A family such as that in Abuelo et al. (1988), with an insertional segment comprising most of 3p (p13→p26, 2.5% of HAL), one could be rather confident that any imbalanced conception would miscarry. The closest viable segment in Schinzel's database is 3pter→p14, and there are only two cases of this listed. A risk of "almost 0%" for an abnormal child could be offered.

Intermediate length segments (1–2% HAL) may imply a risk in the range of 5 to 10%.

The Intrachromosomal Insertion

BIOLOGY

Intrachromosomal insertions, also known as "centromere shifts," are very rare. In their review, Madan and Menko (1992) list only 27 cases. They emphasize that the cytogenetic recognition can be difficult; four out of the 27 had originally been interpreted as paracentric inversions with unbalanced meiotic products. The formation of the intrachromosomal insertion is outlined in Figure 9–8. These insertions can be within-arm or between-arm, and direct or inverted, and they may undergo incomplete or complete synapsis. These differences can have practical consequences, and we need to consider each in turn.

Within-Arm Insertion

A shift of chromatin within the same arm is called, logically enough, a within-arm[2] insertion. Since both segments shift, essentially switching positions, each could be called an "inserted segment." If both segments maintain the same orientation toward the centromere, it is a *direct* insertion. If the orientation of one segment is reversed, it is an *inverted* insertion.[3] In the case of the inverted

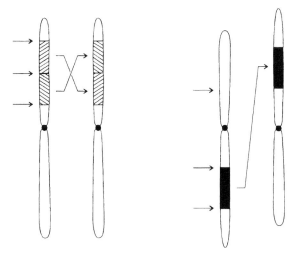

FIGURE 9–8. The formation of the intrachromosomal insertion. *Left,* the within-arm insertion, with the inserted segments crosshatched. *Right,* the between-arm insertion, with the inserted segment in black. Short arrows indicate breakpoints.

insertion, we can distinguish one segment from the other by referring to respective inverted and noninverted segments. In the direct insertion, the shorter of the two segments can be arbitrarily labeled as the inserted segment and the longer as the "noninserted" or "interstitial" segment (Madan and Menko, 1992; Barber et al., 1994); since they are both really insertion segments, we can also speak of the "shorter inserted" and the "longer inserted" segments.

Between-Arm Insertion

The other type is the between-arm[4] insertion, with a segment of chromatin from one arm inserted into a point in the other arm. If we consider the centromere as the fixed reference point of a chromosome, we can regard the centromeric segment as "staying still" while the insertion segment shifts from one arm to the other. This somewhat arbitrary point of view allows us to use the term "inserted segment" unambiguously in the context of the between-arm insertion.

Incomplete Synapsis

Meiosis perforce proceeds in a modified fashion. Consider the *between-arm* shift. In most cases, perhaps, the inserted segments fold out so as to allow a good degree of synapsis of the bivalent, which would include the centromeric segment. One (or any odd number) cross-over within the centromeric segment will produce recombinant chromosomes: one with a duplication of the insertion segment, and the other with a deletion (Figure 9–9). The centromeric segment may be quite long, as a proportion of the whole chromosome, and provide

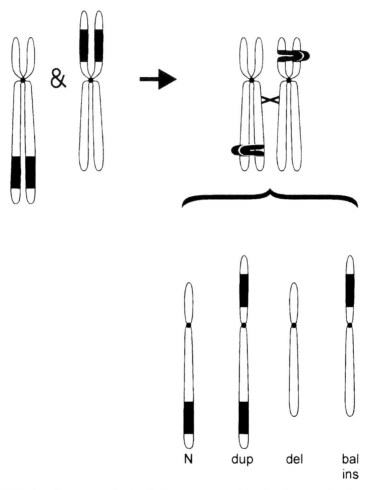

N   dup   del   bal
                                      ins

FIGURE 9–9.   Gamete production following a recombination *between* the sites of re-arrangement in the between-arm intrachromosomal insertion (incomplete synapsis). Based on the ins(5) shown in Figure 9–13. There are four possible types of gamete.

considerable opportunity for cross-over. Thus, the genetic risk is expected to be high; and in theory would approach 50%. In other words, the segregation ratio for the four possible segregant outcomes of normal:balanced insertion:duplication:deletion would be close to 1:1:1:1.

The *within-arm* shift can have a similar folding out of an inserted segment, and its homolog on the normal chromosome, to enable synapsis of the other inserted segment and its homologous region. In Figure 9–10, we depict the shorter insertion segment folded out, with synapsis of the larger inserted segment. (It could have been drawn the other way around.) Recombination within the larger segment will lead, respectively, to duplication and deletion of the shorter segment in the recombinant products passed on to the two resulting gametocytes. Vice versa, if there is synapsis of the shorter inserted segments, followed by recombination, there would be duplication of the larger inserted segment in one gametocyte and deletion of this segment in the other. In theory, the longer the larger segment is, the more likely recombination will be. One might suppose a lesser risk if both segments are short, possibly making crossing-over less likely; but there are, as yet, insufficient data to be sure of this. Certainly, cases are on record of crossing-over taking place in very short inserted segments, in both direct and inverted insertions (Webb et al., 1988; Rethoré et al., 1989; Barber et al., 1994). A greater likelihood for crossing-over in segments more distal from the centromere may also affect the risk.

Complete Synapsis, Direct Insertion

Alternatively, complete synapsis may be achieved. The insertion and the centromeric segments (between-arm shift) or the two insertion segments (within-

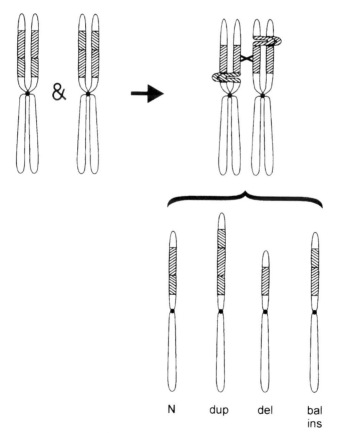

N   dup   del   bal
ins

FIGURE 9–10. Gamete production following a recombination *within* one of the insertion segments of a within-arm intrachromosomal insertion (incomplete synapsis). There are four possible gametic outcomes.

arm shift), and their matching segments on the normal homolog, would need to loop back and forth into each other, forming a double loop (Figure 9–11). Various outcomes are possible from crossing-overs within one or other loop. Considering the *direct between-arm* shift, crossing-over within the *centromeric* segment will lead to recombinant chromosomes deficient or duplicated for the inserted segment (Figure 9–11a,b). If, however, following complete synapsis, there is crossing-over in the *inserted* segment, this will lead to the generation of new recombinant forms: chromosomes that are duplicated for terminal p and deleted for terminal q, or vice versa (Figure 9–11c,d) (e.g., Vekemans and Morichon-Delvallez, 1990).

If complete synapsis is achieved in the *direct within-arm* shift, interestingly enough there is no new category of recombinant form beyond the four which could be generated from incomplete synapsis with folding out of one of the segments. Crossing-over within the longer inserted segment will lead to recombinant chromosomes deficient or duplicated for the shorter inserted segment (Figure 9–11i,j). Vice versa, crossing-over within the shorter inserted segment will lead to recombinant chromosomes deficient or duplicated for the longer inserted segment (Figure 9–11k,l). We illustrate such a case from Webb et al. (1988) in Figure 9–12; equally, this outcome could have arisen from incomplete synapsis, with the longer segments folded out.

Complete Synapsis, Inverted Insertion

Recombination in the inverted *between-arm* insertion, in the setting of complete synapsis, has the same consequences as for the direct insertion as discussed above, provided cross-overs take place within the *centromeric* segment (Figure 9–11e,f). The family illustrated in Figure 9–13 demonstrates this. The recombinant child with a dup(5) could equally have arisen from recombination in a partial synapsis (Figure 9–9) or in a complete synapsis (Figure 9–11f), but in either event the cross-over is within the centromeric segment. The duplication comprises the inverted insertion segment. If, however, the cross-over is in the *inserted* segment, dicentric and acentric products will result, and the compromised conceptus from such a gamete will probably degenerate very early, and may not even implant (Figure 9–11g,h). The same fate awaits conceptions from cross-overs in the inverted *within-arm* shift, if crossing-over happens within the *inverted* segment (Figure 9–11o,p). If crossing-over is in the non-inverted segment, we see the same imbalances (Figure 9–11m,n) as in the direct within-arm shift (Figure 9–11i,j). For example, Rethoré et al. (1989) describe a child with a duplication for the very short segment 5p13.32→14.2 due to a parental inv ins(5)(p13.31p14.3p15.12) with recombination in the even shorter segment 14.3→15.11, reflecting the scenario set out in either Figure 9–11n or Figure 9–10.

The reader may have discerned a pattern in the above construction. Whichever segment recombination takes place in (the active segment, so to say), it is the *other* (passive) segment that comes to be duplicated or deleted. This is logical.

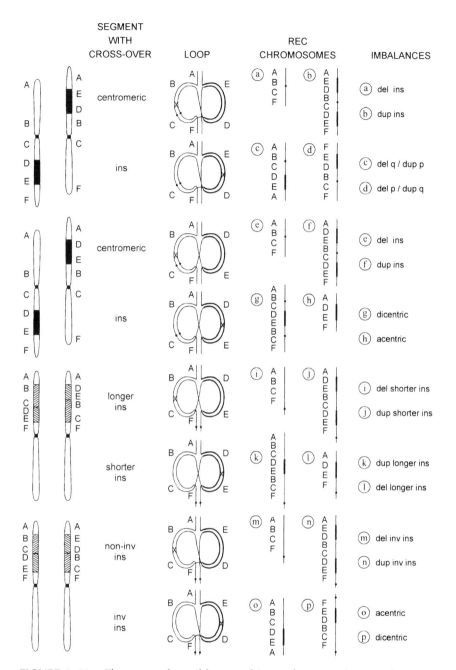

FIGURE 9–11. The range of possible recombinants from crossing-over in one or other insertion loop following complete synapsis of the intrachromosomal insertion. The four panels show, from *above* down, the direct between-arm insertion, the inverted between-arm insertion, the direct within-arm insertion, and the inverted within-arm insertion. The insertion segment 'DE' is shown in thick line in the recombinant chromosomes. Circled letters provide reference points for text comments.

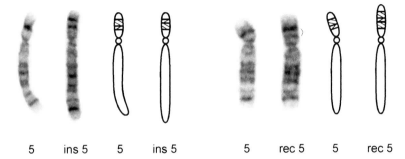

| 5 | ins 5 | 5 | ins 5 | | 5 | rec 5 | 5 | rec 5 |

FIGURE 9–12. Recombination from a direct within-arm shift. Partial karyotypes of an insertion heterozygote mother (*left*) and her recombinant child (*right*). The karyotypes are 46,dir ins(5)(p14.1p14.3p15.1) and 46,rec(5)dup(5p)dir ins(5)(p14.1p14.3p15.1)mat.[5] The child is duplicated for 5p14.3→15.1 (indicated by brace). The recombination may have arisen from crossing-over within band p14.1 at either partial synapsis with ballooning out of segments p14.3→15.1, as in Fig. 9–10, or complete synapsis following double loop formation, as in Fig. 9–11(k). (From the family reported in Webb et al., 1988, courtesy L. E. Voullaire.)

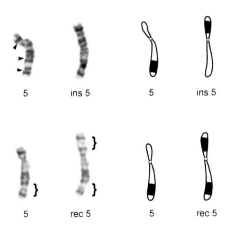

| 5 | ins 5 | 5 | ins 5 |

| 5 | rec 5 | 5 | rec 5 |

FIGURE 9–13. Recombination from an inverted between-arm shift. Partial karyotypes of an insertion heterozygote mother (*above*) and her recombinant child (*below*). The karyotypes are 46,inv ins(5)(p13q33q22), and 46,rec(5)dup(5q)inv ins(5)(p13q33q22)mat. The child is duplicated for 5q22→q33 (indicated by braces). The recombination may have arisen from crossing-over anywhere between 5p13 and 5q22 at either partial synapsis with ballooning out of segments 5q22→q33, as in Figure 9–9, or complete synapsis following double loop formation, as in Figure 9–11(f). (From the family reported in Martin et al., 1985, courtesy N. J. Martin.)

A cross-over will create a new version of the active segment that contains a portion from each contributing chromosome—but it will be the same length as it was before. The other, non-crossing-over segments follow, as it were, passively along.

Abnormal Phenotype In the Carrier

If an abnormal phenotype segregates with the insertion, a causal link is possible. Roberts et al. (1986) describe an apparently balanced inv ins(13)(q21.3q32q31) in four members of a family, of whom three had mental defect and psychiatric disorder. A ''brain locus'' at one of the three breakpoints may have been disrupted or subject to position effect, or there may have been a cryptic imbalance. Alternatively, and given subnormality in some other karyotypically normal relatives, the association could be coincidental.

If the ''critical region'' of the X chromosome is involved, an insertion may, in spite of being balanced, produce gonadal dysfunction in the female (Grass et al., 1981).

GENETIC COUNSELING

The risk of having an abnormal recombinant child, in the 27 families reviewed by Madan and Menko (1992), was 15%, although they considered this quite possibly to be an underestimate. This is an average figure. We may presume a range of from near 50% to zero in the individual case. A high risk is likely if one of the segments is small, and the other long, so that *(1)* there is a high survivability in both the duplicated and deleted state for the small segment, and *(2)* with one long segment, recombination may be more likely. In this situation, a figure of 30 to 40% may be the appropriate one to offer. Given that the partial aneuploid states will involve interstitial regions of the chromosome, very little data, quite possibly none, may be on record for the viability and phenotype of the particular segment; and an educated assessment will have to be made. Risks are presumably less, and possibly zero, if both segments are long (no viable recombinants). They *may* also be less—say, below 10%—if both segments are short, which might weigh against recombination, but we have no firm data to buttress this suggestion. As always, a ''private'' segregation analysis, if the family offers that opportunity, may provide the best estimate of risk. For one specific insertion, Allderdice et al. (1983b) calculated a risk of 31% for female inv ins(9)(q22q34.3q34.1) heterozygotes. One short-segment between-arm shift, 46,dir ins(7)(p22.1p21.4q36.1), with a long centromeric segment for which, from the foregoing, a high risk might have been predicted, in fact produced no liveborn recombinant child in a three generation family, although some first- and second-trimester pregnancy losses may have been due to unbalanced forms (Farrell and Chow, 1992).

NOTES

1. Described also as ballooning out, looping out, folding out, translocation loops.

2. Also called intra-arm, paracentric, and intraradial insertion.

3. If both segments were inverted, the result would be indistinguishable from a paracentric inversion.

4. Also called interarm, pericentric, and extraradial insertion.

5. This karyotype stretches the limits of the short nomenclature, since "dup p" could refer to either 5p14.1 or 5p14.3→15.1. The full nomenclature describes the rearrangement: 46,XX,rec(5)(pter→14.1::15.1→14.3::13.3→qter)dir ins(5)(p14.1p14.3p15.1)mat.

10

Autosomal Rings

Ring chromosomes are uncommon, and it is even more uncommon for a person with a ring (or someone on their behalf) to seek genetic advice about reproductive possibilities. The usual ring phenotype is sufficiently abnormal, with major mental retardation, that procreation is not socially in prospect. But exceptions exist. Remarkably, some persons heterozygous for a ring chromosome seem to be of entirely normal phenotype. Only mild mental retardation, or short stature with minor dysmorphism, characterizes some other cases. It is these categories of normal or mildly abnormal phenotype—in other words, of possible reproductive potential—we particularly consider in this chapter, although at the outset we can state that only a few examples of parental transmission of ring chromosomes are known. About 99% of rings arise sporadically (Kosztolányi et al., 1991). The ring X Turner syndrome variant is noted in Chapter 12.

BIOLOGY

The classic mode of formation of ring chromosomes is breakage in both arms of a chromosome, with fusion of the points of fracture and loss of the distal fragments (Figure 10–1a). In effect, therefore, a partial monosomy for the distal short arm and distal long arm results. Where such a loss of chromatin is cytogenetically detectable, and often when it is not, the clinical picture is one of major dysmorphogenesis and mental retardation. The amount deleted can be very small, and Wintle et al. (1995) describe the smallest recorded deletion in a ring 14 chromosome, comprising no more than 1100 kb of DNA at 14qter, in a phenotypically abnormal r(14) individual. More complicated mechanisms of formation have been described in two individuals with Down syndrome (McGinniss et al., 1992). In one, a rob(21;21), or an i(21q), underwent asymmetric breakage and reunion; and in the other, a small ring was converted by sister chromatid exchange to produce a larger ring. Ramírez-Dueñas et al. (1992) proposed a role of the fragile site at 1p11 in predisposing to an r(1). The r(15)

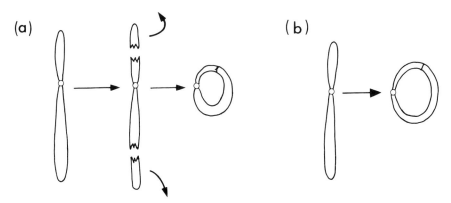

FIGURE 10–1. Formation of a ring chromosome. (*a*) Classic mechanism with deletions in both arms, and fusion of breakpoints and loss of distal segments. (*b*) Telomere-to-telomere fusion.

presents a particular case. If the distal breakpoint is just proximal to the subtelomeric region, loss of a growth factor receptor gene *IGF1R* in 15q26.1→qter may exacerbate, in some but not all, the growth deficiency inherent in the ''general ring syndrome'' effect (Peoples et al., 1995; Nuutinen et al., 1995).

The type of ring that largely concerns us here is the telomere-to-telomere fusion (Coté et al., 1981; Romain et al., 1983b; Kosztolányi, 1987; Wyandt, 1988; MacDermot et al., 1990) (Figure 10–1b). This process entails little or no loss of chromatin, and telomeric and subtelomeric sequences are retained (Pezzolo et al., 1993). In such people the chromosomal constitution is, essentially, balanced. What then may lead to phenotypic abnormality is mechanical disruption of cell division throughout the period of postconceptual growth. This is the consequence of rings becoming entangled, broken, doubled, or otherwise disrupted. (And this, in turn, is due to sister chromatid exchange during the cell cycle before mitosis. The reader can palpably demonstrate this point by constructing a paper chromosome and effecting one or two cross-overs with scissors and tape.) Thus, at mitosis daughter cells arise that are partially or totally aneuploid for the chromosome in question—''dynamic mosaicism.'' These cells may die; some, however, survive in the mosaic state and presumably make an unfavorable contribution to the phenotype. This continuous generation and loss of cells seriously undermines the growth *rate,* although it may not greatly influence the quality of growth. The result is the general ring syndrome—whichever autosome is concerned—of marked growth retardation, borderline to moderate mental deficiency, minor dysmorphogenesis, and, perhaps, intact fertility.

The larger chromosomes (Nos. 1–12) may be particularly prone to this effect and the smaller ones less so: Kosztolányi (1987) refers to labile and stable rings, respectively. Perhaps this is simply a result of their different lengths offering more or less opportunity for sister chromatid exchange to occur. Rings of the smallest chromosomes are, largely or wholly, immune to ring disruption. Thus, a person heterozygous for an r(21) or r(22) could be almost, or apparently entirely, of normal phenotype (Teyssier and Moreau, 1985; Gardner et al., 1986b;

McGinniss et al., 1992). It is this category of telomere-to-telomere fusion that characterizes familial transmission—these persons' phenotypic normality, or near-normality, means that parenthood is entirely possible socially.

At gametogenesis in the 46,r(A) heterozygote (*A* is any autosome) the expectation is, other things being equal, for symmetric disjunction, with 1:1 segregation of the ring and the normal homolog (Figure 10–2). Thus, half of the conceptuses would be entirely normal karyotypically and half would carry the ring. If "dynamic mosaicism" then occurred, these latter may then be lethal in utero, or those surviving to term might have phenotypic abnormality. There are tentative grounds for considering that the ring heterozygote might have an increased risk for nondisjunction, resulting in 2:0 segregation. In this event, with respect to chromosomes 13, 18, or 21, a child with the respective trisomy might be born. So far, this is on record only in the case of a child with ring Down syndrome, 47,+r(21), born to a 46,r(21) parent (Kosztolányi et al., 1991). The r(21) parent is also at risk of having a Down syndrome child due to a recombinant duplication 21 (Howell et al., 1984; Fryns and Kleczkowska, 1987; Miller et al., 1987).

Almost all instances of parent-to-child ring transmission involve the mother as the carrier parent (MacDermot et al, 1990). Probably, spermatogenesis is compromised in the presence of a ring chromosome, and infertility is the consequence for most male heterozygotes. An interesting exception is the family in Mears et al. (1995) in which a phenotypically normal grandfather and father were mosaic for a tiny ring 22 chromosome, 47,XY,+r(22)/48,XY,+r(22),+r(22). A grandchild, also 47,+r(22)/48,+r(22),+r(22) but

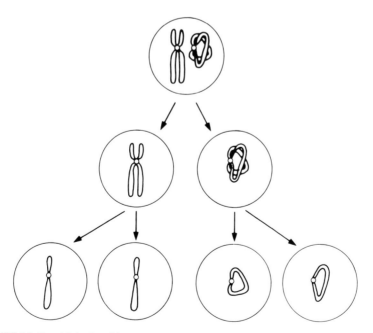

FIGURE 10–2. Meiosis with symmetric segregation in the ring heterozygote.

whose ring chromosomes had increased in size, had "cat-eye syndrome" (see also p. 264).

A small number of families have been recorded with ring chromosome mosaicism in one or both of a parent/offspring pair (Kosztolányi et al., 1991). Jenderny et al. (1993), for example, describe a phenotypically normal mother with 47,XX,+r(18) in only 2/100 cells on blood analysis, the remainder being 46,XX, and who had a daughter with nonmosaic 47,+r(18). Here, a 2:1 meiotic segregation in a segment of the gonad with the 47,+r(18) line presumably produced a disomic gamete. Where both parent and child are 47,+r(A)/46,N, a mitotic loss of the ring in an initially 47,+r(A) conceptus may have produced the 46,N cell line at least in the child.

GENETIC COUNSELING

Certain ring chromosomes are on record as having been transmitted from parent to offspring: chromosomes 11, 14, 15, 17, 18, 20, 21, and 22 (Faugeras and Barthe, 1986; Kosztolányi et al., 1991; McGinniss et al., 1992). In over 90%, the transmitting parent was the mother. Pooling the data (and accounting for ascertainment) gives the following distribution of outcome in 56 pregnancies: 16 offspring with the ring chromosome; 21 who were 46,N, and another 6 normal individuals who were unkaryotyped; and 13 abortions. Thus, somewhat under a half—about 40%—of children of a 46,r(A) parent are also 46,r(A). Hence, the theoretical risk of 50% is substantially borne out in actuality; possibly, the slight shortfall in 46,r(A) offspring may reflect spontaneous abortion of some 46,r(A) conceptions and of any markedly unbalanced recombinant forms.

Except, perhaps, for rings of the smallest chromosome, those offspring inheriting the ring could be expected to suffer from the general ring syndrome at least to the same extent as, and quite probably more severely than, their heterozygous parent. The 46,r(A) parent may be an atypical ring carrier, perhaps with a fortunate pattern of mitotic disruption, to have reached the level of social phenotype that procreation would be likely. In the review of Kosztolányi et al. (1991), about one third of 46,r(A) children were more severely affected mentally than their parent. For example, Bowser-Riley et al. (1981) report a 46,r(14) mother "at the lower end of the normal range" of intelligence who had two retarded 46,r(14) daughters—and a third 46,r(14) pregnancy which was terminated. We have seen a 46,XY,r(4) man, who struggled at school compared with his high achieving siblings but nevertheless holds a managerial job, unwilling to risk a child who might have similar or greater difficulty, but whose wife could not accept prenatal diagnosis with possible termination. They eventually chose artificial insemination with donor sperm.

A person who is mosaic, with a 46,r(A)/46,N karyotype, may or may not be of normal intellect. In any event, the r(A) cell line could include the gonad and thus imply a high risk to have a child who would have the ring chromosome in nonmosaic state, that is, 46,r(A).

In the retarded male, diminished sexual interest and infertility make the question of genetic risk academic. But the retarded female heterozygote for some rings may be functionally fertile (e.g., Donlan and Dolan, 1986), and, in any case, guardians may be concerned about theoretical pregnancy outcomes, whether or not fertility has been established. In some cases sterilization is seen as appropriate (see also Pregnancy and the Mentally Retarded, p. 15).

In the particular case of the r(21) heterozygote, who is often phenotypically normal (Gardner et al., 1986b), there is a small, but as yet unquantified, risk of having a child with Down syndrome due to an uncommon karyotype: 47, +r(21), 46,rob(21q21q) or 46,tan dup(21q21q) (refs. in Kosztolányi et al., 1991). The male with r(21) may be subfertile (Dallapiccola et al., 1986). If, in prenatal diagnosis for a pregnancy of an r(21) heterozygote parent, the same r(21) karyotype were demonstrated in the fetus, based on the slender evidence thus far available, the chance for phenotypic normality would seem to be "substantial," but a (probably mild) degree of abnormality can by no means be excluded. As Kennerknecht et al. (1990) comment, "accurate phenotype-karyotype correlations cannot be made, since there are carriers with a stable ring chromosome who are affected, whereas others with an unstable ring have a normal phenotype and vice versa." Melnyk et al. (1995) report a unique three generation r(21) family in which the (nonmosaic) r(21) persons were of normal appearance and intelligence. In a twin pregnancy of the index r(21) mother, amniocentesis showed a 46,XY karyotype in twin A and a 45,XX,−21/46,XX,r(21) karyotype in twin B. The parents decided to continue the pregnancy, mainly because of concern that the normal twin might be lost in a selective termination, and in due course normal infants were born: twin B had a nonmosaic 46,XX,r(21) karyotype in 80/80 cells on a lymphocyte study, suggesting that the 45,−21 cell line on amniotic fluid culture may have been of extrafetal origin or arose as an in vitro artefact. Possibly, the observations in the case of r(21), and the interpretations put upon them, may also be applicable to the r(22).

11

Complex Rearrangements

Complex chromosomal rearrangements (CCR) occurring in phenotypically normal persons are rare. Three or more chromosomes are involved, and a variety of rearrangements are possible. Translocation segments may involve distal segments, as in the usual reciprocal translocation, or interstitial segments, as in the insertion. An inversion and a translocation, for example, may coexist on the same chromosome. In the phenotypically normal person, the rearrangement is taken to be balanced.

BIOLOGY

Three Major Categories of Complex Chromosome Rearrangement

Three major categories of CCR are recognized. (*1*) The commonest category is the three-way exchange, in which three segments from three chromosomes break off, translocate, and unite (Figure 11–1). Most three-way CCRs are familial, usually transmitted through the mother; although in one of the largest kindreds on record, showing five-generation transmission, three (great)grandfathers must have been CCR heterozygotes (Farrell et al., 1994). (*2*) More complicated CCRs encompass a wide theoretical range, but there are not many actual cases (Bass and Sparkes, 1979; Meer et al., 1981; Kleczkowska et al., 1982; Kousseff et al., 1987; Walker and Bocian, 1987; Lurie et al., 1994; Wang et al., 1994). Most of these are de novo rearrangements. (*3*) The simplest CCR is the ''double two-way exchange'', in which there is a coincidence of two separate simple reciprocal translocations. In a sense, the double two-way exchange is not a ''true'' CCR, and might as well be described as a double or a multiple rearrangement (Kausch et al., 1988; Creasy, 1989; Phelan et al., 1990).

An apparently balanced karyotype may be associated with a normal or an abnormal phenotype. If the individual is phenotypically normal, the chromosome rearrangement is assumed to be truly balanced. These cases are often familial.

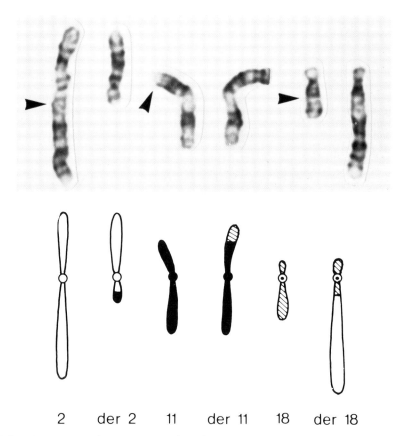

2   der 2   11   der 11   18   der 18

FIGURE 11–1. A three-way complex chromosome rearrangement. Most of 2q is translocated onto 18q; part of 18q is translocated onto 11p; and the tip of 11p is translocated onto 2q.[1] Arrowheads on normal homologs indicate breakpoints. The individual had presented with multiple miscarriages. (From Gardner et al., 1986a, with the permission of the British Medical Association.)

In the phenotypically abnormal individual, presumably some submicroscopic imbalance or other genetic defect exists. These cases characteristically involve a de novo chromosome abnormality. CCRs characteristically originate in male gametogenesis; one "simple" exchange having arisen may then have set the stage for further chromosomal rearrangement (Batista et al., 1994; Lurie et al., 1994).

MEIOSIS

For the purpose of considering meiotic consequences, Kausch et al. (1988) divide CCRs into (1) the three-way exchange as described above, (2) those in which one (or more) chromosome has more than one breakpoint, and (3) those

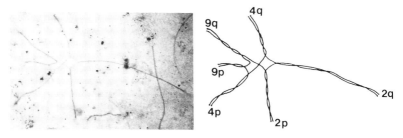

FIGURE 11–2.   The actual appearance of a multivalent at meiosis I. Electronmicrograph of a spermatocyte from a testicular biopsy of a man with a three-way CCR 46,XY,rcp(2;4;9)(p12;q25;p12); line drawing shows component parts of the hexavalent. (From Saadallah and Hultén, 1985, courtesy M. A. Hultén and with the permission of Springer-Verlag.)

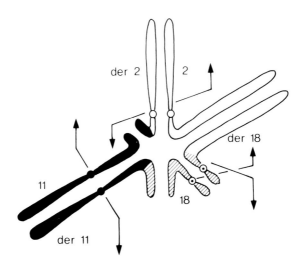

FIGURE 11–3.   Diagrammatic representation of the formation of a hexavalent at meiosis in the three-way 2;18;11 translocation depicted in Figure 11–1. The arrows indicate 3:3 alternate segregation.

with two (or more) independent simple rearrangements. We may refer to these as the three-way CCR, the exceptional CCR, and the double two-way CCR.

Three-way CCR

At meiosis in the three-way CCR heterozygote, the expectation is that the chromosomes involved in the rearrangement will come together and form a multivalent (Saadallah and Hultén, 1985; Figure 11–2). Consider how meiosis would proceed in the rcp(2;18;11) translocation illustrated in Figure 11–1. In theory, a hexavalent configuration would allow full synapsis of homologous segments (Figure 11–3). If disjunction were then symmetric (3:3), up to 20 possible gametic combinations could occur. The two arising from alternate segregation (arrows in Figure 11–3) would be the only ones to be balanced; the remaining 18 would be unbalanced to a greater or lesser degree. Were asymmetric segregation (4:2, 5:1, 6:0) to occur, a great variety of extremely unbalanced gametes would result. However, it appears that, in a number of families, a combination of very early lethality of severely unbalanced conceptuses (occult abortion) and perhaps a tendency to favor symmetric alternate segregation (Walker and Bocian, 1987) implies a reasonable prospect for achieving a normal pregnancy. The risk of having a pregnancy that would go to term but produce an abnormal child reflects the nature of the rearrangement—that is, whether there are possible chromosomal combinations that would lead to aneuploidy for a survivable amount of genetic material. Thus, considering the preceding rcp(2;18;11) example, three unbalanced combinations, one 3:3 and two 4:2, might be expected to be viable (Figure 11–4). Batista et al. (1994), reviewing 29 families with a CCR, determined that an abnormal livebirth is most commonly (78%) due to 3:3 adjacent-1 segregation, followed by 4:2 segregation. Recombination would add yet further possibility of imbalance, but only one instance of this is recorded (Masuno et al., 1993). 4:2 segregation characterizes CCRs in which an acrocentric chromosome is a component. An excess of heterozygotes has been noted amongst the balanced female offspring (Batista et al., 1994).

Exceptional CCR

More complex rearrangements imply an even greater potential range of abnormal gametes. Kausch et al. (1988) calculated a minimum of 70 possible unbalanced gametes due to 4:4, 5:3, 6:2, and 7:1 segregations from an octavalent, in the case of a woman with a five-breakpoint CCR with translocations of chromosomes 1, 2, 5, and 11 and an inversion of No. 1, who had presented with three first trimester miscarriages. Van der Burgt et al. (1992) report a similarly complex de novo balanced CCR (chromosome Nos. 5, 11, 12, 16; five breakpoints

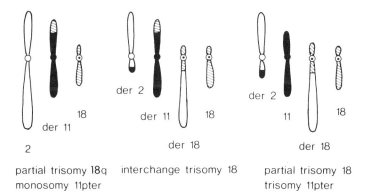

FIGURE 11–4. Three segregant outcomes of meiosis in the rcp(2;18;11) heterozygote shown in Figure 11–1, that might be expected to produce viable but unbalanced offspring. The 3:3 adjacent-1 gamete on the left may be the one most likely to be produced.

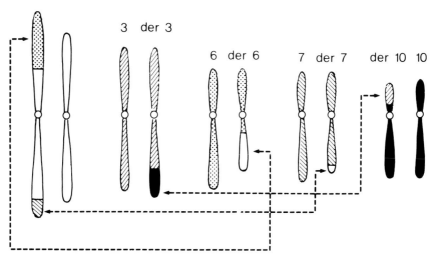

FIGURE 11–5. An extraordinarily complex rearrangement involving three two-way exchanges, with six breakpoints in five chromosomes (see text). (From the family reported in Bass et al., 1985.)

in all) in a mother who had had one miscarriage, one 46,XY child, the index abnormal child, and, as a most unexpected outcome, a de novo 45,rob(13q14q) at prenatal diagnosis in her fourth pregnancy.

One of the most complex cases on record is the CCR with six breakpoints in five chromosomes reported by Bass et al. (1985) and depicted in Figure 11–5. The woman who carried this extraordinary rearrangement had four pregnancies, only one of which miscarried, and two produced offspring with a balanced constitution, though different in each child and different from their mother! Recombination involving the centric segment of chromosome 1 led to a daughter receiving a "new der(1)"—we might also call it a rec(1)—with just the 6p segment being translocated, and a son with a different "new der(1)" having just the 7q segment. A son and a grandson had unbalanced karyotypes, which were different, but each led to partial 7q trisomy. Readers who relish esoteric puzzles may wish to refer to the original paper.

Double Two-Way CCR

Presumably, two separate and independently operating quadrivalents form (Bowser-Riley et al., 1988). Burns et al. (1986) record sperm karyotypes in a man with a double two-way CCR 46,XY,rcp(5;11)(p13;q23.2)rcp(7;14) (q11.23;q24.1) whose wife had had four miscarriages, a child with cri du chat syndrome, and a normal son carrying the rcp(7;14). Only four of 23 sperm analyzed had an overall balanced complement, and the majority (13) had adjacent-1 segregants for one or other translocation. Another five showed 3:1 and (a unique observation) one sperm showed 4:0 segregation. This case is instructive in illustrating the point that different rcps can have different meiotic behavior: for example, 60% of the rcp(5;11) segregants but only 30% of the rcp(7;14) showed alternate segregation.

We referred on p. 83 to a couple each member of which had a simple reciprocal translocation, both happening to involve chromosome 7 (7p in one, 7q in the other). It is a useful exercise to imagine how the chromosomes might be transmitted in this family. The couple could, in theory, have a child with a double two-way CCR who would have a combination of their own karyotypes. Providing fertility were not compromised, this child of theirs in generation II could then, in generation III, have two types of balanced progeny: one with the rcp(7;11) and the other with the rcp(7;22), as in the couple of generation I. We set out this scenario in Figure 11–6. No offspring with a normal karyotype could be produced in generation III unless recombination between the two der(7) chromosomes were to restore a normal chromosome 7.

Very complex rearrangements are generally only seen as de novo cases; the individuals are phenotypically abnormal, and the karyotype may or may not appear balanced. Ten is the greatest number of breakpoints reported in a constitutional CCR, which involved four chromosomes (Muneer et al., 1988). Certainly qualifying as a CCR is the case of Duval et al. (1994): a baby with multiple defects and two unbalanced cell lines with different translocations sharing a common breakpoint at 4q31. A donor segment translocating to more than one recipient chromosomes in this fashion is a "jumping translocation."

Effect Upon Fertility

In several complex rearrangements, in the female at least, gametogenesis can accommodate itself to the complexity thrust upon it, and the heterozygote may be fertile and have pregnancies that produce phenotypically normal children. However, the rule of the greater vulnerability of spermatogenesis to chromosomal complexity seems to apply particularly in the situation of the CCR, and the male heterozygote is often sterile due to spermatogenic arrest (Joseph and Thomas, 1982; Rodriguez et al., 1985), or subfertile (Saadallah and Hultén, 1985). The involvement of an acrocentric chromosome in the CCR may particularly predispose to this male sterility (Gabriel-Robez et al., 1986).

The Cryptic Complex Chromosome Rearrangement

A CCR may be shown, upon detailed cytomolecular study, to have a greater number of breakpoints than had originally been appreciated (Batista et al., 1994). An apparently simple translocation may actually harbor a more complex rearrangement, not detectable on routine cytogenetics but requiring FISH and molecular analysis for its demonstration. At most, this phenomenon is likely to be infrequent among all translocations, and it may in fact be quite rare.

A well-documented example is that of Wagstaff and Hemann (1995). They describe a phenotypically normal father and his two abnormal children, the father and son having an apparently balanced 46,XY,rcp(3;9)(p11;p23) and the daughter apparently 46,XX. On FISH and DNA studies, they could show that

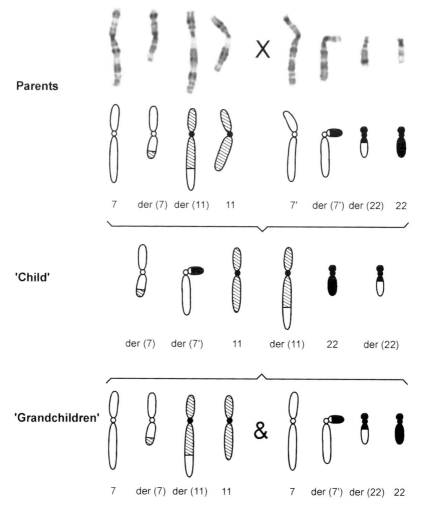

FIGURE 11–6. Theoretical potential pedigree of a couple each of whom carries a simple balanced reciprocal translocation: 46,XY,rcp(7;11)(q22;q23) and 46,XX,rcp(7;22)(p13;q11.2). A child of theirs could have a double two-way CCR combining the two parental karyotypes: 46,rcp(7;11)(q22;q23)rcp(7;22)(p13;q11.2). The original simple translocation karyotypes could be restored in the next generation. The reader can determine how, following one recombination, a 46,N grandchild could be conceived. (Courtesy K. L. Butler.)

the father had a tiny segment of chromatin from the breakpoint in 9p23 removed and inserted into a third chromosome (the long arm of a No. 8) (Figure 11–7). At meiosis, it may have been that a quadrivalent formed from the No. 3 and No. 9 elements, while the two No. 8 homologs synapsed independently as a bivalent. On this interpretation, the two children reflect alternate segregation of the No. 3 and No. 9 elements; with respect to the No. 8s, the rcp(3;9) son inherited his father's normal homolog, so the lack of the 9p23 segment was not

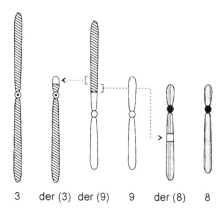

3   der (3) der (9)   9   der (8)   8

FIGURE 11–7. A cryptic complex chromosome rearrangement. On the original cytogenetic study, father and son appeared to have the same simple balanced translocation, 46,XY,rcp(3;9)(p11;p23), and the daughter was 46,XX. DNA and FISH studies showed a CCR, in which a tiny segment within 9p23 had been insertionally translocated into 8q in the father. Brackets and dotted lines show translocation of two separate segments from distal 9p across to 3p and to 8q respectively. After transmission of unbalanced complements (see text), the son had a deletion and the daughter a duplication for the 9p23 segment. (From the family reported in Wagstaff and Hemann, 1995.)

corrected, while the "46,XX" daughter received the No. 8 with the 9p23 insertion. Thus, the son has a del(9)(p23) and the daughter a dup(9)(p23). The pressing question raised by this study is this: do some other apparently balanced simple reciprocal translocations have a cryptic complex rearrangement (p. 92)?

Two abnormalities may coexist on the same chromosome. Bonthron et al. (1993) describe a 45,rob(14q21q) father having an abnormal daughter with apparently the same balanced Robertsonian translocation. Further molecular and FISH study showed, in the child, a de novo microdeletion in the translocation chromosome, in the distal 14q segment. It is an unanswered question whether the link between the translocation and the microdeletion was coincidental or causal.

GENETIC COUNSELING

The male CCR heterozygote who is not otherwise known to be fertile should have a semen analysis to check whether sperm are being produced. For the heterozygote (male or female) who is fertile, a conceptus having either a normal chromosome constitution or the same balanced CCR as the parent would be expected to produce a normal child. But a high proportion of conceptions have an unbalanced karyotype. Gorski et al. (1988) have determined empiric risk estimates. Half of all recognized pregnancies have abnormal outcomes: of these, three-quarters miscarry, and the other quarter result in the birth of a child with multiple malformations. The overall risk to have an abnormal child, expressed as a proportion of all livebirths, is about 20%. The family history may be helpful in determining the probabilities in the individual case of having a normal child, an abnormal child, or a miscarriage. Intuitively, the likelihood for a successful pregnancy would be less for an "exceptional CCR." In some cases, all unbalanced forms might be expected to lead to miscarriage (Creasy, 1989).

It is generally justifiable to advise that, sooner or later, a normal outcome can reasonably be expected. Thus, it is warranted to make continued attempts until a successful pregnancy is achieved. Optimism may need to be guarded; pedigrees exist (e.g., Evans et al., 1984) in which the reproductive history is so unpromising that some years of attempts might be necessary before a normal child is born. In the boy who is a heterozygote, sterility may well ensue.

Bowser-Riley et al. (1988) review the specific case of the double two-way translocation and propose the risk of having an abnormal child to be approximately the sum of the figures derived separately for each rcp; it may be (as they acknowledge) that this would be an overestimate due to nonviability of doubly imbalanced combinations, albeit each on its own might be viable.

When it is determined that viable imbalance is a possibility, prenatal diagnosis is indicated. It is a matter of individual judgment whether this is done in early pregnancy (chorion villus sampling, CVS) or in the second trimester (amniocentesis). Repeated loss of pregnancy, which many CCR couples will have suffered, can be devastating, and individual reactions will vary. On the one hand, if the diagnosis is made early at CVS, an unsuccessful pregnancy can be aborted early. On the other, the woman may prefer to give natural abortion a chance to operate before having amniocentesis at around 14 to 16 weeks; natural selection would have operated on many partial aneuploidies by this time. Morphologic assessment of fetal growth by ultrasonography may allow prediction of upcoming spontaneous abortion.

Advice in the case of a de novo CCR discovered at prenatal diagnosis is given on p. 366.

NOTE

1. In the I.S.C.N. description of the karyotype, the order of chromosomes in the 3-way CCR is as follows: firstly, the lowest number (or X) chromosome; secondly, the chromosome which receives a segment from the first; and lastly, the chromosome donating a segment to the first listed chromosome. Thus, the karyotype for this CCR is written 46,XX,t(2;18;11)(q13;q21.1;p15.3).

12

Parental Sex Chromosome Aneuploidy

There are four major sex chromosome abnormalities. Infertility is practically inevitable in XXY and very common in 45,X and its variants. The other two, XXX and XYY, apparently have little effect on fertility and furthermore are not discernibly associated with any increased risk for chromosomally abnormal offspring. Information on the mosaic forms is less certain.

BIOLOGY

We need briefly to consider why X chromosome aneuploidy is associated with so little phenotypic abnormality compared with autosomal imbalance. The important factor is dosage compensation (see also Chapter 5). Only one X in each cell needs to be fully active, and in the cells of the 46,XX female, one X chromosome is genetically inactivated (lyonization). This inactivation occurs early in embryogenesis. The process originates at an X inactivation center (XIC) within Xq13 and spreads in both directions. The XIC contains the gene *XIST*, which is transcribed only from inactive X chromosomes. This transcript is not translated into protein, but functions as an RNA molecule and localizes to the Barr body (Hendrich et al., 1993). It is thought to be needed for X-inactivation to be initiated but probably not for its maintenance (Brown and Willard, 1994). It is a matter of random chance whether the inactivated X is of maternal or of paternal origin, but once the choice is made, the inactivation pattern remains fixed in all descendants of that cell. An exception is that, during oogenesis, reactivation gives two genetically active X chromosomes.

Certain parts of the X chromosome are not subject to inactivation. The small pseudoautosomal region at the tip of the short arm of the X remains genetically active in the 46,XX female and functions disomically (as also in the 46,XY male, who has copies of the pseudoautosomal region at Xp and Yp) (Rappold, 1993). A number of individual loci in other parts of the X, some of which have homologs on the Y chromosome, escape inactivation and remain active—for

191

example, ZFX/ZFY in Xp22.1 and the ribosomal protein S4 (RPS4) at Xq13 (Ogata et al., 1993; Weil et al., 1993; Ballabio and Willard, 1992). Thus, it is the normal state for them to function disomically in both the 46,XX female and in the 46,XY male. The monosomic (haplo-insufficient) state of these loci in the 45,X or 46,X,del(Yp) female may contribute to the Turner phenotype. A similar mechanism may be the basis of some azoospermic males with deletions in proximal Yq and having a Turner-like somatotype (Barbaux et al., 1995), and in Turner-like neonatal lymphedema with Yq disruption (Erickson et al., 1995). It may be that other loci escaping X-inactivation, but having no Y-borne equivalent, contribute to ovarian development and are compromised in the haplo-insufficient state (Disteche, 1995).

The conceptus with an X chromosome complement in excess of the normal 46,XX or 46,XY accommodates by inactivation of any additional X chromosome. This is nearly successful and, thus, the 47,XXX female and the 47,XXY male have apparently normal in utero survival and a relatively mild postnatal phenotype (see p. 359). The fact that some loci, as noted above, are not subject to inactivation and may therefore function in the disomic, trisomic, or even (in 49,XXXXX) pentasomic states is presumably at least part of the reason for the phenotypic abnormalities associated with these karyotypes.

In females with abnormal X chromosomes the pattern of X inactivation is usually nonrandom, particularly when the imbalance due to the abnormality is "large." In the 46,X,abn(X) karyotype, with one normal X and one abnormal X [abn(X)], the abnormal X is characteristically inactive. However, if the abnormality is a small deletion or a small duplication, the inactivation pattern can be random. In the case of the X-autosome translocation heterozygote, the normal X is usually, but not invariably, inactive (Chapter 5).

Two laboratory procedures require mention. First is the Barr body test (Figure 12–1). This was once a clinically important means of demonstrating the presence of the inactive X chromosome in interphase nuclei of buccal mucosal or other cells. It is no longer used diagnostically because it may mislead interpretation in the case of X chromosome mosaicism or in X,abn(X) karyotypes. Second is the use of late-labeling techniques. Inactive X chromosomes replicate their DNA later in the cell cycle than the other chromosomes. Exploiting this fact, these techniques work on the principle of adding DNA precursor substances (e.g., BrdU, tritiated thymidine) late in the cell cycle and then identifying the precursor cytogenetically (Figure 12–2).

Individuals with low levels of sex chromosome mosaicism, the predominant cell line being 46,N, are encountered occasionally. Might this indicate the possibility of gonadal mosaicism, or does the mosaicism reflect an individual characteristic, such as a predisposition to mitotic and meiotic nondisjunction (Hecht et al., 1984)? In most, at least, we presume it is unlikely that any associated risk for having an abnormal child exists (Horsman et al., 1987). We note in passing that loss of an X or a Y is a common phenomenon in the elderly (Guttenbach et al., 1994a; Catalán et al., 1995).

Meiosis proceeds differently in each of the various sex chromosome abnormalities, and each warrants separate consideration.

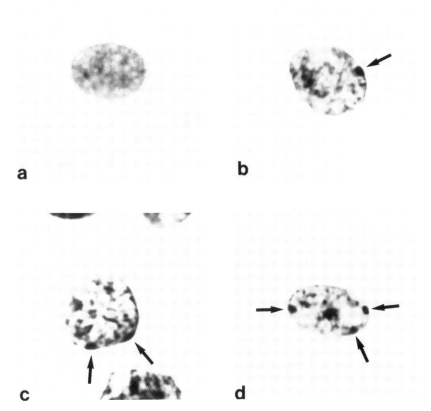

FIGURE 12–1. Buccal mucosal cells from (a) a 45,X female, with no Barr body present; (b) a 46,XX female showing the inactive X as a Barr body; (c) a 47,XXX female showing two Barr bodies; and (d) a 48,XXXX female with three Barr bodies.

XXX

On theoretical grounds, one might expect the three X chromosomes to display 2:1 segregation, with the production of equal numbers of X and XX ova. But this is not the case. No discernible increased risk for chromosomally abnormal offspring of such individuals has been demonstrated. Apparently only normal ova with a single X are regularly produced. It may be that the extra X is lost before meiosis occurs (Neri, 1984) with meiosis then proceeding as in the normal XX female. Alternatively, Hale (1994) proposes a "meiotic quality control" mechanism which eliminates gametocytes containing unpaired sex chromosome univalents.

XXY

Infertility is almost inevitable in Klinefelter syndrome, but remarkable exceptions exist. Terzoli et al. (1992) report an XXY man who had fathered a daugh-

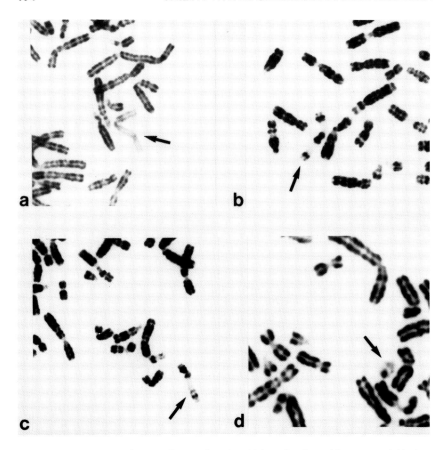

FIGURE 12–2. Partial metaphases showing X inactivation: (*a*) a normal X chromosome, (*b*) an isochromosome of X long arm, (*c*) an X with a short arm deletion, and (*d*) a ring X. BrdU had been added for the last 6 hours of culturing. The inactive chromosomes, replicating at this late time in the cell cycle, incorporate BrdU extensively, and thus are palely stained. The active X stains darkly.

ter, with paternity testing apparently confirming fatherhood, and they quote two other such cases. Undetected XXY/XY mosaicism could account for some of these cases. Cozzi et al. (1994) show that an XXY/XY man, who had had two normal children, produced mostly 23,X and 23,Y sperm, but the frequency of 24,XY sperm (0.9%) was 15 times the usual (0.06%). They propose that a gonadal XXY line produced these 24,XY sperm and that adjacent XY tissue had a sustaining effect to enable spermatogenesis in the XXY cells. Beyond the fact that chromosomally normal children have been recorded, there is no useful information on which to base risk estimates in the extremely rare case of fertility in the XXY male. There may be a risk to have an XXY child; so far, this has never been recorded.

XYY

Meiosis in these men has been studied cytogenetically. The extra Y appears to be eliminated before the spermatocyte forms, and at diakinesis an X–Y bivalent is usually seen (Chandley et al., 1976). Although Speed et al. (1991) found two Y chromosomes in 30% of zygotene/early pachytene nuclei in one subfertile XYY man, as a rule spermatogenesis appears to proceed unhindered. Sperm chromosome analysis shows no differences from the karyotypic range in XY men (Benet and Martin, 1988; Han et al., 1994b). These cytogenetic findings parallel the observation that XYY men have no discernible increase in chromosomally abnormal offspring.

45,X Turner Syndrome

The great majority of women with 45,X Turner syndrome are infertile and do not spontaneously menstruate or develop secondary sexual characteristics. The ovaries appear to be normal in midfetal life but then begin to degenerate. Oocytes disappear at an accelerated rate and, in most cases, are gone by the age of 2 years: "the menopause occurs before the menarche" (Federman, 1987). However, in about 5% of cases spontaneous menstruation does occur, and a very few of these individuals are fertile, although their fertile period may last for only a few years (Baudier et al., 1985; Kaneko et al., 1990; Lippe, 1991). Pregnancy is sufficiently rare (21 cases in the review of Kaneko et al.) to warrant publishing a case report when it happens. Occult X/XX or X/X,abn(X) mosaicism accounts for some of these (see below), but for others, despite much investigation, no cause has been found.

X,abn(X) Turner Syndrome Variants[1]

Turner syndrome variants resulting from an effective partial X monosomy are occasionally associated with fertility—deletion of Xp, deletion of Xq, isochromosome Xq, and large ring X being the major categories (Figure 12–3) (Berkovitz et al., 1983; Kaneko et al., 1990). Presumably a partial synapsis occurs at meiosis, with the intact segment of the abnormal X pairing with the homologous region of the normal X. A 1:1 segregation would be expected, with equal frequencies of gametes carrying either the normal X or the deleted X. Increased in utero lethality of the 46,X,abn(X) conceptus may reflect a different lyonization pattern, with a significant fraction of the abnormal chromosomes being active. Mother–daughter transmission of a del(Xp), and of a del(Xq), are on record (Fitzgerald et al., 1984; Bates and Howard, 1990). Palka et al. (1994) describe an apparently nonmosaic 45,X woman who had an abnormal child with an interstitial Xp deletion, del(X)(p22.2::p11.3). Upon restudy, the mother had one 46,X,del(X) out of 450 cells, allowing the presumption of a somatic–gonadal mosaicism. In a more direct demonstration of gonadal mosaicism, Varela et al. (1991) studied a woman with Turner syndrome

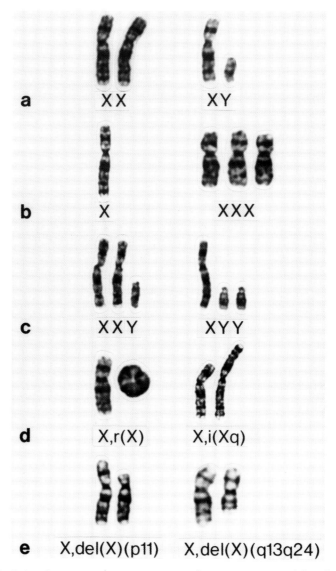

FIGURE 12–3. Some sex chromosome complements: (*a*) normal female XX and normal male XY; (*b*) X and XXX females; (*c*) XXY and XYY males; (*d* and *e*) abnormal chromosomes from females with a ring X, an isochromosome of X long arm, an X short arm deletion, and an X long arm deletion.

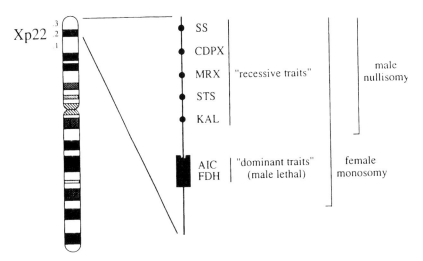

FIGURE 12–4. The position of disease loci on the deletion map of distal Xp. Deletions cause nullisomy in males. Distal deletions may be viable and cause the recessive trait(s); more proximal deletions are probably lethal. In females, an active X with a proximal deletion may express a "dominant" trait. (SS = short stature, CDPX = X-linked chondrodysplasia punctata, MRX = mental retardation, XLI = X-linked ichthyosis, KAL = Kallmann syndrome, AIC = Aicardi syndrome, FDH = focal dermal hypoplasia.) (From Ballabio and Andria, 1992, with the permission of Oxford University Press.) This is one of the most precisely mapped parts of the genome (Ferrero et al., 1995).

and normal menstruation and who had a 46,X,del(X)(p21) daughter. They showed 5/100 cells with 46,X,del(X)(p21) in one ovary, while 100/100 cells from the other ovary, 50/50 fibroblasts, and 100/100 lymphocytes were 45,X. Coto et al. (1995) suggest that many apparently 45,X women actually have a very low level mosaicism, say 1 in 1,000 or less, for a complete or partial Y chromosome.

X Microdeletions and Duplications

X Microdeletions

Small deletions of the X, sometimes too small to be detected on cytogenetics —"microdeletions"—can be transmitted from a 46,X,del(X) mother to a 46,Y,del(X) male conceptus. These male conceptions will be nullisomic for certain loci in the region of the deletion. In the case of a very small deletion, viability may be possible, but the absence of loci will lead to a "contiguous gene syndrome" (Figure 12–4). For example, an Xp22.3 deletion may remove the steroid sulfatase gene, causing ichthyosis, the Kallmann gene, causing hypogonadism and anosmia (inability to smell), the *CDPX* (X-linked chondrodysplasia punctata) gene(s), causing a specific skeletal dysplasia with short stature, punctate calcifications on X-ray, and nasal hypoplasia, and the *OA1* (ocular albinism-1) gene (Ballabio and Andria, 1992; Meindl et al., 1993). Another well-described contiguous gene syndrome is the variable combination of Duchenne muscular dystrophy, retinitis pigmentosa, adrenal hypoplasia, glycerol kinase deficiency, and mental retardation, due to microdeletion within Xp21 (Dunger et al., 1986; Chelly et al., 1986; Francke et al., 1987; Hoffman et al., 1987); the deletion is demonstrable by FISH, enabling accurate recognition of the carrier state in the female (Worley et al., 1995). A retinal gene, the neighboring *DFN3* cochlear gene, and one or more brain genes can be deleted to produce a syndrome of visual loss with choroideremia, deafness with stapes-fixation, and intellectual defect (Merry et al., 1989). In the female carrier, X microdeletions can show selective or random inactivation (Francke, 1984; Wells et al., 1991). Random inactivation may cause nonexpression of a presumed "brain gene" or genes in Xp21 in some parts of the brain, with a degree of intellectual affection in the female carrier (Fries et al., 1993).

X Duplications

In the very rare case of the abnormal X having a duplication of X material, 1:1 segregation in the female heterozygote would be expected. (*1*) Hemizygous XY offspring, in whom the abn(X) is genetically active, have a functional partial X disomy, and are of abnormal phenotype (Steinbach et al., 1980; Schwartz et al., 1986; Schmidt et al., 1991; Rao et al., 1994). If the duplication includes Xp21.1–p21.2, the phenotype may include sex reversal, with ovarian formation and female or ambiguous genitalia, due to disomic expression of a gene *SRVX* (Bardoni et al., 1994; Rao et al., 1994; Arn et al., 1994). Bernstein et al. (1980) record such a case: a mother with the karyotype 46,X,dup(X)(p21-pter) had a severely retarded and malformed daughter, with a female internal genital tract shown at autopsy and karyotypically 46,Y,dup(X). Another daughter, and the grandmother, were 46,X,dup(X), and a subsequent pregnancy was 46,Y,dup(X) at amniocentesis. (*2*) The phenotype in heterozygous daughters is less predictable. If the rule of selective lyonization holds, the abn(X) is consistently inactivated, and normality should be expected. If the rule fails—and in this setting it may—and the normal X is preferentially inactivated, or if inactivation is random, a functional partial pure or mosaic X disomy exists, and this is associated with an abnormal phenotype, of variable degree (Knuutila et al., 1984; Schwartz et al., 1986; Van Dyke et al., 1986).

Sex Chromosome Polysomy

The 48,XXXX female characteristically has diminished ovarian function, and fertility in pure XXXX is on record in only one case (ascertained through a Down syndrome child) (Gardner et al., 1973b). Sterility is presumably invariable in XXXY and XXYY males, who have a further sex chromosome superadded upon the Klinefelter genotype (Borgaonkar et al., 1970).

GENETIC COUNSELING

XXX

XXX mothers have no discernibly increased risk of bearing chromosomally abnormal children. A theoretical increased risk for children with an X aneuploidy has not been demonstrated in practice. Despite reports of chromosomally abnormal children born to XXX women, it should be emphasized, as Dewhurst (1978) and Neri (1984) do, that when biased ascertainment is taken into account, no cases of abnormal offspring have been reported. Neri suggests a risk figure of about 5%; we think this is overly pessimistic and propose an estimate of <1% as more realistic. Both Dewhurst and Neri suggest that prenatal diagnosis is warranted, at least until the picture is clearer. This is a somewhat conservative view, given the fact that *no* strong case has yet been made for any increased genetic risk for sex chromosomal (or autosomal) abnormality. But we acknowledge that uncertainty could be seen as reasonable grounds for seeking the reassurance of prenatal diagnosis. Follow-up of prospective pregnancy data on XXX females detected in newborn population studies should enable the derivation of a definitive risk assessment. Anecdotal evidence indicates that some XXX women face premature ovarian failure, and thus have an early menopause (Villanueva and Rebar, 1983). This evidence can be brought to the attention of these women, so they can choose to have children earlier rather than later in the light of this possibility.

XYY

To our knowledge, there is no report of a discernibly increased risk for the XYY male to have chromosomally abnormal children. Prenatal diagnosis would be discretionary.

45,X Turner Syndrome

Fertility occurs so rarely in Turner syndrome that it is usually appropriate to advise these women that sterility is practically inevitable. However, a 45,X woman who has spontaneous menses may be fertile. The period of fertility is likely to be short-lived; thus, if she wishes to have a child, she should not delay in trying for a pregnancy. Endocrine and ultrasound studies may clarify whether ovulation is occurring.

Kaneko et al. (1990) reviewed the literature on pregnancy outcome in nonmosaic Turner syndrome women (mosaic Turner syndrome is noted under Sex Chromosome Mosaicism below). Thirteen 45,X women had 21 recorded pregnancies. From these, 11 normal children were born. Six miscarried (one with a 45,X karyotype on products of conception), two ended in stillbirth (one with hydrocephalus), one baby born to a 22 year old had Down syndrome, and one infant had a partial cleft palate. This almost 50% rate of abnormal outcome may reflect selective reporting (although *any* pregnancy in a 45,X woman would warrant publication). It may also represent a true risk, and it would be prudent to offer prenatal diagnosis to the pregnant woman with Turner syndrome.

There are now reports of a number of successful IVF (in vitro fertilization) pregnancies in Turner syndrome women, using a donor ovum. We know of one case in which a mother plans to set aside her own ovarian tissue for her daughter's use in due course, should she so wish. Anticipating possible artificial fertility, girls should have hormone treatment from the age of 10 to 12 years in order to avoid uterine hypoplasia (Leclerq et al., 1992). Lippe (1991) discusses the medical implications of pregnancy in Turner syndrome, commenting on an increased rate of caesarean section and exacerbation of underlying hypertension and carbohydrate intolerance.

X,abn(X) Turner Syndrome Variant

Not infrequently, women with incomplete Turner phenotypes due to a 46,X,abn(X) karyotype have normal secondary sexual development, and fertility is likely or proven (Fraccaro et al., 1977; Fryns et al., 1982). The majority of these cases involve deletions of Xp or Xq of quite substantial size, with a phenotypic range from partial Turner syndrome through minor menstrual abnormality (Trunca et al., 1984; Krauss et al., 1987; Tharapel et al., 1993). Premature ovarian failure is likely (Fitzgerald et al., 1984; Bates and Howard, 1990), and this point should be made in the counseling session; an early start on child–bearing may be advisable. Assuming 1:1 segregation, the deleted X will be transmitted in 50% of ova. If the ovum containing it meets an X-bearing sperm, a conceptus with the same karyotype as the mother results. If lyonization is (as in the mother) asymmetric, with consistent inactivation of the abnormal X, a pregnancy going through to childbirth would produce a daughter having a similar phenotype. If the ovum meets a Y-bearing sperm, a zygote with partial nullisomy X results, and will end in early abortion. Viable offspring are in the ratio of 1:1:<1 of chromosomally normal males, normal females, and X,abn(X) females.

Whether or not prenatal diagnosis is chosen in pregnancies of 46,X,abn(X) women depends on their perception of the seriousness of the potential abnormal outcome; it may well also be influenced by how difficult it was to achieve the pregnancy.

X Microdeletion

The carrier can be fertile, and 1:1 segregation with respect to the normal X and the abn(X) would be expected. This implies a 50% risk to have a son affected with the full "contiguous gene syndrome" or a daughter who might display a partial phenotype. There may be an increased fetal loss rate with the 46,Y,del(X) karyotype. Prenatal diagnosis, if chosen, would preferably be a molecular genetic exercise.

Table 12—1 "Occasional" X aneuploidy in women with repeat (2 or more) miscarriages

No. of women	X aneuploid metaphases[a]
86	None
8	47,XXX (1–4)
4	45,X (2–3)
3	45,X (1–3)/47,XXX (1–2)
1	45,X (1)/47,XXX (1)/48,XXXX (1)
1	45,X (1)/49,XXXXX (1)

[a]Numbers in parentheses refer to actual number of abnormal metaphases per 50 or more cells.

Source: From Horsman et al. (1987).

X Duplication

The female carrier has a risk of 50% to transmit the dup(X). If the pregnancy is able to proceed to livebirth, a son would be abnormal due to X disomy. A daughter is not necessarily protected by selective inactivation, and phenotypic abnormality would be possible.

Sex Chromosome Polysomy

Many XXXX women are of low-normal or borderline intelligence, and the questions of fertility and genetic risk may well be raised. In fact, it appears that sterility is usual. XXXY and XXYY men are undoubtedly sterile.

Sex Chromosome Mosaicism

Loss of one X to give an occasional 45,X cell is a normal characteristic of aging in the 46,XX female. Horsman et al. (1987) studied 103 women who had suffered repeat (2 or more) miscarriages; 16% of women had varying types and degrees of X aneuploidy (Table 12–1), but none had more than 10% of cells aneuploid. All of those proceeding to skin fibroblast culture karyotyped 46,XX on this tissue. The total fraction of X aneuploid cells (1.64%) from all the women did not differ significantly from (indeed, was marginally less than) the fraction of 1.78% in an age-matched control population. We may propose the rule that less than 10% of X aneuploidy on blood karyotyping is without reproductive significance in the phenotypically normal woman.

Mosaic Turner Syndrome

Women with a Turner syndrome phenotype and 45,X mosaicism comprise a different category; we may suppose that the 45,X cell line is constitutional and prevalent in much of the soma and gonad. Kaneko et al. (1990) reviewed 117 pregnancy outcomes in 49 cases of X/XX, X/XXX, X/XX/XXX and X/XX/XXX/XXXX mosaicism. For cases with information available, the miscarriage rate was 30%, the stillbirth rate 7%, 43% of babies were normal, and 20% were abnormal. It is probable these abnormality rates are inflated by ascertainment bias; some of the mothers might never have come to a chromosome study if they had not suffered an unfortunate pregnancy outcome. A sex chromosome defect (45,X, X/X,r(X), X/XX, X/XX/XXX or X/XY) was observed in 7% of the children of X/XX women and 23% of the children of X/XX/XXX women; no X/XXX woman had a child with X aneuploidy. This obliges acknowledgment of a causal link in at least some instances, and a ''significant'' and perhaps ''substantial'' risk to have a child with a sex chromosomal defect may apply. We are not yet in a position to define these terms with any precision.

NOTE

1. abn = abnormal

13

Parental Autosomal Aneuploidy

A question of reproduction is usually an academic matter in individuals with functional autosomal aneuploidy. But towards the milder end of the phenotypic range, social and emotional development may be such that forming a stable relationship is possible. Some who lack that degree of maturity may yet have a social freedom that opens the possibility of a sexual encounter. Either on their own behalf, or more likely through the agency of parents or other carers (whose agenda may include sterilization; Karp, 1981; Wolf and Zarfas, 1982), such people may present to the genetic clinic. Ethical issues raised in this context are aired in Chapter 1.

In contrast, some structural imbalances are without discernible phenotypic effect. Deletion or duplication of a small segment of euchromatin, or the presence of an extra structurally abnormal chromosome (ESAC), is occasionally recognized fortuitously in normal and fertile individuals.

BIOLOGY

Parental Trisomy 21

Maternal Trisomy 21

At female meiosis, the three homologs form either a trivalent, or a bivalent and a univalent (Figure 13–1) (Polani et al., 1982; Wallace and Hultén, 1983). (Interestingly, trivalents have also been demonstrated of chromosome 18 at meiosis I of oogenesis in trisomy 18; Cheng et al., 1995). Segregation is then either 2:1, in the case of the trivalent, or 1:1, in the case of the bivalent, with the univalent going randomly to either cell. In either case, the result is disomic (24,+21) and normal (23,N) gametes in equal proportions. Speed (1984) has observed trivalents in about 40% of meiotic cells and a bivalent plus a univalent in the remaining 60%. Cunniff et al. (1991) noted a diminution in the number

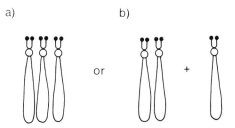

FIGURE 13–1. Possible synapsis of three No. 21 chromosomes: (*a*) as a trivalent and (*b*) as a bivalent and a univalent.

of oocytes in the ovaries of Down syndrome (DS) girls at the time of birth, which could be the cause of a subsequent subfertility.

In a review of the literature, Rani et al. (1990) list 30 reports of pregnancy in DS women. The ratio of DS to normal offspring was 10:17 (there were 3 abortions), not significantly different from a 1:1 ratio, but suggestive of a deficit in trisomic offspring. A reasonable interpretation is that 46,N and 47,+21 conceptions occur with equal frequency, but loss of pregnancy is greater with the trisomic fetuses. About one-third of the 46,N offspring were nevertheless abnormal, which may have reflected paternal or environmental factors.

Paternal Trisomy 21
Schröder et al. (1971) observed in a study of male meiosis in trisomy 21 that spermatogenesis apparently can proceed normally. Two DS males have been documented to have fathered a child (Sheridan et al., 1989; Bobrow et al., 1992; Zühlke et al., 1994), and one other has been implicated (Thompson, 1962).

Parental Trisomy 21 Mosaicism
In practice, it is usually only those individuals with a low percentage of +21 cells who seek genetic advice. These people come to notice because (*1*) their phenotype was subtly suggestive of DS or (*2*) they were studied as phenotypically normal parents of one or two DS children (Uchida and Freeman, 1985). The important factor, if it could only be known, is the degree to which the gonad comprises 46,N and 47,+21 cells. The trisomic cells (see preceding) produce disomic and normal gametes in equal proportion; of course, normal cells, other things being equal, give rise only to normal gametes. Thus, the proportion of abnormal gametes produced depends on the proportion of germ cells that are trisomic. In the limit, the gonad might be fully 47,+21. Any level of correlation between the degree of mosaicism in lymphocytes and gametes is not readily amenable to study. Familial trisomy 21 mosaicism is on record but is exceptional (Werner et al., 1982).

Parental Trisomy 18 Mosaicism

This is extremely rarely recorded in adulthood: only four cases are known (Butler, 1994). Two of the women had a history of miscarriage, one also having a normal child and a stillborn child with trisomy 18. Because of the usual lethality of trisomy 18 in utero the risks obtaining in such women would apply substantially to miscarriage.

Parental Partial Aneuploidy, 46,rea

Barber et al. (1991, 1994) have reviewed the rare circumstance of the same unbalanced karyotype transmitted from parent to child. The usual forms are deletion, duplication, and the derivative chromosome from an unbalanced translocation. Three categories are proposed: *(1)* phenotypically normal parent and child; *(2)* abnormal parent and child; and *(3)* normal parent and abnormal child. Ascertainment in category *(1)* is usually through prenatal diagnosis for maternal age or other fortuitous reason. Wolff et al. (1991) and Moog et al. (1994) each describe a mother and child having an abnormal chromosome 18 with a direct duplication of 18p: the phenotypic normality in the former pair, compared with mild retardation in the latter two, may reflect a slight difference in the amount of duplicated material. The mother in Moog et al. may have been somewhat protected by a minor (20%) 46,XX line. Harmless deletions are documented in 5p14.1→14.3, in 11p12 and in 16q21 (Overhauser et al., 1986, 1994; Barber et al., 1991; Callen et al., 1993). Deletions of G-band dark chromatin may typify the harmless deletion: these regions are poor in CpG islands and thus presumably accommodate fewer genes. One harmless duplication that has caused a certain amount of confusion is dup(15)(q12–q13) (Ludowese et al., 1991; Jalal et al., 1994), which can make the other homolog seem, by comparison, to have a Prader-Willi/Angelman deletion. Barber proposes the expression ''duplication or deletion without phenotypic effect'' for cases in which the additional or missing material is euchromatic. The distinction from a variant chromosome is open to debate, and we comment further on this category in Chapter 15.

Ascertainment of categories *(2)* and *(3)* is usually following referral of a child for a chromosome study. There are uncommon cases of the unbalanced and phenotypically abnormal carrier of a chromosomal rearrangement being functionally fertile and some examples follow. Dhooge et al. (1994) describe a mildly retarded mother with a duplication of segment 8p22–p23.1 (or possibly 8p21.3–p22), whose two children had the same dup(8). Three generation transmission of a dup(7)(p13p12.2) is recorded in association with an unremarkable physical and mild functionally abnormal neurological phenotype (Schaefer et al., 1995). Similarly, a number of instances of familial partial autosomal monosomy due to transmission of a deleted chromosome are on record. Pettenati et al. (1992) record deletion for the segment 8p23.1→pter and provide a family photograph showing unremarkable physical appearances; the del(8p) children had learning and behavioral difficulties. Keppen et al. (1992) describe mild to moderate retardation in a grandmother, mother, and child, each having a deletion of chromosome 5 short arm, p14.3–p13.3 (not with cri du chat syndrome). A severe form of cri du chat syndrome has been documented in mother and child (Martínez et al., 1993; and see p. 16), and a mild form in grandmother, mother and infant daughter (I. M. Winship, pers. comm., 1995). Fukushima et al. (1987) describe a mother and son with a 13q deletion, both with retinoblastoma; curiously, only the child had developmental delay. Loss of a different tumor suppressor gene, the *APC* gene which is the basis of familial adenomatous polyposis, accompanied the del(5)(q22q23.2) in a retarded man, his aunt, and inferentially his retarded mother, causing polyposis in at least the man and his aunt; other family members carried a balanced insertional rearrangement (Cross et al., 1992). Neavel and Soukup (1994) report mother-to-child transmission of "Jacobsen syndrome" (terminal 11q deletion; see p. 279). Cooke et al. (1989) report a father and son with an apparently balanced reciprocal translocation but with a deletion (of about 11Mb) demonstrable on flow cytometry: both displayed minor dysmorphisms and mild intellectual deficit. The chromosome deletion of DiGeorge syndrome can be transmitted from parent to child, with a different clinical picture in each (Stevens et al., 1990; Van Hemel et al., 1995).

Parental Partial Aneuploidy, 47,+ESAC

Genetically Important ESACs

Transmission of an ESAC which contains active genetic material and leads to a functional partial aneuploidy is very rarely observed. Mosaic cases are recorded (Mark et al., 1977; Fryns and Kleczkowska, 1986; Schwartz et al., 1986) and may be associated with a reproductive risk if the abnormal cell line is represented in the gonad. Urioste et al. (1994b) describe a familial unstable supernumerary chromosome with a mother and two daughters having variable manifestations of "cat-eye syndrome" due to 47,+der(22)/46,N. The origin of most ESACs can be determined by FISH. (Partial autosomal aneuploidy resulting from a ring chromosome is dealt with in Chapter 10.)

Genetically Harmless ESACs

ESACs are frequently called "marker chromosomes," but since this term implies that their origin is unknown we prefer the term ESAC. By circular reasoning, the ESAC is regarded as harmless in a phenotypically normal individual; this category of ESAC is also called a B chromosome. They are found by chance in normal people (Ridler et al., 1970) or at prenatal diagnosis (Tsukahara et al., 1986; and see p. 263). Many ESACs are very small and prone to loss during cell division. Consequently, mosaicism and, in the case of a transmitted chromosome, familial mosaicism are seen frequently (Chudley et al., 1983). The majority of these harmless ESACs comprise acrocentric short arm and pericentromeric material or other autosomal pericentromeric chromatin (Callen et al., 1992).

The ESAC would probably form a univalent at meiosis rather than synapsing with whatever chromosome it was derived from. R. H. Martin et al. (1986b) analyzed sperm chromosomes from two men who had a bisatellited ESAC. Slightly less than half the sperm were found to carry it, although the distribution did not differ significantly from 1:1. Interestingly, one man had an excess of sperm disomic for a small chromosome; this may be an exceptional example of interchromosomal effect. Familial ESACs are characteristically maternally transmitted, which could reflect preferential exclusion of the marker in spermatogenesis or, possibly, a reduced male fertility. Jaafar et al. (1994) studied a phenotypically normal man presenting with infertility who had a supernumerary bisatellited heterochromatic chromosome. In most spermatocytes, the ESAC was in close proximity to the X–Y bivalent, and this may have been the cause of the infertility.

GENETIC COUNSELING

Parental Down Syndrome

The risk for the child to have DS is presumably 50%, at least in the case of maternal DS. The other parent is likely to have a degree of mental deficiency, possibly due to a genetic factor. Prenatal diagnosis would of course detect those fetuses with trisomy 21, but the risk of a chromosomally normal fetus having a birth defect or being mentally handicapped could be as high as 30% (Rani et al., 1990). Prevention of pregnancy in those DS women at risk is regarded by many as advisable. In one confirmed case of paternity in a DS man, prenatal diagnosis (with a 46,XY result) was performed (Bobrow et al., 1992). We refer the reader to the discussion in Chapter 1 (p. 15) for a general review of the ethical issues in this setting.

Parental Trisomy 21 Mosaicism

Theoretically the risk for having a child with (nonmosaic) Down syndrome is high—up to 50%. Presumably the risk is related to the proportion of gonadal cells that are trisomic, but this is not accessible information. The proportion seen on lymphocyte analysis offers no real help in this question. One point is clear: it is certainly appropriate to offer prenatal diagnosis.

Parental Partial Autosomal Trisomy Or Monosomy

The risk for a child to have the same defect as the parent is 50%, or very close to it. A lesser risk applies in the case of mosaicism. In the case of a person of only low-normal/borderline intelligence who is functionally fertile, the issue of the risk and possible questions of prenatal diagnosis or sterilization will be difficult to raise (p. 15).

A phenotypically normal individual said to have a partial aneuploidy merits a cytogenetic reevaluation, including the application of high-resolution banding and possibly molecular genetics, to check for the possibility that the supposed aneuploidy is actually a balanced rearrangement that was only partially characterized cytogenetically.

As cytogenetic techniques have become refined, new "defects" are being identified which, upon family study, are revealed as being unusual, but functionally balanced, forms (Barber, 1994). For practical purposes, they can be regarded as variants, rare or possibly even "private" to that family. The counselor must take care that apparently abnormal karyotypes are not overinterpreted and, in doing a family study to clarify a particular unusual chromosome, should see that family members understand the reason for the study. If the "defect" is de novo in an abnormal child, it may well have been the cause of the abnormality; if a parent and other relatives carry the same chromosome (especially if transmitted through both males and females), its probable harmlessness is demonstrated.

The Harmless Extrastructurally Abnormal Chromosome

If an ESAC is judged to be harmless, then on that basis, it would be immaterial whether a parent transmits it to an offspring. Thus, the chance of transmission of up to 50% in the nonmosaic and a lesser likelihood for the mosaic would be academic. Nevertheless, it may be useful to know that, in a particular family, their ESAC has not been associated with any phenotypic abnormality, a point that may be settled by doing a family study; this enables the counselor to offer firm reassurance that those who inherit it in the future will also likely be normal. It would be premature yet to suppose that an associated infertility in the male (Jaafar et al., 1994) is other than coincidental. The single case in R. H. Martin et al. (1986b) of a 47,+ESAC man with increased sperm aneuploidies cannot establish a general risk to 47,+ESAC persons for having chromosomally abnormal offspring; nevertheless, prenatal diagnosis would not be inappropriate in this context.

Real cause for concern arises only when harmlessness cannot be established— for example, in a mosaic individual in whose family no others have the ESAC. A detailed cytogenetic assessment of the chromosome is required and guidelines for estimating risks of phenotypic abnormality are presented in Table 23–5 on p. 370. For an ESAC in which a risk is judged to apply, prenatal diagnosis would be appropriate.

14

The Fragile X Syndromes

Fragile XA syndrome appeared on the cytogenetic scene in the late 1970s; now, in the mid 1990s, it occupies a predominantly molecular genetic stage. But it is entirely appropriate that it retains a place, and indeed a whole chapter, in this book, with the evolution of cytogenetics into "molecular cytogenetics." Fragile XA syndrome is the second most important genetic cause of mental deficiency after Down syndrome and is the most common familial cause. Estimates of population prevalence have ranged widely, and some have been rather high. Current best estimates, in round figures, are as follows: fragile X with full mutation and mental defect, 1 in 4000 males and 1 in 10000 females; female premutation carrier with risk to have a child with a full mutation, 1 in 1000 females; male premutation carrier with risk to have a grandchild with a full mutation, 1 in 5000 males (G. Turner, pers. comm., 1995). A population with a high premutation frequency in unselected women, such as the Québecois with 1 in 259 (Rousseau et al., 1995), may reflect founder effect and/or obfuscation due to premutation-size alleles which have little risk to expand to a full mutation; or perhaps the 1 in 1000 figure is too low. Fragile XE syndrome is rare and is a nondysmorphic form of mild intellectual disability.

BIOLOGY

Fragile XA syndrome is named for the folate-sensitive fragile site, FRAXA, at Xq27.3 (Figure 14–1). There are two other rare fragile sites on the X chromosome distal to FRAXA, named FRAXE and FRAXF. FRAXE is of clinical significance but the associated disorder is yet to be well documented. FRAXF appears to be a harmless variant. FRAXD is a common fragile site, proximal to FRAXA, and is also harmless, and a part of normal chromosome structure.

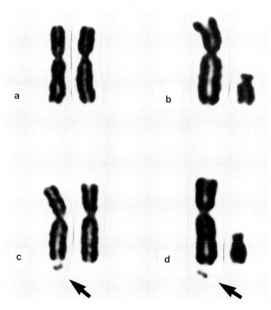

FIGURE 14–1. Plain-stained sex chromosomes from a normal female (*a*) and male (*b*) compared with those of a fragile X female (*c*) and a fragile X male (*d*). The fragile site is arrowed. The segment distal to the fragile site appears as a satellite, as though it is about to break off.

MOLECULAR GENETICS OF THE FRAGILE X LOCI

FRAXA, a Dynamic Mutation

Fragile XA syndrome is a "dynamic mutation" disorder (Sutherland and Richards, 1994). At the fragile site there is a section of DNA comprising the triplet cytosine-cytosine-guanosine (CCG) repeated many times.[1] The fragile site exists in the 5' untranslated region of the *FMR1* (fragile X mental retardation-1) locus which produces a protein product (FMRP) that binds RNA and is necessary for normal brain development and function. Normal X chromosomes have from 6 to about 55 sequentially repeated copies of the CCG triplet. Normal carrier males, sometimes called transmitting males, have approximately 55 to 230 copies of the triplet-repeat ("premutation"). Males with the "full mutation" of more than 230 triplet-repeats (up to about 1000 copies) have fragile XA syndrome (Kremer et al., 1991; Oberlé et al., 1991; Yu et al., 1991). The situation is a little more complex for females, probably because they have two X chromosomes and one of these is inactivated. Female carriers of the premutation do not have fragile XA syndrome, but about half of those with the full mutation are variably mentally impaired (Reiss et al., 1993; Staley et al., 1993; Thompson et al., 1994).

The CCG triplet-repeat sequence, when increased beyond a critical size (in the vicinity of 55 copies), is unstable. *It can change in copy number when transmitted from parent to child.* Thus, a mother with a premutation can transmit a full mutation to her child. A mother with a full mutation will usually transmit a larger (or occasionally a smaller) full mutation to her child. In contrast, fathers only transmit premutations to their children (daughters) regardless of whether they themselves carry a premutation or, very rarely, a full mutation. This process, whereby the initial change to the DNA sequence alters the chance of further changes to it, is termed "dynamic mutation" (Richards and Sutherland, 1992). The change from normal copy number to full mutation is a multistep process, proceeding through premutation steps presumably over several generations, rather than a single event characteristic of classical (or static) mutation.

The varying sizes of the fragile site DNA can be visualized on a Southern blot. Figure 14–2 shows the patterns seen in various types of individual and demonstrates the instability in a family, and further examples are shown in Figure 14–3. If DNA is digested with the enzyme *Pst*I and probed with pfxa3, the normal X chromosome gives a fragment of approximately 1.0 kb. This ~1.0

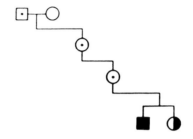

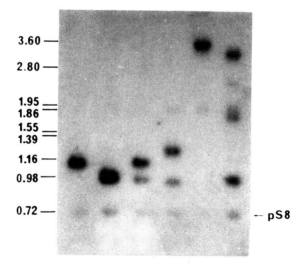

FIGURE 14–2. Inheritance of the fragile XA unstable element in a four-generation lineage from a large affected pedigree. Chromosomal DNA was digested with *Pst*I and probed with pfxa3. The control probe pS8 was included in the hybridization. Pedigree symbols: normal carrier female expressing the fragile XA on cytogenetic study (◑); affected fragile XA syndrome male expressing the fragile XA (■); normal female (○). All carriers (⊙, ▣) are obligate carriers.

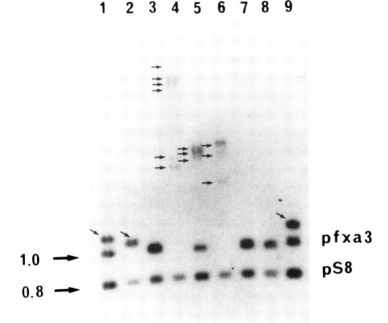

FIGURE 14–3. *Pst*I-digested DNA probed with pfxa3 and pS8. (1) Carrier female, (2) transmitting male, (3) noncarrier female, (4) affected male, (5) carrier female, (6) affected male, (7) noncarrier female, (8) normal male, and (9) carrier female.

kb band represents about 900 bp of DNA flanking the repeat plus the 18 to 165 bp of the actual CCG repeat sequence itself (which amounts to 6–55 triplet-repeats). The DNA fragment from a fragile XA chromosome, having within it the additional copies of the CCG repeat sequence, is larger by this amount. For example, in a person with 230 copies (230 × 3 = 690 bp) of the triplet-repeat—which is about where the premutation merges into the full mutation—the fragment is ~1.6 kb (~900 bp + 690 bp) in size. This is an increase ("amplification") of ~600 bp over the normal size of ~1 kb.

Methylation of the FMR1 Gene

The mechanism by which the CCG repeat causes the molecular pathology which, in turn, leads to the fragile XA phenotype is not yet fully clarified, but hypermethylation appears to play a part (Sutcliffe et al., 1992). The repeat sequence is located within a noncoding portion (5' untranslated region) of the *FMR1* gene (Verkerk et al., 1991). Once there are more than about 230 copies of the repeat, the DNA surrounding the repeat and the repeat itself become hypermethylated. (Methylation is the addition of methyl groups to the C [cytosine] bases in CpG sequences in the DNA molecule.) Hypermethylation is associated with inactivation of the *FMR1* gene containing the triplet-repeat sequence, and it ceases to be transcribed (Pieretti et al., 1991). This lack of *FMR1* gene product (FMRP) is presumed to be the cause of the abnormal phenotype of the fragile XA syndrome (Ashley et al., 1993). Methylated DNA is not cut by methylation sensitive restriction enzymes, and this property can be exploited in the laboratory. Determination of repeat copy number and, if necessary, assessment of methylation as an indicator of the activity state of the gene can be used to predict phenotype.

Methylation status of the triplet-repeat and adjacent DNA in affected males cannot be resolved from the routine FRAXA *Pst*I digestion DNA test (see below). "High functioning" affected males may have amplification values of between 0.6 and 1.0 kb above the normal size. If a more accurate genotype–phenotype correlation is required, analysis of methylation status is done by probing a double digest of *Eco*RI and *Eag*I. *Eco*RI/*Eag*I double digests of DNA from males within this range of amplification values and probed with pfxa3 are shown in Figure 14–4. The probes StB12.3 and Ox1.9 would give an identical result. Interpretation is simpler in males than in females. The normal chromosome of carrier females is also methylated in half the cells, on average, as part of the normal random X-inactivation process.

The rationale for methylation studies is as follows: *Eco*RI gives a normal band size of 5.2 kb. DNA of normal males is unmethylated and gives a 2.8 kb band from *Eco*RI/*Eag*I double digestion. In carrier males the size of these bands is increased by the length of the CCG repeat. However, amplification beyond 230 copies of the CCG repeat is usually associated with methylation. *Eag*I does not cut the methylated DNA, and *Eco*RI/*Eag*I then gives only a band identical to that which would be obtained by *Eco*RI digestion alone (5.2 kb plus the size of the amplification). Males who are mosaic for premutation and full mutation copy numbers of the triplet-repeat give the combination of unmethylated and methylated patterns depending upon the fragment sizes. In females, chromosomes carrying the CCG amplification behave the same as in males, but there are the additional bands contributed by the normal X chromosome. This normal X is randomly inactivated and gives both a 5.2 kb (inactive X) and 2.8 kb (active X) fragment. These patterns have been fully described in Rousseau et al. (1991). More technical aspects of molecular diagnosis are discussed in Mulley and Sutherland (1994).

While methylation may have a role, it is not the only process influencing the function of *FMR1*. In the absence of methylation the gene is transcribed, but the mRNA has difficulty in being translated, and this difficulty increases in proportion to repeat copy number. Feng et al. (1995) analyzed clones of cells having 207, 266, and 285 repeats: these produced, respectively, 24%, 12%, and essentially 0% of the normal amount of the FMR1 protein. Possibly, this reduction in protein is cell type specific and some tissues (for example, chorionic villi) with large unmethylated repeats can still make FMR1 protein.

Two Types of FRAXA Mosaicism

Individuals with full mutations can show somatic instability of the amplified repeat sequence. Different cells in a single tissue can be genetically different, in terms of triplet-repeat length, and genetic differences can exist between tissues. This is manifest as a smear of DNA fragments on Southern blot (Figure 14-3, lanes 4-6).

This instability can lead to two types of mosaicism. While strictly speaking individuals with smears of DNA in the full mutation size range are mosaics (there are different lengths of triplet-repeats), this term is reserved for two specific situations. (*1*) In *mutational mosaicism* there are some cells with full mutations, which are fully methylated, and some cells with premutations, which are unmethylated and functional. The mental phenotype can vary, presumably depending upon the type of mutation predominating in different parts of the brain, and thus the regional activity within neuronal tissues of the *FMR1* gene. Up to 20% of fragile XA syndrome males are mutational mosaics detectable on Southern analysis and some may have an IQ within, but at the lower end of, the normal range. A rare type of mutational mosaic is the individual with some cells containing a normal number of repeat copies (6 to about 55) and others containing premutation or full mutation copy numbers. Polymerase chain reaction (PCR) is a more subtle tool and may indicate the presence of a premutation in a very small fraction of cells in many fragile XA males. De Graaff et al. (1995) could show on brain tissue from an affected male that about 1% of neurons expressed FMRP, and thus presumed that these individual neurons had a genetically active premutation.

In (*2*) "*methylation mosaicism*," the number of repeat copies is characteristic of a full mutation, but the DNA is not methylated in all cells (Figure 14-4, lane 6). This is less common than mutational mosaicism and occurs mostly at the lower end of the range of full mutation copy number. "High functioning" fragile XA syndrome males have been described who are methylation mosaics with full mutations which are partly or completely unmethylated (Hagerman et al., 1994). This diminished DNA methylation correlates with a low level of cytogenetic expression of the fragile XA (less than 5% of metaphases) and possibly a milder phenotype. These males have some FMR1 protein in cultured cells, and this may reflect the in vivo (specifically, brain) situation and explain their "higher functioning" status.

Other Mutational Basis of FRAXA

Almost all fragile XA syndrome is due to triplet-repeat expansion. Very few affected persons (probably less than 1%) have a different mutational basis. A few deletions (Meijer et al., 1994; Hirst et al., 1995) and a single patient with a point mutation (De Boulle et al., 1993) in the *FMR1* gene have been recorded. Apart from these, molecular study of patients with a fragile XA syndrome phenotype has yielded no other mutations, albeit there is some difficulty in identifying nonexpansion cases since they do not manifest the fragile site cytogenetically.

Fragile XE

This fragile site has been much less studied than FRAXA. The mechanism is again a CCG repeat which expands through premutations to full mutations (S. J. L. Knight et al., 1993, 1994; Mulley et al., 1995). The CCG repeat is in

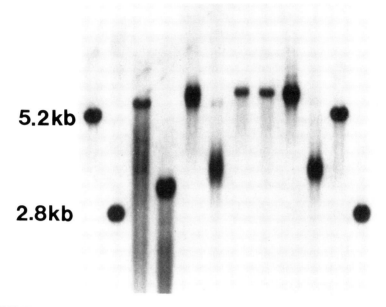

FIGURE 14–4. Restriction patterns for fragile XA males who show methylation differences. *Eco*RI digests are shown in odd-numbered lanes, *Eco*RI/*Eag*I double digests are shown in even-numbered lanes. Normal control male, lanes 1-2 and 11-12. The normal *Eco*RI fragment is 5.2 kb and the normal unmethylated *Eco*RI/*Eag*I fragment is 2.8 kb. Lanes 3 through 10 for affected individuals show fragments of higher than normal molecular weight because of amplification. (Females would exhibit additional complexity because additional methylated and unmethylated bands occur for the normal X chromosome.) The affected individual in lanes 3–4 is unmethylated. Lanes 5–6 is a methylation mosaic, with most of his cells having the *Eag*I restriction site unmethylated, but in some cells it is methylated. The individual in lanes 7–8 is fully methylated; and the one in lanes 9–10 unmethylated. The tissue tested was blood, which may not necessarily reflect methylation patterns in other tissues. (From Loesch et al., 1993, with permission of the American Society of Human Genetics.)

the 5' untranslated region of a gene called *FMR2*, whose 9.5 kb transcript encodes a putative 1302 amino acid protein. *FMR2* transcription is silenced in males with CCG expansion and methylation of the adjacent CpG island (Gecz et al., 1996). Because of its milder phenotype, the diagnosis is less likely to be clinically suspected.

> Gedeon et al. (1995) describe two boys with deletions of part of the *FRAXE* gene, one of whom expresses a truncated FMR2 protein and has FRAXE syndrome, while the deletion in the other is confined to intronic sequences which may or may not affect FMR2 production (Gecz et al., 1996).

Fragile XF
FRAXF is also due to dynamic mutation of a CCG repeat (Parrish et al., 1994), but in this case an apparently harmless one.

CYTOGENETICS

The fragile X chromosomes have a characteristic appearance (Figure 14–5). The fragile sites on the X chromosome are not spontaneously expressed when most standard cytogenetic methods are used. They must be induced by one of the various methods (Sutherland, 1991). These induction methods all lead to a relative deficiency of either thymidine or deoxycytidine at the time of DNA synthesis. Either of these conditions appears to be a requirement for the fragile site expression of fragile X chromosomes.

The fragile Xs are expressed cytogenetically in only a relatively small proportion of cells (10–40% in most fragile X syndrome males) after the cells have been appropriately cultured. The proportion of cells expressing FRAXE and FRAXF may be higher than for FRAXA, especially in females with full mutations. Males with premutations do not express the fragile X cytogenetically; most of those with full mutations do. Some females with premutations express the fragile site in up to 10% of metaphases. This suggests that another requirement for fragile X expression is that the repeat sequence be hypermethylated.

There are four fragile sites recognized cytogenetically on the end of the long arm of the X chromosome (Figure 14–6). Only one, FRAXA in band Xq27.3, is associated with fragile XA syndrome. FRAXD in band Xq27.2 is a common fragile site which can probably be induced on all X chromosomes. It is thus a part of normal chromosome structure and of no pathological significance. It is the only fragile site which can be distinguished from the others by the cytogeneticist, being clearly in band Xq27.2 (Sutherland and Baker, 1992). The other two rare fragile sites are in band Xq28. The more proximal fragile site is FRAXE, and the more distal is FRAXF (Hirst et al., 1993).

GENETICS

FRAXA

Originally it was presumed that the fragile XA syndrome followed standard X-linked recessive inheritance, but atypical properties were soon recognized. The proportion of females with the fragile XA chromosome, or who were obligate carriers of it, and who exhibited features of the syndrome was high (in the order of 35%); and, perplexingly, there were normal male carriers. Segregation patterns of the fragile XA syndrome were examined by Sherman et al. (1984, 1985) when only cytogenetic testing was available. Sherman delineated the paradox, which bears her name, stating that the incidence of fragile XA syndrome is higher in the offspring of daughters of normal carrier males than in the offspring of mothers of these males. Since the discovery of the molecular basis of FRAXA, the transmission of the triplet-repeat sequence has been studied in many families (Rousseau et al., 1991, 1994; Verkerk et al., 1992; Yu et al., 1992) and the inheritance of the syndrome is now well understood. A number of points have emerged:

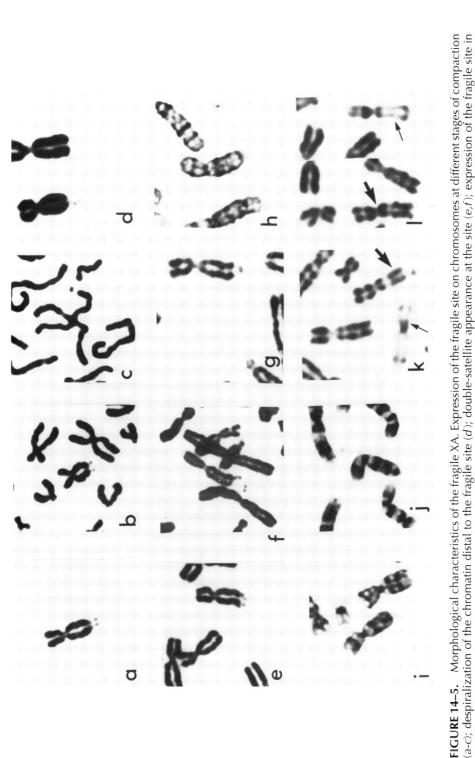

FIGURE 14–5. Morphological characteristics of the fragile XA. Expression of the fragile site on chromosomes at different stages of compaction (a–c); despiralization of the chromatin distal to the fragile site (d); double-satellite appearance at the site (e,f); expression of the fragile site in skin fibroblast metaphase (g); appearance of the fragile X on G-banding (h–j); early replication of the fragile X (thick arrow) by BrdU labeling, with late replication of normal X (thin arrow) in a single metaphase (k); and late replication of the fragile X (thick arrow) by BrdU labeling, with early replication of normal X (thin arrow) from a single metaphase (l). The appearances of fragile XE and fragile XF are identical to those of fragile XA. (Reproduced from Sutherland, 1983, with permission of Academic Press.)

217

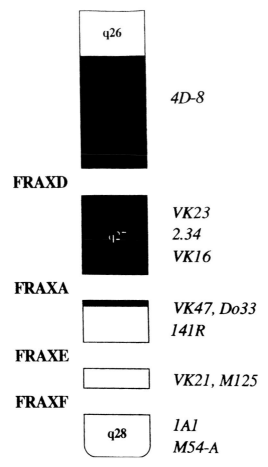

FIGURE 14–6. The fragile sites in distal Xq. FRAXA, FRAXE, and FRAXF are folate-sensitive and can only be distinguished cytogenetically using fluorescence in situ hybridization of the probes shown. FRAXD is a common fragile site. FRAXA, FRAXE, and FRAXF can be distinguished from each other by direct Southern blot diagnosis using specific probes.

1. No new mutation has been observed—that is, no individual with a full mutation has been observed as the offspring of parents with normal numbers of copies of the CCG repeat on their X chromosomes. The mothers of all fragile XA syndrome individuals are carriers of at least a premutation, and where study has been possible, so is a grandparent. Perhaps 80% of all fragile X syndrome in Finland may result from one ancestral mutation in an individual whose descendants went on to colonize northern and eastern Finland in the 16th century (Haataja et al., 1994). The rate of mutation from normal CCG copy number to premutation thus appears to be very low. Morris et al. (1995) provide a mathematical model for a

progression from normal allele→"intermediate" allele→premutation→full mutation at a population level.

2. When the unstable sequence is transmitted by males it characteristically does not increase in size, and may decrease. In males with full mutations, only premutations are seen in sperm (Reyniers et al., 1993).

3. When the unstable triplet-repeat sequence is transmitted by females it usually increases in size (although rare decreases have been reported, and one mother has transmitted a normal gene on her high-risk chromosome due to gene conversion; Vits et al., 1994; van den Ouweland et al., 1994). Women with small numbers of CCG repeats usually show less increase in size than women with larger numbers. Thus, women with less than 70 triplet-repeats ("low-end" premutations) mostly have children who also have premutations (and these offspring are thus normal carrier sons and daughters), although the premutations in these sons and daughters are characteristically larger than those of their mothers. On the other hand, women with "high-end" premutations (90 or more triplet-repeats), and carriers who themselves have a full mutation, virtually always transmit a full mutation (Table 14–2).

4. The mothers of "normal transmitting males" have a smaller number of triplet-repeats than do their grand daughters through these transmitting males. Thus, as per Sherman's observation, these mothers have fewer retarded sons than do the daughters of the transmitting males, and the Sherman paradox is no longer paradoxical (Fu et al., 1991; Rousseau et al., 1991; Yu et al., 1992). This property of FRAXA, displaying increased penetrance of mental defect in the present generation compared with a previous generation, is a form of genetic anticipation.

FRAXE

Not enough fragile XE families have been reported for detailed segregation analyses to be performed. Notably, and in contradistinction to FRAXA, a FRAXE full mutation can be passed from father to daugher (Hamel et al., 1994).

Rare Complexities

We have seen one remarkable family in which both FRAXA and FRAXE are segregating (Mulley et al., 1995). A FRAXE man married a FRAXA heterozygote and they had two daughters, one a FRAXE heterozygote and the other a FRAXE/FRAXA compound heterozygote. The latter, in turn, has had a son with fragile XA syndrome, and FRAXE and FRAXA carrier daughters.

The fragile XA phenotype can coexist with other abnormalities as part of a contiguous gene syndrome. Quan et al. (1995) report a child in whom a deletion in Xq26.3–27.3 removed the *FRM1* and adjacent loci. His phenotypically normal mother showed selective inactivation of the deletion X.

DIAGNOSIS

Opinions differ regarding the relative merits of cytogenetic versus molecular versus immunohistochemical analysis for the ascertainment of index cases of the fragile X syndromes. The availability of good quality cytogenetics and/or molecular diagnosis, Health Service funding structures, and the preferences of individual scientists are factors not without relevance. *Cytogenetics* with fragile site analysis will detect approximately 99% of boys affected with fragile XA as well as FRAXE and FRAXF, but will miss FRAXA in 5 to 10% of mentally retarded females (Tarleton and Saul, 1993). Positive cases then go on to molecular study for FRAXA (and, if the FRAXA study is normal, in laboratories able to offer this complete service, FRAXE and FRAXF). *Molecular* analysis, which has the advantage of combining several samples in one test run and which will detect 100% of cases of FRAXA triplet-repeat expansion, is in some settings the initial diagnostic tool of choice (Oostra et al., 1993), although FRAXE and FRAXF will be missed. *Immunohistochemical* demonstration of FMRP is a new methodology awaiting validation as a diagnostic tool; it will not detect FRAXE syndrome. Since the clinical picture in FRAXA syndrome (and certainly FRAXE) is not necessarily distinguishable with confidence, a conventional cytogenetic study should in any event be done along with the fragile site analysis. Having established the diagnosis in an index case, for all other family members molecular methodology alone is applied to carrier detection, confirmation of diagnosis, and prenatal diagnosis. In our experience only a very small proportion of families have a female index case. Molecular studies may be worthwhile when cytogenetic studies are reportedly normal if there is a family history consistent with a fragile X syndrome.

The American College of Medical Genetics has proposed guidelines for fragile X diagnosis (Park et al., 1994). Noting, as above, the important point that clinical diagnosis can be inconclusive, an initial study in a suspected case should, it is recommended, include both a fragile XA DNA test and a routine cytogenetic evaluation. Once a diagnosis of fragile XA is established in an index case, testing of other family members can then be by DNA alone. Prenatal diagnosis is purely a DNA-based exercise. In many laboratories, fragile site cytogenetics is no longer routinely performed. This policy means that FRAXE would be missed; and it is thus incumbent upon the geneticist to recognize kindreds with a possible X-linked inheritance pattern, and (in those testing negative on FRAXA) to pursue in these selected families a diagnosis of FRAXE, either by fragile site cytogenetics or mutation analysis.

FRAXE

The number of repeat copies characterizing pre-and full mutations of FRAXE remains to be established, and the mutational patterns which characterize intellectual impairment or normality have yet to be clearly determined. The FRAXE mutation can be detected by direct molecular diagnosis. The technique is based on Southern analysis using the probe OxE20 (S. J. L. Knight et al., 1993), similar to the diagnostic protocol used to detect FRAXA. The FRAXE amplification is determined by sizing the *Hind*III fragment (normal size 5.3 kb), and methylation status of the adjacent CpG island is assessed by *Hind*III/*Not*I double digestion (normal size of fragment 2.4 kb). FRAXE carriers are unmethylated at the FRAXA CpG island and have normal numbers of the CCG repeat at that locus.

There are conflicting data about the behavior of the fragile XE mutation. In some families there is a high incidence of female carriers with mental impairment, while in others the females are mostly unaffected. Some males with the fragile site are apparently unaffected. Hamel et al. (1994) suggest there is no premutation (as there is with FRAXA) but the basis for this claim is not clear. They also report two instances of mentally impaired females who have inherited the fragile site from their fathers.

It is likely that the number of copies of the CCG repeat which constitutes a full mutation (i.e., which is associated with hypermethylation) is less than for FRAXA. The full mutation (with DNA methylation) results in the transcriptional silencing of a gene, *FMR2*, in which the FRAXE repeat sequence is located.

FRAXF

FRAXF can be indirectly assumed, in an individual with a cytogenetic fragile Xq28 chromosome, by exclusion of FRAXA and FRAXE. This fragile X chromosome can then be recognized as having no clinical relevance. In a research lab, the FRAXF can be more directly demonstrated by FISH with probes such as those shown in Figure 14–6, or directly by molecular study (Parrish et al., 1994; Ritchie et al., 1994).

CARRIER DETECTION IN FRAXA

Recognition of the FRAXA carrier is, in principle, unequivocal, since the CCG amplification can be directly demonstrated. The probes frequently used, which all yield essentially the same results, are pfxa3, StB12.3 and Ox1.9. The long stretches of CCG repeats in full mutations and many of the premutations are refractory to routine PCR amplification, and so routine diagnosis at the present time is primarily based on Southern analysis. PCR technology is only used to measure the exact CCG triplet-repeat number in those few cases with a fragment size which, on Southern analysis, is near the interface (or region of overlap) between normal polymorphism and premutation. (A protocol for a solely PCR-based diagnosis has been published by Brown et al. [1993] but this has not been widely used and its reliability remains to be assessed.) It is now of largely historic interest that detection of the carrier state could be achieved by genotyping linked DNA markers in order to track the inheritance of the fragile X chromosome through a family (Sutherland and Mulley, 1990).

Different Probes

The simplest detection system uses the probe **pfxa3**. Digestion with a single enzyme, *Pst*I, gives a normal 1.0 kb fragment containing the CCG repeat and detects all premutations and full mutations. Alternative enzymes, such as *Eco*RI alone which gives a 5.2-kb fragment, do not resolve the smaller premutations although they do permit easier visualization of dispersed smears. The pfxa3 probe has been validated on a collection of families previously diagnosed by linkage and cytogenetics (Mulley et al., 1992). Neither **StB12.3** nor **Ox1.9** is able to detect the above mentioned *Pst*I fragment; their sequences do not overlap with the sequences within the *Pst*I fragment containing the actual CCG repeat.

Results of hybridizing pfxa3 to *Pst*I digests are shown in Figures 14–2 and 14–3. The restriction fragment containing FRAXA has a higher molecular weight because of the additional copies of the CCG repeat. The pS8 probe, an anonymous X-linked marker, is used as a control in double hybridization. It detects a 0.8-kb fragment in all individuals and confirms the presence of digested DNA in the track. Probe ratio is adjusted in order to obtain signal intensity approximately equal for each of the probes for DNA from normal individuals. This enables the number of non-fragile XA chromosomes in females to be estimated by inspection of relative intensity of pS8 and pfxa3 fragments. Although such a dosage test is inadequate as a primary diagnostic procedure, it does represent a simple and valuable check to avoid missing carriers with an amplification consisting of a faint smear of fragments. (Affected males have no 1.0 kb band, so there is no difficulty in diagnosis, however dispersed a smear).

GENETIC COUNSELING

As always, good genetic counseling depends upon accurate diagnosis. In the fragile X context, this means the molecular confirmation of the diagnosis of FRAXA and the molecular identification of carriers. Non-FRAXA families, in which fragile X chromosomes have been identified cytogenetically, will require molecular analysis of FRAXE.

RISKS OF HAVING AN ABNORMAL CHILD

FRAXA

We set out the empirical risks to have a child affected with fragile XA syndrome in Table 14–1 and discuss the case with each type of parent below.

Male with Premutation

For a carrier male (''normal transmitting males'') there is, according to current knowledge, no risk to have a mentally impaired child due to the FRAXA gene per se. All his daughters receive the FRAXA gene in its premutation form,

Table 14—1   Empiric risk figures for fragile XA syndrome genetic counseling

	Risk of fragile XA syndrome in a proband's:		
	Son	Daughter	Child of either sex
The proband being a			
Male with premutation or full mutation	0	0	0
Female with premutation[a]	~40%	~25%	~30%
Female with full mutation	~50%	~30%	~40%

[a]Average risks; actual risk depend upon the size of the premutation (see Table 14–2).

whatever its size in terms of triplet-repeats. None receives a full mutation and none, as far as is known, shows somatic expansion. Thus, none would have fragile XA syndrome. All 46,XY sons receive their father's Y chromosome, and obviously his carrier state implies no genetic risk to them.

Male with Full Mutation

Procreation in this group is extremely rarely documented. Retrogression to a premutation in sperm dictates that daughters would be (other things being equal) mentally normal. Sons receive the Y chromosome.

Female with Premutation

The risk to transmit the FRAXA X chromosome is 50%. If it is transmitted, the risk of having a child with fragile XA syndrome (in other words, a child with a full mutation) depends upon the size of the mother's premutation. Fisch et al. (1995) have pooled a large body of data, excluded index cases, and estimated the risk as a function of triplet-repeat number (Table 14–2). The fact that the risk shows, essentially, a consistent proportional rise suggests these figures are broadly valid. Women with "low-end" premutations of less than 60 copies of the triplet-repeat have about a 20% risk of having a child with fragile XA syndrome, while for those with more than 90 copies ("high-end premutation"), the risk is 90 to 100%. The practical conclusion is that for any woman in a fragile XA syndrome family who carries the mutation in any form, except possibly for the very smallest premutations, the risk of having a retarded child is substantial.

A currently unanswerable question is, what is the minimum number of copies that constitutes a premutation. Small premutations in the region of 60 triplet-repeat copies may uncommonly expand directly to a full mutation (Snow et al., 1993; Fisch et al., 1995). Unstable transmission of alleles in the 46 to 50 size range has been reported (Reiss et al., 1994) in families without any history of fragile XA syndrome; and an allele of 51 copies has been stably transmitted for 4 generations in another such family (Snow et al., 1993). "Anchoring" CCT triplets in place of some CCG triplets may characterize stable transmission (Gacy et al., 1995; Zhong

Table 14—2   Risk for fragile X premutation carriers to have a child with a full mutation

Premutation size (number of triplet-repeats)	Number of mothers	Number of offspring	Risk for full mutation
50–59	3	5	0.2
60–69	12	23	0.17
70–79	21	38	0.39
80–89	20	39	0.76
90–99	25	35	0.89
100–109	8	11	0.91
>110	21	33	0.97

Source: From Fisch et al. (1995).

et al., 1995). Our provisional view is that women with alleles of 55 copies or greater should be considered at risk to have a child with fragile XA syndrome. Those with alleles of 45 to 55 copies are very likely not.

Women who are premutation heterozygotes may have a risk of premature menopause and thus, if the choice exists, earlier rather than later childbearing would be advisable.

Female with Full Mutation

Offspring who inherit the fragile XA locus will all have full mutations. Hence, of their children with the fragile XA mutation, all the boys will have fragile XA syndrome, as will about 60% of the girls. (This figure of 60% exceeds the 35% applicable to all female carriers of the fragile XA chromosome since in this example all daughters have full mutations.) The intellectual disability in these affected females is usually less severe than in the male.

Differently Ascertained Families

Families identified through a fragile XA syndrome proband have demonstrable evidence that their mutation causes the phenotype. What risks would apply to a woman with a premutation identified otherwise? This would be particularly difficult to estimate if the premutation is small. There are simply no data available on which to base an answer to this question at present, and until there are it may be advisable to apply the standard fragile X risk figures and to provide prenatal diagnosis.

FRAXE

The fragile XE story is still evolving and referral to a specialist in this area is necessary. For the time being, counseling should include the following caveats: *(1)* The penetrance of mental impairment in males and females is unclear, but may be lower than for fragile XA. *(2)* The severity of mental impairment is less in both sexes than for fragile XA. *(3)* Variation between families appears to be considerable and a detailed family history is particularly important. *(4)* Although the inheritance pattern of fragile XE may be similar to that of fragile XA there are apparently some differences, perhaps the most important being that daughters of fragile XE men can be mentally impaired.

The phenotypic consequences of inheriting a full mutation are unclear. There is some risk of these females being mildly handicapped, as yet unquantified, but probably less than for fragile XA. Some males with full mutations appear to be relatively normal, although not all have had detailed assessments. Nevertheless, we presume the risk of significant intellectual impairment in the male to be substantial, albeit less than 100%. Until the situation becomes clearer it may be best to offer prenatal diagnosis and present what is known to the couples involved. Those wishing to avoid the risk of having a retarded child could justifiably choose to terminate pregnancies if a full mutation in the fetus is identified. We await a more detailed interpretation of findings at prenatal diagnosis, but the picture is likely to be similar to FRAXA.

Fragile XF

Fragile XF appears to be without phenotypic effect and may be an entirely harmless fragile site, although very few FRAXF families have been documented. The counselor will need to consult current literature and seek expert advice.

PRENATAL DIAGNOSIS

FRAXA

Prenatal diagnosis is offered to the female carrier. The essential prerequisite is the molecular confirmation of fragile X carrier status of the mother prior to chorion villus sampling (CVS). Southern analysis requires a larger DNA sample and takes more time to complete than the many PCR based molecular diagnoses now carried out for a range of inherited disorders (Sutherland et al., 1991). Times conservatively quoted for a result from Southern analysis could be 2 to 3 weeks (compared with 2–3 days for PCR-based results). Sufficient DNA must be extracted from the CVS sample for at least one digest (approximately 10 μg) with sufficient additional tissue to initiate a cell culture as a source of back-up DNA. Diagnosis is based on repeat length; methylation status of CVS can be misleading, and nonmethylation of CVS has been associated with methylation in fetal tissues (Castellví-bel et al., 1995). Amniocentesis is not recommended: it is done at a later gestational stage and then takes further time for cell culture to provide enough DNA. We note the concept of preimplantation diagnosis on p. 337.

The possible outcomes of prenatal diagnoses for fragile XA are as follows. Outcomes noted in square brackets are likely only with the carrier of a medium size or "low-end" premutation, that is, <90 triplet-repeat copies (see above and Table 14–2):

1. A normal male fetus (1.0 kb *Pst*I band with pfxa3 probe; triplet-repeat copy number 6–55).

[2.] A male fetus with a premutation (up to 1.6 kb band; approximately 55–230 copies of triplet-repeat) and thus a male carrier is predicted.

3. An affected male fetus with a full mutation (band(s) >1.6 kb size and/ or smear; greater than 230 triplet-repeats). The fragile XA mental retardation syndrome is predicted.

The phenotype of an affected male fetus with copy number mosaicism, that is, a mixture of full and premutations, cannot be accurately predicted from CVS. Although *FMR1* expression will be reduced, knowledge on the effect in critical tissues is lacking; most cases are expected to be at least mildly affected.

4. A normal female fetus (1.0 kb band on pfxa3 probe; triplet-repeat copy number 6–55).

[5.] A female fetus with a premutation (up to 1.6 kb band; approximately 55–230 triplet-repeat copies) and thus a female carrier is predicted.

6. A female fetus with a full mutation (band(s) >1.6 kb size and/or smear; greater than 230 triplet-repeat copies). Mental impairment, of variable degree, is predicted in at least half of full mutation females. There is some evidence that the size of the full mutation may be related to level of intellectual functioning, but the variability is too great for this to have any predictive value.

Linked PCR-based markers flanking and within FRAXA could be used for rapid prenatal diagnosis to exclude the diagnosis of fragile XA syndrome. If it is not excluded, of course Southern analysis is necessary. The linkage approach is more complex because it involves the family rather than the individual as the unit of study, but can be helpful in resolving occasional ambiguous results from Southern analysis.

For male carriers, who will obligatorily transmit the premutation to a daughter, prenatal diagnosis is not an issue according to our present understanding that these daughters have no mental defect due to their FRAXA genotype.

FRAXE

There is no experience in the prenatal diagnosis of FRAXE. We assume the same considerations that apply to FRAXA are relevant. Interpretation of results would be difficult, as discussed above, and expert advice should be sought. The daughters of males with full mutations appear to be at risk of intellectual impairment, but the degree of risk has yet to be determined.

NOTES

1. There is some confusion in the way trinucleotide repeats are expressed (Sutherland and Richards, 1993). Taking the convention that the bases be written in alphabetical order from 5' to 3', the FRAXA repeat is CCG, and the "anchoring triplet" (p. 223) is CCT. Some authors "read" the opposite DNA strand, and write CGG and AGG instead.

15

Variant Chromosomes

Normal chromosomes do not necessarily look exactly alike in different individuals. Some chromosomes show a remarkable degree of variation in their morphology. It is crucial that the cytogeneticist can distinguish normal variation from abnormality. Generally, there is no point in reporting a particular variant to the referring practitioner or to the patient. But it is sometimes necessary to pursue the matter, with family studies, when it is not clear whether a particular finding is a normal variant or an abnormality, or when a previous report has sown a seed of doubt in the patient's mind. The study of normal variants is also a research activity in its own right.

BIOLOGY

Chromosomes show variation in five major areas:

1. Centromeric heterochromatin (C-band) size, position, and staining properties
2. Acrocentric chromosome short arm morphology and staining properties
3. The presence of fragile sites
4. G-band amount
5. Fluorescence intensity

Each of these is considered separately (except for fluorescent intensity polymorphisms, which are usually not striking).

C-Band Size, Position, and Staining Properties

C-band heterochromatin comprises, by definition, permanently inactive DNA (constitutive heterochromatin), and is usually located adjacent to the centromere (*C* for centromeric). It stains darkly on C-banding. The four originally described

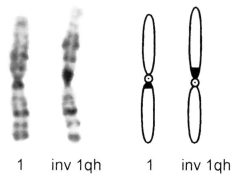

1   inv 1qh   1   inv 1qh

FIGURE 15–1. Chromosome 1 with complete inversion of the heterochromatic region (*right*), alongside its normal homolog. The qh material is now in the proximal short arm. (Courtesy M. D. Pertile.)

variant forms are 1qh, 9qh, 16qh, and Yqh; the differences in size were great enough to have been detected on "solid-stain" chromosomes in the prebanding era. The qh (long arm heterochromatin) regions in chromosomes 1, 9, and 16 are also known as secondary constrictions. C-bands vary in size, and, for those chromosomes in which the material is centromerically placed, there is variation in position relative to the centromere (Craig-Holmes, 1977). The position of the centromere within the C-band positive heterochromatin block of the 1qh, 9qh, and 16qh may vary from one end to the other. Variants at these extremities are sometimes referred to as "inversions" of the heterochromatin. The observed frequencies vary according to the precision of staining and the criteria of the observer (Kaiser, 1988). The most common of these polymorphic inversions— and indeed the most common chromosomal variant in the human race—is the placement of 9q heterochromatin into 9p immediately adjacent to the centromere. In about half of No. 9 chromosomes, a small amount (less than one third) of the heterochromatic block is sited in the short arm. In about 10%, there is a "partial" inversion, with about one third of the heterochromatin in the short arm, inv(9)(p11q12). In 0.6%, all the heterochromatin is in the short arm—a total inversion, inv(9)(p11q13). Partial inversions of the heterochromatic region of chromosome No. 1, inv(1)(p11q12), are quite frequently seen, while total inversions, inv(1)(p13q21), are uncommon enough to be considered as rare heteromorphisms (Figure 15–1).

Whether an "inversion variant" chromosome can influence its own disjunction is speculative. Willatt et al. (1992) observe that in eleven reported cases of the rare mosaic trisomy 9 syndrome, four occurred in the setting of maternal heterozygosity for the inv(9)(p11q12) variant and suggest a causal link; and partial trisomy 9 has been associated with a parental inv(9)(p11q12/3) (Kaiser, 1984; Stamberg and Thomas, 1986). These tiny numbers need to be seen against the background of the hundreds of thousands of inv(9) heterozygotes who have not come to cytogenetic attention for such a reason. Fortuitous coincidence remains a perfectly reasonable explanation.

G banding   C banding   G11 banding α-satellite probe

FIGURE 15–2. A chromosome 20 long-arm variant demonstrated by G-banding and C-banding, G11 banding, and in situ hybridization with a chromosome 20 α-satellite probe (D20Z1) specific for chromosome 20 centromere. Normal No. 20 on left, variant No. 20 on right of each pair. This chromosome was interpreted to be without phenotypic consequence. (From Romain et al., 1991, courtesy D. R. Romain and with the permission of the British Medical Association.)

Variation of C-band material can be demonstrated using other staining techniques, such as Q-banding, which reveals differing intensity of the fluorescence. Most notably, this variation is seen in the C-bands of chromosomes 3 and 4, which range from very dull to very bright. The staining of the C-band material, after one round of replication in BrdU, varies in the pattern of lateral symmetry (Angell and Jacobs, 1978). Heteromorphic staining of the centromeric regions of all chromosomes except No. 8 has been demonstrated using various restriction endonucleases to treat the chromosomes prior to Giemsa staining (Babu et al., 1988). Jabs and Carpenter (1988) showed that the extra C-band material adjacent to the centromere on the short arm of a variant No. 6 is due to increased amounts of a chromosome-specific alphoid DNA repeat sequence.

Other unusual C-band variants are reported for chromosome 3 (Petrovic, 1988), chromosome 5 (Fineman et al., 1989), chromosome 11 (Aiello et al., 1994), chromosome 18 (Pittalis et al., 1994), chromosome 20 with increased C-band material in the short arm (Fryns et al., 1988a), and chromosome 20 long arm (Romain et al., 1991). The 20q variation (Figure 15–2) reflects different amounts of chromosome-specific alphoid DNA. Variation in chromosome 15 α-satellite may confuse the interpretation of a deletion in Prader-Willi and An-gelman syndromes (Delach et al., 1994). A duplication of the centromere itself is a different entity (Callen et al., 1990a). Till et al. (1991), for example, report a duplicated No. 11 centromere and they interpreted this to be of no clinical consequence.

Morphological variants of the Y chromosome are in two categories. *(1) Continuous variation* in the amount of C-band positive heterochromatin can range from a virtual absence, in which case the Y chromosome may appear to be only about half the size of chromosome 22, to a large amount such that the chromosome is about the same size as No. 13. Paternal chromosome study is worthwhile to confirm that very small chromosomes are in fact variants (short Y chromosomes with breakpoints proximal to the Yq11/12 heterochromatin interface are pathogenic deletions; Salo et al., 1995). For very large ones, C-banding is adequate to confirm that the increased size is due to heterochromatin. *(2) Discontinuous variation* in the Y chromosome is expressed as a metacentric appearance, presumably due to pericentric inversion. Satellites on the end of the long arm are another variant; these are presumably due to translocation from one of the acrocentric chromosomes and have been documented to segregate in large kindreds (Genest, 1973) (and see below under NOR Translocation). These discontinuous variants are normally without phenotypic effect but, again, paternal chromosome studies are warranted if there is any doubt.

Acrocentric Short-Arm Morphology

The short arms of the acrocentric chromosomes show a range of morphology, reflecting variation in three components of the short arm: the centromeric heterochromatin, the satellite stalk, and the satellite material (Figures 15–3 and 15–4). A biological role is known only for the stalk, which comprises multiple copies of genes coding for rRNA. The nucleolus is formed by an aggregation of rRNA; thus, the stalk is sometimes called the nucleolar organizing region (NOR). This stalk stains darkly with silver nitrate (Ag-NOR staining) on those acrocentric chromosomes that have an active NOR, and the picture varies from no uptake through marked uptake (darkness) of stain. A newly recognized type of DNA repeat, a 3.3-kb sequence having homology to the repetitive DNA D4Z4 located at distal 4q, is found on the short arms of all the acrocentric chromosomes and has the characteristics of heterochromatin (Lyle et al., 1995).

Length and satellite size and number are distinguishing features. At one extreme, a short arm may seem to be absent; at the other extreme, it may be so long that a D-group chromosome is of C-group appearance, and a G-group chromosome has an F-group resemblance. Molecular analysis of one chromosome 14 with an apparently absent short arm showed loss of satellite III DNA

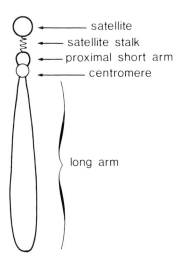

FIGURE 15–3. Diagram of an acrocentric chromosome showing the variable components—satellite, satellite stalk, proximal short arm, and centromere.

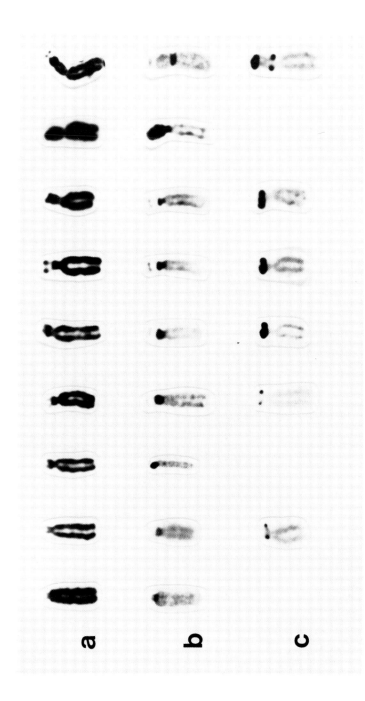

FIGURE 15-4. Variation in the appearance of the short-arm area of D-group chromosomes. The upper row (a) is plain stained, the middle row (b) is C-banded, and the bottom row (c) is silver-NOR stained. Where the same chromosome has been stained by more than one method, they are aligned vertically. Note the variation in morphology from virtually no short arm, on the left, to extensive short arm areas, with and without satellites.

(Earle et al., 1992b). Satellites vary widely in appearance: apparently absent, small or large, and single or double.

In the sense that they cause no phenotypic abnormality, the so-called t(Y;15) and t(Y;22) translocations, in which the C-band material from the long arm of the Y has been translocated onto the short arm of the acrocentric, can be regarded as examples of normal variation (Friedrich and Nielsen, 1972; Cohen et al., 1981; Neumann et al., 1992). Once formed, these variant chromosomes are stable (see also p. 108).

NOR Translocation

The NOR can be translocated to another chromosome, usually to a terminal region. Arn et al. (1995) provide a review, recording examples of this phenomenon in chromosomes 1 through 5, 9, 12, 18, X and Y, and focussing on the particular case of the "satellited 4". These authors discuss a number of routes whereby the abnormal 4ps or 4qs chromosome could be pathogenic; they acknowledge that a lack of consistent phenotype in probands and a normal phenotype in heterozygous parents leaves ascertainment bias as a possible explanation, and we are inclined to accept this as the most probable. Norris et al. (1995) reached the same conclusion in two separate cases involving an interstitial NOR insertion into a Y chromosome at q12 and into a No. 22 at q11.2.

Fragile Sites

A fragile site is a point on a chromosome that is liable to show gaps and breaks. The location of the fragile site is the same in all cells in a particular individual or family (Sutherland and Hecht, 1985). Fragile sites are classified on the basis of their frequency in the population and the conditions of tissue culture that are required to induce them.

In terms of frequency (ignoring fragile XA and fragile XE) there are three categories of fragile site. *(1)* Rare sites are present only in one per several hundred individuals. *(2)* So-called common fragile sites are universal and form part of normal chromosomal architecture. *(3)* Two fragile sites are of intermediate frequency: fra(10q25), seen in 2.5% of individuals, and fra(16q22), seen in 1 to 5% of individuals. Only the rare and intermediate fragile sites are classified as chromosome variants (Figure 15–5). The common fragile sites, being universal, do not vary, although the proportion of metaphases in which they are seen can vary, depending upon conditions, from 0 to 20%. The fragile site at Xq27.3 is not, of course, a normal variant but a pathological change associated with a mental retardation syndrome. This fragile site and others on the end of the long arm of the X chromosome are discussed in Chapter 14.

FRA11B is the fragile site at 11q23.3, within the proto-oncogene *CBL2*, and displays a molecular behavior similar to FRAXA (Jones et al., 1994). Jacobsen syndrome comprises variable deletions of 11q, and there is preliminary evidence

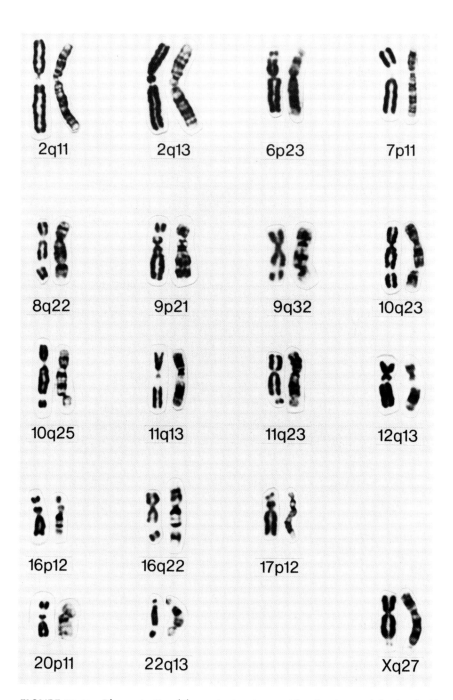

2q11

2q13

6p23

7p11

8q22

9p21

9q32

10q23

10q25

11q13

11q23

12q13

16p12

16q22

17p12

20p11

22q13

Xq27

FIGURE 15–5. The majority of the variant autosomal fragile sites and the fragile X (FRAXA). The chromosome on the left of each pair is plain stained and the one on the right is G-banded.

that mothers of some affected children have a cytosine-cytosine-guanine (CCG) triplet expansion at FRA11B (a premutation or full mutation). The deletion breakpoint in these children is, apparently, at this maternal fragile site. Other cases of Jacobsen syndrome have a breakpoint elsewhere than at 11q23.3 (Penny et al., 1995).

G-Band Variation

The G-band pattern is generally constant, and the relative sizes of G-bands are similar over all human genomes. The degree of compaction of the chromatin will determine the number of bands seen in any metaphase, and even within a metaphase the number of bands on homologous chromosomes may vary (''homolog asynchrony''). True G-band variants exist for chromosomes 9, 15, and 16. Webb et al. (1989) suggested that some of these G-band variants might involve homogenously staining regions. Barber (1994) proposes the expression ''duplication or deletion without phenotypic effect'' for cases in which the additional or missing material is euchromatic; as we note in the chapter on parental autosomal aneuploidy, the distinction between ''variant'' and ''nonpathogenic euchromatic deletion/duplication'' is a subtle one. Before any chromosome with an unusual G-band is determined to be a variant of no pathological significance it should be present in a normal individual, and care needs to be taken to ensure that the chromosome is not involved in some subtle rearrangement such as an insertional translocation. Barber et al. (1991) review possible explanations for phenotypic normality in the context of apparent loss of euchromatin. A question of differential effect according to parent of origin remains open (Bortotto et al., 1990). We list below some ''duplications'' and ''deletions'' that appear to be, in fact, nonpathogenic variants.

Additional Band ("Duplication")

Chromosome 1p21–p31
Zaslav et al. (1993) describe a 1p+ chromosome in a normal mother and daughter with additional presumed euchromatic material in 1p21–p31.

Chromosome 1q42.11–q42.12
Bortotto et al. (1990) describe a chromosome with additional presumed euchromatic material in 1q42.11–q42.12 in a normal mother and son.

Chromosome 9p13
This variant appears to have an extra dark G-band inserted into 9p13. The extra material may be C-band positive or negative (Figure 15–6).

Chromosome 9qh
A variant of chromosome 9 involves a G-band within the C-band heterochromatin (Hoo et al., 1993; Fernández et al., 1994; Conte et al., 1995). Macera et

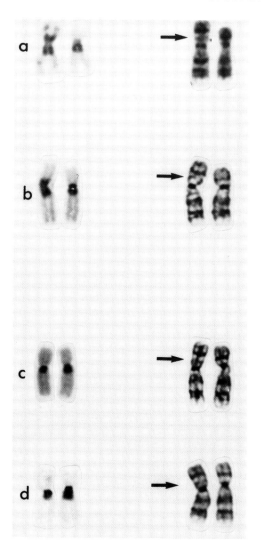

FIGURE 15–6. C-banded and G-banded chromosome pair No. 9 from (*a*) a patient and (*b*) her normal mother, showing an extra dark G-band (arrow) inserted into the middle of band 9p13; (*c*) another patient and (*d*) one of her normal relatives with the same extra G-band (arrow), which in this case is C-band negative. The variant is the left of each pair. (Reproduced from Sutherland and Eyre, 1981, with the permission of Munksgaard, Copenhagen.)

al. (1995) review this heteromorphism and propose that four different types exist, according to the mechanism of formation and the relative positions of the heterochromatin and euchromatin. They suggest that the euchromatic material, potentially containing transcribable genes, is "heterochromatinized" and thus inactivated by virtue of being sandwiched between segments of 9qh.

Chromosome 9q13–q21

Jalal et al. (1990a) reported extra G-band-positive, C-band-negative material in 9q13–q21 in a normal woman. A similar variant was recorded by L. A. Knight et al. (1993) in a normal mother and child.

Chromosome 15q12–q13

Stallard and Van Dyke (1986), Ludowese et al. (1991), and Jalal et al. (1994) report individuals with apparent insertional duplication of 15q12–q13 without any consistent phenotypic effects. The duplicated segment does not include the Prader-Willi/Angelman critical region. This variant may confuse the interpretation of the presence or absence of a Prader-Willi or Angelman deletion (Hoo et al., 1990; Delach et al., 1994). One case of a de novo duplication involving the q11–q13 region presumably *was* the cause of the phenotypic abnormality in the presenting child, and represents a different cytogenetic entity (Clayton-Smith et al., 1993).

Chromosome 16p11.2

There have been a number of reports of a variant of chromosome 16 in which there is an extra G-band-positive, C-band-negative band inserted into 16p11.2 (Thompson and Roberts, 1987; Jalal et al., 1990b; Bogart et al., 1991; Croci et al., 1991; Hasegawa et al., 1992).

Absent Band ("Deletion")

Chromosome 5p14.1→p14.3

Deletions in 5p14.1→p14.3 are apparently harmless (Overhauser et al., 1986, 1994).

Chromosome 11p12

Barber et al. (1991) identified a deletion of band 11p12 at prenatal diagnosis, formally described as del(11)(pter→p13::p1200 *or* p11.2→qter). The normal mother and older child had the same deletion, and its presence was duly confirmed on a blood sample from the normal newborn infant.

Chromosome 11q14.3

We have seen a family in which four normal relatives (grandfather, father, two siblings) of the index case, a child with developmental delay and del(11)(q14.3q14.3), also had the 11q14.3 deletion (pers. comm. S. M. White).

Chromosome 13q21

Couturier et al. (1985) document a del(13)(q21) associated with a normal phenotype, ascertained through miscarriage.

Chromosome 16q21

Witt et al. (1988) identified a chromosome 16 deleted for band q21 in three "entirely normal" members of a three generation family, and Callen et al. (1993) studied the deletion at the molecular level.

SIGNIFICANCE

No significance of variant chromosomes at the level of either cell biology or clinical phenotype is known.

C-band Size

Many studies have purported to show that variant chromosomes involving C-band size and position are associated with congenital malformations, malignant disease, habitual abortion, and infertility. There have equally been many studies that report no such association. Carothers et al. (1982) conclude that "reproductive fitness of carriers of heterochromatic variants of the human karyotype is normal," and that is the view we espouse unless and until persuasive documentation to the contrary is adduced. In the specific case of the inv(9) variants, no increased reproductive risk exists that we can usefully measure or relay to people in whom one is discovered. As for the NOR variants, Hassold et al. (1987) could demonstrate no association with an increased risk for trisomic conception, a possibility that had previously been postulated.

Acrocentric Chromosome Short Arm Morphology

An increased risk to have a child with Down syndrome had previously been proposed for the person with a "double NOR" on an acrocentric chromosome. This was a not unreasonable postulate, given the in vitro cytogenetic observation of "satellite association" and imagining that a similar phenomenon could happen in vivo in meiosis and predispose to aberrant segregation, and that this might be more likely with larger satellites. But the actual observation is, in fact, of no such increased risk (Serra and Bova, 1990).

Fragile Sites

Fragile sites are harmless (except, of course, fragile XA and fragile XE, and, possibly, FRA11B). The fragile sites of rare and intermediate frequency have been described variously as being associated with congenital malformations, sporadic chromosome abnormalities, and a predisposition to malignant disease. But there is no convincing evidence of any of these associations existing other than by chance (Sutherland, 1988). The only note of caution here is that the fragile sites known as the autosomal folate-sensitive group (Table 15–1) have been seen only in heterozygotes. It has yet to be shown that homozygosity for one of these sites is associated with phenotypic normality. Homozygotes for three of the rare folate-insensitive fragile sites (10q25, 16q22, and 17p12) are normal.

MEIOSIS

Variant chromosomes, being normal chromosomes, behave normally at meiosis; and other things being equal, 1:1 segregation occurs. Hence any individual with

Table 15—1 The three groups of rare variant autosomal fragile sites

Folate-sensitive		
1p21.3	7p11.2	11q23.3
2q11.2	8q22.3	12q13.1
2q13	9p21.1	12q24.13
2q22.3	9q32	16p13.11
5q35	10q23.3	19p13
6p23	11q13.3	20p11.23
		22q13
BrdU-inducible		
10q25[a]	12q24.2	
Distamycin A-inducible		
8q24.1[b]	16p12.1[b]	17p12
11p15.1[b]	16q22.1[a]	

[a]Of intermediate frequency.

[b]Recorded in Japanese populations only.

Source: From Sutherland (1993).

a variant chromosome transmits it to, on average, half of his or her offspring. An exception is the autosomal folate-sensitive fragile sites. Unexpectedly, when these are transmitted by a male, only one-quarter of the offspring appear to have them (Sherman and Sutherland, 1986). This may be an effect of unstable DNA sequences, which are amplifications of CCG trinucleotide repeats, and of which these fragile sites are comprised (Nancarrow et al., 1994).

GENETIC COUNSELING

A person carrying a normal variant chromosome has no identified increased risk for having abnormal offspring, abortion, or any other reproductive problem. Some see it as at best pointless and at worst counterproductive even to mention to the individual that a variant chromosome has been found; others feel obliged to pass on the observation. If it is discussed, it must be made clear that it is a normal finding: perhaps interesting, but of no practical importance. There is considerable potential for iatrogenic anxiety, whereas in reality the biology of the supposed "anomaly" has no pathogenetic implication. The counselor may thoroughly understand the presumed harmlessness of a variant chromosome, but the person in whose family it has been discovered may react "non-scientifically". To put a stark setting, the worst possible response might be for a couple to choose to terminate a pregnancy because of an over-interpreted variant chromosome. "Primum non nocere": first do no harm.

For the size variants (C-band and NOR), the point can simply be made that some chromosomes come in short, medium, and long forms, and where a chromosome happens to fit in this continuum is without significance. Some clients may be intrigued to learn that they are of interest to genetic researchers. Likewise, the presence or absence of a variant fragile site is unimportant in terms of reproductive abnormality. There is no apparent relation between fragile sites and mental retardation (Fryns and Petit, 1987). The fact that homozygosity for some nonfolate-sensitive fragile sites (10q25, 16q22, 17p12) is on record and that the individuals studied had no consistent phenotypic abnormality offers further reassurance of the fundamental biological harmlessness of these morphologic curiosities.

Only one tentative exception exists. FRA11B carriers may have a "low" risk to have a child with a de novo deletion of 11q (Jacobsen syndrome). Until this issue is clarified, it may be prudent to offer prenatal diagnosis.

From time to time, children with delayed neurodevelopmental progress with or without minor dysmorphic features are identified as having a subtle deletion or duplication; and in most, of course, the karyotypic abnormality will have been the cause of the phenotypic defect. Occasionally, parental studies will come up with the surprising result that one parent has the same karyotype; and a reinterpretation of "harmless variant" may be made. The counselor will need to make sure that this reinterpretation is well understood and that the label of "chromosome abnormality" does not attach to the child and stifle other clinical investigation.

It is necessary to emphasise (and see Chapter 3) the confusion and misinterpretation that can be due to ascertainment bias. Practically by definition, a child having a chromosome test has to be abnormal; and therefore it follows that a variant chromosome newly discovered in this context is associated with phenotypic defect. Association, however, does not necessarily mean there is a causal link; and if a parent or other relative has the same unusual chromosome it should be seen as being harmless unless otherwise proven, notwithstanding various esoteric scenarios that any imaginative geneticist could devise. One author should, in honesty, acknowledge an early paper which exemplifies this type of error: in this case, an overinterpretation of the clinical relevance of the 1qh variant (Gardner et al., 1974).

Malignant Disease

Persons who have variant fragile sites (we all have the common fragile sites) may be advised, if the question is raised, that there is no evidence that they are at increased risk for developing any malignant disease, notwithstanding suggestions to the contrary. These suggestions have arisen from observations of an apparent correlation between the location of fragile sites and the chromosome bands within which the characteristic breakpoints of some tumor chromosomal rearrangements occur (Hecht and Sutherland, 1984; LeBeau and Rowley, 1984; Yunis and Soreng, 1984). The case for such a correlation is now largely refuted (Simmers et al., 1987; Sutherland and Simmers, 1988; Sutherland, 1988). Families in which rare fragile sites are segregating have no discernible increase in malignant disease.

NORMAL PARENTS WITH A CHROMOSOMALLY ABNORMAL CHILD

16

Down Syndrome, Other Full Aneuploidies, and Polyploidy

In this chapter we consider the case of parents, themselves karyotypically normal, who have had a child, or a pregnancy that aborted, with a full aneuploidy or a polyploidy. Thus, we include the major trisomies (21, 13, 18) and sex chromosome aneuploidies (XXX, XXY, XYY, and 45,X) as well as less commonly seen autosomal aneuploidies and sex chromosome polysomies. The category of polyploidy is substantially devoted to triploidy. In the great majority, these defects arose from an abnormal event during meiosis or (in some triploidy) at conception. In a few, there is a postzygotic generation of aneuploidy. Only in the case of parental gonadal mosaicism, or in the hypothetical setting of an apparent predisposition to nondisjunction, will an increased risk of recurrence apply.

BIOLOGY

Full aneuploidy is presumed in the great majority to be the result of meiotic nondisjunction (p. 26). In practically all cases, nondisjunction occurs at random, with no recognizable individual predisposition. Nondisjunction can happen at any maternal age, but it is more frequent in older mothers (p. 325). (It is moot whether the remarkable case in FitzPatrick and Boyd [1989] reflects simply a maternal age effect in successive pregnancies, or some theoretical constitutional "meiotic weakness": at ages 40, 40, and 43, a woman had pregnancies with trisomy 21, 13, and 18.) Alternatively, an abnormality has arisen in a premeiotic gametocyte, with the parent thus having a "wedge" of gonad that carries the abnormality ("gonadal mosaicism"). Such a parent would, of course, have an increased risk for only the one karyotypic defect. Finally, a small fraction of apparent full aneuploidy may be due to early mitotic nondisjunction in a 46,N conceptus with loss (or restriction to extra-embryonic tissue) of the normal cell line.

Trisomy 21 (Down Syndrome)

Down syndrome is the archetypal chromosome disorder. It was the first medical condition shown to result from a chromosome abnormality. It has for many years been recognized as the most common single known cause of mental retardation and has the highest incidence at birth of any chromosome abnormality. Every counselor can expect to deal frequently with problems relating to Down syndrome and should be familiar with its genetics.

The Down syndrome phenotype—the characteristic facial appearance, body build, and mental defect—is due, in sum, to a triple amount of chromosome 21. It is, in a sense, a "contiguous gene syndrome", but one in which there is an additional dose, rather than a haplo-insufficiency, of an en bloc set of genes. Epstein (1993a,b) reviews what is known of neuronal differentiation, migration, metabolism and physiology that, in sum, cause the "blighted mind" of the individual with Down syndrome, and discusses the principle of gene dosage effects "as the starting point for any potential mechanism" to bring about the phenotype. The catalog of genes coded on chromosome 21 being assembled by several workers will be an entrée to this starting point (Peterson et al., 1994; Chen et al., 1995; Yaspo et al., 1995; Lucente et al., 1995). Certain regions of the chromosome contribute to certain aspects of the phenotype, with the region 21q22.13–22.2 having a predominant influence (Figure 16–1) (Korenberg et al., 1990; Delabar et al., 1993), while regions of low gene content, such as 21q21, may have little effect (Xu et al., 1995). Any gene on 21q influencing neuronal development, such as, for example, the cell membrane potassium channel *GIRK2* which is located in 21q21.1–22.31 (Patil et al., 1995), is a candidate for causing mental defect due to a possible suboptimal function in the triplicated state. Mouse models may cast light (Sweeney et al., 1989; Reeves et al., 1995; Maroun, 1995). Triplication is usually due to the presence of an extra chromosome 21 in all or most cells: in other words, standard trisomy 21 (Figure 16–2). The disorder has a number of other cytogenetic forms. Differences in the source and nature of the genetic errors underlying these various forms require each to be considered separately.

Standard Trisomy 21 Down Syndrome

The great majority (about 95%) of Down syndrome is due to simple trisomy of chromosome 21, and 90 to 95% of these cases reflect a maternal meiotic error. Three-quarters of these maternal errors occur at meiosis I, and one-quarter at meiosis II. Among the small fraction (3–5%) due to paternal errors the ratio is reversed: about one-quarter are from meiosis I and three-quarters are from meiosis II. The remainder reflect a mitotic nondisjunction; notably, these may occur both premeiotically in the germline, or postzygotically (Antonarakis et al., 1992,

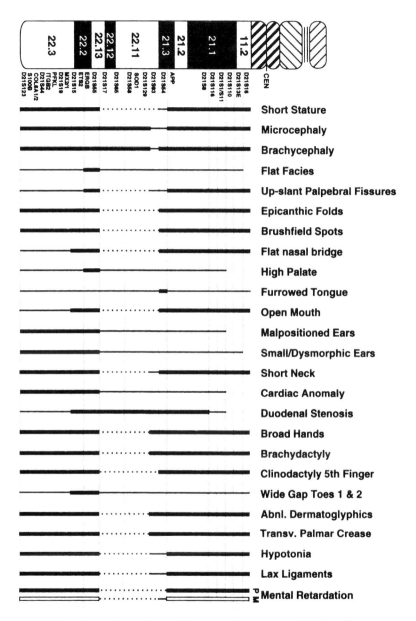

FIGURE 16–1. Phenotypic (trisomic) map of chromosome 21. Thick lines represent regions that must be trisomic to produce the particular trait. Thin-line regions may also contribute to that trait; the contribution of dotted-line regions is less clear. P = profound, M = mild. (From Korenberg et al., 1994, courtesy J. R. Korenberg and with the permission of the National Academy of Sciences of the U. S. A.)

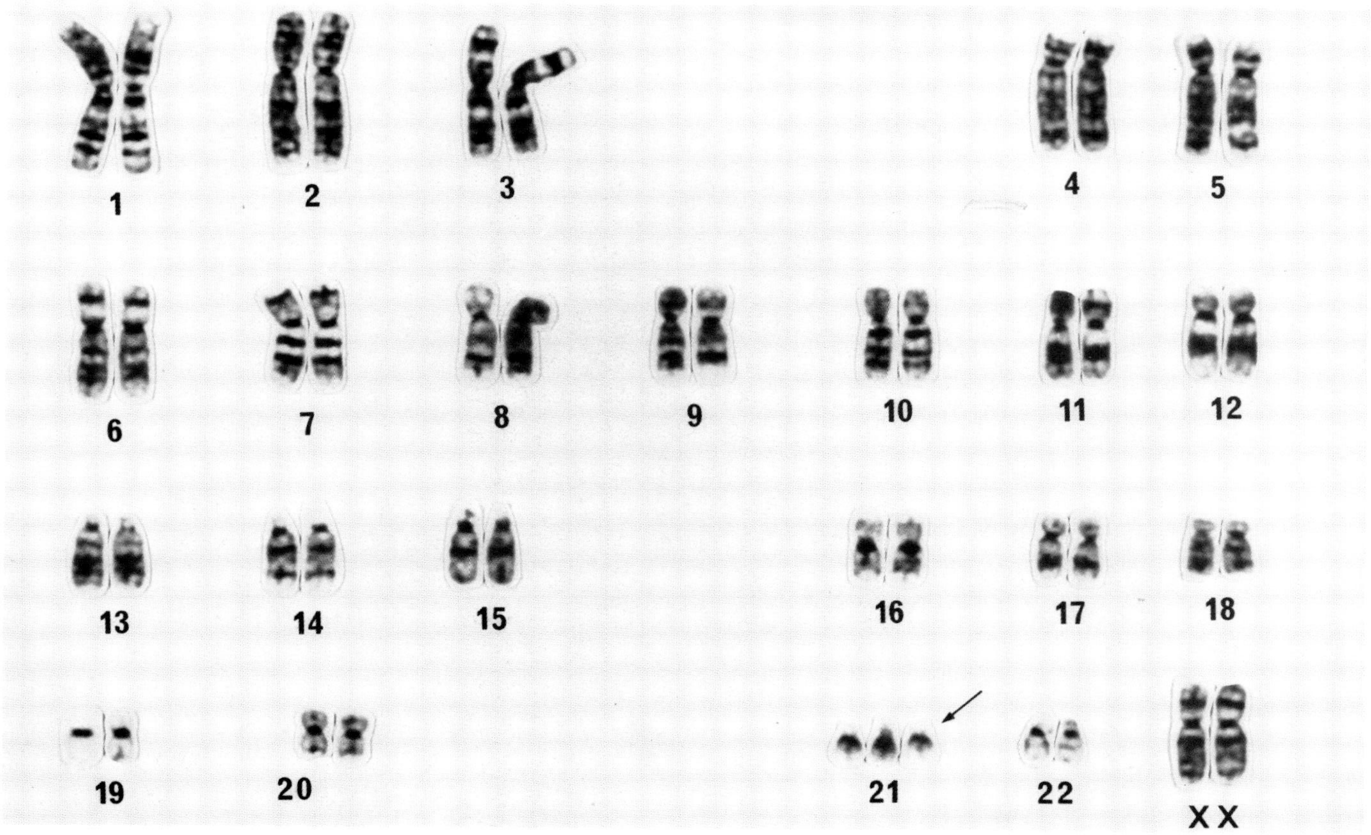

FIGURE 16–2. Karyotype of a child with standard trisomy 21.

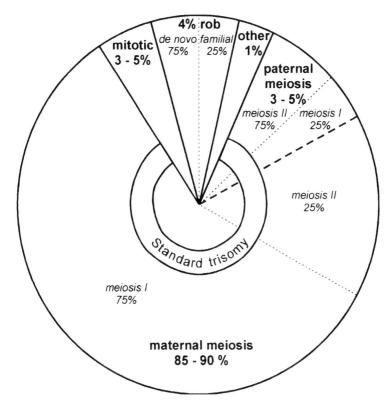

FIGURE 16–3. Origins of trisomy 21 (percentages rounded).

1993a; Sensi and Ricci, 1993; Sherman et al., 1994). Figure 16–3 depicts these proportions graphically. An excess of male Down syndrome individuals has been associated with paternal errors, for reasons that are quite unclear (Petersen et al., 1993). Standard trisomy 21 characteristically occurs as a sporadic event. Only infrequently is more than one sibling affected, and reports of a sibling with some other aneuploidy are likewise infrequent.

What might cause a recurrence of trisomy 21? A trisomy 21 cell population in a parent (gonadal or somatic–gonadal mosaicism) is presumed to be an uncommon cause of the production of disomic 21 gametes, although perhaps less rare than originally thought (Warburton et al., 1987; Sachs et al., 1990; Antonarakis et al., 1993a). A unique example is that of Nielsen et al. (1988), who report a couple having had six documented pregnancies with standard trisomy 21 and five other unkaryotyped pregnancies ending in neonatal death or in abortion. The mother typed 46,N on peripheral blood and 47,+21/46,N in ovarian somatic cells. Even if the actual oocytes were all or nearly all 47,+21 it remains perplexing that no known 46,N conception occurred. Do some individuals, for some biological reason, run an increased risk of producing or carrying a trisomic 21 conception? Pangalos et al. (1992b) addressed this question in a study of 22 families in which trisomy 21 had recurred (in siblings, in second- and in third-degree relatives), applying the tool of DNA polymorphism analysis. Parental gonadal mosaicism was the cause of sibling recurrence in 5 of 13 families (about 40%), but other than this, chance alone was enough to explain the recurrences in most if not all families. Rare families with recurrence of standard trisomy 21 may reflect a genetic predisposition (Mikkelsen, 1966); a chance aggregation remains possible. Sachs et al. (1990) followed 1211 pregnancies at prenatal diagnosis, subsequent to the occurrence of trisomy 21, and observed six recurrences (0.5%). In two of these recurrences, one father karyotyped as 46,N/ 47,+21 on skin analysis only, and one mother showed trisomic cells in 3%, 14%, 44%, and 47% on culture of blood, skin, and each ovary, respectively. Two somatic-gonadal mosaics identified out of 1211 couples—0.08% of 2422 persons—can scarcely justify routine parental karyotyping. We conclude that there is no practicable basis enabling the counselor to identify, ahead of time, those parents whose risk is high, and those whose risk is low, to have a second pregnancy with trisomy 21. The concept of gonadal mosaicism, while a very real one at the level of the biology of recurrence, can be rather academic in day-to-day clinical practice, and we discuss this matter more expansively in Chapter 2.

Estimates of the risk of recurrence are based on empirical data. Warburton et al. (1987) reanalyzed the data of Ferguson-Smith (1983) and Stene et al. (1984), taken from prenatal diagnostic results from the European Collaborative Study of Amniocentesis, and other data, focusing on the age of the mother at the time of birth of her Down syndrome child, the karyotypic outcome of a succeeding pregnancy at amniocentesis, and her age at that pregnancy. They conclude that there are two risk classes: younger (below 30 years) and older mothers. For younger mothers who have had one Down syndrome child, the risk for recurrence at amniocentesis is around 0.8%, with a total risk of a little over 1% when other trisomies are included. Given a 15% natural loss of trisomy 21 fetuses after this stage of pregnancy (Halliday et al., 1995b), the 0.8% figure would reduce to a 0.7% risk to have a liveborn. For mothers who had their Down syndrome child when they were over 30, the overall risk is not discernibly different from the age-specific occurrence figure (see Table 21–1). Subsequent prenatal diagnostic data have given figures which are marginally less but substantially corroborative. Sachs et al. (1990) (see above) in Rotterdam noted 6 recurrences in 1211 pregnancies (3/221 CVS, 3/990 amniocenteses, maternal ages not noted), and J. L. Halliday (pers. comm., 1995) in Melbourne noted 2 in 440 (1/212 CVS, 1/228 amniocenteses, maternal age less than 37), giving an overall recurrence rate for standard trisomy 21 of 0.5%.

A possible link between Down syndrome and Alzheimer disease has been suggested, but it remains unsubstantiated (Katzman and Kawas, 1994). An onset of dementia in middle adult life, over and above the congenital mental defect, is a common observation in Down syndrome, and one Alzheimer susceptibility locus, the β-amyloid precursor protein gene, has its locus on chromosome 21 and may be overexpressed in both conditions (B. T. Lamb et al., 1993). Potter (1991) suggests a tendency to chromosome 21 nondisjunction (mitotic in brain, meiotic in gonad) could be a unitary explanation, and Schupf et al. (1994) propose that "accelerated ageing'' may explain meiotic nondisjunction in some younger (35 years or under) mothers and an increased risk to these women in later life to develop Alzheimer disease. It would be premature to propose that a family history of Alzheimer disease should imply a greater risk to have a Down syndrome child that can usefully be acted upon, and probably damaging to speak of a future risk for Alzheimer disease in the ''younger mother'' of a Down syndrome child, but it does behove the counselor to keep abreast of knowledge and opinion in this controversial area.

When a couple has had two trisomic 21 conceptions, one has to assume an increased risk applies to a subsequent pregnancy. The recurrence may most likely have been due to gonadal mosaicism; a particular parental factor predisposing to nondisjunctional meioses, or simply two chance events, are other possibilities.

Mosaic Down Syndrome

Of individuals with clinical Down syndrome, 47,+21/46,N mosaicism accounts for 2 to 3%. Mosaicism results from a nondisjunction or from an anaphase lag occurring postzygotically. Some individuals with mosaic Down syndrome arise from initially trisomic 21 zygotes, losing a No. 21 at anaphase lag (Figure 2–8c). Others may arise from normal conceptuses, with nondisjunction producing 45,−21/46,N/47,+21 and the 45,−21 line then lost (Figure 2–8a). Whatever the basis, counseling needs to proceed as though the child has standard trisomy 21, recognizing that this will overestimate the risk in some. Genetic counseling for the mosaic individuals themselves is covered on p. 207.

> Pangalos et al. (1994) studied 17 families in which there was a child with mosaic trisomy 21, and 10 children had three No. 21 alleles, indicating their origin from a trisomic conceptus. The No. 21 chromosome subsequently lost to enable formation of the 46,N cell line showed no predilection for being a maternal or paternal homolog. The remaining 7 mosaics had no evidence of a ''third allele,'' and distinction in these between an initially 46,N or 47,+21 conception is not possible.

Isochromosome 21 Down Syndrome

After standard trisomy 21, this is the most common chromosomal category of Down syndrome. It has often been called a 21q21q Robertsonian translocation, but in fact the two 21q components are usually identical and thus isochromosome is the more accurate term, and the karyotype is more accurately 46,i(21)(q10) (Antonarakis et al., 1990; Shaffer et al., 1992). Molecular studies suggest that many of these originate at an early postzygotic mitosis, and this is consistent with the observation that recurrence risk is low. In one series of 112 de novo ''rob(21q21q)'' probands, none of 130 full- and 34 half sibs had Down syndrome (Steinberg et al., 1984). Nevertheless, three of the parents showed a low-grade mosaicism, and presumably their having had an affected child reflected that the 21q21q cell line included the gonad. A small number of recurrences in subsequently born siblings are otherwise recorded (Steinberg et al., 1984; Sachs et al., 1990), and parental gonadal mosaicism can be the basis of such recurrence (Robinson et al., 1994), a point Mark et al. (1977) directly proved in one case: a woman having sequential pregnancies with the karyotype 46,i(21q) herself typed 46,XX,i(21q)/46,XX on ovarian fibroblast analysis (but 46,XX on blood).

Robertsonian Translocation Down Syndrome

Almost all translocation Down syndrome concerns a Robertsonian translocation. Although we discuss this type of translocation in detail in Chapter 6, we review aspects pertinent to translocation Down syndrome here. The Robertsonian translocation may have arisen as a sporadic event (de novo translocation) or may have been transmitted by a carrier parent (familial translocation). One-quarter of Robertsonian translocation Down syndrome is familial and three-quarters is de novo (1 and 3% of all Down syndrome, respectively).

De Novo Robertsonian Translocation Down Syndrome

Both the parents, by definition, have normal chromosomes. The abnormal chromosome may usually arise as a sporadic event in maternal meiosis I, from a chromatid translocation (Petersen et al., 1991). Such mutational events are rare and, in the great majority of families, recurrences are not seen. But gonadal mosaicism remains a possibility. An unique family is described in an erratum (Migeon, 1966) in which there were three translocation Down syndrome sibs, but with two different types of Robertsonian translocation. The so-called rob(21q21q) is, in most cases at least, actually an isochromosome (see above).

Familial Robertsonian Translocation Down Syndrome

One or the other parent (almost always the mother) is a translocation heterozygote and has transmitted the translocation, in an unbalanced state, to the offspring.

Down Syndrome with Reciprocal Translocation

The Down syndrome phenotype is substantially due, as we note above, to a duplication of the chromosome segment 21q22.13–q22.2. A reciprocal translocation involving No. 21, and according to the other participating chromosome and its breakpoint, has the potential to produce, in a gamete from the heterozygote, a duplication for the Down syndrome critical region, whether from 2:2 or 3:1 meiotic segregation. One unbalanced karyotype from the rcp(18q;21q) illustrated in Figure 4–14 is an example, and Scott et al. (1995) describe a child with Down syndrome from a maternal t(12;21)(p13.1;q22.2) that could only be identified with FISH. This is, however, an extraordinarily rare mechanism, the cause of less than 0.1% of Down syndrome.

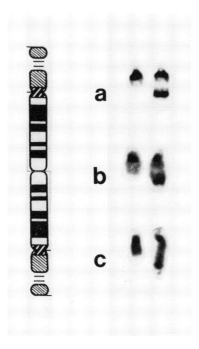

FIGURE 16–4.   The No. 21 chromosomes from three cells (a, b, c) of a patient with the terminal arrangement form of Down syndrome. The rearranged chromosome (*right* of each pair) forms an apparent mirror image of the normal No. 21 (*left*). The ideogram depicts the rearrangement, which at the molecular level may be asymmetrical.

Other Chromosomal Forms of Down Syndrome

A number of chromosomally distinct forms of Down syndrome result from specific structural changes to chromosome 21. The least rare of these is the terminal rearrangement (Figure 16–4) that produces a mirror-image chromosome around the telomeric region (Pfeiffer and Loidl, 1982). The chromosome has two centromeres, one of which is usually inactive, and satellites on both ends. Such chromosomes are always the result of sporadic mutational events, possibly the result of a translocation between sister chromatids (Pangalos et al., 1992a). Down syndrome is seen occasionally in association with other aneuploidies such as 48,XYY,+21; this is known as double aneuploidy. It is the result of either a double event of nondisjunction resulting in one abnormal gamete, or, less likely, separate events in gametogenesis in both parents.

"Interchromosomal effect" has been invoked in standard trisomy Down syndrome in the setting of a parental abnormality not involving chromosome 21 (e.g., a 13;14 Robertsonian translocation); in other words, the rob(13;14) translocation in some way perturbed the distribution of the No. 21s (Couzin et al., 1986). Uchida and Freeman (1986) and Schinzel et al. (1992) have studied

families in which a child with trisomy 21 also had a balanced translocation or inversion, and while in several the translocation or inversion was of paternal origin, the extra chromosome 21 came from the mother. There is no evidence at least for a paternal interchromosomal effect!

Trisomies 18 and 13 (Edwards Syndrome and Patau Syndrome)

These trisomies are much less frequent than Down syndrome (about 1 in 6000 and 1 in 12,000 livebirths, respectively), and both show a maternal age effect. As with trisomy 21, a beginning has been made in the correlative phenotypic mapping of certain segments of chromosomes 18 and 13 (Epstein, 1993b; Boghosian-Sell et al., 1994). In trisomy 18, over 90% reflect a maternal meiotic nondisjunction, which is twice as likely to have been at the second meiotic division; the remainder include cases of postzygotic mitotic errors (Fisher et al., 1995). Recurrence of trisomy 18 has been recorded in single case reports (Pauli et al., 1978). Ferguson-Smith (1983) and Stene et al. (1984) found no recurrences following 99 index pregnancies with trisomy 13, and following 171 cases of trisomy 18, there was one recurrence—and one pregnancy with 46,inv(18). J. L. Halliday (pers. comm., 1995) reviewed data on 148 prenatal diagnoses done in Melbourne from 1986 to 1993 on the grounds of previous trisomy 18 or trisomy 13; there were no recurrences of either trisomy. One case each of 47,XXY and 47,+20/46,N were probably coincidental.

XXY (Klinefelter Syndrome), XXX, XYY

These aneuploidies occur at roughly similar frequencies, about 1 per 1000 of the appropriate sex. About 90% of XXX and about 50% of XXY are due to maternal meiotic errors, and in three-quarters of each of these it is the first meiotic (MI) division that is involved, this MI group showing a maternal age effect. It is noteworthy that almost half of XXY results from a paternal MI error (MacDonald et al., 1994). Manifestly, XYY of meiotic origin must be due to a paternal error, at MII. All three sex chromosomes aneuploidies can have a postzygotic mitotic generation.

45,X Turner Syndrome

In the majority (80%) it is the paternal X chromosome which is absent (Hassold et al., 1991a). The loss may have occurred postzygotically. Kher et al. (1994) reported a unique family with occurrence of 45,X/46,XX in sisters, and in their literature review could find only one instance of 45,X recurrence in sisters. J. L. Halliday (pers. comm., 1995) records 52 prenatal diagnoses done on the basis of previous 45,X: there were no recurrences. (One instance of 47,XXY may have been coincidental.)

Rare Sex Chromosome Polysomies

Polysomies such as XXXX, XXYY, XYYY, XXXY, XXXXX, and XXXXY are very rare. Successive nondisjunctions in one parent, the other contributing a single sex chromosome, is the mechanism in most if not all (Hassold et al., 1990; Deng et al., 1991). Apart from the extraordinary circumstance of (hypothetically) a familial tendency to mosaicism (Bergemann, 1962; Kher et al., 1994), these polysomies arise sporadically. Rare reports of coincidence with some other aneuploidy (Court Brown et al., 1969) may more likely reflect chance than a causal link.

Polyploidy

Triploidy

The chromosome count in triploidy is $3n = 69$, with a double ($2n$) chromosomal contribution to the conceptus from one parent (Figure 16–5). Triploidy can reflect diandry or digyny, with the double contribution coming from the father or mother, respectively. *Diandry* is the consequence of either two sperm simultaneously fertilizing the ovum (dispermy) or of a diploid sperm from a complete nondisjunction in spermatogenesis. *Digyny* may be due to a complete nondisjunction at either the first or the second meiotic division in oögenesis, to retention of a polar body, or to the fertilization of an ovulated primary oocyte. A first meiotic error could be proven in one case of triploidy associated with a maternal translocation (Rochon and Vekemans, 1990).

Triploidy is not uncommon in early pregnancy (1–3% of recognized pregnancies) but almost all (more than 99%) are lost as first trimester miscarriage or second trimester fetal death in utero. The very few diandric triploids that survive to the second trimester show the classic placental phenotype of partial hydatidiform mole (see p. 318) and the fetuses are microcephalic and of relatively normal size. Digynic triploids are more likely to make it to the second trimester, and they develop as a severely growth-retarded fetus with marked head–body disproportion, the head being relatively large, and an abnormally small and nonmolar placenta (McFadden et al., 1993; Miny et al., 1995; Dietzsch et al., 1995). Intrauterine survival may be promoted if there is fetal–placental karyotypic discordance, with the placenta being diploid (Kennerknecht et al., 1993). Exceptional survival to the third trimester is associated with perinatal death (the 5-month survival of one triploid infant being quite extraordinary; Cassidy et al., 1977).

Diploid/Triploid Mosaicism

An initially triploid zygote may "self-correct" by extrusion of a surplus pronucleus at the first mitosis, but then reincorporate it at a subsequent cell division (McFadden et al., 1993). The affected fetus may survive in utero, due to the moderating effect of the diploid cell line (Carakushansky et al., 1994). In most

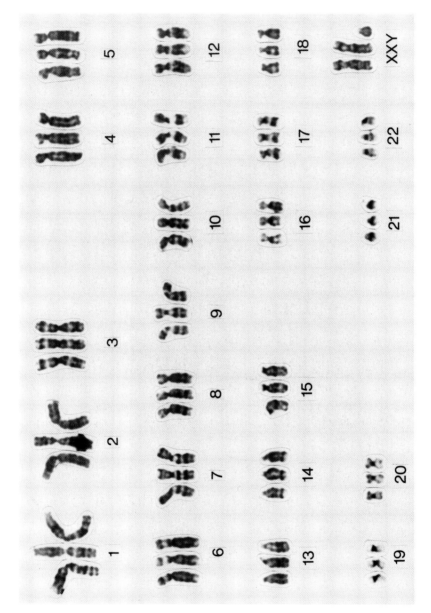

FIGURE 16–5. Karyotype of a 69,XXY triploid fetus (see also Figure 20–4, p. 316).

cases the triploid line is not seen on a blood analysis, and fibroblast culture is necessary. As in some other mosaic states, an irregular pigmentary pattern is characteristic.

Tetraploidy

Tetraploidy ($4n = 92$) in term pregnancy is exceedingly rare. It can occasionally be seen at chorionic villus sampling (CVS) and amniocentesis, in which case it is generally assumed to be artifactual; alternatively, it may reflect a normal tetraploidy of trophoectoderm (Benkhalifa et al., 1993), this being a lineage that contributes to the extra-embryonic tissue obtained at CVS. The usual mechanism for pure tetraploidy may be a normal division of chromosomes but failure of cytoplasmic cleavage at the first division of the zygote; mosaic forms may reflect a similar mechanism at a later mitosis. In one unique case, the mother had tetraploid cells in 6/103 leukocytes and 4/51 skin fibroblasts (Scarbrough et al., 1984). Mosaicism for a 2n and a 4n line has been described in association with severe mental defect, and may only be detectable on skin fibroblast study (Edwards et al., 1994). Sheppard et al. (1982) reported a 92,XXXX spontaneous abortion resembling a hydatidiform mole which may have been due to a trispermic conception.

GENETIC COUNSELING

Down Syndrome

The central requirement for accurate genetic advice in Down syndrome is a knowledge of the chromosomal form in the affected family member. If a child diagnosed as having Down syndrome has died and no chromosome studies were performed, the parents' or the counselee's chromosomes should be checked to exclude the possibility of a familial translocation.

Previous Child with Standard Trisomy 21 (Including Mosaicism)

If the child has standard trisomy 21, or is a 47,+21/46 mosaic, it is unnecessary routinely to study the parents' chromosomes. One can assume, with considerable confidence, that they would type as 46,XX and 46,XY. The questions parents are likely to have include the following:

1. What is the risk for recurrence of Down syndrome in a liveborn child?
2. What is the risk for detection of trisomy 21 at prenatal diagnosis in a subsequent pregnancy?
3. Is there an increased risk for any other type of chromosomal abnormality in a subsequent pregnancy?

Following the material discussed in the Biology section above, the answers are as follows.

1. For a mother under 30 years old at the birth of the Down syndrome child, the risk for recurrence of Down syndrome in a liveborn child is about 0.7% (1 in 150). A woman in her 30s and 40s runs, for practical purposes, the same risk as any other woman of her age (see Table 21–1, p. 327). The cutoff at maternal age 30 is, of course, somewhat arbitrary, but nonetheless reasonable in practice.
2. The likelihood of trisomy 21 being detected at amniocentesis in a mother under 30 is about 0.8% (1 in 130); the mother over 30 has only her age-specific risk (Table 21–2, p. 330).
3. The mother under 30 has an overall risk for chromosomal abnormality including +21 at amniocentesis of marginally above 1%, and marginally less than 1% risk of having a liveborn aneuploid. The mother over 30 has the same risk as her age-specific risk (see Table 21–5, p. 331).

In any event, regardless of the exact figure, the practical point is that the risk for a recurrence of Down syndrome is comfortingly low. Nevertheless, most couples seek the reassurance of prenatal diagnosis in pregnancies after having had a child with Down syndrome. Elkins et al. (1986b) observe that some of these parents declare they would not abort a trisomic 21 fetus, and the counselor needs to be sensitive to possible ambivalent feelings of the parents in this setting.

Two Previous Trisomic 21 Conceptions

One can only offer an educated guess that the risk for a third +21 conception will be increased. If gonadal mosaicism is the cause, a considerable fraction of whichever gonad it is must be involved, since two separate samplings have come from this fraction. A risk in the range of 10 to 20% may be a fair figure to offer.

Isochromosome 21 Down Syndrome

From the 0/164 fraction among siblings of de novo isochromosome 21q Down syndrome in Steinberg et al.'s (1984) series, the risk for recurrence is presumed to be small. Nevertheless, three parents (3%) in this series were demonstrably mosaic, and there is a handful of recurrences otherwise on record; a cautious stance is prudent. A risk figure of 1% or less is a reasonable one to offer.

Previous Child with Robertsonian Translocation Down Syndrome

Obviously, distinction between de novo and familial forms of translocation Down syndrome is crucial; this distinction is made by chromosomal studies of the parents. For the *de novo* translocation, a recurrence risk figure of <1% is applicable (Gardner and Veale, 1974). In the case of *familial* Robertsonian translocation Down syndrome, the genetic risk, for the female carrier, is substantial. The risk to have a liveborn child with translocation Down syndrome is about 10%, while the likelihood to detect translocation trisomy 21 at amniocentesis is about 15%. For the male carrier, the risk to have a child with translocation Down syndrome is small, about 1% (and see Chapter 6).

Previous Child with Non-Robertsonian Translocation Down Syndrome

In the rare instance that translocation Down syndrome is associated with a familial reciprocal translocation, the principles presented in Chapter 4 are to be followed.

Previous Child with Other Chromosomal Category of Down Syndrome

For sporadic structural changes such as the terminal rearrangements, the risks are very low (less than 0.5%). For the double aneuploidies, the risks are the same as the recurrence risks for standard trisomic Down syndrome. Prenatal diagnosis may be justifiable for the reassurance it provides.

Family History of Down Syndrome

There has been some controversy over whether there is an increased risk to second- and third-degree relatives of individuals with standard trisomic Down syndrome for themselves to have offspring with the condition (Tamaren et al., 1983, 1984; ten Kate et al., 1984; Eunpu et al., 1985). There is no conclusive evidence of such an increased risk (Hook, 1992; Pangalos et al., 1992b). The appropriate action in the setting of ''a family history of Down syndrome'' is to determine whether the family member with Down syndrome has standard trisomy 21. If this is the case, the client may be reassured that there is no discernibly increased risk. Nevertheless, a number seek the conclusive reassurance of prenatal diagnosis. If the karyotype of the index case is unknown, the small possibility of a familial translocation should be checked by chromosome study of the counselee.

Trisomy 21 in Products of Conception

The finding of trisomy 21 in products of conception after spontaneous abortion (in those centers where this may routinely be done) presents a problem. Should this, for genetic counseling risk assessment, be regarded as equivalent to having had a child with Down syndrome? From about 10 weeks' gestation through to term, about a third of trisomic 21 conceptions are lost (p. 328), and it may be stochastic events in utero rather than intrinsic genetic differences that distinguish those that abort and those that survive. It may be prudent to err on the side of caution and provide a risk figure as though the abortion had been a liveborn child (see also p. 319).

Trisomy 13 and Trisomy 18

Recurrence of the same trisomy is virtually unknown. Prenatal diagnosis may be offered for reassurance; if any aneuploidy were to be identified, an X or a No. 21 chromosome may actually be more likely than a No.13 or No. 18. It remains to be shown whether a true increased risk, taking maternal age into account, really exists.

XXX, XXY, XYY, 45,X, Other Sex Chromosome Aneuploidy

Likewise, there is no firm evidence (and indeed little soft evidence) that a recurrence risk above the age-specific figure exists. Prenatal diagnosis is discretionary.

Polyploidy

Triploidy

Diandric triploidy associated with partial hydatidiform mole has a 1 to 1.5% risk of recurrence; we discuss this in more detail on p. 320.

Tetraploidy

True (that is, not artifactual) tetraploidy is too rare for a clear picture to have emerged. A postconceptual origin is probably the rule, and thus sporadic occurrence is expected.

17

Structural Rearrangements and Uniparental Disomy

In this chapter we consider the circumstance of karyotypically normal parents who have had a child with a chromosome defect other than a full aneuploidy. The two major categories are (*1*) structural rearrangement and (*2*) uniparental disomy. Under the heading structural rearrangement, we distinguish deletions (partial monosomy) and duplications (partial trisomy). If the rearrangement occurs during meiosis, or at a postzygotic mitosis, we assume a recurrence risk no different from the general population. These cases arise anew—de novo— with the affected child. If, however, the rearrangement arises at a premeiotic mitosis, the parent would be a gonadal mosaic, and an increased risk for recurrence would apply. Usually, no prior distinction between these two possibilities can be made.

We include rearrangements and uniparental disomy in the same chapter for the pragmatic reason that in three important conditions (Prader-Willi syndrome, Angelman syndrome, and Beckwith syndrome) both mechanisms can be causative. Also, for convenience, we include here other causes of these three syndromes, some of which can be familial.

BIOLOGY

Structural Rearrangement

In no area of medical cytogenetics has FISH and molecular technology had more influence than in the delineation of ''partial aneuploidy'' (Ledbetter, 1992). Duplications involving previously unidentified segments can now be defined. Deletions which were at or beyond the limits of light microscopy now yield to dissection by molecular cytogenetics. Previously unseen translocations come to light. Clinical acumen is, if anything, more important: DNA technologies are not (yet!) suitable for screening of every case of "dysmorphism/developmental delay," and clinical diagnosis is necessary to enable a focused molecular-cytogenetic search.

Mosaicism for a structural rearrangement is rarely detected. It requires the agency of a postzygotic event, and two major scenarios warrant consideration: (*1*) A conceptus is chromosomally normal, and at a subsequent mitosis an abnormality is generated which gives rise to a karyotypically abnormal cell line, along with the 46,N line. The karyotype becomes 46,(abn)/46,N. (*2*) Or, from an initially 47,+(abn) conceptus, a postzygotic "correction" with loss of the abnormal chromosome generates a normal cell line, and so the karyotype becomes 47,+(abn)/46,N.

DELETION

Most of the "new" syndromes joining the ranks of partial aneuploidy are due to deletions. The general karyotypic form of an interstitial deletion, in any chromosome *A*, is 46,del(A)(pter→p00::p00→qter) or 46,del(A)(pter→q00::q00→qter). We have traveled a distance from the earliest days of cytogenetics when the first recorded deletion, large enough to be seen on a solid-stained "B group chromosome," was associated with cri du chat syndrome (Lejeune et al., 1963). We have, now, a spectrum from large deletions ("classical cytogenetic deletion syndromes"), through microdeletions detectable only since the use of high-resolution banding, to deletions beyond the range of banding but detected on combined molecular/cytogenetic (FISH) or purely molecular methodology, and deletions which are so small that only a single locus is removed. Here, we shall consider those deletions in which cytogenetic or molecular cytogenetic techniques are important in demonstrating the defect.

Mechanism of Deletion

Numerous mechanisms to generate a deletion can be envisaged. Similar sequences on the same arm within the same chromatid might attach, with the looped out segment then being removed, to give an interstitial deletion. Asymmetric pairing of homologous chromosomes at meiosis could cause nonmatching segments to be adjacent (Chandley, 1989). In order to restore homologous matching, a mismatched segment may be looped out; this segment may, then, be excised, followed by ligation of the chromatids. Or, if the mismatch remains, and the homologs recombine illegitimately, the recombinant products will be reciprocally imbalanced: one with a deficiency, the other with a duplication, such as Kozma et al. (1991) propose for the 17p11.2 deletion of Smith-Magenis syndrome and the dup(17)(p11.2) syndrome (Figure 17–1). Complementary deletion and duplication products may also arise from sister chromatid exchange. A reciprocal translocation arising during gametogenesis could segregate asymmetrically at meiosis I to give a gamete with a derivative

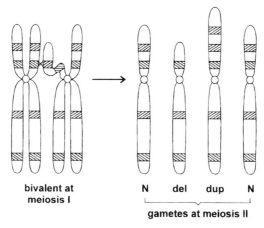

bivalent at   N   del   dup   N
meiosis I
                            gametes at meiosis II

FIGURE 17–1.   One theoretical mechanism to produce a duplication and a deletion. Similar sequences (crosshatched segments) exist at numerous places along the chromosome. Misalignment of two nonhomologous sequences, followed by illegitimate recombination within these two sequences (×), produces recombinant products which are reciprocally imbalanced: one with a duplication of the chromatin between the two sequences (dotted), and the other with a deficiency. The general case is drawn after Chandley (1989). If this were chromosome 17, for example, the dup(17)(p12→p11.2) syndrome and Smith-Magenis syndrome, respectively, could result (Kozma et al., 1991).

deletion/duplication chromosome; Flint et al. (1995) record two possible such examples in "cryptic" rearrangements detected by molecular methodology. Terminal (single breakpoint) deletions, which would lead to loss of the telomere, are apparently rare, although healing with reconstitution of the telomere can occur (J. Lamb et al., 1993; Strathdee et al., 1994). Some regions, such as the Prader-Willi/Angelman segment on chromosome 15, have a propensity to the formation of deletions ("hotspot") (Nicholls, 1993; Christian et al., 1995). We discuss on p. 233 the possibility that a fragile site on 11q may predispose to the genesis of a del(11q) chromosome. An intrinsic predisposition to the production of deletion is illustrated by the male heterozygote for Bloom syndrome (p. 303): his sperm have a high frequency of chromosome breaks (Martin et al., 1994c).

Most de novo deletions are considered to originate at meiosis, and the child is nonmosaic. There are two other possibilities. Firstly, the abnormality may have arisen at a *premeiotic mitosis*, such that the parent is a gonadal mosaic (note that the child would be nonmosaic). Thus, it is usually appropriate to check the parental karyotypes to exclude the possibilities that one may either be a carrier of a balanced rearrangement or a mosaic for the abnormal chromosome (the normal cell line in a phenotypically normal parent being, presumably, predominant). We have referred (p. 42) to the case of an infant with del(18)(q21.3) whose mother had, on a 1000-cell count, 999 cells with 46,XX and one with 46,XX,t(5;18)(p15.3;q21.3); and a few other similar cases are known. Some deletions appear always to be sporadic, and parental karyotyping may be seen as unnecessary. Normal parental karyotypes do not, of course, exclude the possibility of gonadal mosaicism: for example, the two sisters with a chromosome 16 deletion whose parents' karyotypes were normal, described in Hoo et al. (1985). A fuller discussion of gonadal mosaicism is given on p. 42. Secondly, a rearrangement may have arisen at a *postzygotic mitosis*, in which case the child may be a mosaic, generally for a normal and for the abnormal cell line. This category will have no increased risk for recurrence.

A very subtle deletion may submit only to FISH and molecular methodology. Flint et al. (1995) calculate as a tentative figure that about 6% of unexplained mental retardation is due to a very small deletion (in cytogenetic terms) in the gene-rich region subjacent to the telomere: "cryptic subtelomeric monosomy." Such a discovery obliges the search for a very subtle parental translocation. Altherr et al. (1991), for example, describe a child with clinical Wolf-Hirschhorn syndrome with no apparent 4p deletion on standard cytogenetics; but on FISH, not only did the child have a deletion, but the mother carried a balanced translocation. We illustrate a similar case in Figure 22–1.

Contiguous Gene Syndrome

Recollect that loci are arranged in linear order along a chromosome. Often there is no apparent reason for the order: the nonsignificance of the contiguity of two loci has been likened to the unimportance one would attach to Appalachian mountains being next to apple in an encyclopedia. Our genome differs from an encyclopedia in that about a third of all the entries relate to one topic: development of the brain. Many of the other entries (loci) relate to the control of morphogenesis during embryonic life. If a length of chromosome is deleted, a sequence of adjacent (contiguous) genes will be lost. The phenotype resulting from this is a contiguous gene syndrome (Tommerup, 1993). It is very likely that some of the deleted loci will be brain loci, while others could be for anything, but probably including some morphogenesis loci. Thus, we have the classic clinical picture in deletion syndromes of dysmorphism, organ malformation, and intellectual deficit. The deletion produces a monosomy—or "haplo-insufficiency"[1]—for the region of the chromosome that has been removed, and loci in this segment are underexpressed. Some of the loci are beginning to be defined whose haplo-insufficiency contributes to the phenotype in the various deletion syndromes, as noted in individual entries in the Genetic Counseling section, and as illustrated in the particular case of distal 4p haplo-insufficiency in Figure 17–7. A contiguous gene syndrome can be suspected even before a chromosome abnormality has been shown, if two or more rare Mendelian disorders coincide in the one individual. Thus Fryns (1995b) suggests an as yet unseen deletion at 3q22.3-q23 could account for the coexistence of the blepharophimosis/ptosis/epicanthus syndrome and of Langer mesomelic dwarfism in a man with both conditions.

DUPLICATION

Direct and Inverted Intrachromosomal Duplication

The duplication comprises chromatin of the same chromosome and leads to trisomy for the segment concerned. If the linear orientation of a chromosome *A* is maintained, the rearrangement is a *direct duplication*, 46,dir dup(A); if it is reversed, it is an *inverted duplication*, 46,inv dup(A). Possible mechanisms include mismatched pairing of homologs, or of the chromatids of one homolog, which, after recombination or sister chromatid exchange, respectively, can produce countertype duplications and deletions (Van Dyke, 1988); and Hoo et al. (1995) discuss the particular case of the inverted terminal duplication due to U-loop reunion following a two-strand break in a telomeric segment. Compared with other rearrangements, a possibly higher frequency of mosaicism in the dir dup suggests that postzygotic mitosis is the setting in which some arise (Gardner et al., 1994). One particular segment, chromosome 8 short arm, seems particularly prone to inv dup generation, and a concomitant minimal deletion is characteristic (Minelli et al., 1993; Guo et al., 1995). Intrachromosomal triplication, with tetrasomy for the relevant segment, is a variation on the theme (Schinzel et al., 1994b).

Additional Material from Another Chromosome

In other rearrangements, the duplicated material has come from another chromosome. Illegitimate pairing between nonhomologs, followed by crossing-over (presumably within a region of homology), produces reciprocal products which are two derivative chromosomes. In a ''single-segment'' exchange, one of these will have a duplication and the other a deletion. If, then, segregation were asymmetric, gametes with a duplication or with a deficiency would be produced. The karyotype for a duplication in which a segment of, say, chromosome *A* short arm has become attached to the long arm of an essentially intact chromosome *B* has the general form 46,der(B)t(B;A)(q00;p00). J. Zhao et al. (1995) give an example in a child with a ''15p+'' chromosome: molecular and cytomolecular studies showed that the extra segment attaching to 15p came from No. 5 short arm and centromere, so the child's karyotype was actually 46,dic t(5;15)(q11; p11). Other scenarios, with more complex mechanisms, may be imagined. Coles et al. (1992), for example, studied a child with Wolf-Hirschhorn syndrome who had two separate *de novo* rearrangements of the X chromosome with a No. 4 and the Y respectively, and they propose that simultaneous or sequential crossovers happened in a meiotic ''octad'' of four synapsing chromosomes.

Extra Structurally Abnormal Chromosome (ESAC)

Many different ESACs exist, in the general karyotype 47,+ESAC, and they are also known as marker, supernumerary, accessory, and B chromosomes. The

47,+ESAC individual has a duplication (partial trisomy), or in some cases a triplication (partial tetrasomy) of the material comprising the ESAC. The birth prevalence is estimated at 0.14 to 0.72 per 1000. Blennow et al. (1995) record a large Scandinavian experience: of 50 ESACs, almost half were inv dup(15), six were small rings deriving from various autosomes, six were isochromosomes of 18p or 12p, and most of the remainder were harmless ESACs derived from acrocentric chromosomes.

Inverted Duplication 15

One ESAC that warrants special attention is the bisatellited dicentric marker, "inv dup(15)" (Maraschio et al., 1988). These are dicentric chromosomes, sometimes but not necessarily isodicentric. They are also described as dic(15; 15), psu dic(15;15) and iso(15p), but it is less confusing to stick to the most commonly used nomenclature of inv dup (15). They may arise from a U-loop mechanism, as discussed below under Isochromosomes. Webb (1994) divides the inv dup(15) into three groups: (1) very small chromosomes with so little chromatin between the centromeres that the appearance is monocentric; (2) medium-size chromosomes with two distinct centromeres with visible intervening chromatin; and (3) larger chromosomes, greater in size than a G-group chromosome. The very small inv dup(15), in which the additional 15q material is confined to q11, is usually, perhaps always, of no harm per se. The medium- and larger-size chromosomes cause phenotypic defect. Probes for the Prader-Willi/Angelman region in 15q13 are very useful in assessing the amount of material. The presence in trisomic or tetrasomic dosage of the PWS/AS region correlates with abnormality: moderate to severe mental retardation, possibly including epilepsy, autistic behavior, and mild physical defects (Robinson et al., 1993c; Webb, 1994; Leana-Cox et al., 1994; Cheng et al., 1994). A possible influence of imprinting remains open. Abeliovich et al. (1995) report a unique case of a retarded child with three No. 15 chromosomes: a normal homolog, an abnormal homolog with a tandem duplication of segment q11.2-q12, and an inv dup(15). They propose a mechanism whereby an asymmetric exchange firstly produced the tandem duplication and a small centric remnant, and the latter then gave rise to the inv dup(15) by U-type union.

Cat-eye Syndrome

One of the better known ESACs is the inv dup(22)(pter→q11.2) of the "cat-eye syndrome," and Mears et al. (1994) provide a review. The region that is duplicated can vary, and the duplication is not necessarily symmetrical, suggesting that the chromosome can arise from misalignment and exchange over a considerable distance. The critical region comprises, at most, 2.1 Mb (Mears et al., 1995). Most cases arise de novo, but familial transmission is recorded including, remarkably, familial mosaicism (Urioste et al., 1994b). The phenotype appears not to correlate well with the size of the chromosome and indeed the heterozygote may show no signs of the syndrome, although it may be that four copies of the critical region is more likely to produce the phenotype than three (Mears et al., 1995).

Isochromosome

An isochromosome is a "mirror-image" chromosome. Recorded isochromosomes include i(5p), i(8p), i(9p), i(12p) (Pallister-Killian syndrome), i(18p), i(21q), i(22q), and i(Xq). The classical mode of isochromosome formation is by transverse division at the centromere, in a chromosome A, to give an i(Ap) and an i(Aq). A more recently proposed mechanism (Sjöstedt et al., 1989; Sijmons et al., 1993) is that of U-loop formation between replicating DNA strands followed by endoreduplication (Figure 17–2), and other mechanisms are postulated (Lorda-Sanchez et al., 1991; Shaffer et al., 1992; Sijmons et al., 1993; Blennow et al., 1994b). Mosaicism is very frequent, implying that a postzygotic origin is common. The very rare circumstance of recurrence of a nonmosaic isochromosome in siblings presumably reflects the mitotic generation of the abnormality in a parental gonad (Krüger et al., 1987). A scenario for the production of the i(Xq) is noted on p. 155.

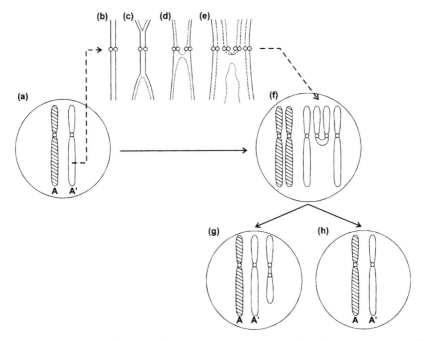

FIGURE 17–2. One theoretical mechanism to produce an isochromosome in a cell (a) entering the S phase of the mitotic cycle. The homolog A', comprising one copy of double-stranded DNA (b), begins replicating DNA (c), and in one replication fork a "U-loop" forms between replicating DNA strands, very close to the centromere (d). Endoreduplication (e) then produces two complete homologs, a dicentric isochromosome, and an acentric fragment which is lost. The cell now has a replicated homolog A, a replicated homolog A', and the isochromosome (f). The daughter cells (g and h) are 47,+i(Ap) and 46,N. After Sjöstedt et al. (1989).

APPARENTLY BALANCED REARRANGEMENT

De novo translocations, inversions, and insertions can appear balanced at the cytogenetic level, but in fact a locus or loci at the breakpoint site(s) is disrupted or deleted and is the cause of an abnormal phenotype. For example, a disruption of the *SOX9* gene is presumably the basis of campomelic syndrome in a case of de novo translocation (Young et al., 1992) and of de novo paracentric inversion (Maraia et al., 1991) involving 17q24.3-25.1. The translocation can be coincidental: Hersh et al. (1995) very reasonably suggested a de novo rcp(1;10) in an infant with thanatophoric dysplasia (TD) might indicate the location of the TD gene, but in fact it has proven to be the fibroblast growth factor receptor-3 locus, which is on another chromosome altogether, at 4p16.3 (Tavormina et al., 1995).

Uniparental Disomy

Uniparental disomy (UPD) causes abnormality when a chromosome segment is subject to genomic imprinting. A segment of chromosome, or perhaps just a single locus, is genetically active, or not active (''silent''), according to whether it had been transmitted from the mother or from the father. Imprintable segments (or loci) function monoallelically. If both segments (or loci) originate from one parent, there will be either biallelic or nulliallelic expression, as the case may be; and this can have untoward consequences. If a chromosome is not imprintable, UPD does not cause abnormality (barring a consequential homozygosity for any recessive gene on that chromosome in the case of uniparental isodisomy).

COMPLETE UNIPARENTAL DISOMY

In complete UPD, both members of a homologous pair come from the one parent. It usually follows restoration of diploidy in an initially trisomic conceptus (Cassidy et al., 1992). In at least the tissue forming the embryo, one of the three trisomic chromosomes is lost, probably by anaphase lag; but, by chance, the discarded chromosome happens to be the one coming from the normal gamete, and so the remaining two are from the same parent (Figure 2–9). Alternatively, although probably very infrequently, UPD may be the consequence of meiotic errors coincidentally in both parents (Figure 2–6c), or of ''correction'' in a monosomic conceptus by replication of the single homolog. In whichever case, the original abnormality will practically always have been a sporadic event, with no discernible increased risk of recurrence: and indeed, as yet not one instance is known of a recurrence of UPD in the setting of normal parental karyotypes. In one UPD, that of chromosome 15, there is a maternal age effect (Robinson et al., 1991; Mascari et al., 1992). Paternal UPD, at least for chromosome 15, may reflect a meiotic II or postzygotic mitotic error (Robinson et al., 1993b).

Infrequently, a 47,+ESAC karyotype may have a coexisting UPD for the same chromosome that the ESAC was derived from; it may be that the zygote from a 23,abn + 23,N → 46,abn conception attempted to correct the imbalance, or at least lessen it, by replication of the normal homolog (James et al., 1995).

Uniparental disomy of chromosome 15, causing Prader-Willi and Angelman syndromes, we discuss below. UPD has been recognized for certain other human chromosomes (Ledbetter and Engel, 1995); those which may cause abnormality are listed below under Genetic Counseling.

Paternal uniparental disomy for the full diploid complement—all 46 chromosomes are of paternal origin—produces the condition of hydatidiform mole, which we discuss in Chapter 20. UPD(mat) for the full diploid complement causes benign cystic ovarian teratoma, an unusual tumor of the ovary in which several embryonic tissues may be represented (Linder et al., 1975). It arises in an unovulated oocyte following failure of the second meiotic division (or possibly fusion with the polar body). In a unique case of parthenogenetic chimerism, a 46,XX/46,XY male child with growth asymmetry had complete maternal isodisomy in the 46,XX cell line and biparental inheritance in the 46,XY line (Strain et al., 1995). Probably, an ovum had completed a mitosis on its own, and then one of its daughter cells received the sperm (for the 46,XY line) while the other underwent diploidization (for the 46,XX line).

SEGMENTAL UNIPARENTAL DISOMY

Segmental UPD arises as the consequence of a postzygotic somatic recombination between the maternal and paternal homolog (Figure 17–3). It can have an effect if the chromosomal arm involved incorporates loci subject to imprinting. If the recombination occurs in a cell after the formation of the inner cell mass (which gives rise to the embryo) the segmental UPD will involve only some cells; in other words, there is mosaic segmental UPD. Beckwith-Wiedemann syndrome is, as yet, the only condition known in which this scenario applies, with the oppositely imprinted and interfunctional insulin-like growth factor 2 (*IGF2*) and *H19* genes on distal 11p being candidates as "BWS loci" (Henry et al., 1993; Weksberg et al., 1993a; Slatter et al., 1994; Weksberg, 1994); in the female, the pattern of X-inactivation may have an intriguing contribution to make in this process (Örstavik et al., 1995).

Prader-Willi and Angelman Syndromes

These syndromes are presumed to be due to the loss or nonfunctioning of a Prader-Willi syndrome (PWS) gene or genes and to the loss or nonfunctioning of an Angelman syndrome (AS) gene or genes, respectively. These genes are located within 15q11–13. *Loss* of these genes is most commonly due to a simple deletion of most or all of the q11–13 segment ("classical deletion"), and whether the phenotype comes to be PWS or AS depends upon which parent contributed the deleted chromosome. *Nonfunctioning* can be due to UPD, with

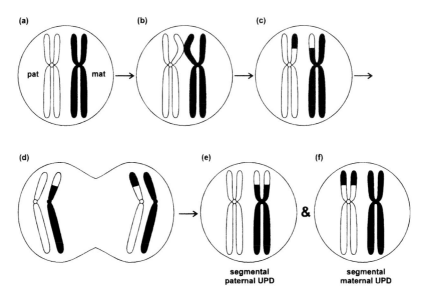

FIGURE 17–3. The genesis of segmental uniparental disomy (in this illustration, UPD of part of the short arm). In one cell of the early conceptus, the paternal and maternal homologs of a chromosome pair (*a*) undergo somatic recombination between the short arms (*b, c*). Segregation at mitosis (*d*) produces daughter cells with segmental UPD: in one (*e*), the short-arm distal segments of both chromosomes are now of paternal origin, and in the other (*f*), they are both of maternal origin. These cells can then be the source of segmentally UPD tissue in a part of the conceptus.

the phenotype according to the parent of origin of the disomic pair of chromosomes. Nonfunctioning may also be caused by absence of, or mutation in, a "15q11–13 imprinting center" that controls resetting of the 15q11–13 imprint (Buiting et al., 1995), or by mutation of a structural AS or (in theory) PWS gene.

A schema for the various molecular defects of PWS and AS is presented in Figure 17–4.

Classical Deletion

The typical deletion removes a substantial segment, about 3 to 4Mb, within 15q11–13 that encompasses the PWS and the AS structural genes and their regulatory sequences, and sequences having a role in the *cis*-regulation of imprinting. Most deletions are of about the same size, whether or not they are detectable cytogenetically; FISH is a more accurate tool than high-resolution cytogenetics (Delach et al., 1994). Normally, the PWS gene(s) is active only on the paternal chromosome, and the AS gene(s) is active only on the maternal chromosome. The deletion characteristically entirely removes both the PWS and AS regions, and adjacent segments of chromosome as well. If the deletion occurs on a paternally originating chromosome, it will cause the PWS phenotype to develop[2]; and a maternal deletion produces AS. In a sense, there is an "unmasking of the silent allele(s)." At least in the case of PWS, a number of loci may contribute to the phenotype, and so the expression "contiguous gene syndrome" is not inappropriate, albeit having a somewhat different sense from its usage elsewhere in this chapter.

Prader-Willi and Angelman syndromes due to deletion, associated with uncommon rearrangement

A deletion removing the PW/AS regions can be due to a translocation or inversion involving chromosome 15. The male carrier of a balanced reciprocal translocation in which one breakpoint is in the region of 15q13 can transmit an unbalanced complement to produce a deletion PWS child (Hultén et al., 1991; Smeets et al., 1992); and the female carrier can have a child with deletion AS (Chan et al., 1993). A de novo unbalanced translocation having a deletion in 15q11–13 would cause PWS, if of paternal origin, and AS, if of maternal origin (Smith et al., 1991; Reeve et al., 1993) (Figure 17–5). A handful of PWS cases have been due to a Y;15 translocation, with breakpoints in Yp and at 15q12–13, having the karyotype 45,X,der(Y)t(Y;15) and deletion of the PW region (Vickers et al., 1994). The 15q11–13 region appears to be prone to asymmetric meiotic recombination in the setting of a balanced parental rearrangement, and there are rare instances of a parent heterozygous for a translocation (Smeets et al., 1992) or inversion (Webb et al., 1992; Chan et al., 1993; Clayton-Smith et al., 1993), which has a breakpoint in this region, producing a deleted gamete and having a PWS or AS child.

Microdeletion

Small or very small deletions (in comparison to the usual size of 3–4 Mb)[3] are the only type of simple deletion associated with sibling recurrence. Very few cases are known of siblings with an Angelman microdeletion (affecting either structural gene or imprinting center), or of a Prader-Willi microdeletion (affecting the imprinting center). Genetic defects such as these, which remove or disable the imprinting center, are the basis of a novel genetic mechanism: the "fixation of an ancestral epigenotype." Saitoh et al. (1992) describe three siblings having AS, with their phenotypically normal mother and grandfather carrying the same 1–1.5 Mb deletion. Presumably, the deletion arose de novo on the grandfather's paternal No. 15 and encompassed only the AS structural and/or controlling gene(s), leaving the PWS gene(s) intact. (Alternatively, there could have been patrilineal transmission of the deletion, harmlessly, for any number of previous generations.) Transmission from the grandfather to the mother was without phenotypic consequence, but upon the mother passing it to her children, the children had AS. Other AS microdeletions involve the imprinting center and can be much smaller, with some in the 10 to 50 kb range. Buxton et al. (1994) studied an AS child with a <200 kb microdeletion which may have removed an AS structural gene, rather than an imprinting element, since the methylation patterns were normal. Siblings with PWS having a very small paternally-originating microdeletion are recorded, for example the three families in Buiting et al. (1995) with deletions of 45 kb, 47 kb and ≥60 kb sizes respectively, involving part of the PWS region. In two of these the deletions were shown in the paternal grandmothers. These deletions could have originated antecedent to the grandmothers, provided subsequent transmission to them had been exclusively matrilineal.

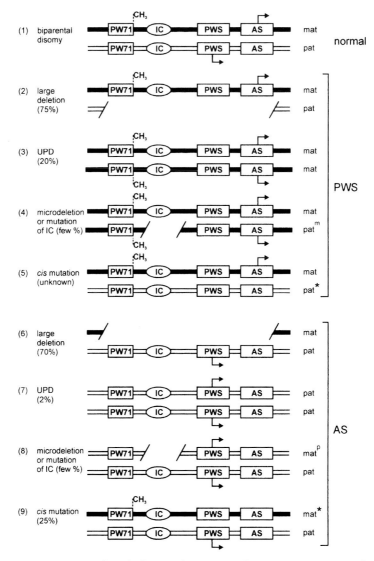

FIGURE 17–4. Normal and abnormal scenarios for genetic activity within the Prader-Willi syndrome (PWS)/Angelman syndrome (AS) region of chromosome 15. An "imprinting center" (IC) controls the functional activation (shown as arrows) of putative PWS and AS gene(s). A "maternally functioning" chromosome is shown as a filled bar, a "paternally functioning" chromosome as an open bar. The actual parental origins are shown at right: mat = maternal chromosome, pat = paternal chromosome, mat^p = "paternally functioning" maternal chromosome, pat^m = "maternally functioning" paternal chromosome, mat* = maternal chromosome with *cis*-mutation, pat* = paternal chromosome with *cis* mutation. Methylation (CH_3) is shown for the PW71 locus (see text). UPD = uniparental disomy. *(1) Normally,* the AS gene(s) are transcribed only from the maternal chromosome, and the PWS gene(s) only from the paternal chromosome, with each chromosome thus functioning appropriately for its parent of origin. In *PWS* there is nonfunctioning of the PWS gene(s) because: *(2)* the PWS gene(s) have been removed by a typical large deletion from the paternal chromosome; *(3)* both chromosomes are of maternal origin; *(4)* a micro-

Uniparental Disomy

The phenotype depends upon the parent of origin of the disomic pair of No. 15 chromosomes. In PWS due to UPD, both No. 15s come from the mother, and so neither of the PWS critical regions is expressed. This functional lack means that the PWS phenotype will arise. In most (80% or more), the UPD had its origin in a maternal meiosis I nondisjunction (Robinson et al., 1993b). Vice versa, in AS due to UPD, both No. 15s are from the father, and neither expresses the AS critical region. Most cases involve a postzygotic (or possibly second meiotic) origin of the extra paternal chromosome (Robinson et al., 1993b). The cytogenetic study in UPD characteristically shows a normal 46,XX or 46,XY karyotype.

Prader-Willi and Angelman syndromes due to uniparental disomy, associated with uncommon rearrangement

Uniparental disomy can result from a variety of rearrangements involving chromosome 15. The male carrier of a rcp(15) could transmit a disomic 15 spermatocyte from 3:1 nondisjunction, with the maternal No. 15 lost, and have a child with UPD AS (Smeets et al., 1992); and vice versa, his carrier sister could likewise have a PWS child. Similarly, a familial nonhomologous Robertsonian translocation in which one of the component chromosomes is a No. 15, which gives a trisomic 15 conception, and with postzygotic loss of the No. 15 from the other parent, would lead to UPD15 with either PWS or AS, according to the sex of the carrier parent (Figure 6–3) (Nicholls et al., 1989; Smith et al., 1993). The same thing could happen if the translocation were de novo. A maternally originating de novo homologous rob(15q15q) (which may actually be a 15q isochromosome), with no No. 15 contributed from the father, would cause PWS (Robinson et al., 1994); and, vice versa, AS would result from a paternal isochromosome 15q (Freeman et al., 1993). Smith et al. (1994) describe AS from asymmetric segregation of a paternal 8;15 translocation (Figure 4–12). The heterozygous father passed on his der(8) and his normal chromosome 15 (thus, paternal UPD), and there was absence of a maternal No. 15. Some PWS children with a 47,+inv dup(15) karyotype may actually have UPD of the two intact No. 15s, and the inv dup (15) is a phenotypically irrelevant relic of the original process of abnormal chromosomal behavior (Robinson et al., 1993d).

---

deletion of or mutation in the IC has fixed a "maternal" imprint status, of no phenotypic effect when transmitted from grandmother to father, and the father then transmitted to the child a "functionally maternal" chromosome; *(5)* a *cis*-acting mutation possibly in a structural PWS gene(s) on the paternal chromosome has prevented its function, the maternal chromosome being normal. In *AS* there is nonfunctioning of the AS gene(s) because: *(6)* the AS gene(s) have been removed by a typical large deletion from the maternal chromosome; *(7)* both chromosomes are of paternal origin; *(8)* a microdeletion of or mutation in the IC fixed a "paternal" imprint status, of no phenotypic effect when transmitted from grandfather to mother, and the mother then transmitted to the child a "functionally paternal" chromosome; *(9)* a *cis*-acting mutation possibly in a structural AS gene(s) on the maternal chromosome has prevented its function, the paternal chromosome being normal. Approximate percentages of each PWS/AS category indicated. Based on Buiting et al. (1995).

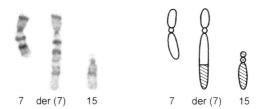

7   der (7)   15   7   der (7)   15

FIGURE 17–5. A (7;15) translocation in which the PWS region is deleted; the child had Prader-Willi syndrome (Jauch et al., 1995). The karyotype is 45,−7,−15,+der(7)(7pter→7q36.3::15q13→15qter). (Courtesy V. Petrovic). Compare and contrast with the similar rcp(8;15) translocation in Figure 4–12, in which the 15q breakpoint is proximal to the PWS/AS region, and so the 45,der(8) carrier parent has a functionally balanced rearrangement.

Nonclassical Deletion, Non-UPD Angelman Syndrome

In about 20 to 30% of AS, there is a normal karyotype, with no classical deletion demonstrable, and with biparental inheritance. Most of these are likely to reflect (*1*) a mutation in an actual AS gene, and a few are due to (*2*) mutations in the imprinting center on the maternal chromosome; these may be point mutations or subtle and as yet undetected microdeletions (Buiting et al., 1995). These two types of mutation can be transmitted by a father in whose child the genetic defect has no effect, since this No. 15 region would in any event carry a paternal imprint and be "silent." But when the daughter of such a man transmits the mutation, neither of her child's No. 15 chromosomes express the AS gene(s), and so the child has AS. If the mutation involves (*1*) an AS structural gene, this defect is "exposed" because the other (normal) No. 15, carrying a paternal imprint, is unexpressed. The methylation test (Driscoll et al., 1992; Dittrich et al., 1992) does not detect these cases. With (*2*) an imprinting center mutation, the imprint on her paternally originating chromosome cannot be erased—there has been "fixation of the ancestral epigenotype"—and so she transmits a "si-

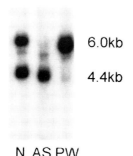

6.0kb

4.4kb

N AS PW

FIGURE 17–6. Molecular testing for Prader-Willi and Angelman syndromes due to UPD or deletion, using a probe that detects a sequence within the PWS and AS region on 15q, in conjunction with a methylation-sensitive enzyme (Dittrich et al., 1992). The normal individual (N) has maternal (6.0 kb) and paternal (4.4 kb) bands. In PWS, there is only a maternal band, and in AS there is only a paternal band (and see text). (Courtesy H. R. Slater.)

lent'' chromosome which is likewise ''exposed.'' The methylation patterns are abnormal (Buiting et al., 1995). In these two mutational types, affected siblings always share the same maternal No. 15, but inheritance of the paternal one is random (Clayton-Smith et al., 1992). Multigenerational transmission has been observed, with AS children born only to carrier daughters of carrier males (Wagstaff et al., 1992; Meijers-Heijboer et al., 1992).

LABORATORY TEST FOR PRADER-WILLI AND ANGELMAN SYNDROMES

An ingenious and elegant procedure which tests the integrity of the PWS/AS region is the use of a probe which maps to the critical region, with a restriction enzyme which does not cut if its cutting site is methylated (methylation-sensitive enzyme) (Driscoll et al., 1992; Dittrich et al., 1992). Such a probe is PW71 (D15S63), used with DNA digested using *Hind*III (cuts regardless of methylation) and *Hpa*II (some methylated sites remain uncut) (Dittrich et al., 1992). In No. 15s of paternal origin, *Hind*III and *Hpa*II both cut, and a 4.4 kb size fragment from 15q11–13 results which can be recognized with the PW71 probe on a standard Southern study. Maternal No. 15s are methylated at the *Hpa*II site, and so only *Hind*III cuts, and a larger 6.0 kb fragment is produced. A normal individual will have, therefore, both a 4.4 kb and a 6.0 kb fragment representing the two parental chromosomes. In PWS, with no paternal critical segment functioning (whether due to deletion, maternal UPD, or imprinting mutation), only a 6.0 kb fragment is seen; on the other hand, a child with AS, who lacks a functioning maternal critical segment (whether from deletion, paternal UPD, or imprinting mutation) shows only the 4.4 kb fragment (Figure 17–6). Note that no distinction can be made from the test result between deletion or UPD as the underlying mechanism. This test detects all cases of PWS (Gillessen-Kaesbach et al., 1995) and AS due to UPD, classical deletion, and imprinting mutation; the more recently developed ''*SNRPN* exon −1'' methylation assay provides an even clearer interpretation (Buiting et al., 1995; Glenn et al., 1996). Newer cytomolecular genetic methodologies may enable further distinction of the different etiologic categories (Knoll et al., 1995).

GENETIC COUNSELING

DELETION

We have mentioned that in most children with deletions, the parents type 46,XX and 46,XY, and the defect is ''de novo.'' The risk for recurrence is very small, but it is not nonexistent. We assume these rare recurrences are due to an occult parental mosaicism, which the routine blood chromosome study could not detect. The abnormal line may be gonadal (confined to gametic tissue) or somatic–gonadal (some somatic tissues involved as well—but not, apparently, blood). The observation of rarity of recurrence allows us to propose the empiric advice that, in the individual case, recurrence is most unlikely. A figure that is appropriate in this setting is ''less than 0.5%''; the counselor should note the converse ''greater than 99.5%'' for a child without the chromosome defect. Nevertheless, in practice many couples advised of a very low risk still request prenatal diagnosis for reassurance; and one can sympathize with this request. If testing is to be based upon cytogenetics alone, care must be exercised in offering prenatal diagnosis of small deletions seen only on high-resolution lymphocyte chromosomes. The technical ability to demonstrate such small changes in amniotic fluid or chorionic villus cells may be limited.

In those deletions where a parent is shown to carry, for example, a balanced translocation, a substantial recurrence risk is probable, and the appropriate chapter should be consulted.

Brief sketches of the major deletion syndromes follow, as well as some less well-known ones, in numerical order of chromosomes. Some gain inclusion because of one specific and striking feature, such as the del(5) syndrome with polyposis. Some which are speculative (Cornelia de Lange syndrome, for example) warrant listing because of their particular interest to the dysmorphologist. We comment in greater or lesser length upon the genetics of each. In some, we make mention of familial transmission; but primarily we are dealing with the case of de novo defects. Chromosomal atlases and catalogs provide greater clinical detail for the various syndromes. In the limit, just about every different deletion, even if only one case is known, could be regarded as a ''new syndrome.''

Chromosome 1

del 1q32–q41: Van der Woude (VdW) Syndrome and Other Defects

A microdeletion in 1q which encompasses the VdW locus and some brain and morphogenesis loci produces a syndrome of lip and palate clefting with ''lip pits'' (VdW syndrome) along with intellectual defect and, if the deletion is extensive enough, other congenital malformations (Bocian and Walker, 1987; Sander et al., 1994). It may be transmissible.

Chromosome 2

del 2q27: Waardenburg Plus Syndrome

The Waardenburg syndrome Type 1 (WS1) of congenital deafness and pigmentary anomalies is due to mutation in, or absence of, the pattern formation gene *PAX3* on one No. 2 chromosome. A deletion which removes *PAX3* and adjacent genes produces a syndrome with the additional features of growth retardation and intellectual deficit (Tassabehji et al., 1994). Other forms of WS reflect defects at different loci, and a deletion of 13q21.2-q32 that removes the endothelin-B receptor gene is associated with WS2 (Van Camp et al., 1995).

del 2q37: Albright-like Syndrome

A syndrome resembling Albright hereditary osteodystrophy (AHO) having a de novo 2q37 deletion has been described by Wilson et al. (1995) and Phelan et al. (1995). This cytogenetic defect should specifically be sought in patients with an AHO morphological phenotype and intellectual deficit, but without the typical endocrine defect.

Chromosome 3

rea 3q26.3: Cornelia de Lange Syndrome

The phenotypic resemblance of Cornelia de Lange syndrome (CDLS) to the distal 3q duplication syndrome raised the question of UPD 3; in fact, there is biparental inheritance of chromosome 3 (Shaffer et al., 1993). Ireland et al. (1991, 1995) report a very typical CDLS patient having a de novo translocation with one breakpoint at 3q26.3, and restudied two "mild" CDLS sibs with a 3q26.3 duplication from a paternal intrachromosomal insertion; and Rizzu et al. (1995) have studied a patient with a maternally inherited paracentric inversion with a 3q27 breakpoint. These observations are suggestive of a "CDLS locus" in this region. Sibship recurrence is rare but not unknown and Krajewska-Walasek et al. (1995) suggest it may be more likely where the "full", severe, phenotype is observed.

Chromosome 4

del 4p: Wolf-Hirschhorn Syndrome

This well-known deletion syndrome of severe mental retardation, identified in the pre-banding era, is one of the few that can, in its classic form, be confidently recognized clinically (Figure 17–7a). Subtle as well as unsubtle deletions occur, and sometimes FISH may be necessary for definitive identification of the former (Altherr et al., 1991). Estabrooks et al. (1994, 1995) document the extent of the deletions at the molecular level, and correlate specific deleted segments with components of the phenotype (Fig. 17–7b). Tommerup et al. (1993a) propose a certain zinc-finger gene which, in the haplo-insufficient state, may contribute substantially to the phenotype. The Pitt-Rogers-Danks syndrome is a variant form—a "syndrome within a syndrome"—in which a *very* small 4p16.3 deletion may produce the essence of the facial gestalt (Clemens et al., 1996). (A more proximal deletion, in 4p15, produces a separate phenotype; Fryns, 1995a). The majority of Wolf-Hirschhorn syndrome occurs de novo, although a few, and including at least one recorded example of Pitt-Rogers-Danks syndrome, are the consequence of parental balanced rearrangement.

Chromosome 5

del 5p: Cri du Chat Syndrome

Deletion can vary from almost all of 5p to just p15-pter (Figure 17–7a). The "*cri*" region has been pinpointed at p15.3 and most other features are due to p15.2 haplo-insufficiency (Overhauser et al., 1994), and deletion of the segment 5p15.3 alone can produce the "cat-like cry" in an otherwise normal child (Gersh et al., 1995). A start has been made on identifying the hundred or so loci that are removed by the deletion (Simmons et al., 1995). One case of recurrence of

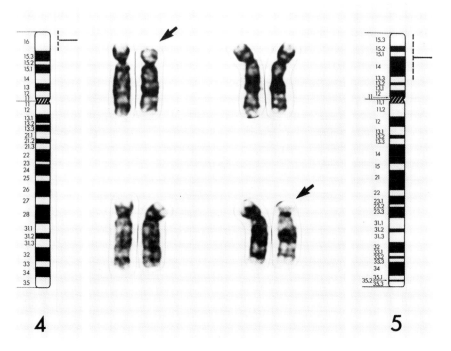

4   5

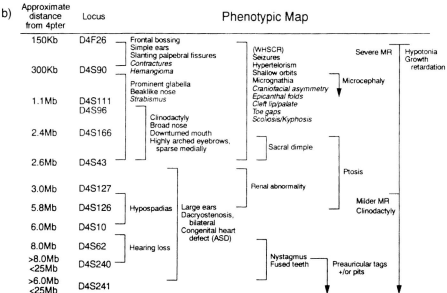

b)

FIGURE 17–7. (a) Chromosomes 4 (*left*) and 5 (*right*) from patients with the Wolf-Hirschhorn syndrome (*center, upper*) and the cri du chat syndrome (*center, lower*). The arrows indicate the deleted chromosomes. The region encompassing the range of deletion is shown on the ideograms. (b) Phenotypic map of distal 4p (4p16→pter) deletions, showing those characteristics of Wolf-Hirschhorn syndrome due to haplo-

276

del(5)(p15.2), identified at prenatal diagnosis, attests to the reality of gonadal mosaicism (Hajianpour et al., 1991).

del 5q21–q22: Polyposis Plus Syndrome

A minor degree of facial dysmorphism and mild to moderate mental retardation are nonspecific features of a syndrome due to deletion of 5q15–q22 or 5q22–q23.2; the unique feature is adenomatous polyposis of the bowel, along with the dental anomalies and subcutaneous lesions of Gardner syndrome (Hockey et al., 1989; Kobayashi et al., 1991). Absence of one *APC* (adenomatous polyposis coli) allele exposes any mutation subsequently occurring in the allele on the intact No. 5; and this, in turn, causes loss of the tumor suppressor function that this locus normally subserves.

Chromosome 7

del 7p13: Greig Cephalosyndactyly Syndrome

This acrocephalopolysyndactyly syndrome, classically inherited as an autosomal dominant, is due to mutation in the *GLI3* locus. Rare microdeletion cases have haplo-insufficiency of *GLI3*, as well as loss of some adjacent brain loci, and the phenotype is combined Greig syndrome plus neurodevelopmental defect (Pettigrew et al., 1991; Fisher and Scambler, 1994).

del 7q11.2: Williams Syndrome

Williams syndrome (WS) is due to a deletion of more than 250 kb within chromosome 7q (Ewart et al., 1993, 1994). The deleted loci include the elastin gene and presumably contiguous brain and morphogenesis loci; degrees of clinical severity may be related to the number of loci deleted. Deletion of the elastin locus alone produces the characteristic cardiac defect in isolation. The WS deletion may equally be of paternal or maternal origin (Brøndum-Nielsen et al., 1994). Kotzot et al. (1995) propose that the demonstration of a deletion by the use of FISH and/or DNA markers mapping to the WS region is now a requirement to confirm the diagnosis; and Lowery et al. (1995) show that almost all (96%) patients with the classic phenotype have an elastin deletion. The great majority of cases are sporadic, and we know of no record of recurrence in siblings of undoubted WS to normal parents. Rare instances of parent to child transmission are recorded (Morris et al., 1993; Sadler et al., 1993; Pankau et al., 1993).

---

insufficiency for specific segments at the molecular level. Mental retardation (MR), hypotonia, and growth retardation presumably have contributory segments throughout the region of deletion. Features in italics may have reduced penetrance. WHSCR = Wolf-Hirschhorn syndrome critical region, ASD = atrial septal defect. From Estabrooks, L. L., Rao, K. W., Driscoll, D. A., Crandall, B. F., Dean, J. C. S., Ikonen, E., Korf, B. and Aylsworth, A. S. (1995). Preliminary phenotypic map of chromosome 4p16 based on 4p deletions. *Am J Med Genet*, 57, 581–586, © Am J Med Genet 1993, courtesy L. L. Estabrooks, and with the permission of Wiley-Liss, Inc., a subsidiary of John Wiley & Sons, Inc.

del 7q21.3: Ectrodactyly Plus Syndrome

One type of split hand and split foot malformation is associated with deletions in 7q21, and loss of one allele at a "digit-formation locus" in this region may be the basis. Loss of contiguous genes encompassed by the deletion may contribute to other less specific dysmorphology and to a diminution of intellectual function (Roberts et al., 1991).

Chromosome 8

del 8q24.11–q24.13: Langer-Giedion Syndrome (Trichorhinophalangeal Syndrome Type II)

This condition is due to a deletion which removes the gene for trichorhinophalangeal (TRP) syndrome type I as well as adjacent brain genes and a bone growth control gene (*EXT1*, which causes exostoses) to give the broader picture of Langer-Giedion syndrome, or TRP syndrome type II (Figure 17–8). Variation in the number of brain loci deleted determines the degree of any associated mental defect (Langer et al., 1984; Lüdecke et al., 1995). Marchau et al. (1993) describe several affected individuals in a family in which the TRP gene was presumed to be deleted or disrupted due to a segregating apparently balanced translocation with one breakpoint at 8q24.

del 8q12.2-q21.2: Branchio-Oto-Renal Plus Syndrome

This microdeletion syndrome is of interest in identifying the location of an autosomal gene for hydrocephalus and of the branchio-oto-renal gene (Haan et al., 1989; Vincent et al., 1994).

Chromosome 10

del 10q11.2: Hirschsprung Disease Plus Syndrome

The locus for the receptor kinase gene *RET* is at 10q11.2. In the haplo-insufficient state, certain neurons may fail to migrate to their proper place in the intestinal wall. Without this nervous control, the segment of bowel is chronically contracted, and this causes a partial or complete obstruction (Hirschsprung disease). The loss of adjacent loci contributes to a wider phenotype (Fewtrell et al., 1994).

Chromosome 11

del 11p13: WAGR Syndrome (Wilms Tumor, Aniridia, Genital Defects, Mental Retardation)

Haplo-insufficiency of the *PAX6* morphogenesis gene causes aniridia (absence of the iris). Loss of one *WT1* allele can comprise the first hit in the sequence of events to cause Wilms tumor, and may also be responsible for the impairment of genital development. These two loci, and presumably some brain loci, are removed in the 11p13 deletion (Figure 17–9).

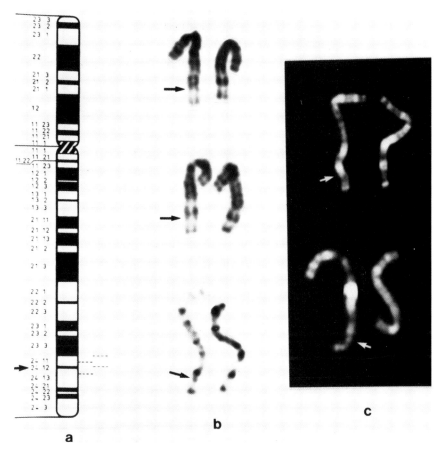

FIGURE 17–8. (a) Ideogram of chromosome 8 at the 850-band stage. The dotted lines denote the postulated sites of breakage and reunion in a patient with the Langer-Giedion syndrome. (b) Three pairs of extended No. 8 chromosomes of the patient, G-banded. Arrows indicate the band 8q24.12 on the normal homolog. (c) Two pairs of chromosome 8 prepared as in part b, but stained with quinacrine. The arrows indicate the band 8q24.12 on the normal homolog. (Reproduced from Bowen et al., 1985, with the permission of Expansion Scientifique Française.)

del 11q23: Jacobsen Syndrome
This syndrome is of particular interest because a specific rare fragile site (*FRA11B*) at 11q23.3 may predispose to the generation of the deletion (Jones et al., 1994).

Chromosome 13

del 13q14: Retinoblastoma Plus
This deletion removes the *RB* locus on one chromosome, and loss of, or change in, the second locus on the normal No. 13 comprises the classic ''second hit'' of the process of initiation of tumorigenesis. Bilateral tumors are characteristic.

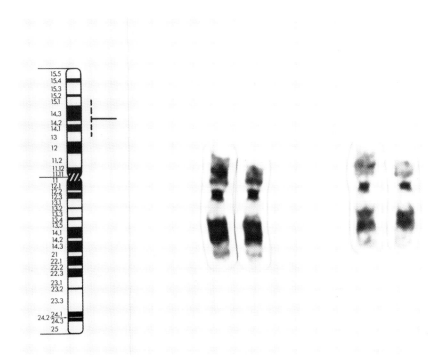

FIGURE 17–9. Chromosome pair 11 from two cells of a patient with aniridia and Wilms tumor showing a deletion (indicated on the ideogram) of part of the short arm.

Dysmorphism and intellectual compromise can variably accompany the eye defect, according to the extent of loss of contiguous genes (Figure 17–10).

Chromosome 15

del 15q11–13: Prader-Willi Syndrome, Angelman Syndrome
See below under Conditions with More than One Cytogenetic Basis.

Chromosome 16

del 16p13.3: α-Thalassemia and Mental Retardation
This is one of two α-thalassemia and mental retardation (ATR) syndromes (the other being an X-linked Mendelian condition). In the del(16p) ATR syndrome there is monosomy for a segment including the α chain globin loci and some brain loci. This can be a true terminal deletion, with "healing" of the single breakpoint by the addition of telomeric sequences (J. Lamb et al., 1993).

del 16p13.3: Rubinstein-Taybi Syndrome
This syndrome has a distinctive phenotype, and the facies and the broad thumbs are very characteristic. In a minority of cases a deletion can be seen on FISH

using a cosmid probe, RT1 (Figure 17–11). The basic defect is haplo-insufficiency for (or mutation in) a gene *CREBBP* (cyclic AMP-regulated enhancer binding protein) which may then lead to a generalized dysregulation of expression in a number of target genes, and thus it is a single locus disorder rather than a contiguous gene syndrome (Petrij et al., 1995). This does not entirely square with the observation that the psychomotor defect may be more severe in those cases with a FISH-detectable deletion (Breuning et al., 1993; Masuno et al., 1994). The range of severity may simply reflect a variable expressivity of the abnormal genotype; the case of identical twins with Rubinstein-Taybi syndrome having rather different neuro-behavioral phenotypes supports this suggestion (Preis and Majewski, 1995).

Chromosome 17

del 17p13.3: Miller-Dieker Syndrome

A deletion of the brain morphogenesis gene *LIS1* produces lissencephaly (''smooth brain''), a severe neuronal migration defect (Reiner et al., 1993). Loss of adjacent loci adds in defects of other systems and characteristic dysmorphogenesis, and this constitutes the Miller-Dieker karyotype and phenotype (S. A. Ledbetter et al., 1992) (Figure 17–12). The diagnosis may be confirmed with a commercially available FISH probe, by analysis of a polymorphic marker map-

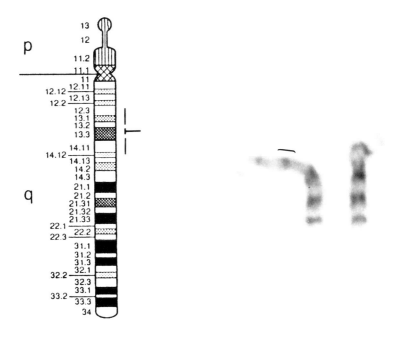

FIGURE 17–10.   A small deletion of chromosome No. 13, from a woman who had had bilateral retinoblastomas as a child and who has a mild intellectual deficiency and minor facial dysmorphism. The karyotype is 46,XX,del(13)(q12q14). The deleted chromosome is on the *right*; the segment q12-q14 is indicated on the intact chromosome, *left*. Her parents and brother karyotyped normal. (Courtesy L. V. Hills.)

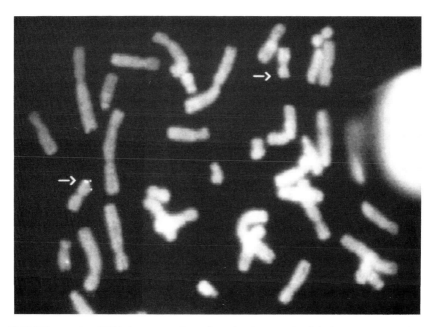

FIGURE 17–11.   FISH demonstration of a submicroscopic deletion at 16p13.3 in a child with Rubinstein-Taybi syndrome, using the probe RT-1. One homolog shows normal hybridization (arrow, *left*), while the deletion chromosome fails to hybridize (arrow, *right*). (Courtesy E. Baker.)

ping to the region, or by direct *LIS1* mutation testing (Mantel et al., 1994; Pilz et al., 1995). One instance of affected sibs was due to the mother carrying a pericentric inversion 17 (Greenberg et al., 1986).

del 17p11.2: Smith-Magenis Syndrome
This syndrome of dysmorphology and mental defect can have the particular characteristics of disturbed sleep pattern, diminished pain sensitivity and self-destructive behavior although there is quite a range of clinical phenotype (Colley et al., 1990; Greenberg et al., 1991). Candidate genes which, being haplo-insufficient, may contribute to the SMS phenotype are small nuclear RNA U3 (*SNU3*) (Chevillard et al., 1993), the human homolog of the *Drosophila flight-less-I* gene (Chen et al., 1995), and a microfibril-associated glycoprotein *MFAP4* (Z. Zhao et al., 1995). FISH may be necessary to diagnose cases in which the deletion is at the limit of cytogenetic resolution (Juyal et al., 1995).

The possibility of parental gonadal mosaicism is not negligible. Zori et al. (1993) have reported a SMS child whose (phenotypically abnormal) mother was 46,XX,del(17)(p11.2–12)/46,XX. This case, along with a few other SMS cases that reflect at least somatic mosaicism (Gardner et al., 1994), and the view of Moncla et al. (1993) that this region of No. 17 may be a hotspot for rearrangement, suggest that a considerable fraction of these deletions may be mitotically generated; although it is noteworthy that one case in which mosaicism had been proposed on high-resolution cytogenetics in fact proved to be nonmosaic on

FISH (Juyal et al., 1995). Albeit no case of recurrence is on record, a risk figure of about 1% may be appropriate to offer. Prenatal diagnosis is now achieved primarily by molecular methodology, using markers such as D17S29 and D17S71, which are deleted in all SMS cases (Moncla et al., 1993).

Chromosome 18

del 18p, del 18q

Quite substantial deletions of chromosome 18 short arm and long arm (Figure 17–13) were recognized in the early days of medical cytogenetics; the small size of this chromosome facilitated recognition of these deletions on "solid-stain" cytogenetics (De Grouchy et al., 1964, 1966). Three decades later, Silverman et al. (1995) could focus on the detail of the breakpoints at a molecular level. Kline et al. (1993) have reviewed patients with different terminal 18q deletions and assembled a preliminary karyotype-phenotype correlation.

Chromosome 20

del 20p11.2: Alagille Syndrome

The characteristic features of this syndrome are stenosis of the peripheral pulmonary arteries and insufficient development of bile ducts within the liver (thus, "arteriohepatic dysplasia"), along with certain eye and skeletal defects and a

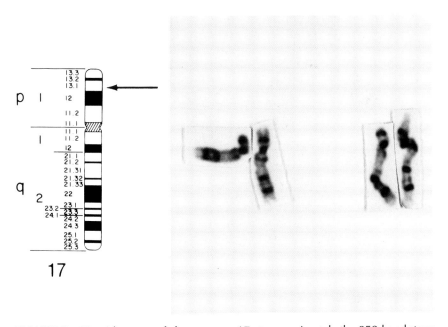

FIGURE 17–12.   Ideogram of chromosome 17 at approximately the 850-band stage with breakpoint at p13.1 arrowed. G-banded chromosome pair 17 from a patient with Miller-Dieker syndrome and deletion of 17p13.1. The deleted chromosome is on the left of each pair. (From Stratton et al., 1984, with the permission of Springer-Verlag.)

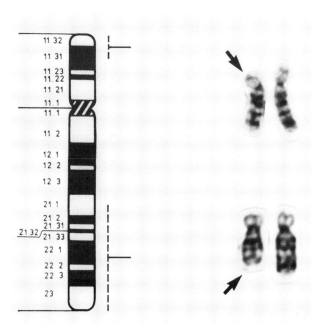

FIGURE 17–13. Chromosomes from patients with deletion of chromosome 18p and 18q. The arrows indicate the deleted chromosomes, and the regions encompassing the range of deletion are shown on the ideogram.

distinctive facies. Autosomal dominant inheritance is characteristic (Hol et al., 1995), but a cytogenetic deletion is detectable in a minority (Schnittger et al., 1989; Zhang et al., 1990, Teebi et al., 1992). It remains an open question whether contiguous genes are deleted or whether there may be just a single Alagille locus (Spinner et al., 1994; Elmslie et al., 1995).

Chromosome 21

del 21q: Partial Monosomy 21
A variety of 21q deletions exist, and this allows an assessment of the contribution of different haplo-insufficient segments to the observed range of phenotype; deletion of the segment encompassing the *APP* (amyloid precursor protein) and *SOD1* (superoxide dismutase-1) loci is particularly important (Chettouh et al., 1995). Most cases are sporadic, but some have occurred in the setting of a parental balanced translocation (Huret et al., 1995).

Chromosome 22

del 22q11.21–q11.23: DiGeorge/Shprintzen Velocardiofacial Syndrome
These two conditions, originally regarded as separate entities, came together when deletions in the same region were shown to underlie both (Scambler, 1993; D. I. Wilson et al., 1993a) (Figure 17–14). This may be the most common

human site of deletion. There is a range of phenotype (Motzkin et al., 1993; Lindsay et al., 1995b), and, in the familial case, a parent can, for example, show mild features of the condition or have a predominantly Shprintzen facial and palatal phenotype, with a child showing a characteristic DiGeorge cardiac and endocrine phenotype (Stevens et al., 1990; Desmaze et al., 1993). Psychiatric disorder can be associated, and Demczuk et al. (1995) record that a hemizygous father of a child with DiGeorge syndrome himself had psychiatric illness but no physical abnormality. Goodship et al. (1995) report monozygous twins having a de novo deletion and each presenting a characteristic facies and nasal speech, but who differed in their neurodevelopmental progress and only one of whom had a heart defect, which attests to the phenotypic variability that can flow from the same deletion on the same background genotype. Other variant clinical forms exist (Seaver et al., 1994; Franke et al., 1994; McDonald-McGinn et al., 1995), and increasing clinical experience may lead to a better recognition of more subtly dysmorphic cases. Several candidate genes have been proposed (Morrow et al., 1995; Wadey et al., 1995) of which the most promising may be *DGCR3* (Budarf et al., 1995). It remains to be shown whether different phenotypes all have provenance in the one locus or in the same group of loci, or if they reflect deletions of different sets of contiguous genes.

About 90% of cases are de novo, and it remains to be clarified whether there

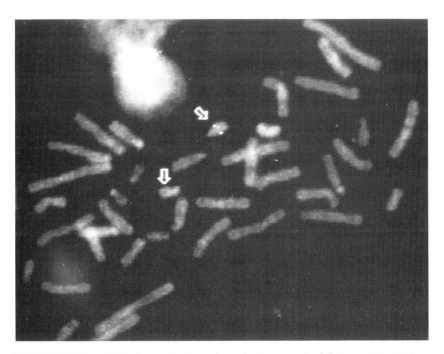

FIGURE 17–14. FISH demonstration of a submicroscopic deletion at 22q11 in a child with velocardiofacial (Shprintzen) syndrome, using a DiGeorge critical region probe. One homolog shows normal hybridization (arrow, *left*) while the deletion chromosome fails to hybridize (arrow, *right*).

is an excess of maternally originating deletions (Demczuk et al., 1995; Morrow et al., 1995). Presumed parental gonadal mosaicism has been described (Eydoux et al., 1995), and prenatal diagnosis using FISH may be considered in a subsequent pregnancy to cover this possibility (Driscoll et al., 1993); the use of microsatellite markers within the DiGeorge critical region may prove a more efficient analytical tool (Morrow et al., 1995).

The DiGeorge phenotype may not always reside in a demonstrable 22q genetic defect. No deletion is identified in about one fifth, at least with current methodology (Lindsay et al., 1995a). Maternal diabetes may be an uncommon cause of the condition (T. A. Wilson et al., 1993b).

Chromosome X

Chromosome X deletions are discussed in Chapter 12.

DUPLICATION

Intrachromosomal Duplication, 46,dup

Theoretically, parental gonadal mosaicism may be more likely in the *direct* duplication (46,dir dup) than in most rearrangements, with a parent being 46,N/46,dir dup. Most, however, are presumed to arise truly de novo. Accommodating the possibility of parental gonadal mosaicism, a recurrence risk figure around 1% (rather than the <0.5% we suggest for most rearrangements) may be appropriate. For the *inverted* duplication, 46,inv dup, we assume a low (<0.5%) recurrence risk. (Extremely rarely, an inverted duplication may, in fact, be due to recombination within a parental paracentric inversion [p. 153]. Paracentric inversions can be difficult to detect, and a careful and directed search may be appropriate.)

While there are certainly very many individual duplication cases on record, rather fewer duplication phenotypes have acquired eponymic (or acronymic) status than with deletions and we do not provide a catalog comparable to the listing of deletion syndromes above. One potential candidate as a duplication syndrome, the CHARGE (coloboma, heart, choanal atresia, retardation, genital, ear) association with dup(14)(q22–q24.2), might be more likely due to a microdeletion at one of these breakpoints, since most other dup(14q) cases do not have this phenotype (and in any event, CHARGE is genetically heterogeneous) (North et al., 1995).

Interchromosomal Rearrangement with Duplication, 46,rea

The great majority of these rearrangements arise de novo, presumably from illegitimate meiotic recombination. The possibility of parental gonadal mosaicism warrants consideration of prenatal diagnosis; we assume a low (<0.5%) recurrence risk.

Extra Structurally Abnormal Chromosome, 47,+ESAC

Parental mosaicism is not excluded by normal lymphocyte karyotypes. Although a risk for recurrence will be "small" (which we cannot precisely define, although we presume a low single-digit % figure), prenatal diagnosis is appropriate. In the specific case of the common *inv dup (15),* mosaicism is a well recognized possibility, and parental karyotyping is important. Normal parental karyotypes imply a low (<0.5%) recurrence risk; indeed, we know of no record of inv dup(15) recurrence.

Isochromosomes

A couple having had a child with isochromosome mosaicism (karyotype 47,+i/ 46,N) can be given very reassuring advice. Very likely, the karyotype at conception was 46,N, with the isochromosome generated postzygotically (e.g., Figure 17–2). Two specific categories are dealt with elsewhere: the mosaic or nonmosaic isodicentric 15, usually referred to as inv dup (15) (above), and de novo nonmosaic isochromosome 21q Down syndrome (p. 249).

Complex Abnormality

Theoretically, a complex defect might be less likely to arise at a premeiotic mitosis, and thus parental gonadal mosaicism would be most exceptional. The risk of recurrence may be of the order of no more than 0.1%.

DE NOVO "APPARENTLY BALANCED" REARRANGEMENT

We know of no instance of recurrence of a de novo "apparently balanced" translocation, inversion, or insertion in which the abnormal chromosome in the affected child was considered to have been causally related to an abnormal phenotype.

Uniparental Disomy

Uniparental disomy has been recognized for most chromosomes (Table 17–1, and Table 2 in Ledbetter and Engel, 1995). For some there is no apparent phenotypic consequence. For others there may be: and we list below some of the proposed syndromes of UPD. Kalousek and Barrett (1994) caution that phenotypic defect may have been due to an accompanying placental trisomy rather than to the UPD itself.[4] No instance of recurrence of full UPD for a particular chromosome with a 46,XX or 46,XY karyotype is known, and we assume there to be no discernibly increased recurrence risk. UPD for the entire chromosome set (hydatidiform mole) is exceptional in that recurrence is recorded (p. 320). Segmental UPD arising postzygotically, and which is karyotypically 46,XX or

Table 17—1 Chromosomes for which
UPD has been reported

Chromosome	Number of reported cases
2	1
4	1
5	1
6	1
7	5
10	1
11	14
13	1
14	8
15	47
16	10
21	3
22	6
X	3
Total	102

Source: Modified from Kalousek and Barrett (1994).

46,XY, we presume to imply no increased risk. (UPD due to rearrangement would have a risk according to the nature of the specific rearrangement.)

Chromosome 2
A single case report of maternal uniparental heterodisomy 2 documents intrauterine and postnatal growth retardation but normal neurodevelopmental progress and absence of malformations; the UPD had probably arisen as a postzygotic ''correction'' following trisomy 2 due to maternal meiosis I nondisjunction (Harrison et al., 1995).

Chromosome 6
The very rare condition of neonatal diabetes may, in some cases, be due to UPD 6 (Abramowicz et al., 1994; Temple et al., 1995).

Chromosome 7
Growth retardation is a feature of maternal but not paternal UPD 7, and may be a cause of Silver-Russell syndrome (Höglund et al., 1994; Kotzot et al., 1995).

Chromosome 11
Complete paternal UPD 11, following post-zygotic ''rescue'' of trisomy 11, has been associated with severe intrauterine growth retardation (Webb et al., 1995). See also below under Conditions with More than One Cytogenetic Basis (Beckwith-Wiedemann syndrome).

Chromosome 14
UPD 14 is considered to produce different syndromes according to the maternal or paternal origin of the disomy (Temple et al., 1991; Wang et al., 1991; Pentao

et al., 1992; Antonarakis et al., 1993b; Donnai, 1993; Healey et al., 1994). One example of phenotypic normality with UPD 14(mat) is on record (Papenhausen et al., 1995). In the setting of parental chromosomal normality, two karyotypic classes can be envisaged, one of which has been reported in a few cases, while the existence of the second is yet to be proven. (*1*) An apparently balanced de novo Robertsonian translocation, for example, 45,rob(13;14)(q10;q10). A meiotic origin is likely, but parental gonadal mosaicism cannot be excluded. In a future pregnancy, prenatal diagnosis would be discretionary. (Familial Robertsonian translocations are discussed in Chapter 6.) (*2*) An apparently normal karyotype in which the probable mechanism has been the postzygotic "correction" of an initially 47,+14 conception. The initial error was a meiotic nondisjunction. Recurrence would be, in theory, the remotest possibility.

Chromosome 15
See below under Conditions with More than One Cytogenetic Basis (Prader-Willi syndrome and Angelman syndrome).

Chromosome 16
A supposed syndrome of UPD 16 associated with intrauterine growth retardation may in fact be due to placental dysfunction consequent upon mosaic or complete trisomy 16 in the placenta (Kalousek et al., 1993; Kalousek and Barrett, 1994), although the possibility of an effect due to imprinting remains open (Whiteford et al., 1995).

Chromosome X
UPD X(pat) in one child with low-level 45,X/46,XX mosaicism was associated with marked short stature and possible gonadal dysfunction and otherwise "only a few indistinct Turner stigmata" (Schinzel et al., 1993). UPD X(mat) is apparently without effect (Avivi et al., 1992). Chu et al. (1994) propose a parent-of-origin effect in 45,X Turner syndrome.

Conditions with More Than One Genetic Basis

Chromosome 11: Beckwith-Wiedemann Syndrome

1. Uniparental Disomy 11
Most (about 85%) BWS arises sporadically, and, in a quarter or more of these cases, it is due to a mosaic segmental paternal UPD for distal 11p15 (Slatter et al., 1994). The UPD presumably causes a functional imbalance of the imprint status of the two No. 11 chromosomes. Hemihyperplasia is a clinical indicator of this category. Normally, there is an even mix of methylation at the *H19* locus, but in paternal UPD 11p the methylation index is >0.6, and this has been proposed as a simple confirmatory laboratory test (Reik et al., 1994). There is no known instance of recurrence of segmental UPD 11, and, as a postzygotic

event, we assume no increased risk would apply. (Some sporadic BWS with biparental disomy may have a similar functional basis, in which an "epigenetic accident" affecting the ovum or early conceptus leads to the expression of the *H19-IGF2* domain on the maternal chromosome 11 taking on a paternal pattern; Reik et al., 1995).

2. Balanced 11p Rearrangement

A reciprocal translocation or an inversion with one breakpoint in distal 11p can, if transmitted by a mother, lead to BWS (Weksberg et al., 1993b; Tommerup et al., 1993b; Elliott and Maher, 1994). The breakpoint is either close to (but not actually within) the *IGF2* locus at 11p15.5 or more proximally at 11p15.4. Speculatively, the rearrangement may have a "position effect" that alters the imprint status of the (or a) BWS gene on the maternally transmitted translocation chromosome. The female carrier will have an approximately even risk of transmitting the normal chromosome, or of the balanced translocation state. Imbalanced possible outcomes need to be assessed individually as for any translocation (Chapter 4).

3. Mendelian Mutation

Autosomal dominant BWS is recognized from the pedigree structure (vertical transmission, offspring only of female heterozygotes are affected, normal cytogenetics) (Moutou et al., 1992). Careful review of the pedigree is necessary to identify mildly affected individuals bearing in mind the amelioration of phenotype with time (Hunter and Allanson, 1994; Elliott et al., 1994). Phenotypic differences from sporadic BWS suggest the possibility of a different molecular pathogenesis in the familial form, and more than one locus may be involved (Weksberg et al., 1993a; Cohen, 1994; Nyström et al., 1994). An imprinting mutation is a possibility (Reik et al., 1995). The risk of transmitting a BWS gene is 50%; if it is transmitted, the BWS phenotype may be incomplete (*forme fruste*) or barely discernible.

4. Distal 11p Duplication

If the duplication chromosome is of paternal origin (Brown et al., 1992; Krajewska-Walasek et al., 1994), double expression of an 11p locus or loci may bring about the BWS phenotype. Functional trisomy of nonimprinted 11p segments may contribute to the phenotype. Kubota et al. (1994) describe a unique BWS case in which the distal 11p segment of a paternally originating de novo X-11 translocation escaped inactivation. See above under Duplication for comments on recurrence risk, according to the cytogenetics of the duplication.

Chromosome 15: Prader-Willi Syndrome

1. Classical Deletion q11–q13

About two-thirds to three-quarters of PWS is due to the simple deletion 46,del(15)(q11–13), in which 3 to 4 Mb of DNA is removed (Nicholls, 1993). The deletion is of paternal origin. No case of recurrence of PWS due to a classical deletion is on record. This empiric observation of zero recurrences out of some thousands of ''trials'' underscores the considerable unlikelihood of significant paternal gonadal mosaicism for the deletion observed in his PWS child. This is the basis of the substantial optimism that can be offered to parents in terms of any further pregnancies. A figure of around 0.1% may be a fair one to offer for the risk of recurrence, and the grounds for prenatal diagnosis are not pressing. In the context of CVS, note that the PW71 imprint is not expressed in chorionic villus, and that chorionic villus tissue is not suitable for high resolution cytogenetics. The PW71 methylation test can, however, be applied to amniotic fluid cells (H. R. Slater, pers. comm., 1995). The *SNRPN* exon -1 test (Glenn et al., 1996) may prove superior in prenatal diagnosis.

2. Uniparental Disomy 15
About 20% of PWS is due to maternal UPD 15 from a mother who is 46,N. We know of no recorded instance of recurrence of UPD PWS in a 46,N couple and would otherwise assume, on theoretical grounds, any increased risk in a future pregnancy to be negligible, the modest maternal age effect notwithstanding.

3. Uncommon Cytogenetically Detectable Rearrangement
The nature of the rearrangement (see the Biology section) and the parental karyotypes will determine the recurrence risk in each type. Prenatal diagnosis for the detection of a deletion or of UPD requires FISH or molecular methodology respectively.

4. Exceptional Defect
These rare cases of possible mutations in or microdeletions of the imprinting center will require individual expert advice. They can be suspected if a child is true to type clinically but there is neither classical deletion nor UPD demonstrable. Assuming the father carries the genetic defect, there is a high recurrence risk, namely, 50%. The problem is that some of these genetic defects may not be recognized as such; the methylation strategy described above, along with high-resolution cytogenetics, for example, in a child with an imprinting center defect, would give a result not distinguishable from UPD. New methodologies will surely be developed (Knoll et al., 1995). Very few imprinting-mutation cases are presently known (Buiting et al., 1995), although with the more widespread use of sophisticated technology, further examples will come to light.

Chromosome 15: Angelman Syndrome

1. Classical Deletion q11–q13
As for PWS, about two-thirds to three-quarters of AS is due to a large deletion, encompassing 3 to 4 Mb (Kuwano et al., 1992). No case is recorded of recurrence of a typically sized deletion and thus we presume, as for classical deletion-PWS, a very low recurrence risk. The comments on prenatal diagnosis in PWS (see above) apply similarly here.

2. Uniparental Disomy 15

AS due to paternal UPD 15 is rare (Saitoh et al., 1994), perhaps only 1 to 2% of all AS. Interestingly, the AS phenotype may be somewhat milder in UPD 15, and in some children it was only after an EEG showed typical findings that the diagnosis was suspected (Bottani et al., 1994). No recurrence is on record (Chan et al., 1993), and we assume on theoretical grounds no increased risk would exist.

3. Non-classical Deletion, Non-UPD

AS in which both a classical deletion and UPD have been excluded may be due (*1*) to a mutation in the (or a) AS gene itself, or (*2*) to loss (by microdeletion) or disabling (by mutation) of an imprinting center carried on the maternal No. 15 chromosome that prevents functioning of the AS gene(s) (see Biology section above). If a mother has had more than one affected AS child, the presence of a defect within one of these categories is actually demonstrated. A history of an AS child born to a female relative is also indicative (Meijers-Heijboer et al., 1992; Wagstaff et al., 1993). The risk for recurrence, assuming the maternal carrier state, is 50%.[5] In the case of an imprinting center defect, the methylation test is abnormal; this could be the basis of prenatal diagnosis at amniocentesis.

If the nonclassical deletion non-UPD AS child is a sporadic case, the picture is rather less clear (Saitoh et al., 1994). Without sophisticated study, we cannot be sure if this is due to the mother being a carrier of a structural or imprinting center mutation or microdeletion, if there has been a fresh mutation with the child, or whether some other mechanism has been operative. Analogous to PWS, an imprinting center defect would not be distinguishable from UPD simply on methylation testing and high-resolution cytogenetics. If the AS case is an only child, or if other children have the other maternal 15q11–13 haplotype, maternal heterozygosity for a mutation remains entirely possible. The risk is high (we cannot say exactly how high, but it may be close to 50%), and—if the clinical diagnosis is confidently based—prenatal diagnosis as for the known carrier (see above), with appropriate caveats, may be considered. If, on the other hand, a normal sib shares the same maternal 15q11–13 haplotype as the AS child, fresh mutation in the AS child is possible. In this setting, the empiric risk figure would be smaller; how much smaller we cannot presently say. Disconcertingly, maternal somatic-gonadal mosaicism for a microdeletion has been recognized (R. D. Nicholls, pers. comm., 1995). Alternatively, a genetically different basis for the child's condition—which is thus actually an AS phenocopy—could exist. This question of genetic heterogeneity remains open (and is crucially dependent upon accurate clinical diagnosis; Williams et al., 1995). However, the universal sharing of maternal No. 15 haplotypes in familial AS, so far, does indicate that at least much (and quite possibly all) ''nonclassical deletion non-UPD AS'' is due to abnormality at a locus or loci within the q11–13 region. This is a complex issue, and the counselor will need to keep abreast of current knowledge.

4. Uncommon Cytogenetically Detectable Rearrangement

The nature of the rearrangement (see the Biology section), and the parental karyotypes, will determine the recurrence risk in each type.

NOTES

1 This word can be, and is, used in the context of a single locus: for example, haplo-insufficiency of the peripheral myelin protein *PMP-22* locus, due to deletion of about 1.5 Mb of DNA within 17p11.2 that contains this gene, produces the peripheral neuropathy "hereditary pressure-sensitive palsy." It is usually applied in cytogenetics to the more recently delineated "microdeletion" syndromes, but can in principle refer to the classical syndromes with larger deletions. By the same token, the expression "triplo-excess" could be, but is not, used in the context of the duplication syndromes; and neither do we speak of the normal state as "diplo-sufficiency."

2 An aide-mémoire: *Pra*der-Willi due to *Pa*ternal *del*etion.

3 Thus, "microdeletion" in this context refers to a deletion that is smaller than the usual "classical PWS/AS microdeletion." A word like micromicrodeletion, or picodeletion, would have been clumsier, but perhaps less confusing.

4 Other possible explanations for phenotypic abnormality associated with UPD are mosaicism with a residual trisomic cell line in those cases resulting from postzygotic correction of trisomy, and fortuitous coincidence.

5 Since the mutation operates in *cis*, the affected chromosome can, in principle, be tracked by linked markers flanking the region. This would require that a DNA sample be available from the mother's AS child, or from an unaffected child of hers, in order to give the phase of linkage. If, at prenatal diagnosis, the high-risk marker-haplotype is transmitted (without recombination), it is probable the child would have AS, and conversely, transmission of the low-risk haplotype would indicate an unaffected child. However, an incomplete knowledge of the relative position of the mutation, along with a possible increased recombination rate within the 15q11–13 region (Robinson and Lalande, 1995; Christian et al., 1995), oblige considerable circumspection in this context.

18

The XY Female, the XX Male, and the True Hermaphrodite

The idea of an XY female and an XX male may seem a contradiction in terms. Yet to those who have studied the mechanics of sexual differentiation, perhaps what is more remarkable is that most of the time there is a clear association between being XX and female and being XY and male. The XX and XY embryo are built on a fundamentally similar outline plan, and only subsequently do certain modifications evolve. If at any point in this sequential process some genetic instruction is faulty, inappropriate, or cannot be acted on, the proper direction of sexual development may proceed imperfectly. In the extreme, the opposite path is taken. This latter state is the particular subject of this chapter.

BIOLOGY

Somewhat simplified, the fundamental plan of the genital tract is that bilateral gonads connect with bilateral paired internal ducts (Müllerian and Wolffian), which enter a midline genital sinus, opening at the perineum. This opening is buttressed on each side by labioscrotal folds and capped above by a phallus. Otherwise uninfluenced, the gonad inherently develops into an ovary, and the duct system develops into fallopian tubes and uterus. The genital sinus remains as an opening (the vagina), flanked and surmounted by labia and clitoris. But if a Y chromosome is present—or at least that part of the Y that contains *SRY*, the *s*ex-determining *r*egion *Y* gene, otherwise known as the testis-determining gene (Sinclair et al., 1990)—this inherent plan is modified. The *SRY* gene encodes a DNA-binding protein that initiates a cascade of activation of genes elsewhere in the genome that causes the primordial gonad to develop into a testis. Presumed examples of such genes are sex-reversing loci *SRVX* at Xp22.11–p21.1 (Arn et al., 1994), *SOX9* on 17q, and *DSS* at Xp21.3 (see below). The testis secretes hormones and influences the genital tract to masculinize. A vas deferens forms from the duct system. The phallus enlarges. The labioscrotal folds fuse in the midline and accommodate the descending testes.

XX Male

"XX males" arise either from the presence of Y material (rarely visible cytogenetically) or from the inappropriate activity of a gene that is normally switched on only after Y-originating genetic instruction. In about three-quarters of cases, the *SRY* gene is present, usually the consequence of an abnormal exchange between the X and Y during gametogenesis in their fathers (Weil et al., 1994; Wang et al., 1995). These are referred to as *SRY*⁺ XX males, the remainder being *SRY*⁻. The phenotype in the *SRY*⁺ XX male is similar to that of Klinefelter syndrome, presumably reflecting the similar basic genotypes of active X + inactive X + *SRY* in the two conditions; however, the XX male differs in being of normal height and of unimpaired intelligence (Ferguson-Smith et al., 1990). In these *SRY*⁺ XX males a more accurate designation would be 46,X,der(X)t(X; Y)—or more fully 46,X,der(X)t(X;Y)(p22.3;p11.2)—albeit the exchange is not usually visible on standard cytogenetics, and so we also refer to this entity in the section on the X;Y translocation (Chapter 5). Some XX males are actually XXY/XX mosaics in whom the XXY cells are difficult to demonstrate (Wachtel, 1994). XX males in whom no Y chromosomal material is demonstrable often have ambiguous external genitalia (Mittwoch, 1992).

45,X Male

We refer to this very rare disorder on p. 111. Most, in fact, have a "molecular translocation" of the *SRY* gene to an autosome or to the X chromosome (and might therefore be thought of as a type of Y;autosome or X;Y translocation), while a few are actually X/XY mosaics (de la Chapelle et al., 1986; Abbas et al., 1990; Weil, et al., 1993).

XY Female

XY Pure Gonadal Dysgenesis (Swyer Syndrome)
In its rare *familial* form, the classic modes of inheritance are apparent X-linked recessive and Y-linked. (*1*) In the X-linked forms (distinction from an autosomal form may not be possible), the XY female has a perfectly normal Y chromosome, with a normal *SRY* testis-determining gene; presumably, there is a mutation in an X-linked (or autosomal) gene controlling a later event in the testis developmental pathway. (*2*) In the Y-linked form, there is a mutation in *SRY*. In some Y hemizygotes, the mutant gene has nevertheless been able to reach a threshold of operation and to induce testis development, while in others it has not. Thus, for example, an XY male with a mutation in *SRY* may be a normal fertile man, while his XY child may be a daughter. The threshold is all-or-nothing: partial expression, that is, intersex, does not result (Jäger et al., 1992). A father may be a gonadal mosaic for an *SRY* deletion: Barbosa et al. (1995)

report two sisters with XY gonadal dysgenesis (one with gonadoblastoma) having deletion of *SRY*, but their father showed a normal *SRY* result; there were three other normal sisters and six normal brothers. Similarly, Schmitt-Ney et al. (1995) describe two XY sisters and a half-sister whose father was shown to be mosaic for an *SRY* mutation.

Sporadic occurrence is usual, and in about 10 to 20% of these the *SRY* gene has a de novo mutation which abolishes its function of testis determination (Hawkins, 1994). XY females with an intact *SRY* gene presumably have a mutation in one of the other genes in the testis-determining pathway.

The gonad in the XY female is dysgenetic and is seen as a "streak" gonad. (An extraordinary case is reported in Cussen and MacMahon [1979], of an XY girl from whose dysgenetic gonad an XY oocyte was obtained.) The genital tract feminizes. The lack of female sex hormones causes failure of normal pubertal development. Gonadoblastoma, a premalignant neoplastic change in the dysgenetic gonad, is common (Verp and Simpson, 1987). Amenorrhea and failure of pubertal development are the usual complaints that lead these girls to seek medical advice.

Complete Androgen Insensitivity Syndrome (Testicular Feminization)

Here, the defect lies further down the developmental path. The gonad becomes a testis, and produces testicular secretions, but the genital tract, internal and external, is resistant to the effects of these secretions. The inheritance is X-linked recessive, and in about 75% a defect in the androgen receptor gene at Xq11–13 is demonstrable (Morel et al., 1994). The individual who is 46,XY appears externally very much as a female, but there is amenorrhea and pubic and axillary hair is absent. Internally, the vagina is short, and only remnants of the uterus and tubes are to be seen. Malignancy of the gonad is uncommon but has been recognized (Rutgers and Scully, 1991).

XY Female with Extragonadal Defects

A number of rare conditions exist in which sex reversal coexists with physical, metabolic, and/or mental defect. One of these is *campomelic dysplasia with sex reversal,* a complex dominantly inherited syndrome of skeletal dysplasia (campomelia refers to long bone bowing) and other malformations; XY sex chromosomes can be associated with a female genital tract development. The usual cause is a mutation within the *SOX9* gene (in 17q24.3–25.1), one of the genes operating on the sexual differentiation pathway and which also influences limb bud mesenchymal development (Wagner et al., 1994); another cause is deletion in an apparently balanced translocation with haplo-insufficiency at the locus. A significant recurrence risk applies, on the order of 5%, which may include the etiologies of mildly affected transmitting parent, parental gonadal mosaicism, recessive phenocopy, and familial rearrangement involving 17q (Mansour et al., 1995).

A syndrome of *dosage sensitive sex reversal* inheres in a locus *DSS* at Xp21.3, a double dose of which in the 46,dup(X),Y genetic male leads to imperfect feminization; the abnormal phenotype otherwise presumably reflects a functional partial Xp disomy (Bardoni et al., 1994).

Steroid enzyme deficiencies comprise a very rare cause of female genital development in the genetic male. Defects of enzymes in the biochemical pathway of steroidogenesis perturb the production of androgenic hormones and cause defects in other steroid hormones (glucocorticoid, mineralocorticoid) that have crucially important physiological roles. Inheritance is autosomal recessive. We refer the reader to Zachmann (1994) for a full discussion.

Other Rare Forms of Gonadal Agenesis and Dysgenesis

In *XY (or XX) gonadal agenesis*, the gonads are absent, and the external phenotype is female. Presumably, an autosomal ''gonad development locus'' is involved in this very rare recessive condition (Mendonça et al., 1994). The distinct condition ''XX gonadal dysgenesis'' concerns, presumably, a different locus, in that females only are affected (Aittomäki, 1994); and the *embryonic testicular regression sequence*, which affects only males and comes under the rubric of XY gonadal dysgenesis (Marcantonio et al., 1994), has yet another genetic basis. There are rare disorders of *gonadal agenesis and extragonadal defects*, such as the syndrome of Kennerknecht et al. (1995) of agonadism in XY sisters with mental retardation, short stature, and several minor anomalies.

True Hermaphroditism

True hermaphroditism generally presents as a problem in determining the sex of a newborn infant—in other words, genital ambiguity. The formal definition of true hermaphroditism is that the gonads comprise both ovarian and testicular elements: there may be a testis and an ovary, or one or both may be an ovotestis. Interestingly, the most common karyotype is 46,XX, and almost all lack Y-chromosome sequences (Fechner et al., 1994). XX true hermaphroditism is unusually prevalent among Bantu-speaking Blacks in Southern Africa; Spurdle et al. (1995) excluded the presence of *SRY*, and of uniparental disomy X, in 16 out of 16 individuals studied. Inappropriate activation of the testicular developmental cascade at a post-*SRY* stage, in some parts of the gonad, is the likely basis in these SRY^- cases. Most of the remainder are accounted for by 46,XY and 46,XX/46,XY karyotypes; other sex chromosome mosaic or chimeric states are rare (Simpson, 1978; Green et al., 1994). The rare SRY^+ 46,XX cases may develop testicular and ovarian tissue according to whether the *SRY*-bearing X, or the normal X, is active in that part of the developing gonadal tissue (McElreavey et al., 1992; Fechner et al., 1994). Rare familial 46,XX cases may reflect the agency of a gene, whether autosomal or X-linked, that induces the testis developmental cascade to proceed at a post-*SRY* stage (Kuhnle et al., 1993). One 46,XY case had a post-zygotic mutation in *SRY* with SRY^+/SRY^- gonadal mosaicism (Braun et al., 1993). Presumably the SRY^+ line was responsible for the testicular elements in the gonad as was the SRY^- line for the ovarian elements.

GENETIC COUNSELING

XX Male

Given that many XX boys are not diagnosed until after childhood, by which time the parents are likely to have completed their family, requests for advice about recurrence will be rare. Some cases may be recognized at amniocentesis following discordant karyotypic and ultrasonographically observed genital sex, or following the birth of a boy who was predicted to have been a girl. The great majority of cases occur as a sporadic event, and the likelihood of recurrence is small. Given the rarity of the condition, sufficient data are not at hand to define exactly how small the likelihood is. In the absence of a family history of XX male or XX hermaphroditism, the figure probably lies in the range of 0.1 to 5%, and likely closer to 0.1% than to 5%. Molecular studies in some cases may permit a distinction between a sporadic case and one whose father's X chromosome contains an *SRY* gene, the latter implying a high genetic risk. It may be appropriate to consider prenatal diagnosis in the *SRY*$^+$ case. If the fetus is 46,XX, testing for *SRY* along with an ultrasonic assessment of external genital morphology should distinguish the affected case.

XY Pure Gonadal Dysgenesis

Typical XY gonadal dysgenesis, when *familial*, is classically inherited as an X-linked recessive. The risk to the known female heterozygote to have an affected child is, as for any X-linked recessive condition, 25%. She cannot be distinguished on any phenotypic basis, but only on her position in the pedigree as an obligate carrier. The risk to other female relatives is given by Bayesian analysis. Although the XY female phenotype is close to that of a normal female, some couples may want to consider prenatal diagnosis. The use of cytogenetics (XY) and ultrasound morphology (female external genitalia) would, presumably, allow detection of the condition.

Identification of a paternal *SRY* mutation would allow the counselor the rare opportunity to apply principles of Y-linked inheritance to risk estimation, incomplete penetrance of these mutations implying a figure below 50%. The specific mutation could be tested for at prenatal diagnosis.

Couples electing not to consider prenatal diagnosis (or to continue a pregnancy in which a positive diagnosis has been made) should know of the importance of two factors in managing these girls. *First*, the psychosexual orientation of these individuals is female. But with secondary sexual characteristics developing incompletely, and infertility being invariable, their self-image is vulnerable. In discussing the condition with parents, the counselor should note the importance of using language that reinforces their view of themselves as girls and women and avoid using such terms as "genetic male." It may be explained to them, beginning in simple terms in childhood, that a genetic factor prevented their ovaries from developing normally (Goodall, 1991). Pubertal development can be enhanced with hormonal treatment or, if the result is unsatisfactory, augmentation mammoplasty may be considered. Pregnancy has been achieved with in vitro fertilization and a donor ovum (Bianco et al., 1992). *Second*, there is a risk of neoplastic change in the dysgenetic gonad. A gonadoblastoma arises in around half of cases of familial XY gonadal dysgenesis. The gonadoblastoma itself is noninvasive, but it is often associated with malignant elements, most commonly dysgerminoma, which do invade. Thus, and given that the gonad does not usefully contribute in terms of hormone production, early (first decade) gonadectomy is advisable (Troche and Hernandez, 1986; Verp and Simpson, 1987).

Advice on the recurrence risk in the *sporadic* case is less straightforward. If a de novo *SRY* mutation is demonstrated, only paternal testicular mosaicism—which has, actually, been observed—could imply an increased risk for recurrence; a figure of <5% may be appropriate in this circumstance.

The rare syndromes of XY femaleness and extragonadal defects each need to be judged on their individual merits.

Complete Androgen Insensitivity (Testicular Feminization)

This condition is inherited as an X-linked recessive trait, and the risk of recurrence follows classic Mendelian principles. The carrier may be identified and prenatal diagnosis accomplished by direct mutation testing of the androgen receptor (AR) gene, or by linkage with an intragenic polymorphism (Quigley et al., 1992; Sultan et al., 1993; Morel et al., 1994). Issues relating to prenatal diagnosis are discussed in Morel et al. (who make the interesting but unsurprising point that incomplete forms can imply a worse burden than the complete form, with partially virilized males—"Reifenstein syndrome"—having "considerable psychological distress and poor function in their adult life"). Similar considerations with respect to gender orientation in the XY girl, as discussed in the preceding section, apply to complete androgen insensitivity. The risk for neoplastic change in the gonad is less (2–5%) in the case of testicular feminization; thus, some propose gonadectomy may reasonably be delayed to allow spontaneous pubertal feminization (Jones, 1978; Verp and Simpson, 1987).

True Hermaphroditism

Recurrence of true hermaphroditism within a family is on record, but it is rare. In some cases, the cytogenetics (46,XY, 46,XX/46,XY or other mosaic karyotype) or molecular genetics (*SRY* mutation not present in father) may allow a more secure reassurance of nonrecurrence. A positive family history would, of course, imply a high risk.

19

Chromosome Instability Syndromes

A defect of DNA repair underlies the chromosome instability syndromes, also known as chromosome breakage syndromes (Bartram, 1980; Bridges and Harnden, 1982; Taylor and McConville, 1992). Thus, they can be described as mutagen-hypersensitivity syndromes. The "instability" refers to the predisposition of the chromosomes to undergo rearrangement or to display other abnormal cytogenetic behavior. Their inclusion in this book is warranted in that special cytogenetic techniques have a role in clinical diagnosis and prenatal diagnosis.

The classic chromosome instability syndromes are Fanconi pancytopenia syndrome, ataxia-telangiectasia, and Bloom syndrome. The main cytogenetic features are listed in Table 19–1. They are Mendelian conditions, and in each the mode of inheritance is autosomal recessive. There is genetic heterogeneity in Fanconi syndrome, with cells homozygous for one mutation able to correct in vitro cells homozygous for another mutation ("complementation"). Heterozygotes for the three conditions may have an increased cancer susceptibility (Heim et al., 1992). We briefly note two other very rare mutagen-hypersensitivity syndromes, the Nijmegen breakage syndrome and the "ICF syndrome." Although no defect of DNA repair is known, Roberts syndrome, in which a cytogenetic anomaly (heterochromatin repulsion) may be a confirmatory diagnostic test, also rates a mention in this chapter.

Chromosome instability has been reported in certain other conditions including progeria, Rothmund-Thomson syndrome, Gorlin syndrome, Shwachman syndrome and the *v*ertebral, *a*nal, *c*ardiac, *t*racheal, *e*sophageal, *r*enal, and *l*imb (VACTERL) plus hydrocephalus association (Hecht and McCaw, 1977; Kaiser-McCaw, 1982; Szamosi et al., 1985; Tada et al., 1987; Wang et al., 1993), but they have yet to be accorded the status of an actual chromosome instability syndrome. Rare or unique families with various conditions have been associated with chromosomal instability (e.g., Webster et al., 1982; Byrne et al., 1984; Wegner et al., 1988; Tommerup et al., 1993c; Woods et al., 1995). In some other cancer-predisposing disorders such as Cockayne syndrome, xeroderma pigmentosum, and hereditary nonpolyposis colon cancer, DNA repair mechanisms

Table 19—1   The three classic chromosome instability syndromes

	Cytogenetic features	Prenatal diagnosis	References
Fanconi anemia	Increased spontaneous and inducible chromosome breakage	Yes	Auerbach et al., 1986; Auerbach, 1993; Giampietro et al., 1994
Ataxia-telangiectasia	Increase in chromosome breaks, presence of clones with translocations having specific breakpoints in 7, 14, and X; may be normal	Yes	Shaham et al., 1982; Schwartz et al., 1985; Gatti et al., 1993; Savitsky et al., 1995
Bloom syndrome	Increased spontaneous and inducible SCE; increase in spontaneous chromatid breakage with production of symmetrical quadriradials	Yes	Ray and German, 1981; Weksberg et al., 1986; German, 1993; Howell and Davies, 1994

are faulty, but no abnormality is manifest at the cytogenetic level. Heterochromatin repulsion may also characterize Baller-Gerold syndrome (Huson et al., 1990). We do not discuss these conditions further, other than to note that atypical forms of Fanconi anemia may account for some of them.

GENETICS

All of the classic chromosomal breakage syndromes, as well as the Nijmegen breakage syndrome and the ''ICF syndrome'', are of autosomal recessive inheritance, and the recurrence risk, for parents who have had one affected child, is one in four.

LABORATORY DIAGNOSIS AND PRENATAL DIAGNOSIS

Fanconi Anemia/Pancytopenia Syndrome

This uncommon disorder of protean manifestation is the least rare of the breakage syndromes. Originally described as a disorder of short stature, characteristic facies, and certain malformations along with progressive bone marrow failure, the picture has now widened (Schroeder et al., 1989; Auerbach, 1993; Giampietro et al., 1994). Chromosomes show a range of abnormalities, including an increase in chromosome breakage, both spontaneously and, in particular, upon exposure to DNA cross-linking agents (Figure 19–1); the fault may lie in a propensity to aberrant cleaving of DNA at specific sites (Laquerbe et al., 1995). The increase in chromosome breakage after exposure of cells to the cross-linking agent diepoxybutane (DEB) provides a reliable diagnostic test (Auerbach et al., 1985; Auerbach, 1987, 1993).

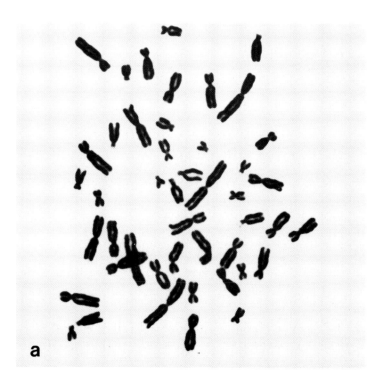

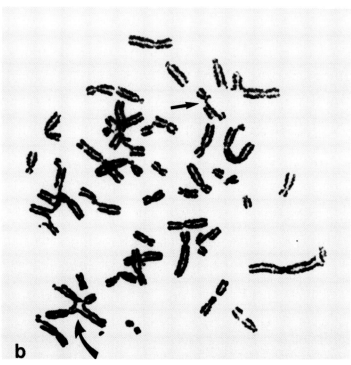

FIGURE 19–1. Metaphase from (*a*) a control and (*b*) a patient with Fanconi anemia after exposure to diepoxybutane. Note the high level of chromatid breakage in the patient metaphase. One chromatid break is shown (straight arrow), and a quadriradial figure is indicated (curved arrow).

There are at least four genetic complementation groups for Fanconi pancytopenia syndrome, groups A, B, C, and D. The gene for one of these (*FACC*, complementation group C) has been cloned (Strathdee et al., 1992a, b), and maps to 9q22.3. Group C comprises about 8 to 14% of all Fanconi syndrome, with different *FACC* mutations causing different degrees of disease severity (Verlander et al., 1994; Gibson et al., 1994). The FAC protein may have roles in controlling the cell-cycle control factor p53 and in influencing DNA activation (Liebetrau et al., 1995). The *FACA* locus, accounting for about two-thirds of all FA, maps to 16q24.3, and the *FACD* locus maps to 3p22-p26 (Pronk et al., 1995; Whitney et al., 1995).

Prenatal diagnosis by mutation detection will be possible in some cases of complementation group C Fanconi syndrome. Otherwise, DEB-induced chromosome breakage in amniotic fluid or chorionic villus cells provides a satisfactory approach (Auerbach et al., 1986).

Ataxia-Telangiectasia

Ataxia-telangiectasia (AT) is a rare disease characterized by cerebellar ataxia, oculocutaneous telangiectasia, immunodeficiency, and increased cancer predisposition with sensitivity to ionizing radiation and radiomimetic chemicals (Shiloh, 1995). The cytogenetic hallmarks of AT are: *(1)* the frequent presence of nonrandom rearrangements of chromosomes 7, 14, and occasionally X in T lymphocytes; nonspecific chromosome breakage in fibroblasts; normal chromosomes in bone marrow; *(2)* telomeric fusions in some persons (these are not tissue specific); *(3)* increased vulnerability of chromosomes when cells are exposed to ionizing radiation and radiomimetic chemicals such as bleomycin (Kojis et al., 1991).

At least most, and probably all AT is due to homozygosity or compound heterozygosity for a recessive gene *ATM* (AT mutated) whose locus is at 11q22.3 (Savitsky et al., 1995). This locus homogeneity had been somewhat obscured by the existence of ''complementation groups'' assigned according to in vitro cellular phenotypes in response to radiation; in fact, different complementation groups can have the identical genotype. The *ATM* gene appears to have key roles in the control of the cell cycle, response to DNA damage, and in pathways mediating immune responses of the lymphocyte.[1]

Prenatal diagnosis is in principle possible by using flanking markers (Gatti et al., 1993) or by direct mutation analysis on chorionic villus tissue or amniocytes. The molecular approach will, surely, supplant the cytogenetic methodology based upon a variety of cellular markers and in vitro response to irradiation as outlined by Auerbach (1987) and Llerena et al. (1989).

Bloom Syndrome

Bloom syndrome (BS) is a rare disorder which has its highest prevalence in Ashkenazi Jews but occurs in many other ethnic groups. It is characterized clinically by proportionate short stature, a characteristic facies, sun sensitive skin rash, immunodeficiency, and a marked susceptibility to cancer (German, 1993). Infertility seems to be invariable in the male; females have difficulty conceiving, but a few have given birth (Martin et al., 1994c). BS shows no complementation and is presumably due to a single gene (Weksberg et al., 1988). This gene has been mapped to 15q25-qter by the elegant approach of determining the region of isodisomy in a child with BS and concomitant Prader-Willi syndrome due to uniparental disomy 15 (Woodage et al., 1994).

The diagnostic cytogenetic finding in this condition is a markedly increased level of spontaneous sister chromatid exchange (SCE). The normal is 6 to 10 per cell; in BS, it is more than 50 per cell (Figure 19-2). In lymphocyte cultures there can be a mixture of cells with high and normal SCE frequencies whereas fibroblasts always show high SCE levels (Weksberg et al., 1986). The other cytogenetic abnormality is an increased incidence of spontaneous chromatid aberrations, giving the classic symmetrical quadriradial configuration. Intriguingly, this effect can manifest in the haploid state, with the heterozygous male producing an excess of sperm with chromosome breaks and rearrangements (Martin et al., 1994c).

Prenatal diagnosis should be possible with cytogenetics (Weksberg et al., 1988). Although about 16 at-risk pregnancies have been monitored, only one affected fetus has yet been diagnosed (German, pers. comm., 1994; Howell and Davies, 1994). For the affected individual's reproductive outlook (in those few surviving to adulthood), the standard Mendelian advice, with consideration of the likelihood of the spouse being heterozygous, applies. Three women with BS have had a normal child; the affected males are infertile (German, 1993).

Nijmegen Breakage Syndrome

This very rare syndrome of microcephaly, immune deficiency, and risk for lymphoreticular malignancy shares with ataxia-telangiectasia certain cytogenetic features (preferential involvement of chromosomes 7 and 14 in rearrangements) and radiation hypersensitivity (Taalman et al., 1983). Complementation studies show it to be a distinct disorder (Jaspers et al., 1988).

Roberts Syndrome

Roberts syndrome (RS) is a syndrome of craniofacial abnormalities and limb defects, usually severe (Maserati et al., 1991). Intellect is normal. It has been interpreted as a human mitotic mutation syndrome which leads to secondary developmental defects (Van Den Berg and Francke, 1993). Most affected individuals (about 80%) exhibit a chromosomal phenomenon known as "heterochromatin repulsion" (HR) (also referred to as premature centromere separation); those not showing this sign may represent a different complementation group (Allingham-Hawkins and Tomkins, 1995). There is an abnormality of sister chromatid apposition around the centromeres, particularly noticeable for those chromosomes with large blocks of heterochromatin (Figure 19–3). It is best seen in plain stained or C-banded chromosomes; G-banding obscures the phenomenon (Van Den Berg and Francke, 1993).

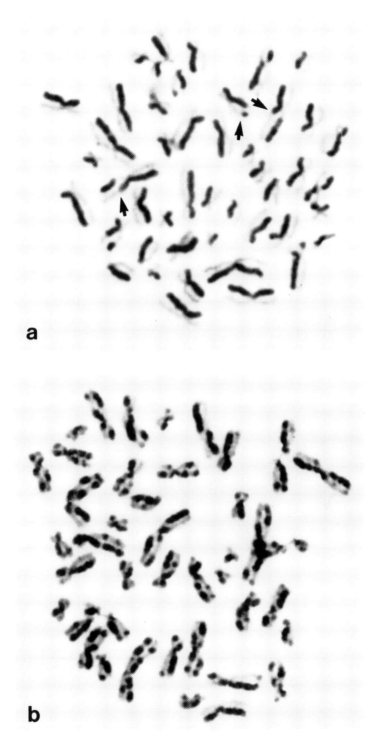

FIGURE 19–2. Metaphase from (*a*) a control and (*b*) a patient with Bloom syndrome, showing very high sister chromatid exchange (SCE) in the latter. Three points of SCE are indicated (arrows) on the control metaphase.

305

Prenatal diagnosis by HR can only be inclusive; absence of HR would not necessarily exclude RS in a pregnancy at risk. A combination of cytogenetics (on chorion villus or amniotic fluid cells) and ultrasound should detect most cases (Stioui et al., 1992). However, the case of Van Den Berg and Francke (1993) is salutary: ultrasound anomalies (decelerating growth of long bones and multiple cysts in one kidney) were not detected until 31 weeks' gestation and the mildly affected infant had growth retardation and hemangioma.

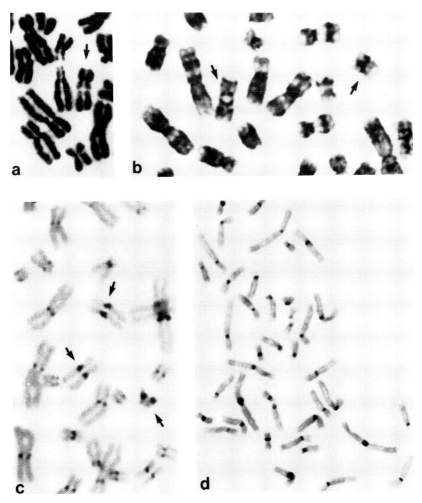

FIGURE 19–3. Unusual appearance of the chromosomes in Roberts syndrome: puffing at the centromeres (a, b); a C-banded preparation showing separation of the heterochromatic segments (c) is compared with a C-banded preparation from a control showing the normal centromere appearance (d). (Reproduced from Mann et al., 1982, with the permission of the British Medical Association.)

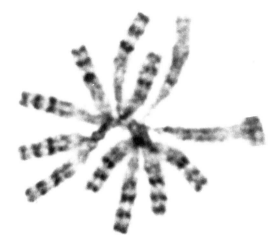

FIGURE 19–4. A "windmill" multiradial No. 1 chromosome in the ICF syndrome. From Sawyer, J. R., Swanson, C. M., Wheeler, G. and Cunniff, C. (1995). Chromosome instability in ICF syndrome: formation of micronuclei from multibranched chromosomes 1 demonstrated by fluorescence in situ hybridization. *Am J Med Genet*, 56, 203–209, © Am J Med Genet 1995, courtesy J. R. Sawyer, and with the permission of Wiley-Liss, Inc., a subsidiary of John Wiley & Sons, Inc.

ICF (Immunodeficiency, Centromeric Instability, Facial Anomalies) Syndrome

The extremely rare ICF syndrome is characterized by immunodeficiency, an unusual facies, growth and developmental retardation, and a most remarkable tendency of certain chromosomes, mostly Nos. 1, 9, and 16, to form "windmill" multiradials by interchange within heterochromatic regions, possibly a consequence of hypomethylation of satellite DNA (Smeets et al., 1994; Miniou et al., 1994; Sawyer et al., 1995) (Figure 19–4). Franceschini et al. (1995) document the variability of the phenotypic range. No case of prenatal diagnosis is on record.

NOTE

1. It is proposed that AT heterozygotes have a predisposition to cancer, with possibly a three to fourfold increased risk in general, and a fivefold risk for breast cancer in women (Savitsky et al., 1995). Now that the gene has been identified, the nature of this risk should become clearer.

REPRODUCTIVE FAILURE

20

Pregnancy Loss and Infertility

Human conception and pregnancy is both a vulnerable and a robust process. Vulnerable, in that a remarkably large proportion of all pregnancies are chromosomally abnormal, with the great majority of these aborting; robust, in that more than 99% of the time, a term pregnancy results in a chromosomally normal baby. The human species is comparatively inefficient at producing gametes. But the cost is not horrendous; it is measured largely in terms of miscarriage. The occasional chromosomally abnormal child is, relatively speaking, an exceptional outcome—the tip of the iceberg (Figure 20–1).

BIOLOGY

Chromosome Abnormality in Gametes and Conceptions

How may we study the cytogenetics of pregnancy? Before conception, the gamete whose chromosomes are most readily analyzable is the sperm. Sperm karyotyping is done with the ''humster'' (human sperm + hamster ovum pseudofertilization) test, and chromosome counts can be made directly on sperm using fluorescence in situ hybridization (FISH) analysis. The mean frequency of aneuploidy is estimated at 3 to 4% from sperm karyotyping, with another 10% having structural chromosome abnormalities (Martin et al., 1991). Sperm chromosome analysis by FISH is an evolving technique, prone to artifactual confounding, and a clear picture is yet to be drawn (Williams et al., 1993; Miharu et al., 1994; Guttenbach et al., 1994b,c; Martin et al., 1994a; Bischoff et al., 1994). Using three-color FISH (which distinguishes diploidy and disomy), diploidy (46,XY, 46,XX, 46,YY) is seen in 0.1 to 0.5% of sperm, while disomy rates for chromosomes X, Y and 1 are in the range 0.04 to 0.4%, 0.01 to 0.1%, and 0.2% respectively (Chevret et al., 1995).

The chromosomes of the oocyte can be examined in ova following induced ovulation. Such data are scanty, and subject to some doubt; the

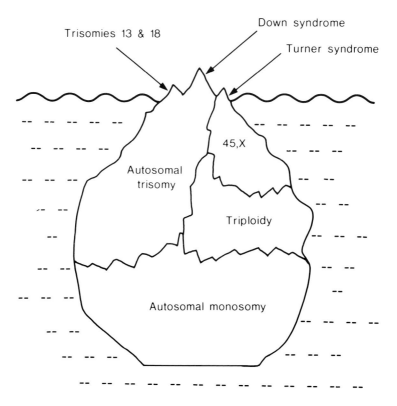

FIGURE 20–1.   The iceberg of chromosomal pregnancy loss.

women sampled are of older maternal age, the process of stimulating ovulation might itself cause nondisjunction, and the oocytes analyzed are those which failed to fertilize (''leftover oocytes'') (Hook, 1992; Hassold et al., 1993). Pellestor (1991) reviewed 14 studies: the frequency of aneuploidy ranged from 3% to 57%, and the three largest series showed somewhat better agreement (21%, 24%, and 27%). Kamiguchi et al. (1993) consider these figures artifactual overestimates; their improved technique gave the lower rate of 11%. Hassold et al. (1993) note that in four studies of unstimulated oocytes (which may better reflect nature) aneuploidy rates were 1.5%, 0%, 3%, and 20% respectively.

An aneuploid gamete (nullisomic or disomic) will lead to an aneuploid conceptus (monosomic or trisomic). Two gametes that are coincidentally nullisomic and disomic will engender uniparental disomy at conception. A diploid gamete, meeting a normal gamete, will give rise to a triploid conceptus. Triploidy may also result from dispermy (two sperm fertilizing the one ovum). An abnormal cell division occurring after the time of fertilization (post-zygotic) can give rise to mosaicism.

Our knowledge of the frequency of chromosome abnormalities in early human conceptions[1] has come mainly from the analysis of ''spare'' preimplantation embryos produced at in vitro fertilization, possibly unrepresentative material. Zenzes and Casper (1992) reviewed the small body of literature. In four studies, chromosome abnormalities were identified in from 23% to 40% of embryos. The 24 abnormals included monosomy, trisomy, double trisomy, haploidy, multiple nullisomies, mosaic monosomy/trisomy, diploid/triploid mosaicism, and tetraploidy (and two with 47,XXY).

Nonimplantation and Occult Abortion

Some genetic imbalances are so devastating that even the first few cell divisions are fatally compromised, leaving the conceptus unable to implant. Most, perhaps almost all, very early conceptions that undergo spontaneous developmental arrest are likely to be chromosomally abnormal (Munné et al., 1994). Polyploidy, including mosaic polyploidy, and autosomal monosomy are frequent. Some imbalances may allow development to the blastocyst stage, with transient implantation, but the conceptus is then cast off some time within the first 2 weeks. There may be little or no perturbation of the menstrual cycle, although the woman may feel pregnant. This is "occult abortion" (Miller et al., 1980; Craft et al., 1982).

Miscarriage (Spontaneous Abortion)

Further on in pregnancy, we have a much better idea of how many conceptuses are chromosomally abnormal and what the abnormalities are. Of all recognized pregnancies, about 10 to 15% end in clinical miscarriage ("spontaneous abortion"), mostly in the first trimester. Embryonic/fetal tissue recovered from the products of conception may be successfully cultured and karyotyped. Around half such abortuses have a chromosome abnormality (Figure 20–2). The two most common are 47,+16 and 45,X. All the trisomies, except for 47,+1, have been seen, and they account for about 60% of all abnormalities. Mosaic autosomal trisomy is uncommon. Monosomy X and polyploidy (mostly triploidy) account for approximately 20% and 15%, respectively. Structural rearrangements constitute most of the remainder.

The great majority of these chromosomally abnormal pregnancies abort at between 8 and 16 weeks' gestation. A few may remain beyond this time and be lost as a later abortion (presenting clinically as intrauterine fetal death) or as a perinatal death (i.e., stillbirth or early neonatal death). A representative of this latter group is 47,+18. Among liveborn babies, only 1 in 250 has an unbalanced chromosome abnormality. Thus, there has been a very effective natural selection against those large numbers of gametes and conceptions that were abnormal (Figure 20–3).

A fetus may or may not be identifiable in the products of conception collected at the time of spontaneous abortion due to chromosomal abnormality. Sometimes growth arrest occurs, with perhaps just an amorphous nubbin of tissue to be found within an otherwise fluid-filled gestational sac (blighted ovum or empty sac). In one small study of miscarriage with blighted ovum or missed abortion,

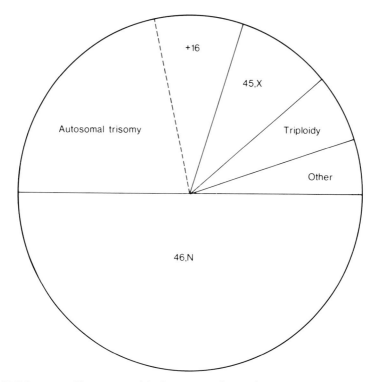

FIGURE 20–2. Chromosomal findings in products of conception from spontaneous abortion. (After Kajii et al., 1980.)

culture of chorionic villi showed aneuploidy in 19 out of 19 cases (Sorokin et al., 1991). In other miscarriages, recognizable fetal parts are present, but with greater or lesser morphological distortion (e.g., Figure 20–4). Warburton et al. (1991) provide a graphic catalog of embryonic/fetal phenotypes from their material of about 1300 karyotypically abnormal spontaneous abortuses collected over a 12-year period in New York State. What actually leads to expulsion of the conceptus from the uterus may be the declining vascular and endocrine function of the placental tissue, with decidual necrosis (i.e., death of tissue) finally causing uterine irritation and contraction (Rushton, 1981). Thomas (1995) suggests that genomic imprinting—"a phenomenon in search of a reason"— might be a mechanism that facilitates the detection and rejection of a trisomic embryo. If an abnormal twin dies the normal twin may ensure continuation of the pregnancy, and only a parchment-like vestige (*fetus papyraceous*) remains, preserved in the uterus along with the normal twin. In the specific case of monosomy X, Canki et al. (1988) document four different phenotypes: sac with no umbilical cord site; sac with umbilical cord having a fragment of embryonic tissue at its end; deformed embryos of 12–13 weeks' gestation but only 7 weeks developmental age; and second trimester fetuses with cystic hygroma and other tissue fluid accumulation, several having vascular defects.

A ''vanishing twin'' has plausibly been proposed in the study of a pregnancy in which two cell lines were identified at CVS, 46,XX and 47,XY,+9. Amniocentesis gave a 46,XX result, and a normal girl was subsequently born. Analysis of a fibrotic area of the placenta gave the same two karyotypes, 46,XX and 47,XY,+9 (Falik-Borenstein et al., 1994). The likely explanation is that a 47,XY,+9 co-conceptus died, and the fibrotic placental tissue was the only remnant.

Confined Placental Mosaicism

A chromosome abnormality may be present in a pregnancy but not involve the embryo/fetus. In the first week postconception, only a few cells are destined to give rise to the embryo proper; thus a postzygotic nondisjunction leading to the establishment of, say, a trisomic cell line may contribute to the growth of only the extraembryonic membranes (chorion and amnion). Therefore, the placenta may come to be aneuploid, while the fetus is normal (''confined placental mosaicism''). A trisomic placenta may be structurally and functionally abnormal, possibly leading to loss of the (normal) fetus, although this is controversial (see p. 354). The presence of a normal cell line in the placenta, the fetus being abnormal, may promote survival in some aneuploidies (monosomy X, trisomy 18) (Held et al., 1992; Harrison et al., 1993; Robinson et al., 1995a). Trisomy

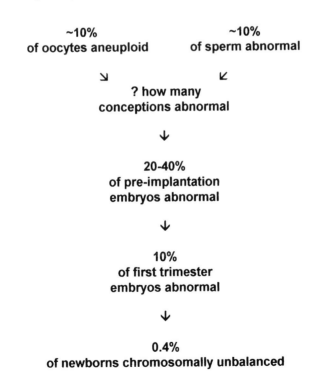

~10%
of oocytes aneuploid

~10%
of sperm abnormal

? how many
conceptions abnormal

↓

20-40%
of pre-implantation
embryos abnormal

↓

10%
of first trimester
embryos abnormal

↓

0.4%
of newborns chromosomally unbalanced

FIGURE 20–3. The frequency of chromosome abnormalities at gametogenesis and during pregnancy, demonstrating the effectiveness of natural selection.

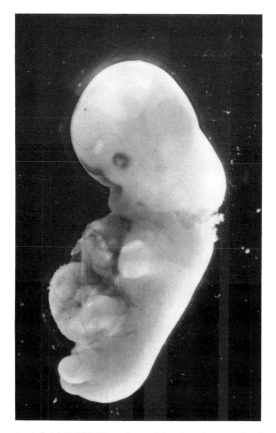

FIGURE 20–4.   A triploid (69,XXY) embryo. The face has no landmarks other than eyes and a single opening. The anterior trunk is open, with the heart and liver visible. Spontaneous abortion occurred at 18 weeks' gestation, but the length is that of 6 to 7 weeks' gestation. The disrupted tissue at the neck was the site of biopsy for the cytogenetic analysis.

20 may be a particular aneuploidy that can involve the amnion, the fetus and chorion being chromosomally normal (Baldinger et al., 1987).

Parental Chromosomes

The vast majority of chromosomally abnormal pregnancy loss occurs to chromosomally normal parents, and the chromosome abnormality is presumed to have arisen, as a sporadic event, in gametogenesis. Maternal meiosis I may be the most vulnerable stage. Hassold et al. (1993) studied trisomic miscarriages in couples and concluded that randomness rather than individual biological predisposition lay behind these nondisjunctions. Sperm chromosome studies show no significant differences in aneuploidy rates between fertile and subfertile men (Miharu et al., 1994). Drugan et al. (1990b) proffered tentative evidence to the contrary: in a group of 305 couples having had recurrent miscarriage and currently pregnant, the incidence of aneuploidy (monosomy X, trisomies 13, 18, 21) at amniocentesis or at birth was a little higher than in a control group.

For the small group of people who are heterozygous for a chromosomal rearrangement, pregnancy loss occurs with a much higher frequency, this loss being the usual reason for their coming to cytogenetic analysis. In around 2 to 5% of couples in which the woman has had two or more spontaneous abortions, one or other of the couple, more often the woman, is a translocation or inversion carrier (Campana et al., 1986; Bourrouillou et al., 1986; Castle and Bernstein, 1988). Simpson et al. (1989) suggest there may be a biased selection in some studies, and in a purely obstetric–gynecologic referral base in which a karyotype is done as a first-up investigation, the fraction may be rather less, around 0.5%. The translocation is more often reciprocal than Robertsonian.

Hydatidiform Mole

Hydatidiform mole is an abnormal pregnancy that is, in a sense, a male chromosomal disorder: there is either a completely paternal karyotypic origin (two haploid paternal sets, $2n = 46$) or an additional male haploid set (one maternal and two paternal haploid sets, $3n = 69$). The chorionic villi undergo a degenerative hydropic (fluid-filled) change, looking rather like grapes (hence, *hydatidiform*; the word *mole* means mass); this phenotype is marked ("complete mole") when the genetic origin is completely paternal, and attenuated ("partial mole") in the presence of a maternal haploid contribution.

Complete Mole

The complete form usually has the karyotype 46,XX looking, at first sight, like a normal female karyotype. This is due, in most, to a doubling of the chromosomal complement of a (normal) 23,X sperm, while a minority are dispermic (Lawler et al., 1991). Rare 46,XY moles are of dispermic origin. In consequence, the mole's nuclear genome is of entirely paternal origin: a complete uniparental paternal disomy ("uniparental diploidy"). Moles due to doubling of a sperm complement are entirely homozygous; in other words, they have a complete uniparental isodisomy. Perhaps this doubling represents an attempt by the sperm, albeit a forlorn one, to correct the situation when it enters an "effectively empty egg," that is, an ovum in which the integrity of the nuclear structure has broken down. This nuclear failure occurs more often at the beginning and end of reproductive life in the female (Bagshawe and Lawler, 1982); complete mole is more common in the early teenager and in women in their 40s.

The complete mole usually presents with vaginal bleeding, and ultrasonography shows a vesicular pattern of the placenta reflecting the swollen villi. There is a widespread and marked hyperplasia of the trophoblast, and no fetal elements are identifiable. The incidence of complete mole is about 1 in 2000 diagnosed pregnancies, although regional variations exist (La Vecchia et al., 1985; Jeffers et al., 1993; Palmer, 1994).

There is a small but significant risk of recurrence, and there are several recorded observations of women having had three or more complete moles. Edwards et al. (1990) studied a couple who had had four pregnancies, over 8 years, all four being complete moles; 14 oocytes fertilized in vitro showed abnormal behavior of the pronuclei, which may have reflected an intrinsic defect of the second meiotic spindle.

Partial Mole

An additional paternal haploid chromosome set is the basis of most cases of partial mole. This is triploidy, 69,XXX or 69,XXY, which is the result of a normal ovum fertilized either with two sperm (dispermy) or with a diploid sperm (Lawler et al., 1991; McFadden et al., 1993). The double paternal contribution is referred to as "diandry." Partial moles have a focal and not so pronounced trophoblastic hyperplasia and hydatidiform change of some villi, and the placenta is abnormally large. It is underdiagnosed and may occur in as many as 1 in 700 pregnancies (a figure Jeffers et al., 1993, derive from a review of all 2251 spontaneous abortions occurring in the catchment population of a Dublin hospital over a 3 year period during which there were 19,457 recorded pregnancies). The usual presentation is of threatened, incomplete, or missed abortion; fetal development, in the very few cases proceeding far enough for this to be assessed, is characterized by a relatively normal growth pattern (McFadden et al., 1993). If the triploidy is confined to the placenta, it is possible for the pregnancy to proceed successfully to the birth of a 46,N child (Sarno et al., 1993).

> The placenta in triploidy due to "digyny," from a diploid ovum, is nonmolar and abnormally small, and the fetal phenotype is of a severe growth retardation of the body with relative sparing of head size. Extremely rarely, such pregnancies may continue through to the third trimester; the baby inevitably is stillborn or dies very early. The different phenotypes of diandric and digynic triploidy may reflect a parental imprinting effect (McFadden et al., 1993; Haig, 1993).

An uncommon variant type of partial mole has a normal diploid karyotype, with both maternal and paternal contributions (Vejerslev et al., 1991); uniparental disomy at critical loci with overexpression of paternal alleles may be the basis (Lage et al., 1992).

GENETIC COUNSELING

Miscarriage (Spontaneous Abortion)

People who have had one or two miscarriages generally do not come to a genetic clinic, nor would it be appropriate for them to do so. Their physician or obstetrician will have advised them that this loss will very likely be part of the 15% or so of all pregnancies that miscarry, and the chance of a successful pregnancy in the future would be good. But having three miscarriages requires investigation. To use the jargon, such couples have had "multiple abortions" or "recurrent miscarriage."

The usual gynecological investigations and a chromosome analysis of the couple should be done at this point. If a chromosomal rearrangement is identified, this could well be the underlying cause (Gadow et al., 1991), but it might be a fortuitous discovery. The precise nature of the rearrangement (consult the appropriate chapter), the reproductive history of any others in the family who have it, and the presence or absence of gynecological pathology allow one to determine whether it was virtually certainly the cause, highly likely, or just a possible cause.

Most couples, however, karyotype as 46,XX and 46,XY. In most centers, cytogenetic analysis of abortus material is not routinely done, and so chromosomal normality or abnormality is not usually able to be demonstrated. This is not unreasonable, since demonstration of an abnormality (prior likelihood, 50%) generally makes no practical difference to management (which is not to say that the woman might not find it helpful to have an actual cause shown for the pregnancy loss), and culture of products of conception is time–consuming and expensive. Warburton et al. (1987) concluded that "repeat abortion is much more likely to be due to factors leading to loss of chromosomally *normal* [our italics] conceptions. Thus, when parental karyotypes are known to be normal, [previous recurrent abortion] should not be an indication for prenatal diagnosis". This viewpoint is consonant with the conclusion of Hassold et al. (1993), although not of Drugan et al. (1990b), noted above.

Some laboratories do offer routine karyotyping of "products of conception." If an aneuploidy for chromosome 13, 18, 21, or X is identified, in the setting of normal parental karyotypes, it may be that this is equivalent to having had a child with such a trisomy. Otherwise, Warburton et al. (1987) and Morton et al. (1987) conclude that a chromosomally abnormal abortion, the parents being chromosomally normal, implies minimal or no increased genetic risk for a future pregnancy. Perhaps only in the case of trisomy 21 should prenatal diagnosis in a subsequent pregnancy actually be recommended (notwithstanding, some couples are likely to request prenatal diagnosis for reassurance in the setting of a documented previous aneuploid miscarriage).

Infertility

Infertility comprises the inability to achieve conception or the inability to sustain a pregnancy through to livebirth (the latter known also as "infecundity"). Many causes exist involving the male (Skakkebæk et al., 1994) and the female (Healy et al., 1994) partner. A blood chromosome test is an important part of an infertility investigation, particularly in the azoospermic or severely oligospermic male of whom 12% are karyotypically abnormal (De Braekeleer and Dao, 1991). Sex chromosomal defects include XXY and XXY/XY in the male, and Turner syndrome and its variants in the female. The XX male and XY female are rare (Chapter 18). Autosomal abnormalities are infrequently seen as a cause of infertility (p. 24). Complex rearrangements (Chapter 11) and rings (Chapter 10) often present an insurmountable obstacle to cell division in the spermatocyte, resulting in azoospermia. (Oogenesis is apparently less vulnerable.) Likewise, the reciprocal translocation (especially when an acrocentric is involved) and the inversion may be associated, though infrequently, with spermatogenic arrest (Chapters 4 and 8). Some Robertsonian translocations may be associated with male infertility; it is unclear, in an individual case, whether the association is causal or fortuitous (Chapter 6). Translocation between a sex chromosome and an autosome, particularly when an X breakpoint is in the critical region, is a rarely identified cause of infertility (Chapter 5).

Intrinsic fertility cannot be restored in these azoospermic men and anovulatory women. Demonstrating a chromosomal cause of the infertility is useful because it provides an explanation and prevents the disappointment resulting from undergoing fertility treatment that has no chance of success. Artificial insemination using donor semen in the case of male infertility, and possibly in vitro fertilization (IVF) using donor ova for female infertility (Bianco et al., 1992), may be appropriate means of achieving the desired goal of having a child (discussed further vis-à-vis Turner syndrome, p. 200).

Chandley and Cooke (1994) suggest as much as 10% of azoospermia may be due to cytogenetically visible deletions or microdeletions involving Yq11.23. Loss of a gene YRRM, or more probably DAZ (deleted in azoospermia; Reijo et al., 1995), both of which are Y chromosome RNA recognition motif genes, may be the crucial defect. Molecular analysis of YRRM and DAZ may come to be a routine part of male infertility investigation. Other Y-borne loci controlling aspects of testicular structure and function within this region may also have a role (Kobayashi et al., 1994). If a Y-linked defect produces oligospermia, rather than complete failure of spermatogenesis, IVF with microinjection of sperm into an oocyte may be a means to achieve pregnancy. Couples choosing this option should know that, in this context, a male child might be predicted to have the same type of infertility (Liebaers et al., 1995). A possible small increased risk for a sex chromosome aneuploidy following sperm injection is the subject of debate (Liebaers et al., 1995, et seq.).

Hydatidiform Mole

Berkowitz et al. (1994) report a 27 year experience in following 1205 women having had a complete mole and 149 having had a partial mole (not distinguishing diandric and digynic partial moles). Given the different genetic etiologies, it is interesting (and suggests an underlying similar genetic predisposition) that the risk of recurrence is similar for either type of mole and that a recurrence can be either of the same or of the other type. The risk figure is 1 to 1.5%. Ultrasonographic surveillance is advisable in a future pregnancy and consideration can be given to cytogenetic testing and to beta hCG (human chorionic gonadotrophin) testing (Cole, 1994).

In Berkowitz et al.'s (1994) series, 24 women having previously had two molar pregnancies had yet another, for a risk figure of 20% to have a third mole. Multiple recurrence of partial mole may be characteristic of the diploid, biparental category (Vejerslev et al., 1991; Sunde et al., 1993; Jeffers et al., 1993). Kircheisen and Schroeder-Kurth (1991) report three sisters having had seven molar pregnancies between them, both complete and partial, and none with a normal child; and the woman having had four successive complete moles in Edwards et al. (1990) is noted above in the Biology section. There is no increased risk for other abnormal pregnancy outcome, and in particular the incidence of congenital malformations is no greater.

Malignancy

A major aspect of management is that the *complete mole* may undergo neoplastic transformation into a choriocarcinoma (gestational trophoblastic tumor). When a mole is diagnosed, prompt evacuation of the uterus is necessary; if preservation of fertility is not a concern, hysterectomy may reduce the risk of gestational trophoblastic tumor (Goldstein and Berkowitz, 1994). Choriocarcinoma associated with a complete mole has a better prognosis than when it follows a term pregnancy; perhaps the completely paternal (i.e., foreign) origin of the mole-originating tumor explains this difference (Surti et al., 1980). The malignant potential of the mole may lie in the expression of paternal genes which are normally unexpressed; this in turn may be a consequence of "relaxation of imprinting" (Mutter et al., 1993; Ariel et al., 1994). Chemotherapy, either at the time of evacuation of complete mole or for "persistent gestational trophoblastic tumor" following the index pregnancy, seems to be without untoward effect in a subsequent pregnancy.

It may be that triploid *partial mole* implies no long-term sequelae, but follow-up remains appropriate until this picture becomes clearer. Diploid partial mole may have a risk in terms of subsequent malignant potential (Jeffers et al., 1993).

NOTE

1. In utero life is divided into three periods: pre-embryonic (the first 3 weeks), during which the morula, blastocyst, and presomite embryo form; embryonic (to the end of the eighth week) when the body form and organs are constructed; and fetal (from 8 weeks to term), characterized by growth and changes in proportion rather than the appearance of new features (Williams and Wendell-Smith, 1969). Often the word fetal is used loosely to refer to the entire period. Conceptus, in theory, applies to any stage, but it generally refers to early pregnancy.

PRENATAL DIAGNOSIS

21

Parental Age Counseling and Screening for Fetal Trisomy

The maternal age association in Down syndrome was known long before the chromosomal association. In 1909 Shuttleworth recorded that ''with regard to parentage . . . the outstanding point is the advanced age of the mother at the birth of the child . . . the next point that strikes one is the large proportion of Mongol children that are lastborn, often of a long family.'' He considered that either age or parity could be an etiologic factor. Subsequently, Penrose (1934) demonstrated that it was the mother's age that was the key factor. Paternal age is also increased, but simply because most couples are about the same age. Hassold et al. (1993) comment that ''The association between increasing maternal age and trisomy is arguably the most important etiologic factor in human genetic disease. Nevertheless, we know almost nothing about its basis.'' Likewise, Sherman et al. (1994) state ''. . . increasing maternal age is one of the most important factors in human reproductive failure, as well as being a leading contributor to mental retardation among live-borns.'' Phillips et al. (1995) conclude that it is actual chronological age that is important, not ''reproductive age,'' that is, the distance in time from approaching menopause.

The maternal age effect in Down syndrome—whatever it may be—operates upon oogenesis, predisposing to nondisjunction of chromosome 21 at both meiotic divisions (Hassold et al., 1993; Antonarakis et al., 1993a); we comment upon the mechanics in more detail in chapters 2 and 16. In more general terms, segregation of some other chromosomes is vulnerable to the maternal age effect and thus ''older women'' who are pregnant run an increased risk for having a pregnancy with 47,+13, 47.+16, 47,+18, 47,XXX, and 47,XXY, as well as 47,+21. For chromosome 16 and the X chromosome, the maternal age effect appears to disturb only the first meiotic division (Hassold et al., 1993); indeed, in trisomy 16 the nondisjunction is invariably due to maternal first meiotic nondisjunction. There is also a slight maternal age association with some categories of 47,+ESAC (extra structurally abnormal chromosome) (Hook and Cross,

1987a) and with Prader-Willi syndrome due to maternal uniparental disomy (Robinson et al., 1991). Advanced maternal age is the most common indication for prenatal diagnosis.

Definition of Older Maternal Age

How old is "older," and what is "advanced" maternal age? The age of 35 years has commonly been taken as a threshold. Hook (1994) points out that this cutoff reflected merely an apparent quantum jump at age 35 if one looked at the original risk calculations, which were based on 5 year intervals. If we were a six-fingered species, and used a duodecimal system, presumably 36 would have been the boundary! When, as is now the case, risks are calculated by single year intervals, no sudden changes are seen, and there is a smooth upward progression in risk. These more precise data are certainly necessary. Firstly, we can give women in each age category their own specific risk figure, enabling them to make an informed decision for or against prenatal diagnosis. Secondly, in some screening programs for fetal trisomy (see below), the mother's age-related risk is an important datum to be included, along with the various laboratory test results, to derive her overall risk estimate. Thirdly, we can make rational decisions about an appropriate cutoff age in age-based prenatal diagnosis programs: the balancing of what society can afford, what society regards as desirable, and what constitutes a level of risk that warrants intervention (Hook, 1994; Ganiats et al., 1994). Thus, in some jurisdictions 37 is now regarded as a more suitable cutoff age at which the choice of prenatal diagnosis can be offered.

DERIVATION OF RISK FIGURES

Down Syndrome

Hecht and Hook (1994) have critically reviewed maternal age data vis-à-vis Down syndrome from a number of sources, and they consider published Swedish and Belgian data most likely to be complete. From these data, they derive risk figures at maternal ages from 15 to 50, using different regression criteria. We have used the regression for maternal ages 20 to 45 as the basis of the age-related figures presented here (Table 21–1). For higher maternal ages in particular, these data may not take into account an influence of modern obstetric practice in promoting survival of a trisomic fetus, and we therefore append (for ages 37–42) the more recently derived data of Halliday et al. (1995b) from Victoria, Australia. Their figures are marginally higher than Hecht and Hook's, and we may perhaps extrapolate that mothers of whatever age, having good obstetric care in the late 20th century, are at slightly greater risk to have a liveborn Down syndrome baby than their own mothers may have been a generation previously.

Table 21—1   Maternal-age-specific risks for trisomy 21 at livebirth

Maternal age (years)	Prevalence at livebirth ‰	Prevalence at livebirth 1 in	Maternal age (years)	Prevalence at livebirth ‰	Prevalence at livebirth 1 in	1 in[a]
15–19	0.64	1560				
20	0.65	1540	36	3.57	280	300
21	0.66	1520	37	4.59	220	220
22	0.67	1490	38	5.98	170	165
23	0.69	1450	39	7.84	130	125
24	0.71	1410	40	10.4	97	90
25	0.74	1350	41	13.8	73	70
26	0.78	1280	42	18.3	55	50
27	0.83	1200	43	24.5	41	40
28	0.90	1110	44	32.8	30	
29	0.99	1010	45	44.1	23	
30	1.12	890	46	59.3	17	
31	1.29	775	47	79.7	13	
32	1.52	660	48	107	9	
33	1.83	545	49	145	7	
34	2.24	445	50	195	5	
35	2.81	355				

Source: Taken from Table 4, third column, of pooled estimates in Hecht and Hook (1994).

[a]The italicized figures are from Halliday et al. (1995b), and represent more recent unpooled data, modeled to the best fit. Figures are rounded.

Other Aneuploidy

The figures for Down syndrome are of most interest, as this condition (*1*) produces a major mental handicap, (*2*) implies a major burden for parents in that survival well into adult life is now the norm, and (*3*) is the most common single chromosome defect. But the data for other aneuploidies are not without relevance. Women seeking advice on their age-related risk should, of course, know about Down syndrome; but they should know also that some other rather uncommon trisomies (13 and 18) might be detected, which usually cause early death with invariable profound brain defect, and that, on the other hand, there are some age-related sex chromosome aneuploidies (XXX, XXY) that have much milder, but not trivial, effects. Tables 21–3 and 21–4 set out age-related risk estimates for these other categories of aneuploidy. There is also the possibility, irrespective of maternal age, that some other type of chromosome defect might exist. Table 21–5 sets out the risk of any chromosomal defect, whether maternal-age associated or not, being detected at prenatal diagnosis. To put these figures into some perspective, we remind the reader that the prevalence of unbalanced chromosomal abnormality in the whole newborn population is approximately 0.4%, or 1 in 250 (Table 1–3). Some counselors use the livebirth risk figures while others prefer to offer the risk that the defect would be discovered at prenatal diagnosis.

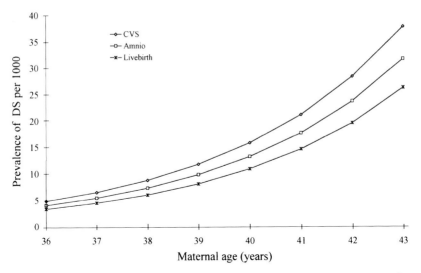

FIGURE 21–1. Prevalence of Down syndrome for maternal ages 36 to 43 at three "windows of observation": the time at which CVS is done (about 10 weeks), amniocentesis (14 to 18 weeks), and at livebirth. From Halliday et al. (1995b). (Courtesy J. L. Halliday.)

Risk and Gestational Stage

The prevalence of chromosome abnormality is greater at the time of prenatal diagnosis than at term. A trisomic conceptus is more likely to be lost following intrauterine death of the fetus than a normal conceptus. Thus, looking through the three windows of observation—chorion villus sampling (around 10 weeks), amniocentesis (about 14–18 weeks), and term—the frequency of chromosomal abnormality, for a particular maternal age, progressively reduces. At 10 weeks, not only is there a greater proportion of potentially viable abnormalities that would subsequently miscarry, but also a number of lethal abnormalities that would inevitably abort (Hook et al., 1988). From the number of trisomic 21 fetuses existing at the time of CVS, Halliday et al. (1995b) estimate the losses in the whole cohort thereafter from spontaneous abortion (and see Figure 21–1). In the time frames CVS→amniocentesis, amniocentesis→20 weeks, and 20 weeks→livebirth, the relative loss rates over and above the background are 17%, 13%, and 5% respectively. Overall, the excess loss rate is about a third. Hook et al. (1995) take the approach of determining the absolute loss rate in women who have had a +21 result at amniocentesis, and who decide to continue with the pregnancy. The rate falls progressively from about 50% for those diagnosed at 14–17 weeks and levels off at 16% after 27 weeks. For trisomies 13 and 18, the spontaneous abortion rate from amniocentesis→livebirth is 43% and 68%, respectively (Hook, 1983). A factor which may influence survival in trisomy 18 and 13 is placental mosaicism. If a proportion of placental tissue is chromosomally normal, there may be less compromise of placental function (Kalousek et al., 1989). For XXX and XXY, there appears to be little or no selective loss in the latter part of pregnancy. (Note how little the figures differ in the amniocentesis and livebirth columns in Table 21–4.) Concerning the likelihood for detection of fetal trisomy 21 at chorionic villus sampling or amniocentesis, Hook (1992) has summarized and tabulated maternal-age risk figures from several sources. We list these risk figures for age of the mother and according to timeframe in pregnancy in Table 21–2. Comparable figures are published in Snijders et al. (1994a).

No Parental Age Effect in Some Defects

There is no discernible increasing risk with increasing maternal age for the following chromosomal abnormalities: de novo rearrangement, XYY, triploidy, and unbalanced karyotype due to transmission of parental translocation. For monosomy X the risk lessens with increasing maternal age. There is no parental age effect in Down syndrome due to a paternal nondisjunction (Hook, 1986, 1987; Hatch et al., 1990), and increased paternal age is not of itself an indication for chromosomal prenatal diagnosis.

SECULAR CHANGES IN MATERNAL AGE DISTRIBUTION AND DOWN SYNDROME PREVALENCE

Changing maternal age profiles in a population will influence the birth prevalence of Down syndrome. In New Zealand in the 1920s, for example, about 45% of all mothers were aged 30 and over, and about 90% of all Down syndrome babies (at least those surviving to the 1960s to have a chromosome study) were born to mothers in this age group. Over the next four decades, family planning practices became gradually more widespread. By the late 1960s, most women were completing their families while still in their 20s, and "older mothers" made much less contribution to the overall birth rate. Only 20% of all mothers were 30 and over; and the proportion of all Down syndrome babies born to this age group had fallen to 53% (Gardner et al., 1973a). We suppose, therefore, that the birth prevalence of Down syndrome in New Zealand progressively fell over the period 1920 to 1970. Hook (1992) has reviewed the prevalence of Down syndrome in various parts of the world during the early 1980s alongside the proportions of mothers aged 35 and older. The former Czechoslovakia had the lowest proportion, 3.6%, of older mothers, and Northern Ireland, at 11.1%, the highest. As expected, observed rates of Down syndrome births showed a relationship, with 1.06‰ in Czechoslovakia and 1.60‰ in Northern Ireland. In the 1980s and 1990s, there has been a reversal of the maternal age trend in some parts of the world. In South Australia, for example, after falling to a trough around 1975 to 1978, the fraction of mothers over age 35 years has progressively risen, and the birth prevalance of Down syndrome was anticipated to rise from a low point of about 0.9‰ in the late 1970s to greater than 1.5‰ in 1990 to 1994 (Staples et al., 1991). In Israel, maternal age dipped in 1978 to a low of 8% of Jewish mothers being 35 or older and rose to 17% by 1992 (Shohat et al., 1995).

Table 21—2 Maternal-age-specific risks for trisomy 21 at prenatal diagnosis, for maternal ages in the mid 30s to 49

Maternal age (years)[a]	Prevalence at CVS			Prevalence at amniocentesis		
	‰	1 in	1 in*	‰	1 in	1 in*
33				2.4	420	420
34				3.1	320	320
35	4.2	240		4.0	250	280
36	5.7	175	205	5.2	190	250
37	7.5	135	155	6.7	150	180
38	10	100	115	8.7	115	135
39	13	75	85	11	89	100
40	18	56	65	15	69	75
41	24	42	45	19	53	55
42	32	32	35	24	41	40
43	42	24	25	31	32	30
44	56	18		40	25	
45	75	13		52	19	
46	~100	10		67	15	
47	~130	8		86	12	
48	~180	6		111	9	
49				144	7	

[a]Age at time of procedure (CVS or amniocentesis).

Source: Taken from Tables 20.8 and 20.10 in Hook (1992).

The italicized figures are from Halliday et al. (1995b). Figures are rounded.

Table 21—3 Maternal-age-specific risks for trisomies 18 and 13 at amniocentesis and livebirth

Maternal age (years)[a]	Trisomy 18		Trisomy 13	
	Amniocentesis	Livebirth	Amniocentesis	Livebirth
35	1 in 2000	1 in 3330	1 in 5000	1 in 3330
36	1400	2500	3300	3330
37	1000	2000	2500	2500
38	700	1670	2000	2500
39	500	1250	1250	2000
40	360	1000	910	2000
41	260	830	670	1670
42	180	630	480	1430
43	130	500	2000	?1430
44	210	?500	2000	?1430
45–49	210	?500	2000	?1430

[a]Age at time of amniocentesis or birth, respectively.

Source: Taken from Table 20.4 and 20.7 in Hook (1992). Figures are rounded.

Table 21—4 Maternal-age-specific risks for 47,XXX and 47,XXY at amniocentesis and at livebirth

Age	XXX			XXY		
	Amnio	Livebirth		Amnio	Livebirth	
	‰	‰	1 in	‰	‰	1 in
33		0.4	2500		0.4	2500
34		0.5	2000		0.4	2500
35	0.4	0.5	2000	0.5	0.6	1650
36	0.5	0.6	1650	0.6	0.7	1450
37	0.7	0.8	1250	0.8	0.9	1100
38	0.9	0.9	1100	1.1	1.1	900
39	1.1	1.1	900	1.4	1.4	700
40	1.4	1.3	770	1.8	1.7	600
41	1.8	1.6	630	2.4	2.2	450
42	2.2	1.9	530	3.1	2.7	370
43	2.8	2.2	450	4.1	3.4	300
44	3.6	2.7	370	5.4	4.3	230
45	4.5	3.2	310	7	5.4	180
46	5.7	3.8	260	9	6.8	150
47	7	4.5	220	12	8.5	120
48	9	5.5	180	15	11	95
49	11	6.5	150	20	13	75

Source: Taken from data in Tables 20.4 and 20.7 in Hook (1992). Figures are rounded.

Table 21—5 Maternal-age-specific risks for all unbalanced chromosomal abnormalities at chorionic villus sampling[a] and at amniocentesis[b]

Maternal age[c]	Chorionic villus sampling		Amniocentesis	
	%	1 in	%	1 in
33			0.5	200
34			0.6	160
35	0.9	115	0.8	120
36	1.2	85	1.0	100
37	1.5	65	1.2	80
38	2.0	50	1.5	65
39	2.5	40	2.0	50
40	3.5	30	2.5	40
41	4.5	22	3	33
42	6.0	17	4	25
43	7.5	13	5	20
44	10	10	6	17
45	13	8	7	14
46	~17	6	9	11
47	~23	4	10	10
48	~30	3	10	10
49			10	10

[a]Including invariably lethal defects.

[b]Including those for which there is no maternal age effect.

[c]Age at time of procedure.

Source: Taken from "averaging" data in Tables 20.7 and 20.8 (amniocentesis), and from Table 20.10 (CVS) in Hook (1992). Figures are rounded, the 47 and older data considerably so (see Hook for discussion of differences in 47 and older data from different studies).

The prevalence is also influenced by the use of prenatal diagnosis and selective pregnancy termination. In Denmark, Hook observes that with 7.1% of mothers 35 and over, a rate of 1.35‰ was to be expected; but in fact the Down syndrome prevalence is 1.02‰. He presumes, therefore, that prenatal diagnosis has led to a 25% reduction in prevalence. Likewise, in England and Wales, 14% of potential Down syndrome births were avoided by selective abortion over the period 1974 to 1987, reducing the birth prevalence from 12.6 to 10.8‰ (Cuckle et al., 1991). The South Australian figures noted above are estimates of the birth prevalences had termination not been used; in fact, the actual prevalences have been, and will be, less.

Population prevalence (the number of Down syndrome persons, of all ages, per 100,000 population) is to be distinguished from birth prevalence (the number of Down syndrome babies per 1000 newborns, usually over a specified period of time). While the birth prevalence (also called birth incidence) may have fluctuated in different parts of the world in different periods of this century, other factors are influencing prevalence. Survival is less than that of the normal population; most deaths occur in the first year of life, and the death rate increases in the mid 40s (Baird and Sadovnick, 1989). Survival rates are changing due to improvements in medical care, a major factor being the increasing utilization of heart surgery.

MATERNAL SERUM SCREENING FOR FETAL TRISOMY

Accessibility to health care is an important issue. Would it be desirable, or feasible, to make definitive prenatal diagnosis (amniocentesis or CVS) for trisomy 21 available to every pregnant woman, whatever their age? As for feasibility, as of now, no. With current cytogenetic technology, culture of a sample from all (or most) women would require more staff and laboratory wherewithal, and more dollars to fund it, than could realistically be justified. According to the way the sums are done (and if this costing approach is accepted), a maternal age can be calculated beyond which the costs of testing outweigh the costs of maintaining a handicapped child who will make little or no economic contribution him or herself. In most jurisdictions, younger mothers will not have direct access, as a right, to state-funded amniocentesis or chorionic villus sampling. (Private testing is another matter.) Nevertheless, it is these younger mothers who produce most Down syndrome babies. Their age-specific risks are, of course, less; but pregnant women in their late teens, 20s and early 30s greatly outnumber "older mothers."

Screening Methodologies

The above being so, pressure existed to determine a means to screen out the pregnancies in the younger population that are at increased risk for Down syndrome; and these mothers could, then, go on to have the definitive diagnostic test (namely, amniocentesis). Screening would, by definition, have to use a simple procedure, such as taking a blood sample. The first such tool to be applied was second trimester maternal serum alphafetoprotein (AFP) measurement, and subsequently other biochemical indices have been discovered. Three of these (AFP, estriol, chorionic gonadotrophin)—hence, the "triple test"—were developed to provide, along with a consideration of maternal age and gestational stage, a separation of women into those at increased risk and those at an intermediate or lesser risk. Serum AFP and estriol are somewhat lower in mothers carrying a trisomy 21 fetus, and chorionic gonadotrophin (hCG) is somewhat higher. Latterly, the free beta component of hCG and AFP together present a better distinction (Macri et al., 1994). Presumably, these differences reflect biochemical perturbation in the trisomic fetoplacental unit. Other indices are being assessed and may in due course be added to or supplant one or some of these analytes (Agrawal et al., 1994). One of these is serum PAPP-A (pregnancy-associated plasma protein A), which may have a place in earlier pregnancy screening, during 8 to 14 weeks (Macintosh et al., 1994); free beta hCG and AFP testing may also be applicable in early pregnancy (Berry et al., 1995). Urine may prove preferable as a test sample (Cuckle et al., 1995). Because the range of analyte levels in mothers of normal babies and in mothers of Down syndrome babies overlaps, a clear-cut answer is not forthcoming: merely an adjustment of the woman's prior risk based on age. Trisomy 18, although having a low prior risk and not of itself justifying screening, can efficiently and usefully be detected in conjunction with Down syndrome screening (Palomaki et al, 1995).

The analysis is rather complex, and computer programs have been developed for the purpose. If it is determined that a woman's risk is greater than that of a certain cutoff, she is offered amniocentesis. If a high cutoff were chosen (say 1 in 100), most trisomy 21 pregnancies would be missed. If a lower cutoff (say 1 in 300) were chosen, too many women would come to have an amniocentesis. If, for the sake of argument, a cutoff of 1 in 200 were selected (this is about the same as the risk for a 37-year-old mother), this will dictate, using the "triple test" for the whole pregnant population, a detection rate of 62% and a false positive rate of 3.6% (Wald and Cuckle, 1992).[1]

Interpretation of Screening Results

What do these figures mean? A little epidemiology is in order. Imagine a group of 10,000 mothers, of all ages. Assuming a birth prevalence for Down syndrome of 1.2‰, we can take it that 12 would give birth to a baby with Down syndrome. Screening, according to the above scenario, will detect 62% of these, that is, seven; and 360 amniocenteses (3.6% of 10,000) will have a normal result. Of the 9640 women screening as "low-risk", 5 will nevertheless have a Down syndrome baby. Putting these figures in the conventional format, we have:

	Baby with DS	Baby without DS	Total
Test shows "increased-risk"	7	360	367
Test shows "low-risk"	5	9628	9633
	12	9988	10,000

The *sensitivity* (detection rate) of the test is 7/12 (60%). Thus, 40% of women with a trisomic 21 fetus will be missed by the test. The *positive predictive value* of the test is only 7/367 (1.9%). Thus, 98.1% of women giving an "increased risk" result will *not* have a Down syndrome baby. The *negative predictive value* is 9628/9633 (99.95%); in other words, a "low-risk" result means a 99.95% chance for an unaffected baby.

The interpretation of a maternal blood test result to the patient is fraught with potential for confusion. The major pitfall is that what some laboratories call a "screen-positive" test is sometimes understood by the woman and her medical adviser to mean that Down syndrome is very likely. As we showed above, *the great majority of women testing "positive" will yet go on to have a normal baby.* Some damage has been done, in more than one part of the world, because people have not understood, explicitly or intuitively, the concept and relevance of a low positive predictive value. Women have gone on to amniocentesis believing that they are carrying an abnormal baby. Albeit a normal amniocentesis result may, in due course, assuage their concern, it was a false concern in the first place and should not have arisen. Some doctors who have occasional patients with "screen-positive" results who then proceed to amniocentesis have been perplexed when, again and again, none returns a chromosomally abnormal test. Counselors doing this sort of work need a clear understanding of these issues; women can scarcely give informed consent if their advisers cannot give clear information (Smith et al., 1995).

A new test has to prove its worth, and some will be doubtful that a blood test which analyzes indirect effects of fetal trisomy, and which gives merely an altered risk estimate rather than a clear-cut answer, is a secure basis for reassurance. Haddow et al. (1994) offer some comfort on this point in their study of over 5000 women 35 and older who were having an amniocentesis. There were 54 Down syndrome pregnancies and had screening been offered, 48 of these (89%) would have tested "high-risk." This high detection rate went with a high false positive rate (25%); a high false positive rate is more acceptable in an older age group, in which all women might otherwise have had an amniocentesis. Maternal attitudes (is this a "last-chance pregnancy"?) and perceptions (what figure constitutes a high risk?) are important. Beekhuis et al. (1994) assessed the response to a "screen-positive" result in women aged 30 to 35, 36 to 37, and 38+; the older women in whom a "screen-positive" test result gave, nevertheless, a risk figure less than that of their prior maternal age risk mostly decided against amniocentesis. Whether serum screening will come to be the first step for any pregnant woman, irrespective of age, remains to be seen (Kellner et al., 1995). A difficulty with serum screening is the inherent delay in receipt of the test result in those women who do go on to amniocentesis compared with those who have amniocentesis first off. The development of rapid analyses on uncultured amniocytes (Cacheux et al., 1994; Pertl et al., 1994; Van Opstal et al., 1995) may, if the technology is established, have the obvious advantage of lessening the wait. Same-day or next-day exclusion or confirmation of trisomy 21 may become a reality.

These various issues are canvassed in considerable detail in *Screening for Down's Syndrome* (Grudzinskas et al., 1994), and the interested reader is referred to this definitive document. In particular, Macintosh's essay ''Perception of Risk'' provides a very readable and practical commentary for the counselor.

NOTE

1. In a pregnancy in which gestation has been confirmed by ultrasound scan. If unscanned, the figures are 54% and 4%, respectively. (See Table 32.9 in Wald and Cuckle, 1992).

22

Prenatal Diagnostic Procedures

The means to diagnose the fetal karyotype has provided medical cytogenetics with one of its major areas of application. The discovery of an abnormality allows the option of termination or, later in the pregnancy, a more suitable obstetric management (Platt et al., 1986; Rochelson et al., 1986). The main indications for prenatal cytogenetic diagnosis are increased age of the mother, parental heterozygosity for a chromosome rearrangement, the birth of a previous child with a chromosome defect, abnormal maternal blood chemistry indicating an increased risk for fetal trisomy 21 (p. 332), and intrauterine growth retardation and/or fetal malformation detected on ultrasonography.

Certain major ultrasonographic defects are fairly specific (Gagnon et al., 1992; Boyd and Keeling, 1992; Nicolaides et al., 1993): for example, holoprosencephaly predicts trisomy 13, fetal hydrops/cystic hygroma predicts monosomy X or trisomy 21, and an endocardial cushion defect or duodenal atresia predicts trisomy 21. The relatively minor sign of a ''nuchal lucency'' (actually, this separation of the skin from the underlying tissue can extend from the occiput down to the lower back) indicates an increased risk for fetal trisomy: thicknesses of 3 mm, 4 mm, 5 mm and $\geqslant$6 mm are associated with a 3- 18- 28- and 36-fold increased risk, respectively, for fetal trisomy 21, 18, or 13 (Pandya et al., 1995). Vintzileos and Egan (1995) provide tables for the risk of trisomy 21 according to the presence of various ultrasonographic markers and in the context of a given maternal age or triple-screen result. Choroid plexus (CP) cysts, if isolated and small (<3 mm), imply little if any increased risk (Duff et al., 1994). Gupta et al. (1995) offer a figure of 1 in 150 that a fetus with isolated CP cysts would have a chromosomal aneuploidy, mostly trisomy 18, and only 1 in 880 would have Down syndrome (the latter figure not different from the background population risk). However, larger cysts in the company of other abnormalities are a pointer to an increased risk for fetal aneuploidy (Snijders et al., 1994b), and in the review of Gupta et al. (1995) the risk for a chromosome abnormality in the presence of CP cysts and other ultrasonographic fetal anatomic defects was very high, 1 in 3. Single umbilical artery as an isolated finding may not warrant prenatal karyotyping (Khong and George, 1992) although lacking, as yet, definitive evidence of the innocuousness of this sign, it remains a discretionary option (Saller and Neiger, 1994).

Parental anxiety, for a variety of reasons, is a not uncommon "soft" indication for prenatal diagnosis (PND). Chromosomes are sometimes studied when PND is performed for another diagnostic purpose—neural tube defect, metabolic abnormality, or molecular analysis for a Mendelian disorder. Although there may be no specific cytogenetic indication, some maintain that, having subjected the woman to an invasive procedure and the pregnancy to risk of miscarriage, any information on the well-being of the fetus that can reasonably be obtained ought to be. The availability of resources, the policies of health care providers, and the willingness of patients to pay are factors that may determine whether a chromosome study is done in a "nonchromosomal" PND.

Since the early 1970s, PND of chromosome disorders has been carried out routinely by means of culture of amniotic fluid cells obtained by amniocentesis at about 16 weeks of pregnancy. There are now a number of approaches to PND during the first and second trimesters of pregnancy, which range from preimplantation diagnosis (following in vitro fertilization), through chorion villus sampling (CVS), early amniocentesis (prior to 16 weeks), placental biopsy, and fetal blood sampling. Naturally, parents are anxious to have results as early as possible. A desire for an early result needs to be balanced against a number of considerations which can include complexity of the procedure, both clinically and in the laboratory, procedural trauma and risks, reliability of results, cost, and the prior risk for a fetal abnormality.

Preimplantation Diagnosis

This is a costly and technically demanding procedure, done in the context of in vitro fertilization, in which the results may not be totally reliable, and postimplantation genetic change such as mosaicism would remain a possibility. There is, of course, the advantage of having a result even before the pregnancy is in utero; only a genetically normal embryo is implanted. Only couples with a high genetic risk, and for whom termination would not otherwise be acceptable, might be suitable for this approach.

The world experience is minuscule. Less than 30 normal babies have been born following preimplantation diagnosis, and mostly for conditions other than a chromosomal abnormality (Black, 1994; Delhanty, 1994). Pregnancy rates are 22% per cycle, or 28% per embryo transfer. Sex determination has been used for couples at risk of an X-linked disorder; separation of X and Y sperm can improve the chance for an XX conception. Some single-gene disorders are testable using PCR. In principle, aneuploidy would be demonstrable on FISH, but in practice detection is very difficult when only one or two nuclei are available for study. Mosaicism may be not uncommon in early cleavage blastocysts, so there may be a risk for "confined blastomere mosaicism" (Delhanty, 1994). For technical and biological reasons, fragile X preimplantation diagnosis would be very difficult to achieve (Black, 1994), although Dreesen et al. (1995) suggest it may become possible to identify a low-risk embryo by using closely linked markers which can be amplified by PCR. If the technology were to advance, it might in due course prove useful in couples at high risk for unbalanced conceptions, but scarcely for fertile couples at relatively low genetic risk. As yet, it is an experimental procedure at an early stage of development.

Chorionic Villus Sampling (CVS)

CVS became popular in the mid 1980s and by 1992 an estimated 150,000 procedures had been done worldwide (Kuliev et al., 1992); in the United Kingdom in 1993 to 1994, 4663 CVS procedures were done compared to 37,803 amniocenteses (Howell, 1994). The usual time for a CVS procedure is at 10 to 11 weeks.[1] If a defect is identified, and abortion is chosen, this can be a more private matter, and the termination procedure is an operative intervention (curettage or suction evacuation of the uterus). Parents are more likely to make a choice for abortion when the diagnosis has been made in the first trimester (Verp et al., 1988). The main disadvantages are a slightly higher risk to cause a miscarriage than with amniocentesis (1% compared to 0.5%, over the background rate) and a higher likelihood of equivocal diagnostic results (Chapter 23); these issues need to be pointed out. CVS is generally the procedure of choice for couples with a medium to high genetic risk (>5%). It is the necessary procedure for fragile X diagnosis, since this requires a sufficient amount of DNA for a Southern blot analysis. For prenatal diagnoses using special techniques such as FISH, and which may take some time to complete, CVS is preferable. For couples with a relatively low genetic risk, CVS remains an option.

> *Direct, short-term, and long-term CVS* Chorionic villi can be analyzed directly (same day), after short-term culture (next day or two), or after long-term (a week or two) culture. Trophoblast cells are the source of the population studied at direct and short-term CVS culture. These cells are no longer extant (if they have not already been removed by trypsinization at sample receipt) after the first few days, and it is the mesenchymal core of the villus which provides the cells that are analyzed at long-term culture (and see Figure 23–3).

In the early 1990s there were disconcerting reports of an increased incidence of transverse limb deficiencies and tongue and jaw defects ("oromandibular-limb hypogenesis") following early (before 10 weeks) CVS. This association was not observed in some jurisdictions but supported in others, and the issue remains controversial (Halliday et al., 1993; Silver et al., 1994; Brambati, 1995; Olney et al., 1995). Thrombosis in or spasm of the embryonic limb bud vasculature has been suggested as a cause; this is plausible speculation, but speculation nonetheless (Ibba et al., 1994; Hibbard et al., 1994). A prudent response is to confine CVS procedures to no earlier than the 9th week from the date of the last menstrual period (Kuliev et al., 1992). A factor due to a different vascular mechanism is feto-maternal transfusion following transabdominal CVS, which may lead to a reduction in fetal blood flow and which might be an uncommon cause of fetal loss (Brezinka et al., 1995).

Early Amniocentesis

In the latter 1980s early (10–13 weeks) amniocentesis was introduced as an alternative to CVS (Lockwood and Neu, 1993; Kerber and Held, 1993). In a carefully controlled comparison, Nicolaides et al. (1994) found a 2 to 3% additional fetal loss rate in early amniocentesis and, possibly, a higher incidence of talipes amongst subsequently born children. They considered CVS to be the better procedure but acknowledged that early amniocentesis does have a place.

"Standard" Amniocentesis

Transabdominal amniocentesis, done at about 16 (usual range 14–18) weeks gestation, has been the standard cytogenetic prenatal diagnostic procedure for over a quarter of a century. It has a very high degree of safety to both mother and infant: maternal complications, or fetal injury due to direct trauma, are practically unknown. The risk for maternal Rh immunization (Rh negative mother, Rh positive fetus) can be prevented by antibody injection. The only significant complication is a procedure-related fetal loss rate of about 0.5%. The cytogenetic results are highly reliable. The only biological sources of error are, firstly, that maternal rather than fetal cells, or a mixture, are sampled, which may happen in at most 1% of cases (Benn et al., 1983). Since the maternal cells are unlikely to comprise all of the sample, most instances of contamination in at least a 46,XY pregnancy will be recognized. The rare birth of a boy, after the prediction of a girl, would be obvious; in the case of a normal daughter the error would pass unnoticed. Secondly, fetal mosaicism may go undetected, since only a limited number of cells can feasibly be examined. Very few examples of this error are recorded.

> Amniotic fluid culture has a high success rate. Persutte and Lenke (1995) have suggested that in the infrequent instance of failure of amniotic cells to grow, for no obvious reason, there is a substantial risk for fetal aneuploidy (13% of 32 cases). If this finding is confirmed, a policy of vigorously pursuing such failures, and offering a repeat procedure, would be advisable.

The obvious disadvantage of 16 week amniocentesis is that the results are not to hand until 18 weeks. If the reason for the amniocentesis had been an "increased-risk" result from maternal serum screening, the procedure may not be done till 17 to 18 weeks, aggravating this difficulty. If a result cannot be available by 20 weeks, another procedure (fetal blood sampling, placental biopsy) may be worth considering.

Fetal Blood Sampling

Fetal blood is aspirated by direct puncture of a blood vessel in the umbilical cord, and a cytogenetic result is obtained in only a few days. Originally, fetoscopy was required, and this had a high (5%) fetal loss rate. Now, cordocentesis under ultrasound guidance is a considerable improvement, and has a loss rate of less than 2%. Fetal blood sampling is particularly applicable in the case of midtrimester diagnosis when structural defect has been identified at ultrasonography: quick knowledge of the fetal karyotype is needed because the likelihood for an abnormality is considerable, and since most ultrasound diagnoses are made at around the 18 week mark, time is of the essence. It has a role in settling the issue of mosaicism on amniotic fluid culture (Gosden et al., 1988; Shalev et al., 1994).

Placental Biopsy

In principle, this is the same as a direct-culture CVS: tissue from the fetal component of the placenta, the chorionic villi, is sampled. It is usually performed in the late second and third trimesters, when a rapid result is needed (Constantine et al., 1992). Because of the inherent inaccuracy in a direct or short-term culture (see p. 349), placental biopsy is second-best to fetal blood sampling, in terms of the correctness of the result, but it is a more straightforward procedure and has a lesser risk to cause loss of the pregnancy.

Rapid Amniocyte Karyotyping

Yet another technique of use in the context of the necessity for a quick result is rapid karyotyping from amniotic fluid, which may yield a result within 4 to 6 days (Claussen, 1980; Claussen et al., 1994). Fetal defect on ultrasound, increased-risk maternal screen result (especially if delayed), and simply late presentation of the pregnant woman are suitable indications. The methodology is not widely available.

Future Possibilities

The earlier, the more easily, and the quicker, the better. Several new methodologies for prenatal diagnosis are in an investigational phase, and some of these may, eventually, be sufficiently developed that they become standard techniques. The October 1995 issue of *Prenatal Diagnosis* reviewed the current state of non-invasive or ''minimally invasive'' methodologies, with particular reference to fetal cell isolation from maternal blood, and from transcervical sampling (Adinolfi, 1995).

Fetal Cell Isolation from Maternal Blood

This has been tried for many years (Schroder and de la Chapelle, 1972), but the advent of polymerase chain reaction (PCR) for analysis of DNA using an automated DNA sequencer and of FISH for chromosome analysis from a small number of cells has given impetus (Bianchi et al., 1992; Mansfield, 1993). Fetal cells of various types are present in the maternal circulation from the first trimester (Simpson and Elias, 1993). Separation is difficult, and while a pure fetal cell preparation cannot be obtained, various approaches are being developed to obtain enriched fractions (Zheng et al., 1995; Simpson et al., 1995; Andrews et al, 1995). Nucleated erythrocytes had seemed a promising source, but in fact pregnancy of itself induces maternal production of these cells (Slunga-Tallberg and Knuutila, 1995). The U.S. National Institute of Child Health and Development has launched a multicenter feasibility trial which should be completed in 1997. Trophoblast cells may enter the maternal circulation, and Johansen et al. (1995) have done preliminary work on isolation methodologies.

FISH and Uncultured Cells

FISH can be applied to interphase nuclei with chromosome-specific probes to detect a single, double, or triple dose of a particular chromosome (Bryndorf et al., 1994a,b; Philip et al., 1994; Van Opstal et al., 1995). Thus, the need for culture would be bypassed, whether the cells were from amniotic fluid, CVS, or fetal blood, offering earlier diagnosis and a considerable saving in laboratory time and expense and thus a wider availability of prenatal diagnosis. A limitation is that only those specific aneuploidies being tested (the major autosomal trisomies and possibly sex chromosome aneuploidies) could be detected; a normal result would not necessarily mean a normal fetal karyotype. The American College of Medical Genetics (1993) has promulgated a policy statement on this issue.

Cystic Hygroma and Pleural Effusion Fluid

Cystic hygroma, in particular, has a strong association with fetal aneuploidy. Fluid from cystic hygroma and pleural effusion contains lymphocytes, and these cells can be cytogenetically analyzed within the time frame of a few days. In one small series, three out of four cystic hygroma analyses showed aneuploidy (trisomy 21, monosomy X) (Costa et al., 1995).

Cervical Washings

Trophoblast cells may be shed from the placenta and enter the endocervical canal, and can be collected for analysis by endocervical irrigation and aspiration, or by cytobrush. This would be advantageous in giving an early (7–10 weeks) sample, and via a simple procedure (Adinolfi et al., 1995; Bahado-Singh et al.,

1995; Ishai et al., 1995; Rodeck et al., 1995; Tutschek et al., 1995). The practical value remains to be assessed.

QUALITY OF CYTOGENETIC RESULTS

Blood lymphocyte culture followed by high-resolution banding gives the best-quality cytogenetics. The quality from any other tissue is almost never as good. Mostly, this is not a serious problem in prenatal diagnosis, since this is primarily aimed at detecting complete aneuploidy. It is important that both patient and doctor realize that very subtle chromosome abnormalities, which could have a serious consequence, may escape detection, regardless of the procedure chosen. In the absence of a known risk factor, microdeletion syndromes may not be detected at routine prenatal diagnosis. Of course, if a subtle parental rearrangement is known, the cytogeneticist knows precisely what to look for and can apply a specific focus, possibly resorting to FISH and chromosome painting to provide a clear picture (Figure 22–1).

"PRIMUM NON NOCERE"

"First, do no harm" is a frequently quoted precept. Yet, practically inevitably, having a prenatal diagnostic procedure causes anxiety. Rothman (1988), in her book *The Tentative Pregnancy* is particularly critical of what she sees as a medicalized distortion of the normal process of being pregnant. Hodge (1989) describes her personal experience of "Waiting for the Amniocentesis," and we reproduce her letter in full:

I drafted the following letter to the editor one week before I expected to hear the results of my amniocentesis:

"I am 40 years old and 19 weeks pregnant with what will presumably be my third child. I am on the basic science faculty of a medical school. When I teach medical students about amniocentesis, I occasionally mention the difficulty for the woman of having to wait until well into the second trimester to receive her results.

"I am in that situation myself now, awaiting my results. And before experiencing it, I was unprepared for two phenomena. One was just how difficult the wait is. Pregnancy is always a time of waiting, but now time has slowed down to an extent I did not anticipate. The other, more disturbing phenomenon is how the waiting has affected my attitude toward the pregnancy. At many levels I deny that I really am pregnant until after we get the results. I ignore the flutterings and kicks I feel; I talk of if rather than when the baby comes; I am reluctant to admit to others that I am pregnant. I dream frequently and grimly about second-trimester abortions. In some sense I am holding back on bonding with this child-to-be. This represents an unanticipated negative side effect of diagnostic amniocentesis. And all this, even though my risk of carrying a chromosomal abnormality is less than 2 percent.

"I presume I am not alone in these reactions, yet I have not seen this problem mentioned in the literature, nor did my physician or genetic counselor discuss it with me. I am writing now to bring it to the attention of clinicians with pregnant patients undergoing

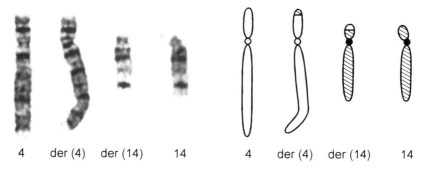

4   der (4)   der (14)   14   4   der (4)   der (14)   14

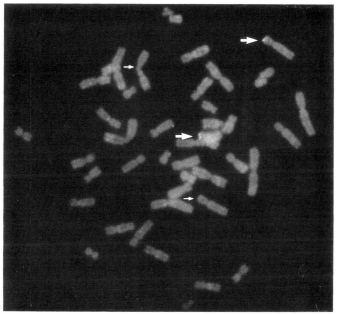

FIGURE 22–1.   A rcp(4;14)(p16.3;p12), not discernible on G-banding (*above*), in which very small segments of distal 4p, and of 14p distal to the nucleolar organizing region, have exchanged position. FISH with 4pter probe (*below*) enables a clear distinction. This shows signal on the normal 4 (larger arrow, above) and the der(14) (larger arrow, below). The der(4) and the normal 14 are indicated by smaller arrows. (Courtesy Y. Hull).

diagnostic amniocentesis. I suggest to both clinicians and their patients that, when weighing the relative risk and benefits of prenatal diagnosis performed later (amniocentesis) as compared with earlier (chorionic villus biopsy), they not underestimate the negative effects of a 4½ month wait before the woman knows if she is really pregnant.''

The next day, before I had mailed this letter, I received the results, and unfortunately they were the dreaded ones: trisomy 21. I have since then had the grim second-trimester abortion. From my current perspective of grief and shock, I encourage clinicians to help their patients avoid the denial described in my letter. My husband and I spared ourselves no pain by holding back emotionally. It has become a cultural expectation that one will keep one's pregnancy a secret until one has had the "all clear" from the amnio. One reasons, "If we get a bad result, we won't have to tell anyone." But I now believe that reasoning is wrong. After our bad result, my husband and I did tell everyone. Sympathy and support from our friends, family, and colleagues have helped us to survive the ordeal of aborting a wanted pregnancy. By keeping the loss a secret, we would have cut ourselves off from such support when the feared outcome did happen."

Not every couple will react this way—some preferring to keep their personal affairs private—but some will. The counselor needs to acknowledge these criticisms, and to rise to the challenge of providing a sympathetic and skilful service to their clients, according to their varying responses to deciding to have, to undergoing, and to waiting for the results of prenatal diagnosis, and then supporting those who do get an abnormal result. Primum non nocere may be a counsel of perfection; a more practical injunction is that inevitable harms be anticipated, recognized, minimized, and coped with. These issues are addressed in detail in *Prenatal diagnosis The human side* (Abramsky and Chapple, 1994).

NOTE

1. Note that this refers to 10 to 11 weeks after the last menstrual period; the true conceptual age is usually 2 weeks less than this, that is, 8 to 9 weeks.

23

Chromosome Abnormalities Detected at Prenatal Diagnosis

Generally, people who chose to have prenatal diagnosis (PND) are concerned about some specific chromosomal condition, the most common of which is Down syndrome in the context of increased maternal age. The major categories of unexpected chromosomal abnormality are (*1*) a sex chromosome aneuploidy, (*2*) some autosomal trisomy other than +21, (*3*) polyploidy, (*4*) a structural rearrangement, (*5*) an extra structurally abnormal chromosome, and (*6*), for each of the foregoing, mosaicism. In fact, an unexpected abnormality may be more likely than the "expected" one: for example, in Victoria, Australia during 1993, out of nearly 3000 prenatal diagnostic procedures for advanced ($\geqslant 37$ years) maternal age, 1.4% gave a result of trisomy 21, whereas 2.9% showed other chromosomal abnormalities (J. L. Halliday, pers. comm., 1995).

To some extent, the possibility of "other abnormalities" should be raised at counseling before PND. But when an abnormality is actually discovered, it is of course necessary to discuss in detail with the couple the implications of this particular abnormality and to help them decide on a suitable course of action (Engel et al., 1981; Robinson et al., 1992). In transmitting the information, the counselor is obliged to be clear and accurate about the particular aneuploidy and to take care that the parents' autonomy in the decision-making process is not compromised. A decision for or against termination is the immediate one to be made. Engel et al. (1981) list these factors influencing the parents' decision: their philosophy of life, their religious views, their socioeconomic status, and whether this was a first or wanted pregnancy or a later, unplanned pregnancy. Outlines of the clinical consequences of these abnormalities follow, to serve as a basis for these decisions. The grayest area is sex chromosome aneuploidy. In Denmark, J. Nielsen et al. reported in 1986 that approximately 80% of prenatal diagnoses of sex chromosome aneuploidy are followed by the choice of abortion. In an English/Finnish study, termination (in about 60% overall) was mostly chosen in the case of the XXY and 45,X karyotypes, by younger parents with fewer previous children, and in all cases in which an ultrasonographic defect was identified (Holmes-Siedle et al., 1987).

Holmes-Siedle et al. (1987) and Robinson et al. (1989) note that a choice to continue a pregnancy is more often made when the information has been transmitted by a clinical geneticist/genetic counselor. Robinson et al. reports decisions to terminate for XYY, 45,X, XXX, and XXY karyotypes in 32%, 44%, 35% and 45% respectively, (total 38%), in their own material, compared with 57%, 74%, 56%, and 75%, respectively (total 67%), from a review of published series (Verp et al., 1988). Marteau et al. (1994, pers. comm., 1995) assessed different approaches of obstetricians, geneticists, and genetic nurses in England and Wales to the prenatal diagnosis of Klinefelter syndrome. These professionals were asked whether they counsel nondirectively (''try to be as neutral as possible, covering both positive and negative aspects''), directively for termination (''encourage termination'' or ''try to be as neutral as possible but overall convey more negative than positive aspects of the condition''), or directively against termination (''encourage parents to carry to term'' or ''try to be as neutral as possible but overall convey more positive than negative aspects of the condition''). The greatest differences were that more genetic nurses would counsel non-directively (70% compared to 42–47% geneticists and obstetricians), and more obstetricians would counsel in favor of termination (27% compared to 9% geneticists and 2% genetic nurses). Fairly similar proportions would counsel in favor of continuing the pregnancy (31% obstetricians, 44% geneticists, 28% genetic nurses). Marteau et al. (1994) raise the question whether a decision for or against termination depends upon which type of health professional a woman consults; a predicament Drugan et al. (1990a) try to avoid by having both a physician and a genetic counselor present at the consultation. Drugan et al. (1990a) found that 93% of parents having a prenatal diagnosis with a ''poor prognosis'' (autosomal trisomy, unbalanced translocation, 45,X with major ultrasonographic defects) chose pregnancy termination, while only 27% of parents given a ''questionable prognosis'' (sex chromosome aneuploidy, 45,X with normal ultrasonography, de novo apparently balanced translocation or inversion) took this course. They make the interesting observation that ultrasound visualization of fetal defects ''in a society dominated by the television screen'' can be useful in helping parents better grasp the implications of the diagnosis.

MOSAICISM: CONSTITUTIONAL, CONFINED, AND PSEUDO

Mosaicism is the bane of cytogenetic prenatal diagnosis (but a better understood bane than it once was). Firstly, chromosomal mosaicism detected in chorion villus sampling (CVS) or amniocyte culture does not necessarily truly reflect a constitutional mosaicism of the embryo. A chromosomally abnormal cell line may exist only in extraembryonic tissues (chorion, amnion), and the embryo is 46,N. This is ''confined placental mosaicism'' (CPM). CPM is much more likely to be encountered at CVS than at amniocentesis. Or, embryonic and extraembryonic tissues are all 46,N, and the abnormality arose during tissue culture in vitro (''cultural artifact''). This is ''pseudomosaicism'' (this expression is sometimes erroneously used in referring to CPM). Secondly, when mosaicism does truly involve the embryo, we usually cannot offer a firm prediction of what effect this may have on the phenotype. At the outset, we should state that true mosaicism of the fetus is very infrequently observed, and *the great majority of mosaicism identified at prenatal diagnosis does not presage an abnormal baby*. It is important to keep this perspective in talking with parents (according to the particular attributes of the mosaicism, as we go on to discuss) and avoid causing any more anxiety than that which, inevitably, an ''abnormal'' result brings.

Applied Embryology

Interpreting mosaicism obliges an understanding of the earliest events of development of the conceptus (Figures 23–1, 23–2, and 23–3). Bianchi et al. (1993) provide a scholarly and important reevaluation of early human embryology in this context. The zygote undergoes successive mitoses to produce a ball of cells (*morula*) (Figure 23–1,1). The morula then cavitates to produce an inner cyst and becomes the spherical *blastocyst* (this is happening at the beginning of the second week) (Figure 23–1,2). The shell of the blastocyst is comprised of trophoblast, and this tissue becomes the outer investing layer of the chorionic villi. The inner cell mass protrudes into the blastocystic cavity, and it will give rise to the embryo. It comprises two different cellular layers, the epiblast and the hypoblast.

The *hypoblast* forms the spherical primary yolk sac (whose roof is, transiently, the ''ventral'' surface of the embryo). The yolk sac gives rise to the extraembryonic mesoderm, sandwiched between itself and the outer cytotrophoblast, giving a three-layered sphere, and then it involutes and disappears, to be replaced by the secondary yolk sac. The mesodermal cells now invade the blastocystic cavity (Figure 23–1,3), and this mesodermal mass is in turn cavitated to produce the extraembryonic celom, such that there are outer and inner layers of extraembryonic mesoderm. The outer layer, underlying the trophoblast, gives rise to the mesenchymal core of the chorionic villus, and the inner layer becomes the outer surface of the amniotic membrane. The amniotic cavity enlarges at the expense of the extraembryonic celom (Figures 23–1,5 and Figure 23–2) and eventually obliterates it (by the end of the first trimester), with the mesodermal layer of the amnion fusing with the mesodermal layer of the chorion.

The *epiblast* gives rise to the amniotic cavity, the floor of which is the ''dorsal'' (ectodermal) surface of the embryo, and its roof is the amnion, these being continuous at their margins. Thus, the embryonic integument and the inner surface of the amniotic membrane—which are the source of the embryonic and amniotic epithelial cells present in amniotic fluid—have the same lineage. At the beginning of the third week, the primitive streak arises from the epiblast, and this in turn gives origin to both endoderm and intraembryonic mesoderm. Thus, endoderm and intraembryonic mesoderm are closely related developmentally to ectoderm; and, importantly, the extra- and intraembryonic mesoderms have different origins. Endoderm gives origin inter alia to urinary tract and lung epithelia, desquamated cells from which contribute to the cellular population of amniotic fluid.

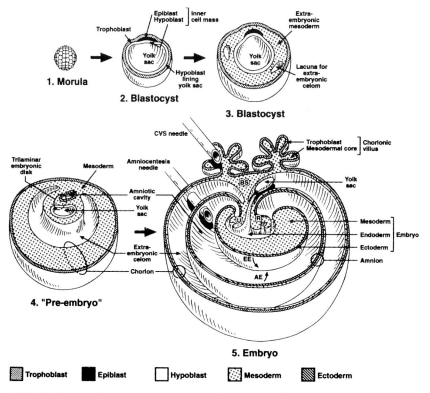

1. Morula

2. Blastocyst

Trophoblast

Epiblast | Inner
Hypoblast | cell mass

Yolk sac

Hypoblast lining yolk sac

3. Blastocyst

Extra-embryonic mesoderm

Yolk sac

Lacuna for extra-embryonic celom

4. "Pre-embryo"

Trilaminar embryonic disk

Mesoderm

CVS needle

Amniocentesis needle

Amniotic cavity

Yolk sac

Extra-embryonic celom

Chorion

5. Embryo

Trophoblast
Mesodermal core } Chorionic villus

Yolk sac

Mesoderm
Endoderm } Embryo
Ectoderm

Amnion

▨ Trophoblast ■ Epiblast ☐ Hypoblast ▨ Mesoderm ▨ Ectoderm

FIGURE 23–1. Developmental origins of tissues sampled at prenatal diagnosis (simplified). *(1)* Morula, 3 to 4 days postconception. *(2)* Cross-section of blastocyst at beginning of second week, showing outer rim of trophoblast, the inner cell mass comprising epiblast (black) and hypoblast (white), and the yolk sac cavity lined by an inner rim of cells of hypoblastic origin. *(3)* Blastocyst toward end of second week. The hypoblastic cells of the yolk sac have given rise to extraembryonic mesoderm. Lacunae are beginning to appear in this mesoderm, and these will coalesce to form the extraembryonic celom. *(4)* Pre-embryo, with extraembryonic celom cavitating the extraembryonic mesoderm, and the much smaller spaces of the amniotic cavity and the yolk sac. Note that the embryonic mesoderm (middle layer of the trilaminar embryonic disk) arises from the *epiblast,* and thus has a different lineage from the extraembryonic mesoderm. *(5)* Composite embryo/early fetus. (Rotation has reversed the relative positions of the yolk sac and amniotic cavity.) The three embryonic tissue types (ectoderm, mesoderm, endoderm) all had origin from the epiblast. Amniotic epithelium (AE) can shed into amniotic cavity. Embryonic epithelium both from its ectodermal surface (EE) and from endodermal derivatives (respiratory and urinary tracts, R and U) are cast off into, or pass into, the amniotic cavity. Chorionic villi comprise mesenchymal core (of extraembryonic mesodermal origin), gloved by trophoblast. Extraembryonic and embryonic mesoderms are continuous at the body stalk (BS).

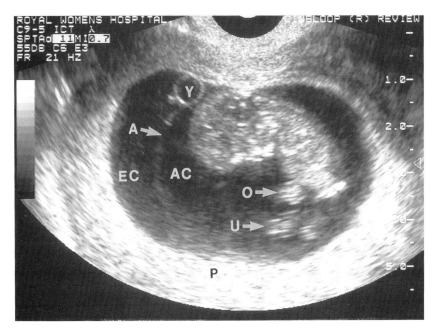

FIGURE 23–2. Ultrasound picture of embryo at 10 weeks' gestation, showing amnion (A), amniotic cavity (AC), extraembryonic celom (EC), umbilical cord (U), "physiological omphalocele" (O), yolk sac (Y), and placenta (P). (Courtesy H. P. Robinson.)

Amniocentesis, therefore, is a procedure which samples cells having origin from the epiblast of the inner cell mass, and these cells closely reflect the true constitution of the embryo. CVS, on the other hand, samples more distantly related cells: trophoblastic cells (direct and short-term culture), which were the first lineage to differentiate from totipotent cells of the morula; and villus core cells (long-term culture), which reflect the rather more recently separated lineage of the extraembryonic mesoderm. Trophoblast cells are very rapidly dividing, for the crucial task of providing tissue to make an attachment to the uterine wall (which happens at the beginning of the second week), and this may endow a greater vulnerability to mitotic error. The differing origins of tissues sampled by different means are set out in Figure 23–3.

The resolution of mosaicism in the cytogenetics laboratory and in its clinical interpretation can differ for CVS and amniocentesis, and we will consider them separately. In terms of the laboratory result, we can apply to both CVS and amniocentesis the concept of different levels of in vitro mosaicism, originally developed for amniocentesis by Worton and Stern (1984) and refined by Hsu et al. (1992), as follows:

Level I

A single abnormal cell is seen ("single cell mosaicism"). With near certainty this is cultural artifact and may be resolved as set out in Tables 23–1 and 23–2.

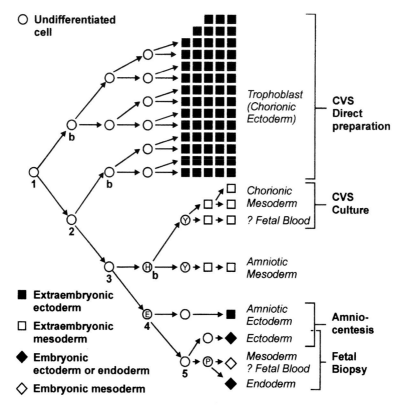

FIGURE 23–3. Diagram of cell lineages arising from differentiation in the very early conceptus. The fertilized egg (1) produces a trophoblast precursor (1b) and a totipotent stem cell (2) which in turn forms another trophoblast precursor (2b) and a stem cell (3) that produces the inner cell mass. The inner cell mass divides into stem cells for hypoblast (3b) and epiblast (4). The epiblast cell(s) (5) produces embryonic ectoderm and primitive streak, and the latter is the source of embryonic mesoderm and endoderm. The cell lineages sampled at various prenatal diagnostic procedures are indicated at right. E, epiblast; H, hypoblast; P, primitive streak; Y, yolk sac. (From Bianchi, D. W., Wilkins-Haug, L. E., Enders, A. C. and Hay, E. D. (1993), Origin of extraembryonic mesoderm in experimental animals: relevance to chorionic mosaicism in humans, *Am J Med Genet*, 46, 542–550, © Am J Med Genet 1993, courtesy D. W. Bianchi, and with the permission of Wiley-Liss, Inc., a subsidiary of John Wiley & Sons, Inc.)

Level II

Two or more cells with the same chromosomal abnormality in a dispersed culture in a single flask, or a single abnormal colony in an in situ culture (i.e., possibly or probably just a single clone). This form of mosaicism—"multiple-cell mosaicism"—is almost always pseudomosaicism. A course of action to resolve this cytogenetically is given in Tables 23–1 and 23–2.

Level III

Two or more cells or colonies with the same chromosome abnormality, distributed over two or more flasks. This is likely to be a true mosaicism.

Table 23—1 Proposed guidelines for workup of possible pseudomosaicism/mosaicism

Flask method[a]	In situ method[b]
A. Indications for extensive workup	
(1) Autosomal trisomy involving a chromosome 21, 18, 13, 8, or 9 (SC, MC)	(1) Autosomal trisomy involving a chromosome 21, 18, 13, 8, or 9 (SCo, MCo)[b]
(2) Until further decision, autosomal trisomy involving a chromosome 12, 14, 15, 20, or 22 (SC, MC)	(2) Until further decision, autosomal trisomy involving a chromosome 12, 14, 15, 20, or 22 (SCo, MCo)
(3) Unbalanced structural rearrangement (MC)	(3) Unbalanced structural rearrangement (MCo)
(4) Marker chromosome (MC)	(4) Marker chromosome (MCo)
B. Indications for moderate workup	
(5) Extra sex chromosome (SC, MC)	(5) Extra sex chromosome (SCo, MCo)
(6) Autosomal trisomy involving a chromosome 1, 2, 3, 4, 5, 6, 7, 10, 11, 16, 17, or 19 (SC, MC)	(6) Autosomal trisomy involving a chromosome 1, 2, 3, 4, 5, 6, 7, 10, 11, 16, 17, or 19 (SCo, MCo)
(7) 45,X (MC)	(7) 45,X (SCo, MCo)
(8) Monosomy (other than 45,X) (MC)	(8) Monosomy (other than 45,X) (SCo, MCo)
(9) Marker chromosome (SC)	(9) Marker chromosome (SCo)
(10) Balanced structural rearrangement (MC)	(10) Balanced structural rearrangement (MCo)
	(11) Unbalanced structural rearrangement (SCo)
C. No additional workup	
(11) 45,X (SC)	
(12) Unbalanced structural rearrangement (SC)	(12) Balanced structural rearrangement (SCo)
(13) Balanced structural rearrangement (SC)	(13) Break at centromere with loss of one arm (SCo)
(14) Break at centromere with loss of one arm (SC)	(14) All single cell abnormalities

[a]SC = single cell (single flask); MC = multiple cells (single flask).

[b]SCo = single colony (single dish); MCo = multiple colonies (single dish).

Source: From Hsu et al. (1992).

The distinction is not quite as clear as this in practice, but it is a useful working definition. Some allow level III to include more than one colony in only a single flask; this could reflect an "overinterpreted level II" if two or more colonies in the one flask had arisen from a single cell whose progeny migrated and established separated colonies. Welborn and Lewis (1990) offer a rather more detailed classification to account for the complexity that is, in practice, encountered.

Table 23—2   Nature of additional laboratory workup to resolve mosaicism issues

Flask method[a]	In situ method[b]
Moderate workup	
Examine extra 10 cells from first flask in which the abnormal cell(s) was found	Examine extra 12 colonies from different culture vessels
Extensive workup	
Examine extra 10 cells from second flask and 20 cells from a third flask	Examine extra 24 colonies from multiple vessels, not including the initial vessel in which the abnormal colony(ies) was found

[a]Based upon routine analysis of 10 cells in each of 2 culture flasks which contain 12 or more colonies before harvest.

[b]Based upon routine analysis of 10 to 16 colonies from more than 1 culture vessel.

Source: After Hsu et al. (1992).

Chorionic Villus Culture

Karyotypic differences between cytotrophoblast, villus stroma, and fetus are seen in 1 to 2% of CVS procedures done at the 10 to 11 week mark (Kalousek et al., 1989; Simoni and Sirchia, 1994). Mosaicism from an early mitotic error can give rise to *confined* mosaicism (confined to placenta, or to fetus) or to *generalized* mosaicism (present in both fetus and placenta). The extreme form is complete discordance, with a nonmosaic 46,N karyotype in fetus and nonmosaic aneuploidy in CVS, or vice versa. If a mitotic error (a nondisjunction or an anaphase lag) happens in (*I*) a trophoblastic cell, this will give rise to mosaicism confined to this category of chorionic villus tissue. Because of its high rate of cell division, the mosaicism is detectable in direct and short-term cultures. A mitotic error occurring in (*II*) extraembryonic mesoderm produces confined placental mosaicism affecting the villus stroma and is detected in long-term CVS cultures. A mitotic error in (*III*) an early inner cell mass stem cell, without affecting the hypoblast, could produce an abnormal fetus with normal short-term and long-term CVS cultures—a true false negative. This is scarcely ever observed. An error in (*IV*) a totipotent cell about to contribute to the inner cell mass, and affecting both epiblast and hypoblast, would lead to karyotypic abnormality in both fetus and CVS stroma, with normal CVS trophoblast. Finally, (*V*) an initially trisomic conception in which ''correction'' (see below) occurs in the cell about to give rise to the epiblast would give a trisomic placenta (trophoblast and villus core) and a disomic embryo. If the correction occurred a little later, during epiblast formation, there would be true mosaicism of the embryo.

The above scenarios for confined mosaicism are set out as types I to V in Table 23–3. Mosaicism detected on laboratory analysis in cytotrophoblast but not in stroma will usually be confined placental mosaicism, type I, and require no further action. (Many laboratories have ceased routine direct and short-term cultures, and thus for them a question of type I CPM no longer arises.) Mosaicism identified in stroma may be confined or generalized. The distinction between confined (placental) mosaicism type II, generalized (fetal-

Table 23—3   Types of confined mosaicism at CVS (see also text)

Type	CVS direct or short-term culture	CVS long-term culture	Embryo/fetus	Relative frequency
I	Abnormal or mosaic	Normal	Normal	50%
II	Normal	Abnormal or mosaic	Normal	25%
III	Normal	Normal	Abnormal or mosaic	Almost 0%
IV	Normal	Abnormal or mosaic	Abnormal or mosaic	10%
V	Abnormal or mosaic	Abnormal or mosaic	"Normal" (disomic)	15%

Source: After Bianchi et al. (1993).

placental) mosaicism types IV and V, and in vitro artifact can be difficult to make. It may be appropriate to follow the process outlined for amniotic fluid culture in table 23–1 for the flask method in order to help resolve level II mosaicism; level III mosaicism very probably reflects a true mosaicism, at least of the placenta (these *levels* I to III of in vitro mosaicism are not to be confused with the five *types* I to V of in vivo placental–fetal mosaicism noted above).

Level II Mosaicism

In the case of level II mosaicism, which is seen in 1 to 2% of CVS, Fryburg et al. (1993) conclude that it "has little clinical significance." In a collaborative U.S. study of 11,473 CVS procedures, level I or II mosaicism was recorded in 181, followed up cytogenetically in 24, and in none of these was fetal mosaicism confirmed (D. H. Ledbetter et al., 1992).

Level III Mosaicism

Level III mosaicism (seen in about 1% of CVS) is a different matter. Management at this point (which will be around 12–13 weeks) is aimed at demonstrating, as much a possible, fetal normality; or, if it so transpires, at confirming a true fetal mosaicism. Amniocentesis, along with detailed ultrasonographic assessment of fetal morphology, is called for. (It is too early in the pregnancy for fetal blood sampling.) In Fryburg et al.'s (1993) series, of 20 level III CVS diagnoses, termination was chosen in seven cases (mosaic trisomies 5, 7, 9, 13, 16, 18, 21), with karyotypic confirmation post-termination in four (trisomy 5, 13, 18, 21). Of the seven proceeding to livebirth and followed up (mosaic trisomies 2, 7, 9, 16, 21, tetrasomy 7, and X/XX), clinical and karyotypic study of the newborns, and of some as infants, revealed no abnormality (except that one baby died suddenly at 18 days), although in three cases placental biopsy showed the trisomy (chromosomes 7, 9, 16). From these small numbers, one would conclude that most level III mosaicism, albeit a true mosaicism, is confined to the placenta—a conclusion similarly reached by D. H. Ledbetter et al.

(1992). With respect to the major "viable autosomes," of five cases of level III trisomy 21 mosaicism in Ledbetter et al., three appeared to reflect confined placental mosaicism, but two did show a true fetal 47,+21/46,N mosaicism; in Fryburg et al. (1993), as noted above, three diagnoses of mosaicism for trisomies 13, 18, and 21 were confirmed post-termination in the abortus. In the diagnosis of 47,+5/46 in Fryburg et al.'s series that led to termination, 2/55 testis cells were +5, but no amniocytes, muscle, lung, or skin cells, and the authors ask, "Could this have been an isolated problem restricted to the testis or would other tissues also have been involved? Would development have been normal?"— questions that can be more generally applied to any case of level III mosaicism. Klein et al. (1994) provide a partial answer in one example, a child born of a pregnancy in which trisomy 8 was observed in 81% of CVS cultured cells, 0% of amniotic fluid cells, and in 60% of a placental biopsy at delivery: the child had 4% and 1% mosaicism on bloods at 2 and 7 months of age and 0% on a skin fibroblast study, and was normal in appearance, growth, and developmental progress at age 30 months. (A trisomic chromosome other than No. 8 might have had a less benign effect.) Of course, fetal morphologic defect shown on ultrasonography indicates the very substantial probability of a major degree of true fetal mosaicism, and the choice of immediate termination is appropriate, such as Guichet et al. (1995) report in a case of 50/50 normal/trisomy 8 mosaicism. A specific concern in CPM type V, in which the trisomy involves an imprintable chromosome (e.g., 14, 15), is uniparental disomy of the embryo following "correction" by postzygotic loss of the additional chromosome, while the placenta remains partly or wholly trisomic (Kalousek and Barrett, 1994; Sirchia et al., 1994; Webb et al., 1995) (see Figure 2–9, and p. 32). In the particular case of 47,+15/46 or 47,+15 diagnosed at CVS, and if a 46,N karyotype is shown at the subsequent amniocentesis, a Prader-Willi/Angelman methylation test (p. 291) can be applied to the cultured amniotic fluid cells. A CVS diagnosis of trisomy 16 followed by a normal karyotype at amniocentesis raises concern about an abnormal fetal phenotype due either to an effect of UPD, or to placental dysfunction (see below) (Whiteford et al., 1995). Other uniparental disomies, such as UPD 10(mat), seem to be without phenotypic effect per se (Jones et al., 1995). We return, nevertheless, to our earlier statement: levels I and II mosaicism imply a minimal risk to the fetus, and only in level III mosaicism should the counselor imply to the patient a major and potentially serious concern.

If a cytogenetically abnormal cell line (mosaic or nonmosaic) is confined to the placenta, does this have any implication for placental function? While some reports pointed to an association with pregnancy loss (Johnson et al., 1990; Wapner et al., 1992) and intrauterine growth retardation (Kalousek et al., 1991; Kalousek, 1993), inferentially due to the placental karyotypic defect, other studies have produced conflicting conclusions (Wolstenholme et al., 1994; Roland et al., 1994). Apparently, at least for most trisomies, a placenta that is trisomic in part or in whole retains nevertheless a sufficient or nearly sufficient level of function, and as a general rule the (46,N) fetus is satisfactorily supported (Simoni and Sirchia, 1994). Placental trisomy 16 may be an exception (Vaughan et al., 1994; Kalousek and Barrett, 1994; Wolstenholme, 1995). Schuring-Blom et al. (1993) describe FISH as a means to determine the extent of this type of aneuploidy in the term placenta.

Mosaicism confined to the fetus, with a normal placental karyotype (type III mosaicism, as above), has almost never been encountered (Pindar et al., 1992). Thus, a normal long-term CVS result practically certainly means a chromosomally normal baby.

Amniotic Fluid Cell Culture

A mitotic error in epiblast may produce mosaicism of both embryonic and amniotic tissue, or it may be confined to the amniotic membrane. An in vitro cell division defect causes artifactual pseudomosaicism. Separating confined mosaicism and pseudomosaicism from true fetal mosaicism is critical, but by no means straightforward. The distinction is, in the first instance, based upon the number of abnormal cells seen, and whether one or more than one presumptive abnormal clone exists, according to the three levels I through III set out above. Level I mosaicism is seen in 2.5 to 7% of amniocenteses, level II in 0.7 to 1.1%, and level III in about 2 per 1000 amniotic fluids (Wilson et al., 1989).

Once the laboratory studies are completed, the cytogeneticist will provide an opinion about the level of mosaicism, taking into account technical aspects of the cultures. There is generally no point, and indeed it could be counterproductive, to report level I mosaicism to the consultand. Liou et al. (1993) studied fetal blood karyotypes from nine pregnancies where there had been a level I mosaic result at amniocentesis, and in none was the mosaicism confirmed. Some level II mosaicism and all level III mosaicism do, however, require to be conveyed to the patient, *carefully and clearly interpreted.*

Level II Mosaicism

Liou et al. (1993) studied fetal blood karyotypes from 70 pregnancies where there had been a level II mosaic result at amniocentesis, and this was confirmed in only 1 (1.4%), in which there was a true 47,+21/46 karyotype; this very low fraction is consistent with Worton and Stern's (1984) observation of 138 cases in none of which was the mosaicism confirmed in the aborted fetus or infant— nor was any abnormal phenotype noted that could be ascribed to the mosaicism. The nature of the "mosaic chromosome" is important. If it is one that has been recorded, in life, in the nonmosaic trisomic state, or in the mosaic state, concern is justifiable. This includes, for example, mosaic trisomies 8, 9 (Saura et al., 1995), 13, 18, and 21 and mosaic isochromosomes 12p and 18p. Albeit true mosaicism for some other trisomies (e.g., 5, 7, 10, 12, 14, 15, 16, 17, 19, and 22; Von Koskull et al., 1989; Sciorra et al., 1992a; Jenkins et al., 1993; Garber et al., 1994) has been observed in the malformed fetus in a pregnancy advancing well into the third trimester or in an abnormal liveborn child, these cases are so rare that a level II amniotic fluid mosaicism is still much more likely due to artifact than a true significant fetal mosaicism. High-resolution ultrasonography provides helpful information in this context. If further cytogenetic investigation is judged desirable—and for many, the reassurance of a very low risk will have been sufficient—fetal blood sampling (if available) is generally the procedure of choice (although note that not all mosaicism is necessarily present in blood, i(12p) being a particular example). A result can be obtained in a few days, and a large number of cells (hundreds) are available for a "mosaic count." A 46,N result from fetal blood sampling and normal ultrasonography should be seen as very substantially (almost 100%) reassuring. Is there any point in repeating the amniocentesis? While the same result as obtained the first time would effectively exclude a cultural artifact (converting a level II to a level III mosaicism; Worton and Stern, 1984), it could also represent a resampling of a confined abnormality; and in any event a normal result does not invalidate the previous abnormal one.

Strictly speaking, no amount of investigation could ever completely exclude the possibility of a true mosaicism of the fetus, albeit the distribution of the abnormal cell line may be rather limited and of minor, minimal, or negligible phenotypic consequence. We have seen, for example, a case of level II 47,XX,+13/46,XX mosaicism at amniocentesis followed by fetal blood sampling at which 100/100 cells were 46,XX, and a cord blood sample from the newborn baby showed 47,XX,+13 in 3 out of 100 cells; the baby looked normal and was developing satisfactorily on review at age $5\frac{1}{2}$ months (M. B. Delatycki et al., in prep.). Rare similar examples exist to disquiet the counselor (Terzoli et al., 1990; Vockley et al., 1991), but a sense of perspective should be kept: for each autosome, only the tiniest number of level II mosaicisms (zero for most chromosomes) have turned out to reflect, in fact, a true and significant mosaicism of the fetus.

Level III Mosaicism

Even if further prenatal studies were to give normal results, an important risk remains that a true fetal mosaicism exists, and this could be associated with a significantly abnormal phenotype. Liou et al. (1993) checked fetal blood karyotypes from 55 pregnancies where there had been a level III mosaic result at amniocentesis, and the mosaicism was confirmed in 22 (40%). This contrasts somewhat with Shalev et al. (1994), who confirmed a fetal mosaicism in only 3 out of 23 cases of "true" amniotic fluid culture mosaicism: possibly some examples of colony mosaicism in their study may have reflected in vitro seeding of a single ("level I") cell. Of 19 pregnancies in this study having a 46,N fetal blood karyotype and proceeding to full term, all produced phenotypically and karyotypically normal infants. Hsu et al. (1992) record their's and others' experience with respect to trisomies for individual autosomes, and these findings are set out in Table 23–4. Some mosaicisms need a particularly circumspect appraisal: in the specific case of trisomy 12 mosaicism, for example, Petrella and Hirschhorn (1990) comment that further prenatal studies "often fail to contribute information that would be helpful toward decision-making and in some cases may lead to the wrong diagnosis", and Wyandt et al. (1990) and Frohlich and Falk (1991) echo this sobering assessment. Mosaicism for ESACs appears to carry a greater risk than for autosomal trisomy (Table 23–4). Ultrasonography provides useful adjunctive, but not necessarily definitive, evidence.

Table 23—4 Outcomes of true (level III) autosomal trisomy mosaicism diagnosed at amniocentesis[a]

Chromosome	Number of prenatal diagnoses[b]	Number abnormal per cases with information[c]
2	4	4/4
3	1	0/1
4	1	1/1
5	3	0/3
6	3	0/3
7	2	0/1
8	11	1/10
9	20	10/16
11	1	0/1
12	13	2/11
13	15	5/11
14	4	2/3
15	4	1/4
16	3	0/3
17	5	0/4
18	15	6/7
20	103	11/101
21	60	17/24
22	9	4/8

[a]Chromosomes not listed (1, 10, 19) were not seen in mosaic trisomy.

[b]References to individual cases in Hsu et al. (1992). Causal link in some uncertain.

[c]Observed post abortion, fetal demise, or birth.

Source: After Hsu et al. (1992).

One should always attempt to confirm a diagnosis of mosaicism, either on multiple fetal samples following pregnancy termination or on cord blood, cord, amnion, and perhaps urine epithelial cells in an infant (Sutherland et al., 1973). Such follow-up studies are likely to confirm that level III mosaicism reflects the fetal chromosome constitution in around 50% of cases involving an autosome, in 90% with a sex chromosome, and in 80% with an ESAC (Hsu and Perlis, 1984). A post-termination study that did *not* confirm the abnormality could cause parents very great distress, and a decision needs to be made with them beforehand as to whether they would be given such a result.

Jewell et al. (1992) describe an extraordinary case of mosaicism detected at prenatal diagnosis with very different tissue distributions. A dup(12) chromosome was present in 87% of amnion cells, 60% of fetal blood, but only in 2% of chorionic villi and 0% of chorionic membrane. Kingston et al. (1993) provide a similar remarkable (and disconcerting) example. Amniotic fluid cells had 3% with an additional abnormal chromosome, a sample of fetal blood showed all cells 46,N, and several tissues taken post-termination had various fractions of mosaicism, including brain with 88% of cells aneuploid. These cases are instructive in emphasizing that the proportions of abnormal cells in one tissue can not be taken as indicative of proportions elsewhere; but they are also exceptional cases and may not apply to the generality of mosaicism.

SEX CHROMOSOME ANEUPLOIDY

The main conditions are XXY, XXX, XYY, and 45,X. Two of these (XXY and 45,X) may be firmly predicted in terms of an abnormality of development of the reproductive system. Children with Klinefelter and Turner syndrome are almost certainly going to be infertile. Robinson et al. (1986) offer a useful commentary concerning raising this issue with parents. Parents of children predicted to be infertile might feel a sense of loss—a "sadness and regret about their child's anticipated loss and about their own loss of grandchildren" and "concern about their children's wholeness and, by extension, their own." Robinson et al. encourage open discussion between parents and children to allow the best possible adaptation to this situation. Parents may take some comfort from knowing that infertility is by no means an uncommon problem in the general population.

The picture for intellectual and psychological functioning is less clear-cut for each of the four conditions. Earlier adult studies defining a strong association with mental deficiency and psychological disturbance were contaminated by ascertainment bias (and counselors' personal experience is more likely to have been with those children whose problems were sufficiently severe that they came to medical attention). Children identified in newborn populations screened for cytogenetic abnormalities and subsequently followed up constitute a group unbiased in their ascertainment although perhaps subject to other but less important biases (Puck, 1981). Data from the study of such children in several American and European cities, followed from infancy through childhood, adolescence, and young adulthood now give a reasonably clear picture of the natural history of the more common sex chromosome aneuploidies (Evans et al., 1990a). In general, it seems probable, as Hook (1979) had proposed, that some sex chromosome aneuploidies influence brain function in such a way that the development of intellectual capacity, emotional maturity, and speech and language skills are affected to some extent, but none of these effects necessarily occurs, none is specific to sex chromosome aneuploidy, and some may be amenable to corrective intervention. There is considerable overlap with the XX and XY population! Robinson et al. (1992) studied a group of children with sex chromosome abnormalities who had been diagnosed prenatally and whose parents had made informed decisions to continue the pregnancies. This group of children (aged 7–14 years at the time of the study) were performing developmentally as well as their siblings and are doing better at school and in peer relations than a group that was diagnosed postnatally. Robinson et al. (1992) comment that the better performance of the prenatally diagnosed may be due to their high socioeconomic status and a supportive environment provided by families that had made a conscious decision to continue the pregnancies; others have noted that children with some sex chromosome aneuploidies are more vulnerable to the effects of instability and dysfunction in the family than are their 46,XX and 46,XY siblings (Stewart et al., 1990; Bender et al., 1993).

We next outline the predicted outlook for the more commonly encountered sex chromosome aneuploidies. For more detail, the reader should consult the document "Children and Young Adults with Sex Chromosome Aneuploidy" that we referred to above (Evans et al., 1990a).

XXY (Klinefelter Syndrome)

Almost certainly, the child becomes a sterile adult, and while penile size is usually normal the testes will be small (4–6 ml, cf. normal >12 ml). Androgen deficiency can be managed by replacement therapy with testosterone; some recommend it from age 12 years for all XXY boys (Winter, 1990), whereas others remain to be convinced that it is beneficial (Ratcliffe et al., 1990; Stewart et al., 1990). It may be that treatment induces a more masculine body habitus, improved self-esteem, vitality, ability to concentrate, and sexual interest (Nielsen, 1990; Winter, 1990). Onset of puberty is not delayed. Gynecomastia may be present, transiently, in 50%; if it persists, it can be treated surgically. IQ is diminished by some 10 to 15 points, and a particular impairment in language expression is common. Learning difficulty at school is to be expected. Of 13 XXY boys studied by Walzer et al. (1990), 11 had persistent reading and spelling problems. Bender et al. (1993) note that a deficit in verbal fluency and reading with XXY is "the most homogeneous and consistent cognitive impairment found in any sex chromosome abnormality group," and may reflect a specific dysfunction of the left cerebral hemisphere. Nielsen and Wohlert (1991) followed six Danish XXY boys from birth to ages 15 to 19: all but one needed remedial teaching, and their career plans were carpenter, draughtsman, gardener, unskilled laborer, mechanic, and undecided. Walzer et al. (1990) refer to the specific characteristics of a lowered level of motor activity, a pliant disposition, and a cautious approach to new situations; thus, in the classroom setting, they are perceived as "low-key children, well liked by their teachers, and presenting few behavioral management problems." Stewart et al. (1990) comment that "XXY boys are unlikely to reach a level of personal and social development that is consistent with their family background." In a summary of psychosocial adaptation from several studies, recurring adjectives to describe the XXY personality were "shy," "immature," "restrained," "reserved"; in general the formation of peer relationships has been poor, although some young men report having had a girlfriend (Robinson et al., 1990). We note above the ameliorative effect of growing up in a stable and supportive family.

XXX

Physical development of the XXX female is generally unremarkable, although there is a tendency toward tallness. Gross and fine motor skills are likely to be somewhat impaired, and children are awkward and poorly coordinated. Pubertal development and fertility appear uncompromised. The major concerns relate to intelligence and language; the effects on IQ score are greater for XXX than any of the other three major aneuploidies. Full scale and verbal IQ is reduced by some 20 points (Netley, 1986; Bender et al., 1993). Language comprehension and use of speech are impaired in over half the cases. Learning difficulty is likely and many will benefit from additional remedial teaching, but few require education outside the mainstream. In one small study of 11 girls, 9 needed special-education intervention, and one was placed in a class for retarded children (Bender et al., 1993). There is no obvious increased risk for behavioral problems. Difficulty in forming interpersonal relationships is not unusual, although many do have boyfriends. These observations notwithstanding, Robinson et al. (1990) comment that ''we continue to receive positive reports from parents of young 47,XXX daughters who were diagnosed prenatally.'' As with XXY, they suggest a vulnerability of these children to stress and the desirability, therefore, of a supportive environment.

XYY

The multicenter prospective study documented in Evans et al. (1990a) reviewed progress in 39 boys and young men. The particular physical attribute of the XYY male is increased stature. Sexual activity is normal, and fertility is apparently uncompromised. While IQs are in the normal range, they are usually lower than those of sibs or controls, and about half of XYY boys have a mild learning difficulty. Motor proficiency may be impaired. It may be that the aneuploidy causes a minor and subtle impairment of neurologic maturation, leading to some features of minimal brain dysfunction (Theilgaard, 1986). Perhaps the major concern is in psychosocial adaptation: these boys can have a low frustration tolerance, and are prone to temper tantrums in childhood progressing to aggressive behavior as teenagers, and they need help to learn to cope with this. The vignettes from the series of Ratcliffe et al. (1990) of ten Scottish subjects who had left school give an idea of what XYY young men are capable of: one runs a market stall, two are chefs, and the others are a private in the army, a waiter, a supermarket assistant, a video shop assistant, a technician, a laborer, and one is training as a painter and decorator. The functioning of the family may be as much an ingredient as the karyotype in psychosocial development.

45,X (Turner Syndrome)

Unlike the foregoing aneuploidies, 45,X has a very high in utero lethality, peaking at around 12 to 15 weeks' gestation. Spontaneous abortion follows amniocentesis-detected 45,X in three-quarters of cases (Hook, 1983). But some survive pregnancy and are born as infants with Turner syndrome. Robinson et al. (1990) provide a useful and practical outlook: (1) The child will most likely be short, with an average adult height of 145 cm (4 feet 9 inches). A useful increment can be achieved with growth hormone treatment (Rosenfeld et al., 1992). (2) Sterility is almost certain: ''counseling about the expectations and future management of the patient with Turner syndrome who is diagnosed before puberty needs to include the very high possibility of gonadal failure and infertility, but not its inevitable occurrence'' (Lippe, 1991). A few have a spontaneous onset of puberty, but progress may arrest at any stage; if menstruation does occur, it is irregular. Childbearing via ovum donation may be successful in some cases

(p. 200). *(3)* Certain physical defects are associated, of which the major are neck webbing and coarctation (narrowing) of the aorta. *(4)* ''Mental retardation is not to be expected. IQ is variable, spans a wide range, and is usually lower than that of her sibs.'' *(5)* Some delay in neurodevelopmental progress in infancy, and some learning difficulty in school are to be anticipated, and should be managed no differently from a 46,XX girl with the same problems. *(6)* ''A supportive environment that provides stimulation and encouragement is of considerable importance''. *(7)* ''Variability among 45,X girls is considerable; and precise predictions about any child's prognosis are not possible.'' Pavlidis et al. (1995) review sexual functioning in women with Turner syndrome and suggest strategies to avoid possible difficulties.

Sex Chromosome Polysomy

Linden et al. (1995) review the phenotypes of 48,XXXX, 48,XXXY, 48,XXYY, 48,XYYY, 49,XXXXX, 49,XXXXY, 49,XXXYY, 49,XXYYY, and 49,XYYYY. In each, variable intellectual compromise or frank mental retardation is characteristic, the more so in karyotypes with four or more X chromosomes. While the authors' comment is well taken that a general perception of seriousness of phenotypic abnormality may have been overstated due to ascertainment bias, and indeed they describe normal (but low) IQs in some of the $2n = 48$ karyotypes, it remains true that most have substantial handicap due to intellectual deficit and abnormal behavior.

Sex Chromosome Mosaicism

XX/XY

This is usually pseudomosaicism, resulting from the growth of maternal cells in a 46,XY pregnancy (Worton and Stern, 1984). Obviously, it is normally undetected if the fetus is female. Level III XX/XY mosaicism, curiously enough, is most likely to indicate a phenotypically normal female fetus in whom the XY source is unknown, particularly when the XX cells predominate (Worton and Stern, 1984); a male ''vanished twin'' is a theoretical possibility. Ultrasonography with respect to fetal external genital morphology may be helpful.

X/XY

Patients found to have 45,X/46,XY mosaicism range in phenotype from females with classical Turner syndrome through infants with ambiguous genitalia to normal but infertile males. By contrast, most instances of X/XY detected at PND—in other words, cases whose ascertainment was unbiased—and going through to birth result in a normal male infant. Hsu (1989) found in a series of 54 prenatal diagnoses that in 90% a phenotypically normal male child is born but comments that ''the 10% risk of an abnormal outcome still deserves much of our attention.'' Similarly, from a study of 92 prenatally diagnosed cases, Chang et al. (1990) concluded that 95% will have normal male genitalia. There were no data on development on X/XY children beyond the age of

4 years; up to that age, the phenotypic range in 23 patients was normal. Of 14 pathology studies on fetuses post-termination, two were found to have ovotestes and one had a "precancerous" lesion. Concerning this risk for neoplasia of the gonad, Müller and Skakkebæk (1990) provide guidance on tumor surveillance and management; the actual risk may inhere in the presence of a gene *GBY* (GB = gonadoblastoma) on the Y chromosome (Salo et al., 1995). The placenta may have been the origin of the 45,X line in some X/XY (and X/XYY) mosaicism (McFadden and Kalousek, 1989), although most cases will show 45,X cells on postnatal follow-up (Chang et al., 1990).

Other Sex Chromosome Mosaicism

The karyotypes most frequently seen are 45,X/46,XX, 47,XXY/46,XY, 45,X/47,XXX, and 47,XXX/46,XX. It appears that the great majority of cases of true sex chromosomal mosaicism of these types are associated with concordant (Y→male, no Y→female) and normal genital development (Hsu and Perlis, 1984; Wheeler et al., 1988). In general, IQ is not discernibly affected in X/XX, X/XXX, X/XX/XXX, and XXX/XX mosaicism; verbal IQ may be slightly lowered in XXY/XY (Netley, 1986; Bender et al., 1993). Hsu et al. (1992) report that of 98 cases with X/XX mosaicism in which the pregnancy outcome was documented only 8 had some features of Turner syndrome. Koeberl et al. (1995) record twelve cases of 45,X/46,XX mosaicism detected at amniocentesis, with the percentage of 45,X cells in ten of these being in the region of 20–70%. Postnatal studies (blood and/or skin) confirmed the mosaicism in nine (with the percentage of 45,X being lesser in all but one), while in three of the children no 45,X cells were seen. None showed growth retardation postnatally and in none would a clinical suspicion of Turner syndrome have arisen. Two cases of presumed early ovarian dysfunction, one of these also having urogenital anomalies, might reflect an effect of the karyotype; it is possible some of the remaining cases could also manifest abnormal ovarian function at a later age. The abnormal neurology in one of the twelve is of uncertain significance. Mosaicism with a large ring X or an isochromosome for the X long arm, 45,X/46,X,r(X) and 45,X/46,X,i(Xq), respectively, would lead to variant Turner syndrome.

As with X/XY, the X/XYY mosaic state is (necessarily) abnormal in postnatally ascertained cases, but three prenatally diagnosed cases had an apparently normal male phenotype, at least on fetal or newborn assessment (Pettenati et al., 1991). Mosaicism for a 45,X and a 46,X,dic(Y) (isodicentric Y) cell line is associated, at least at postnatal diagnosis, with a wide phenotypic range, often with genital ambiguity and usually with short stature (Tuck-Miller et al., 1995).

NONMOSAIC AUTOSOMAL TRISOMY

Trisomies 13 and 18 (and rarely 8, 9 and 22) are practically the only nonmosaic autosomal trisomies besides +21 that are detected at amniocentesis. Others occur but virtually all miscarry before the usual time of amniocentesis. Chorion villus sampling (CVS), on the other hand, is done at a gestational stage when a number of trisomies destined to abort have not yet done so.

Trisomies 13 and 18

There is a high likelihood (43% for +13 and 68% for +18; Hook, 1983) of spontaneous abortion after amniocentesis, and presumably it is somewhat higher if detection is by CVS. But the outlook for a liveborn child is so bleak, with inevitable profound mental deficiency, barely a vestige of social response in those few who survive beyond early infancy, and a requirement for full nursing care (Smith et al., 1989b; Singh, 1990; Van Dyke and Allen, 1990), that termination is sought by the majority of couples. Those who decide to maintain the pregnancy should know of the high perinatal and early infant mortality, the high likelihood of congenital malformation, and the extreme rarity of survival beyond infancy. Many would regard life-sustaining emergency surgery to the newborn as inappropriate (Bos et al., 1992).

Trisomy 21

It is hardly necessary that we record the predicted Down syndrome phenotype. Marteau et al. (1994) appraised the views of obstetricians, geneticists, and genetic nurses regarding the prenatal diagnosis of Down syndrome and recorded some striking differences. The respective proportions who would counsel nondirectively (see definitions above) were 32%, 57%, and 94%, and the respective proportions counseling directively in favor of termination were 62%, 40%, and 7%. About 6% of obstetricians would counsel directively in favor of continuing the pregnancy, but practically no geneticists or genetic nurses would.

Other Autosomal Trisomy

Never (almost) do other nonmosaic true fetal trisomies survive through to a stage of extrauterine viability. Kuhn et al. (1987) could muster only 20 recorded cases (half being trisomy 9). Miscarriage is virtually inevitable, usually within the 8- to 14-week gestation range. If natural abortion has not already occurred by the time the chromosomal result is received, termination may be seen as appropriate.

MOSAIC AUTOSOMAL TRISOMY

We discuss above the question of distinguishing true fetal mosaicism from confined mosaicism and pseudomosaicism. Hsu et al. (1992) have compiled data on the prenatal diagnosis of autosomal trisomy mosaicism at amniocentesis and pregnancy outcome, as set out in Table 23–4. Mosaicism for chromosomes 18 and 21 frequently predicts fetal abnormality. Trisomy 13 mosaicism predicts abnormality in about half of cases (but see the commentary on p. 356). The high incidence of fetal abnormality associated with mosaic trisomy 9 (Saura et al., 1995) and 22 accords with knowledge of these mosaic states postnatally. Concerning other trisomies, we refer the reader to Hsu et al.'s original paper. A question may arise that trisomy could convert to UPD (p. 32), and UPD 15 Prader-Willi syndrome is the classic example. A unique case is that of Harrison et al. (1995), who report UPD 2 in the 46,XY child of a pregnancy in which true trisomy 2 mosaicism (13/40 cells) was shown at amniocentesis and at placental sampling after delivery; growth retardation was documented, but neurodevelopmental progress was normal. Some true trisomies may be quite benign; for example, trisomy 7 may be a normal finding in renal proximal tubule cells (Knuutila et al., 1995), and perhaps these cells contribute to the amniotic cell population via the fetal urine.

Mosaic Trisomy 20

This is a special case. Trisomy 20 may exist harmlessly in amnion cells, the fetus being chromosomally normal; it may exist as a true fetal mosaicism, yet be associated with an apparently normal phenotype; and, uncommonly, a true mosaicism may cause phenotypic defect (Holzgreve et al., 1986; Hsu et al., 1991; Brothman et al., 1992). In certain fetal regions in which the trisomy may exist, in particular kidney and gut, the imbalance apparently has no discernible untoward effect. In those physically normal infants followed up, child development for at least the first few years of life has been normal (Hsu et al., 1987). In a small minority, the trisomic cell line may be more widespread and lead to variable and nonspecific malformation. It was originally thought that this latter group may be identifiable at the time of PND in having most (over 60%) of the amniotic cells trisomic, but subsequent experience has not validated this impression (Hsu et al., 1991). Fetal blood sampling is not helpful, as the trisomic cells do not appear in blood.

Autosomal Isochromosome Mosaicism

Isochromosomes arise somatically, at least most of the time, and thus the mosaic state is usual. This being so, discovery of 47,+i/46,N is always a concern, even at a level II mosaicism. In the Pallister-Killian syndrome, the 12p isochromosome can vary from being in the majority of cells sampled, to none at all. Bernert et al. (1992) showed in one example 100% of short-term CVS cells and 10% of amniotic fluid cells having the 47,+i(12p) karyotype; the pregnancy was terminated. Horn et al. (1995) report a pregnancy in which CVS gave a 46,XY result on direct (17 cells) and cultured (8 cells) analysis (and 28 further cells on a retrospective study), and the abnormal newborn baby was 46,XY on a peripheral blood study (100 cells counted); at 18 months, a clinical diagnosis of Pallister-Killian syndrome was made, and the karyotype on skin fibroblast culture was 47,XY,+i(12p)/46,XY, with 85% of cells having the isochromosome. Sijmons et al. (1993) document 47,XY,+i(5p) in only 1/217 cells at short-term CVS culture; the dysmorphic and neurologically compromised child had the 5p isochromosome in 3/31 lymphocytes and 12/14 skin fibroblasts. An i(20q) identified at amniocentesis may be a benign finding, possibly reflecting a confined placental mosaicism, and although no case is yet known of a child with an abnormal phenotype, the reported cases are very few and a firm prediction of normality cannot presently be offered (Richkind et al., 1991; Djalali et al., 1992; Donnenfeld and Kershner, 1993).

POLYPLOIDY

Close to 100% of the time, *triploidy* aborts spontaneously, but in some cases not until the pregnancy is well advanced. This being so, termination is appropriate when triploidy is diagnosed. Cassidy et al. (1977) describe the emotional turmoil suffered by the family when a triploid infant, predicted to die immediately, survived for the extraordinary period of five months. Sarno et al. (1993) report a unique case of complete placental/fetal discordance with triploidy on CVS and a normal diploid karyotype on amniocentesis and fetal blood sampling with the birth of a normal baby; such a possibility warrants consideration where triploidy on CVS accompanies an ultrasonographically normal fetus. *Tetraploidy* seen at PND, in the context of normal ultrasonography, may be artifactual, or possibly a vestige from the blastocystic stage of normally occurring trophoblastic tetraploidy (Benkhalifa et al., 1993). In either case, a 46,N fetal karyotype is to be expected (Kohn and Robinson, 1970; D. H. Ledbetter et al., 1992; Teshima et al., 1992a). However Edwards et al. (1994), having observed true normal/tetraploid mosaicism in two severely retarded individuals, do caution that a tetraploid cell line is not absolutely certain to be an innocuous finding.

STRUCTURAL REARRANGEMENT

Structural rearrangements are seen in about 1 in 1000 cytogenetic prenatal diagnoses (Warburton, 1991). It is a matter of urgency to do parental chromosome studies to distinguish between a familial or a de novo rearrangement in the fetus. If one parent is discovered to have the same apparently balanced rearrangement identified at PND, there is no firm evidence for an increased risk of fetal abnormality; but a small (perhaps <1%) risk *may* apply due to a defect beyond the limits of routine cytogenetic resolution (see p. 92).

De Novo "Apparently Balanced" Structural Rearrangement

A major difficulty is posed by the rearrangement which, at the level of cytogenetic analysis, is ''apparently balanced.'' But even with the highest resolution banding and an apparently balanced karyotype, a submicroscopic abnormality (deletion or duplication, or gene disruption) may still be present (Rosenberg et al., 1994; Wagstaff and Hemann, 1995; Tsuji et al., 1995). On postnatal observation, one can be wise after the event. Considering, for example, the specific case of the de novo inversion identified in an abnormal individual, the association of the breakpoint and a known locus can lead to the reasonable conclusion that the cytogenetic abnormality was the cause of that abnormal phenotype (p. 137). If there has been a consistent picture with other rearrangements involving the same region, such as a case of de novo inv(7)(p22q21.3) with a particular split hand/foot malformation also seen with some other 7q21.3–22 rearrangements (Cobden et al., 1995), again the presumption of a causal relationship may reasonably be made. In a normal person, presumably an apparently balanced rearrangement really is balanced.

Naturally, prenatal inference is less clear. Nevertheless, we should emphasize the observation that most de novo inversions, and likewise most reciprocal translocations, occur with normal babies (see below). Presumably, these normal cases reflect breakpoints in DNA that does not code for a gene.

Warburton (1991) has conducted a review of major laboratories in the U.S.A. and Canada over a 10-year period and collected data based on more than a third-of-a-million procedures. A de novo translocation was identified in about 1 in 2000 amniocenteses, a Robertsonian translocation in about 1 in 9000, and an inversion in 1 in 10,000. Given the imperfection of outcome assessment (lack of longterm follow-up, inadequacy of fetal pathology) the derived figures may underestimate the true risk. The difference between the risk figures for translocations and inversions may be more apparent than real.

De Novo Apparently Balanced Reciprocal Translocation

In Warburton's study, serious malformations were identified in 6.1% of pregnancies with a *de novo* simple reciprocal translocation, either at elective termination or at livebirth. This is some 3% above the background 3% risk for malformation and/or serious functional defect that applies to all pregnancies. Thus, we may draw the inference that in about 3% of these de novo translocations the chromosomal defect was causative. It remains moot whether "3%", or a somewhat higher figure, say 5%, should apply to the overall risk for not only major malformation but also substantial functional deficit. Normal ultrasonography would be considerably, but not definitively, reassuring.

Very few de novo whole-arm translocations are recorded, "although the existing examples suggest an optimistic prognosis can be given" (Farrell and Fan, 1995).

A de novo apparently balanced complex chromosome rearrangement probably has a high risk for intellectual impairment and physical malformation, although prospective data are very meager. In the series of Sikkema-Raddatz et al. (1995), 2 out of 4 children followed up after prenatal diagnosis had at least neurodevelopmental defect, while 2 were normal as young children.

In the case of a de novo X-autosome translocation, there are the additional possible complications of gonadal dysgenesis if the breakpoint is within the critical region of the X chromosome, of the unpredictability of the patterns of inactivation with the possibility of severe abnormality, and of a Mendelian disorder if the breakpoint is within a gene (e.g., Bodrug et al., 1990; Punnett, 1994; Seller et al., 1995) (see also Chapter 5). Evans et al. (1993) could actually show normal dystrophin on a fetal muscle biopsy following detection at amniocentesis of an apparently balanced rcp(X;1) with the X breakpoint at p21, and so predicted the child would not have Duchenne/Becker muscular dystrophy; and their prediction proved to be correct. A de novo Y-autosome translocation is likely to be associated with a normal phenotype if the breakpoints are in proximal Y long arm and the short arm of an acrocentric; abnormality is probable if the autosome concerned is not an acrocentric (see also Chapter 5).

De Novo Robertsonian Translocation

The additional risk for phenotypic defect associated with a de novo balanced Robertsonian translocation is very small, and less than 1%; the 95% confidence limits of this estimate encompass 0%. That this risk figure is very small is not surprising, since the formation of the Robertsonian translocation classically does not disrupt unique-sequence DNA. Some of the ''less than 1%'' might be due to UPD of the particular chromosome (e.g., Bricarelli et al., 1994), for a rob in which one or both of the component chromosomes is subject to imprinting, viz., a No. 14 or No. 15. Consideration can be given to molecular analysis to check for this presumably rare possibility, if there is access to this technology.

De Novo Apparently Balanced Inversion

The risk for phenotypic abnormality is 9.4%, which is 6 to 7% over and above the background risk. Inversions of the X, pericentric or paracentric, may produce gonadal insufficiency in the female (Dar et al., 1988; Dahoun et al., 1990) and, in theory, Mendelian disease in the male if a locus is disrupted. (Note that an ''inversion'' detected in this setting may in fact be an unbalanced translocation.)

De Novo Apparently Balanced Insertion

Only one case is recorded of a de novo apparently balanced interchromosomal insertion detected prenatally (Hashish et al., 1992). The child proved to be phenotypically normal. One could not unreasonably extrapolate from the de novo apparently balanced reciprocal translocation (two breakpoints) to suggest that the risk for the interchromosomal insertion (three breakpoints) might be similar or possibly a little greater. Perhaps 5% is a fair figure to offer for the risk of ''unspecified malformation and/or intellectual deficit''. A de novo intrachromosomal ins(X) may produce gonadal insufficiency but an otherwise normal phenotype (Grass et al., 1981).

De Novo Unbalanced Structural Rearrangement

For any de novo structural rearrangement in which cytogenetic imbalance can be demonstrated, serious phenotypic abnormality is highly likely. Molecular methodology may be applied to certain subtle suspected defects, such as a possible Prader-Willi/Angelman deletion (Toth-Fejel et al., 1995). With an X-autosome translocation, albeit the pattern of inactivation may lessen the effect, a significant defect remains very probable (Couillin et al., 1992; Kubota et al., 1994; Kulharya et al., 1995).

Mosaicism for a Structural Rearrangement

The arrangement may be an apparently balanced translocation, an unbalanced translocation, or some other category of rearrangement. The great majority of *balanced* translocation mosaicism is level I or II, and is pseudomosaicism due to in vitro change; in terms of implications for fetal phenotype, it can be disregarded. Some breakpoints (6p21, 13q14) are preferentially involved in pseudomosaicism for a balanced rearrangement (Benn and Hsu, 1986). True mosaicism for this type of structural change is very rare (Fryns and Kleczkowska, 1986). Hsu et al. (1992) identified 15 examples (among 601 mosaic amniocenteses) showing at least one cell line with a balanced rearrangement, and in no case had phenotypic abnormality been observed.

As for the *unbalanced* rearrangement, Hsu et al. (1992) record 34 cases with at least one cell line having an unbalanced rearrangement (thus, presumed to be a true mosaicism); in follow-up studies, phenotypic abnormality was noted in about 50% and cytogenetic confirmation in 65%. Each rearrangement needs to be considered on its merits: thus, 47,+i(12p)/46 predicts the Pallister-Killian syndrome, while 47,+i(20q)/46 is associated with a favorable outcome and a karyotypically normal baby (as noted above).

EXTRA STRUCTURALLY ABNORMAL CHROMOSOME (ESAC)

ESACs are a heterogeneous group. They have been described variously as marker, supernumerary, accessory, and B chromosomes (Hook and Cross, 1987a). Some are quite harmless, and associated with phenotypic normality (the B chromosome), and others are not. ESACs are encountered in about 1 in 2500 prenatal diagnoses, frequently in mosaic form with a normal cell line (Warburton, 1991). Upon the discovery of an ESAC at prenatal diagnosis, an urgent parental chromosome analysis is required.

While fetal ultrasonography is, of course, indicated, in fact in Warburton's (1991) series only about one third of those with significant abnormality were likely to have been identified in this way. Improvements in ultrasound experience and technology since may have increased the rate of detection. It is not clear what reduction to the risks in Table 23–5 could be offered in the presence of a normal ultrasound examination. What is clear, however, is that with a reasonable level of cytogenetic characterization of ESACs and ultrasound examination it is possible to categorize most fetuses as being either at high risk of abnormality or at a relatively low risk (less or much less than 5%). Brøndum-Nielsen and Mikkelsen (1995) report a 10-year experience in Glostrup during which nine de novo ESACs were identified. In seven cases, termination of pregnancy was chosen with some of these showing defects at pathological examination; and in the two pregnancies continuing, one infant with a minute acrocentric-derived ESAC was normal at birth, while one with a ring-like 17 was "slightly retarded" at age 2 years.

Familial ESAC

Interpretation in the case of a familial ESAC is usually straightforward. If one parent is also 47,+ESAC and phenotypically normal, it can be assumed that no discernibly increased risk for fetal abnormality exists (Tsukahara et al., 1986; Brøndum-Nielsen and Mikkelsen, 1995). When the parent has the ESAC in mosaic state, prediction for the fetus is more difficult: the chromosome could be potentially harmful, but the parent might have been protected by a particular tissue distribution. In this situation, recourse to the risks outlined in Table 23–5 may be the best approach. If the ESAC is revealed as being a small derivative chromosome from 3:1 malsegregation, one parent being a balanced translocation carrier (Stamberg and Thomas, 1986), serious phenotypic abnormality is almost certain.

De Novo ESAC

For the nonfamilial ESAC the risks to the fetus are not so easy to quantify. Series of liveborn children with ESACs are mostly seriously biased by ascertainment in favor of phenotypic abnormality. Series of prenatally diagnosed fetuses are deficient in that there is usually only a short-term follow-up of liveborn children, while pathological assessments following termination can only show major structural malformations. Warburton (1991) estimated a risk for abnormality detectable at fetal pathology study or in the immediate newborn period of 15% for nonsatellited ESACs and 11% for those with satellites; this begs the question whether intellectual abnormality might not come to light in future years. Perhaps surprisingly, mosaicism appears not to alter the risk for abnormality.

ESAC Heterogeneity

Lumping ESACs into a group is rather like putting Down, Edwards, and Patau syndromes into a single trisomy category. Precise characterization is necessary, and this requires C-banding, Ag-NOR staining, distamycin A/DAPI staining, and, in particular, FISH. This has allowed some estimates of genetic risk for specific chromosomes, particularly in terms of developmental abnormality with subsequent intellectual handicap. On this basis, and with reference to Warburton (1991), we have produced a table of risks (Table 23–5) which can be used for counseling. These figures need to be put into the usual perspective of a 2 to 3% background risk of major malformation or functional handicap.

A number of ESACs have been reasonably well characterized cytogenetically and have recognized phenotypic outcomes (p. 263–265). Among these are the

Table 23—5   Approximate risks of fetal abnormality following prenatal detection of an ESAC, depending upon level of its characterization

ESAC	Risk
i(18)p	100%
i(12)p	100%
idic(22)	100%
der(X) without XIST	100%
Multiple ESACs	95%
Larger der(15), breaks distal to q11.2 (> No. 21 in size)	95%
Distamycin A/DAPI-negative rings	80%
Satellited acrocentrics with euchromatin	80%
Without satellites[a]	15%
Any, not further characterized[a]	13%
Satellited[a]	11%
Small, mostly C-band positive	5%
Smaller der (15), breaks proximal to q11.2 (< No. 21 in size)	5%
der(Y)	<5%
"dots"	<5%
Small distamycin A/DAPI-positive rings	<5%
der(X) with XIST	<5%
Small bisatellited, single centromere	<2%

[a]Excludes i(18)p and i(12)p.

Source: From Warburton et al. (1991).

inv dup (15), discussed below; the **i(18p)** which leads to a well defined syndrome (Callen et al., 1990b); the **i(12p)** which results in the Pallister-Killian syndrome; and the bisatellited **inv dup(22)** ESAC which causes cat eye syndrome (in which, notably, the severity of the phenotype does not correlate with the extent of the duplication/triplication; Mears et al., 1994).

Inv Dup(15)

Almost half of all ESACs are inv dup (15)s. These are frequently dicentric and bisatellited although one of the centromeres may be suppressed. The smallest ones (smaller than chromosome 21) appear to be the harmless, but larger ones result in the "inv dup(15) syndrome"; we discuss this in more detail on p. 264. Leana-Cox et al. (1994) draw attention to an "urgent need for long-term follow-up of prenatally diagnosed cases"—"although we report a significant association between the presence of the PWS/AS region and abnormal phenotype, . . . our data are heavily weighted [by ascertainment bias]." Rare inv dup(15)s have been associated with UPD 15 or 15q11–13 deletion (Spinner et al., 1995), and it may be warranted to check for this possibility.

Ring ESAC

Another group of ESACs with a high likelihood of causing phenotypic abnormality are small distamycin A/DAPI negative ring chromosomes. These originate from a variety of chromosomes and contain euchromatin (Callen et al., 1992; Plattner et al., 1993; Blennow et al., 1994a). In one case, an ESAC ring (of chromosome 6) was associated with UPD 6 (James et al., 1995).

Sex Chromosome ESAC

ESACs derived from sex chromosomes are a special group. Der(Y) chromosomes are unlikely to cause phenotypic defect in a 47,XY,+der(Y) male fetus, but in a female fetus (sometimes with 45,X/46,X,+der(Y) mosaicism) they can be associated with abnormality of genital tract differentiation. Large ring X chromosomes are noted under Other Sex Chromosome Mosaicism (above). The "tiny ring X syndrome" with the karyotype 45,X/46,X,r(X) has a functional X disomy and is associated with a severe phenotype of physical and mental defect (Migeon et al., 1994).

APPENDIXES

Ideograms of Human Chromosomes, and Haploid Autosomal Lengths

HAPLOID AUTOSOMAL LENGTH

To determine the (quantitative) amount of a particular segmental imbalance, as a fraction of the haploid autosomal length (HAL), multiply (*1*) the fraction of the whole chromosome that this segment comprises by (*2*) the HAL of the whole chromosome. The fraction is readily estimated by placing a millimeter rule against the ideograms overleaf (or by reference to the relative distances between borders of bands listed in Table 1 in Francke, 1994). The HAL of the autosome concerned is taken from Table A–1.

For example, what proportion of the HAL does the segment 4q25→qter constitute? First, the segment comprises 41% of the length of chromosome 4: running a millimeter rule alongside the ideogram of chromosome 4 in Figure A-1, the whole chromosome is 109 mm and the segment is 45 mm, and 45/109 = 41%. Second, from the table, chromosome 4 is 6.30% of the total HAL. Thus, 41% of 6.30% = 2.6% of HAL.

Table A—1 The percentage of HAL that each autosome constitutes

Chromosome	Percentage of HAL	Chromosome	Percentage of HAL
1	8.44	12	4.66
2	8.02	13	3.74
3	6.83	14	3.56
4	6.30	15	3.46
5	6.08	16	3.36
6	5.90	17	3.25
7	5.36	18	2.93
8	4.93	19	2.67
9	4.80	20	2.56
10	4.59	21	1.90
11	4.61	22	2.04

Source: From Daniel (1979).

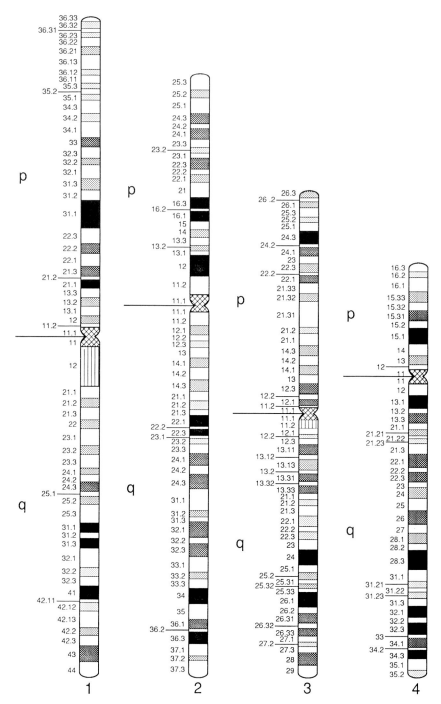

FIGURE A–1. These depictions represent the bands that can be distinguished at a very high level (850 band) of cytogenetic resolution. Different shadings and lengths

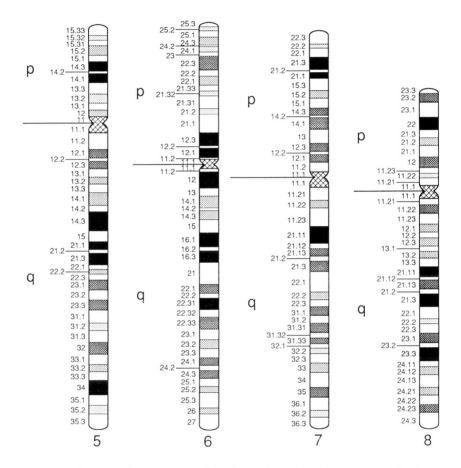

of bands reflect actual intensities and lengths as observed by the cytogeneticist. (From Francke (1994), Digitized and differentially shaded human chromosome ideograms for genomic applications, *Cytogenetics and Cell Genetics,* 65, 206–219, 1994, courtesy U. Franke and with the permission of S. Karger.)

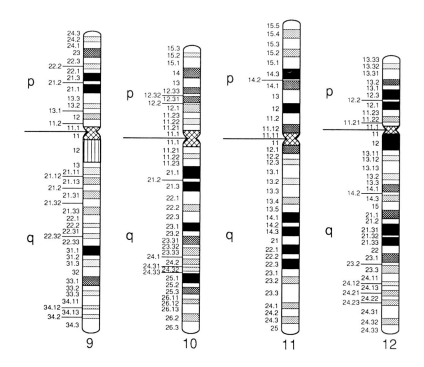

FIGURE A—1 (continued)

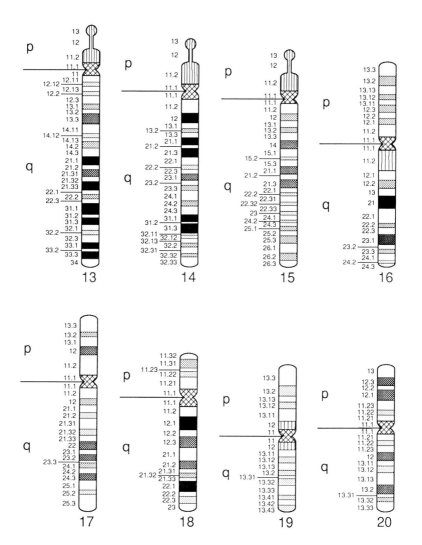

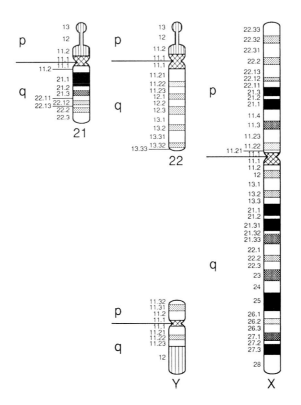

FIGURE A—1 (continued)

Cytogenetic Abbreviations and Nomenclature

The description of chromosomal constitution in most laboratory reports and in most case reports in the literature follows an internationally accepted format: the International System of Cytogenetic Nomenclature (ISCN, 1995).[1] First, the diploid number is given. Second, the sex chromosome constitution is given. Thereafter, any abnormality or variant is described. Certain abbreviations are used, as listed below. In structural rearrangements, the position of breakpoints is given by reference to the band involved: short or long arm (p or q), region, and band or subband(s) within that band. The region is denoted by a digit, 1 through 4; the band by a digit, 1 through 8; and the subband(s) by digit(s) following a "decimal point." The centromere is p10 or q10. Illustrative examples of commonly described karyotypes follow.

ABBREVIATIONS

add	Additional material of unknown origin
del	Deletion
der	Derivative chromosome
dic	Dicentric chromosome
dup	Duplication
fis	Fission (at the centromere)
fra	Fragile site
h	Secondary constriction
i	Isochromosome
ins	Insertion
dir ins	Direct insertion
inv ins	Inverted insertion
inv	Inversion

ish   In situ hybridization
mar   Marker chromosome
mat   Maternal origin
minus (−)   Loss of a whole chromosome
mos   Mosaic
p   Short arm
pat   Paternal origin
plus (+)   Gain of a whole chromosome
q   Long arm
r   Ring
rcp   Reciprocal translocation
rea   Rearrangement
rec   Recombinant chromosome
rob   Robertsonian translocation
solidus (/) Separates cell lines in describing mosaics
stk   Satellite stalk
t   Translocation
ter   Terminal (end of chromosome arm)
upd   Uniparental disomy

SOME EXAMPLES OF CYTOGENETIC NOMENCLATURE

Normal

46,XX   Normal female
46,XY   Normal male
46,XX,9qh+   Normal female, additional material in heterochromatic
                         region of chromosome 9 long arm
46,XY,Yqh−   Normal male, deletion of material from heterochro-
                         matic region of Y long arm
46,XY,fra(10)(q23.3)   Normal male, fragile site on chromosome 10 long arm
                         at subband 23.3

Abnormal

Sex Chromosome Aneuploidies

45,X   Monosomy X (Turner syndrome)
47,XXY   Klinefelter syndrome
47,XXX   Triple X female
47,XYY   XYY "syndrome"
48,XXXX 49,XXXXY   Two of the more common types of polysomy X
47,XXY/46,XY   Mosaic Klinefelter syndrome
45,X/46,XX   Mosaic Turner syndrome

Autosomal Aneuploidies

47,XY,+21	Trisomy 21 (Down syndrome)
47,XX,+21/46,XX	Mosaic Down syndrome
47,XX,+18	Trisomy 18 (Edwards syndrome)
47,XY,+13	Trisomy 13 (Patau syndrome)
47,XX,+8/46,XX	Mosaic trisomy 8
47,XY,+16	Trisomy 16
45,XX,−21	Monosomy 21

Polyploidies

69,XXY	Triploidy
92,XXXX	Tetraploidy

Rearrangements

Deletions

46,XX,del(4)(p15)	Deletion No. 4 short arm (Wolf-Hirschhorn syndrome)
46,XX,del(5)(p13)	Deletion No. 5 short arm (cri du chat syndrome)
46,XX,del(18)(q12)	Deletion No. 18 long arm

Translocations

46,XX,t(4;12)(p14;p13) *or* 46,XX,rcp(4;12)(p14;p13)	Reciprocal translocation between chromosome 4 and 12, with breakpoints at p14 in chromosome 4 and p13 in chromosome 12
46,XY,der(12)t(4;12)(p14;p13)mat	Unbalanced complement, having received derivative No. 12 in place of normal 12 from translocation carrier mother
47,XX,+der(22)t(11;22)(q23;q11)pat	Unbalanced complement having received derivative 22 as a supernumerary chromosome from translocation carrier father

Robertsonian Translocations

45,XY,der(14;21)(q10;q10) *or* replace der with rob	"Balanced" carrier of monocentric fusion Robertsonian translocation between chromosomes 14 and 21
46,XY,der(14;21)(q10;q10)mat,+21 *or* replace der with rob	Unbalanced complement, having received (14;21) Robertsonian chromosome as well as a "free" No. 21 from mother (the karyotype of translocation Down syndrome)

Inversions

46,XX,inv(3)(p23q27)   Inversion (pericentric) of chromo-
                                     some 3, breakpoints at p23 and
                                     q27
46,XY,rec(3)dup(3p)inv(3)(p23q27)mat Recombinant chromosome has been
                                     transmitted from mother carrying
                                     inversion chromosome 3. There is
                                     duplication of the short arm seg-
                                     ment distal to p23; and deletion of
                                     the long arm segment distal to q27
46,XY,inv(11)(q13q22)   Inversion (paracentric) of chromo-
                                     some 11, breakpoints at q13 and
                                     q22

Insertions

46,XY,dir ins(10;8)(q21;q21.2q22)   Direct insertion of segment q21.2→q22
                                     of chromosome 8 into q21 of chro-
                                     mosome 10. Segment has original ori-
                                     entation to centromere, namely, q21.2
                                     is proximal and q22 distal
46,XX,inv ins(2)(p13q31q21)   Inverted insertion of segment q31→q21
                                     into band p13. Segment has opposite
                                     orientation to centromere, namely, q31
                                     is proximal and q21 distal

Other

46,XX,r(15)   A ring chromosome of No. 15
46,X,i(Xq)   An isochromosome of the X long arm
46,XX,add(19)(p13)   Additional material of unknown origin attached to
                      band p13 of chromosome 19
46,XY,upd(15)mat   Uniparental disomy for a maternally derived chromo-
                      some 15
46,Y,fra(X)(q27.3)   Male with a fragile site in subband 27.3 on the X long
                      arm
1(pp)(qqqqqqqqqq)   Multiradial of No. 1 comprising two short arms and
                      ten long arms (see Figure 19–4).

NOTE

1. The 1995 I.S.C.N. came into our hands only as this book was going to press. While this appendix and some of the text is up to date, much "old fashioned" nomenclature remains in the body of the book. We make no apology: the reader consulting any paper published prior to the dissemination of the new nomenclature will need to understand both the old and the new.

Determining 95 Percent Confidence Limits, and the Standard Error

CONFIDENCE LIMITS

The "Exact Confidence Limits for p" tables in Documenta Geigy (1982, pp. 89–102) are a useful source of data on confidence limits for the sizes of sample geneticists generally collect. Suppose in a kindred—ascertainment bias having been suitably accounted for—5 of a total of 54 offspring of translocation carriers were abnormal and 49 were phenotypically normal. The frequency for abnormality from this particular sample is 9.3% (5/54). Checking in Documenta Geigy under $N = 54$, $x = 5$, we see that the 95% confidence limits are given as 3.08 to 20.30%. In other words, we may take it as close to being sure that the true risk lies in the range 3 to 20%.

STANDARD ERROR

The standard error (SE) is calculated from the simple formula

$$SE = \sqrt{\frac{a(n-a)}{n^3}}$$

where a = the number of abnormals, and n = the total number of offspring after ascertainment correction (Stengel-Rutkowski et al., 1984). Thus, for the preceding example

$$SE = \sqrt{\frac{5(54-5)}{54^3}}$$

$$= 0.039$$

And thus the risk is given as $9.3 \pm 3.9\%$.

References

Abbas, N., Novelli, G., Stella, N. C., Triolo, O., Corrado, F., Fellous, M., Chery, M., Gilgenkrantz, S. and Dallapiccola, B. (1990). A 45,X male with molecular evidence of a translocation of Y euchromatin onto chromosome 1. *Hum Genet*, **86**, 94–98.

Abe, T., Morita, M., Kawai, K., Misawa, S., Kanai, H., Hirose, G. and Fujita, H. (1975). Transmission of a t(13q22q) chromosome observed in three generations with segregation of the translocation D$_1$-trisomy syndrome. *Hum Genet*, **30**, 207–215.

Abeliovich, D., Dagan, J., Werner, M., Lerer, I., Shapira, Y. and Meiner, V. (1995). Simultaneous formation of inv dup(15) and dup(15q) in a girl with developmental delay: origin of the abnormal chromosomes. *Eur J Hum Genet*, **3**, 49–55.

Abeliovich, D., Yagupsky, P. and Bashan, N. (1982). 3:1 meiotic disjunction in a mother with a balanced translocation, 46,XX,t(5;14)(p15;q13) resulting in tertiary trisomy and tertiary monosomy offspring. *Am J Med Genet*, **12**, 83–89.

Abramowicz, M. J., Andrien, M., Dupont, E., Dorchy, H., Parma, J., Duprez L., Ledley, F. D., Courtens, W. and Vamos, E. (1994). Isodisomy of chromosome 6 in a newborn with methylmalonic acidemia and agenesis of pancreatic beta cells causing diabetes mellitus. *J Clin Invest*, **94**, 418–421.

Abramsky, L. and Chapple, J. (eds.) (1994). ''Prenatal diagnosis. The human side.'' Chapman and Hall, London.

Abuelo, D. N., Barsel-Bowers, G. and Richardson, A. (1988). Insertional translocations: report of two new families and review of the literature. *Am J Med Genet*, **31**, 319–329.

Adinolfi, M. (1995). Non- or minimally invasive prenatal diagnostic tests on maternal blood samples or transcervical cells. *Prenat Diagn*, **15**, 889–896.

Adinolfi, M., Sherlock, J., Tutschek, B., Halder, A., Delhanty, J. and Rodeck, C. (1995). Detection of fetal cells in transcervical samples and prenatal diagnosis of chromosomal abnormalities. *Prenat Diagn*, **15**, 943–949.

Agrawal, Y. P., Ylikangas, P., Parviainen, M. T. and Penttilä, I. M. (1994). Flow cytometric method to measure urea-resistant alkaline phosphatase from blood neutrophils for use in the prenatal screening of Down's syndrome. *Prenat Diagn*, **14**, 1141–1149.

Aiello, V., Ricci, N., Palazzi, P., D'Agostino, G., Azzini, G. and Calzolari, E. (1994). New variant of chromosome 11. *Am J Med Genet*, **50**, 294–295.

Aittomäki, K. (1994). The genetics of XX gonadal dysgenesis. *Am J Hum Genet*, **54**, 844–851.

Al-Gazali, L. I., Mueller, R. F., Caine, A., Antoniou, A., McCartney, A., Fitchett, M. and Dennis, N. R. (1990). Two 46,XX,t(X;Y) females with linear skin defects and congenital microphthalmia: a new syndrome at Xp22.3. *J Med Genet*, **27**, 59–63.

Allderdice, P. W., Ali, M. and McAlpine, P. J. (1991). Complementation by two non-homologous recombinant chromosomes 3. *Am J Med Genet*, **39**, 396–398.

Allderdice, P. W., Browne, N. and Murphy, D. P. (1975). Chromosome 3 duplication q21→qter deletion p25→pter syndrome in children of carriers of a pericentric inversion inv(3)(p25q21). *Am J Hum Genet*, **27**, 699–718.

Allderdice, P. W., Aveling, J. V., Eales, B. A., Lewis, M. J., McAlpine, P. J., Ross, J. B. and Simms, R. J. (1983a). Familial t(X;Y)(p223q11) associated with short stature in 4 male and 5 female carriers, and with X-linked ichthyosis and anhydrosis in 4 male carriers. *Am J Hum Genet*, **35**, 124A.

Allderdice, P. W., Eales, B., Onyett, H., Sprague, W., Henderson, K., Lefeuvre, P. A. and Pal, G. (1983b). Duplication 9q34 syndrome. *Am J Hum Genet*, **35**, 1005–1009.

Alley, T. L., Gray, B. A., Lee, S.-H., Scherer, S. W., Tsui, L.-C., Tint, G. S., Williams, C. A., Zori, R. and Wallace, M. R. (1995). Identification of a yeast artificial chromosome clone spanning a translocation breakpoint at 7q32.1 in a Smith-Lemli-Opitz syndrome patient. *Am J Hum Genet*, **56**, 1411–1416.

Allingham-Hawkins, D. J. and Ray, P. N. (1995). FRAXE expansion is not a common etiological factor among developmentally delayed males. *Am J Hum Genet*, **56**, 72–76.

Allingham-Hawkins, D. J. and Tomkins, D. J. (1995). Heterogeneity in Roberts syndrome. *Am J Med Genet*, **55**, 188–194.

Almeida, J. C. C. D., Llerena, J. C., Gomes, D. M., Martins, R. R. and Pereira, E. T. (1983). Ring 13 in an adult male with a 13:13 translocation mother. *Ann Génét*, **26**, 112–115.

Altherr, M. R., Bengtsson, U., Elder, F. F. B., Ledbetter, D. H., Wasmuth, J. J., Mc-Donald, M. E., Gusella, J. F. and Greenberg, F. (1991). Molecular confirmation of Wolf-Hirschhorn syndrome with a subtle translocation of chromosome 4. *Am J Hum Genet*, **49**, 1235–1242.

American Academy of Pediatrics, Committee on Bioethics (1990). Sterilization of women who are mentally handicapped. *Pediatrics*, **85**, 868–871.

American College of Medical Genetics (1993). Prenatal interphase fluorescence in situ hybridization (FISH) policy statement. *Am J Hum Genet*, **53**, 526–527.

Andrews, K., Wienberg, J., Ferguson-Smith, M. A. and Rubinsztein, D. C. (1995). Enrichment of fetal nucleated cells from maternal blood: model test system using cord blood. *Prenat Diagn*, **15**, 913–919.

Angell, R. R. (1991). Predivision in human oocytes at meiosis I: a mechanism for trisomy formation in man. *Hum Genet*, **86**, 383–387.

Angell, R. R. (1995). Meiosis I in human oocytes. *Cytogenet Cell Genet*, **69**, 266–272.

Angell, R. R. and Jacobs, P. A. (1978). Lateral asymmetry in human constitutive heterochromatin: frequency and inheritance. *Am J Hum Genet*, **30**, 144–152.

Angell, R. R., Xian, J., Keith, J., Ledger, W. and Baird, D. T. (1994). First meiotic division abnormalities in human oocytes: mechanism of trisomy formation. *Cytogenet Cell Genet*, **65**, 194–202.

Antonarakis, S. E., Adelsberger, P. A., Petersen, M. B., Binkert, F. and Schinzel, A. A. (1990). Analysis of DNA polymorphisms suggest that most de novo dup(21q) chromosomes in patients with Down syndrome are isochromosomes and not translocations. *Am J Hum Genet*, **47**, 968–972.

Antonarakis, S. E., Avramopoulos, D., Blouin, J.-L., Talbot, C. C. and Schinzel, A. A. (1993a). Mitotic errors in somatic cells cause trisomy 21 in about 4.5% of cases and are not associated with advanced maternal age. *Nature Genet*, **3**, 146–149.

Antonarakis, S. E., Blouin, J.-L., Maher, J., Avramopoulos, D., Thomas, G. and Talbot, C. C. (1993b). Maternal uniparental disomy for human chromosome 14, due to loss of a chromosome 14 from somatic cells with t(13;14) trisomy 14. *Am J Hum Genet*, **52**, 1145–1152.

Antonarakis, S. E., Petersen, M. B., McInnis, M. G., Adelsberger, P. A., Schinzel, A. A., Binkert, F., Pangalos, C., Raoul, O., Slaugenhaupt, S. A., Hafez, M., Cohen, M. M., Roulson, D., Schwartz, S., Mikkelsen, M., Tranebjaerg, L., Greenberg, F., Hoar, D. I., Rudd, N. L., Warren, A. C., Metaxotou, C., Bartsocas, C. and Chakravarti, A. (1992). The meiotic stage of nondisjunction in trisomy 21: determination by using DNA polymorphisms. *Am J Hum Genet*, **50**, 544–550.

Ariel, I., Lustig, O., Oyer, C. E., Elkin, M., Gonik, B., Rachmilewitz, J., Biran, H., Goshen, R., de Groot, N. and Hochberg, A. (1994). Relaxation of imprinting in trophoblastic disease. *Gynecol Oncol*, **53**, 212–219.

Arn, P., Chen, H., Tuck-Muller, C. M., Mankinen, C., Wachtel, G., Li, S., Shen, C.-C. and Wachtel, S. S. (1994). SRVX, a sex reversing locus in Xp21.2→p22.11. *Hum Genet*, **93**, 389–393.

Arn, P. H., Younie, L., Russo, S., Zackowski, J. L., Mankinen, C. and Estabrooks, L. (1995). Reproductive outcome in 3 families with a satellited chromosome 4 with review of the literature. *Am J Med Genet*, **57**, 420–424.

Ashley, C. T., Wilkinson, K. D., Reines, D. and Warren, S. T. (1993). FMR1 protein: conserved RNP family domains and selective RNA binding. *Science*, **262**, 563–566.

Ashley, T. (1990). Prediction of mammalian meiotic synaptic and recombinational behavior of inversion heterozygotes based on meiotic breakpoint data and the possible evolutionary consequences. *Gentica*, **83**, 1–7.

Auerbach, A. D. (1987). Prenatal diagnosis of mutagen-hypersensitivity syndromes. *Curr Prob Dermatol*, **16**, 197–209.

Auerbach, A. D. (1993). Fanconi anemia diagnosis and the diepoxybutane (DEB) test. *Exp Hematol*, **21**, 731–733.

Auerbach, A. D., Min, Z., Ghosh, R., Pergament, E., Verlinsky, Y., Nicolas, H. and Boué, J. (1986). Clastogen-induced chromosomal breakage as a marker for first trimester prenatal diagnosis of Fanconi anemia. *Hum Genet*, **73**, 86–88.

Auerbach, A. D., Sagi, M. and Adler, B. (1985). Fanconi anemia: prenatal diagnosis in 30 fetuses at risk. *Pediatrics*, **76**, 794–800.

Augusseau, S., Jouk, S., Jalbert, P. and Prieur, M. (1986). DiGeorge syndrome and 22q11 rearrangements. *Hum Genet*, **74**, 206.

Avivi, L., Korenstein, A., Braier-Goldstein, O., Goldman, B. and Ravia, Y. (1992). Uniparental disomy of sex chromosomes in man. *Hum Genet*, **51**, A11.

Ayukawa, H., Tsukahara, M., Fukuda, M. and Kondoh, O. (1994). Recombinant chromosome 18 resulting from a maternal pericentric inversion. *Am J Med Genet*, **50**, 323–325.

Babu, A., Agarwal, A. K. and Verma, R. S. (1988). A new approach in recognition of heterochromatic regions of human chromosomes by means of restriction endonucleases. *Am J Hum Genet*, **42**, 60–65.

Bagshawe, K. D. and Lawler, S. D. (1982). Unmasking moles. *Br J Obstet Gynaecol*, **89**, 255–257.

Bahado-Singh, R. O., Kliman, H., Feng, T. Y., Hobbins, J., Copel, J. A. and Mahoney, M. J. (1995). First-trimester endocervical irrigation: feasibility of obtaining trophoblast cells for prenatal diagnosis. *Obstet Gynecol*, **85**, 461–464.

Baird, P. A. and Sadovnick, A. D. (1989). Life table for Down syndrome. *Hum Genet*, **82**, 291–292.

Baldinger, S., Millard, C., Schmeling, D. and Bendel, R. P. (1987). Prenatal diagnosis of trisomy 20 mosaicism indicating an extra embryonic origin. *Prenat Diagn*, **7**, 273–276.

Balkan, W., Burns, K. and Martin, R. H. (1983). Sperm chromosome analysis of a man heterozygous for a pericentric inversion of chromosome 3. *Cytogenet Cell Genet*, **35**, 295–297.

Balkan, W. and Martin, R. H. (1983). Segregation of chromosomes into the spermatozoa of a man heterozygous for a 13;21 Robertsonian translocation. *Am J Med Genet*, **16**, 169–172.

Ballabio, A. (1995). MLS, Aicardi and Goltz syndromes: how many genes involved? *Am J Med Genet*, **59**, 100.

Ballabio, A. and Andria, G. (1992). Deletions and translocations involving the distal short arm of the human X chromosome: review and hypotheses. *Hum Mol Genet*, **1**, 221–227.

Ballabio, A. and Willard, H. F. (1992). Mammalian X-chromosome inactivation and the *XIST* gene. *Curr Opin Genet Dev*, **2**, 439–447.

Barbaux, S., Vilain, E., Raoul, O., Gilgenkrantz, S., Jeandidier, E., Chadenas, D., Souleyreau, N., Fellous, M. and McElreavey, K. (1995). Proximal deletions of the long arm of the Y chromosome suggest a critical region associated with a specific subset of characteristic Turner stigmata. *Hum Mol Genet*, **4**, 1565–1568.

Barber, J. C. K. (1994). Euchromatic heteromorphism or duplication without phenotypic effect? *Prenat Diagn*, **14**, 323–324.

Barber, J. C. K., Ellis, K. H., Bowles, L. V., Delhanty, J. D. A., Ede, R. F., Male, B. M. and Eccles, D. M. (1994). Adenomatous polyposis coli and a cytogenetic deletion of chromosome 5 resulting from a maternal intrachromosomal insertion. *J Med Genet*, **31**, 312–316.

Barber, J. C. K., Mahl, H., Portch, J. and Crawfurd, M. d'A. (1991). Interstitial deletions without phenotypic effect: prenatal diagnosis of a new family and brief review. *Prenat Diagn*, **11**, 411–416.

Barbosa, A. S., Ferraz-Costa, T. E., Semer, M., Liberman, B. and Moreira-Filho, C. A. (1995). XY gonadal dysgenesis and gonadoblastoma: a study in two sisters with a cryptic deletion of the Y chromosome involving the SRY gene. *Hum Genet*, **95**, 63–66.

Bardoni, B., Zanaria, E., Guioli, S., Floridia, G., Worley, K. C., Tonini, G., Ferrante, E., Chiumello, G., McCabe, E. R. B., Fraccaro, M., Zuffardi, O. and Camerino, G. (1994). A dosage sensitive locus at chromosome Xp21 is involved in male to female sex reversal. *Nature Genet*, **7**, 497–501.

Bartram, C. R. (1980). DNA repair: pathways and defects. *Eur J Pediatr*, **135**, 121–128.

Bartsch, O., König, U., Petersen, M. B., Poulsen, H., Mikkelsen, M., Palau, F., Prieto,

F. and Schwinger, E. (1993). Cytogenetic, FISH and DNA studies in 11 individuals from a family with two siblings with dup(21q) Down syndrome. *Hum Genet*, **92**, 127–132.

Bartsch, O., Petersen, M. B., Stuhlmann, I., Mau, G., Frantzen, M., Schwinger, E., Antonarakis, S. E. and Mikkelsen, M. (1994). ''Compensatory'' uniparental disomy of chromosome 21 in two cases. *J Med Genet*, **31**, 534–540.

Bass, H. N. and Sparkes, R. S. (1979). Two balanced translocations in three generations of a pedigree: t(7;10)(q11;q22) and t(14;21)(14qter-cen-21qter). *J Med Genet*, **16**, 215–218.

Bass, H. N., Sparkes, R. S., Lessner, M. M., Fox, M., Phoenix, B. and Bernar, J. (1985). A family with three independent autosomal translocations associated with 7q32→7qter syndrome. *J Med Genet*, **22**, 59–63.

Bates, A. and Howard, P. J. (1990). Distal long arm deletions of the X chromosome and ovarian failure. *J Med Genet*, **27**, 722–723.

Batista, D. A. S., Pai, G. S. and Stetten, G. (1994). Molecular analysis of a complex chromosomal rearrangement and a review of familial cases. *Am J Med Genet*, **53**, 255–263.

Baudier, M. M., Chihal, H. J., and Dickey, R. P. (1985). Pregnancy and reproductive function in a patient with nonmosaic Turner syndrome. *Obstet Gynecol*, **65** (Suppl.), 60S-64S.

Baumann, W., Zabel, B. and Holl, M. (1984). Inversion péricentrique familiale du chromosome X [inv(X)(p11q28)]. *Ann Génét*, **27**, 106–108.

Beekhuis, J. R., De Wolf, B. T. H. M., Mantingh, A. and Heringa, M. P. (1994). The influence of serum screening on the amniocentesis rate in women of advanced maternal age. *Prenat Diagn*, **14**, 199–202.

Bell, J., Dunlop, R. and Bryan, J. (1991). Another paracentric inversion of chromosome 18. *Am J Med Genet*, **39**, 238.

Bender, B. G., Linden, M. G. and Robinson, A. (1993). Neuropsychological impairment in 42 adolescents with sex chromosome abnormalities. *Am J Med Genet*, **48**, 169–173.

Benet, J. and Martin, R. H. (1988). Sperm chromosome complements in a 47,XYY man. *Hum Genet*, **78**, 313–315.

Benkhalifa, M., Janny, L., Vye, P., Malet, P., Boucher, D. and Menezo, Y. (1993). Assessment of polyploidy in human morulae and blastocysts using co-culture and fluorescent in-situ hybridization. *Hum Reprod*, **8**, 895–902.

Benn, P. A., and Hsu, L. Y. F. (1986). Evidence for preferential involvement of chromosome bands 6p21 and 13q14 in amniotic fluid cell balanced translocation pseudomosaicism. *Clin Genet*, **29**, 116–121.

Benn, P. A., Schonhaut, A. G. and Hsu, L. Y. F. (1983). A high incidence of maternal cell contamination of amniotic fluid cell cultures. *Am J Med Genet*, **14**, 361–365.

Bergemann, E. (1962). Manifestation familiale du karyotype triplo-X. Communication préliminaire. *J Génét Hum*, **10**, 370–371.

Berkovitz, G., Stamberg, J., Plotnick, L. P. and Lanes, R. (1983). Turner syndrome patients with a ring X chromosome. *Clin Genet*, **23**, 447–453.

Berkowitz, R. S., Bernstein, M. R., Laborde, O. and Goldstein, D. P. (1994). Subsequent pregnancy experience in patients with gestational trophoblastic disease. New England trophoblastic disease center, 1965–1992. *J Reprod Med*, **39**, 228–232.

Bernardi, G. (1989). The isochore organization of the human genome. *Annu Rev Genet*, **23**, 637–661.

Bernert, J., Bartels, I., Gatz, G., Hansmann, I., Heyat, M., Niedmann, P. D., Rehder, H., Waldenmaier, C. and Zoll, B. (1992). Prenatal diagnosis of the Pallister-Killian mosaic aneuploidy syndrome by CVS. *Am J Med Genet*, **42**, 747–750.

Bernstein, R. (1985). X;Y chromosome translocation and their manifestations. In "Progress and topics in cytogenetics" (A. A. Sandberg, ed.), Vol. 6B. A. R. Liss, New York, pp. 171–206.

Bernstein, R., Jenkins, T., Dawson, B., Wagner, J., Dewald, G., Koo, G. C. and Wachtel, S. S. (1980). Female phenotype and multiple abnormalities in sibs with a Y chromosome and partial X chromosome duplication: H-Y antigen and Xg blood group findings. *J Med Genet*, **17**, 291–300.

Berry, E., Aitken, D. A., Crossley, J. A., Macri, J. N. and Connor, J. M. (1995). Analysis of maternal serum alpha-fetoprotein and free beta human chorionic gonadotrophin in the first trimester: implications for Down's syndrome screening. *Prenat Diagn*, **15**, 555–565.

Bianchi, D. W., Mahr, A., Zickwolf, G. K., Houseal, T. W., Flint, A. F. and Klinger, K. W. (1992). Detection of fetal cells with 47,XY,+21 karyotype in maternal peripheral blood. *Hum Genet*, **90**, 368–370.

Bianchi, D. W., Wilkins-Haug, L. E., Enders, A. C. and Hay, E. D. (1993). Origin of extraembryonic mesoderm in experimental animals: relevance to chorionic mosaicism in humans. *Am J Med Genet*, **46**, 542–550.

Bianco, S., Agrifoglio, V., Mannino, F., Cefalu, E. and Cittadini, E. (1992). Successful pregnancy in a pure gonadal dysgenesis with karyotype 46,XY patient (Swyer's syndrome) following oocyte donation and hormonal treatment. *Acta Eur Fertil*, **23**, 37–38.

Bickmore, W. A. and Sumner, A. T. (1989). Mammalian chromosome banding—an expression of genome organization. *Trends Genet*, **5**, 144–148.

Biesecker, L. G., Rosenberg, M., Dziadzio, L., Ledbetter, D. H., Ning, Y., Sarneso, C. and Rosenbaum, K. (1995). Detection of a subtle rearrangement of chromosome 22 using molecular techniques. *Am J Med Genet*, **58**, 389–394.

Bischoff, F. Z., Nguyen, D. D., Burt, K. J. and Shaffer, L. G. (1994). Estimates of aneuploidy using multicolor fluorescence in situ hybridization on human sperm. *Cytogenet Cell Genet*, **66**, 237–243.

Black, S. H. (1994). Preimplantation genetic diagnosis. *Curr Opin Pediatr*, **6**, 712–716.

Blennow, E., Bui, T.-H., Kristoffersson, U., Vujic, M., Annerén, G., Holmberg, E. and Nordenskjöld, M. (1994a). Swedish survey on extra structurally abnormal chromosomes in 39 105 consecutive prenatal diagnoses: prevalence and characterization by fluorescence *in situ* hybridization. *Prenat Diagn*, **14**, 1019–1028.

Blennow, E., Telenius, H., de Vos, D., Larsson, C., Henriksson, P., Johansson, O., Carter, N. P. and Nordenskjöld, M. (1994b). Tetrasomy 15q: two marker chromosomes with no detectable alpha-satellite DNA. *Am J Hum Genet*, **54**, 877–883.

Blennow, E., Nielsen, K. B., Telenius, H., Carter, N. P., Kristoffersson, U., Holmberg, E., Gillberg, C. and Nordenskjöld, M. (1995). Fifty probands with extra structurally abnormal chromosomes characterized by fluorescence in situ hybridization. *Am J Med Genet*, **55**, 85–94.

Blouin, J.-L., Avramopoulos, D., Pangalos, C. and Antonarakis, S. E. (1993). Normal phenotype with paternal uniparental isodisomy for chromosome 21. *Am J Hum Genet*, **53**, 1074–1078.

Blouin, J.-L., Binkert, F. and Antonarakis, S. E. (1994). Biparental inheritance of chromosome 21 polymorphic markers indicates that some Robertsonian translocations t(21;21) occur postzygotically. *Am J Med Genet*, **49**, 363–368.

Bobrow, M., Barby, T., Hajianpour, A., Maxwell, D. and Yau, S. C. (1992). Fertility in a male with trisomy 21. *J Med Genet*, **29**, 141.

Bocian, M. and Walker, A. P. (1987). Lip pits and deletion 1q32→41. *Am J Med Genet*, **26**, 437–443.

Bocian, E., Mazurczak, T. and Stanczak, H. (1990). Paracentric inversion inv(18)(q21.1q23) in a woman with recurrent spontaneous abortions. *Am J Med Genet*, **35**, 592–593.

Bodrug, S. E., Roberson, J. R., Weiss, L., Ray, P. N., Worton, R. G. and Van Dyke, D. L. (1990). Prenatal identification of a girl with a t(X;4)(p21;q35) translocation: molecular characterisation, paternal origin, and association with muscular dystrophy. *J Med Genet*, **27**, 426–432.

Bogart, M. H., Bradshaw, C. and Jones, O. W. (1991). Prenatal diagnosis of euchromatic 16p+ heteromorphisms in two unrelated families. *Prenat Diagn*, **11**, 417–418.

Bogart, M. H., Fujita, N., Serles, L. and Hsia, Y. E. (1995). Prenatal diagnosis of a stable de novo centric fission: a case report. *Am J Med Genet*, **59**, 36–37.

Boghosian-Sell, L., Mewar, R., Harrison, W., Shapiro, R. M., Zackai, E. H., Carey, J., Davis-Keppen, L., Hudgins, L. and Overhauser, J. (1994). Molecular mapping of the Edwards syndrome phenotype to two noncontiguous regions on chromosome 18. *Am J Hum Genet*, **55**, 476–483.

Bonthron, D. T., Smith, S. J. L., Fantes, J. and Gosden, C. M. (1993). De novo microdeletion on an inherited Robertsonian translocation chromosome: a cause for dysmorphism in the apparently balanced translocation carrier. *Am J Hum Genet*, **53**, 629–637.

Borgaonkar, D. S., Mules, E. and Char, F. (1970). Do the 48,XXYY males have a characteristic phenotype? *Clin Genet*, **1**, 272–293.

Bortotto, L., Piovan, E., Furlan, R., Rivera, H. and Zuffardi, O. (1990). Chromosome imbalance, normal phenotype, and imprinting. *J Med Genet*, **27**, 582–587.

Bos, A. P., Broers, C. J. M., Hazebroek, F. W. J., van Hemel, J. O., Tibboel, D., Wesby-van Swaay, E. and Molenaar, J. C. (1992). Avoidance of emergency surgery in newborn infants with trisomy 18. *Lancet*, **339**, 913–917.

Bottani, A., Robinson, W. P., DeLozier-Blanchet, C. D., Engel, E., Morris, M. A., Schmitt, B., Thun-Hohenstein, L. and Schinzel, A. (1994). Angelman syndrome due to paternal uniparental disomy of chromosome 15: a milder phenotype? *Am J Med Genet*, **51**, 35–40.

Boué, A. and Gallano, P. (1984). A collaborative study of the segregation of inherited chromosome structural rearrangements in 1356 prenatal diagnoses. *Prenat Diagn*, **4** (Special Issue), 45–67.

Bourrouillou, G., Colombies, P. and Dastugue, N. (1986). Chromosome studies in 2136 couples with spontaneous abortions. *Hum Genet*, **74**, 399–401.

Bourrouillou, G., Dastugue, N. and Colombies, P. (1985). Chromosome studies in 952 infertile males with a sperm count below 10 million/ml. *Hum Genet*, **71**, 366–367.

Bowen, P., Biederman, B. and Hoo, J. J. (1985). The critical segment for the Langer-Giedion syndrome: 8q24.11→q24.12. *Ann Génét*, **28**, 224–227.

Bowen, P., Fitzgerald, P. H., Gardner, R. J. M., Biederman, B. and Veale, A. M. O. (1983). Duplication 8q syndrome due to familial chromosome ins(10;8)(q21; q212q22). *Am J Med Genet*, **14**, 635–646.

Bowser-Riley, S., Buckton, K. E., Ratcliffe, S. G. and Syme, J. (1981). Inheritance of a ring 14 chromosome. *J Med Genet*, **18**, 209–213.

Bowser-Riley, S. M., Griffiths, M. J., Creasy, M. R., Farndon, P. A., Martin, K. E.,

Thomson, D. A. G., Larkins, S. A., Johnson, R. A. and Watt, J. L. (1988). Are double translocations double trouble? *J Med Genet*, **25**, 326–331.

Boyd, P. A. and Keeling, J. W. (1992). Fetal hydrops. *J Med Genet*, **29**, 91–97.

Brahams, D. (1987). House of lords upholds decision to sterilise 17-year-old mentally handicapped girl. *Lancet*, **1**, 1099–1100.

Brambati, B. (1995). Chorionic villus sampling (early and late). In "Diseases of the fetus and newborn" (2nd edn.) (G. B. Reed, A. E. Claireaux and F. Cockburn, eds.). Chapman and Hall, London, pp. 1077–1082.

Brandriff, B., Gordon, L., Ashworth, L. K., Littman, V., Watchmaker, G. and Carrano, A. V. (1986). Cytogenetics of human sperm: meiotic segregation in two translocation carriers. *Am J Hum Genet*, **38**, 197–208.

Brandriff, B., Gordon, L. A., Crawford, B. B., Schonberg, S. A., Golabi, M., Charzan, S., Golbus, M. S. and Carrano, A. V. (1988). Sperm chromosome analysis to assess potential germ cell mosaicism. *Clin Genet*, **34**, 85–89.

Braun, A., Kammerer, S., Cleve, H., Löhrs, U., Schwarz, H.-P. and Kuhnle, U. (1993). True hermaphroditism in a 46,XY individual, caused by a postzygotic somatic point mutation in the male gonadal sex-determining locus (*SRY*): molecular genetics and histological findings in a sporadic case. *Am J Hum Genet*, **52**, 578–585.

Breuning, M. H., Dauwerse, H. G., Fugazza, G., Saris, J. J., Spruit, L., Wijnen, H., Tommerup, N., van der Hagen, C. B., Imaizumi, K., Kuroki, Y., van den Boogaard, M.-J., de Pater, J. M., Mariman, E. C. M., Hamel, B. C. J., Himmelbauer, H., Frischauf, A.-M., Stallings, R. L., Beverstock, G. C., van Ommen, G.-J. B. and Hennekam, R. C. M. (1993). Rubinstein-Taybi syndrome caused by submicroscopic deletions within 16p13.3. *Am J Hum Genet*, **52**, 249–254.

Brezinka, C., Hagenaars, A. M., Wladimiroff, J. W. and Los, F. J. (1995). Fetal ductus venosus flow velocity waveforms and maternal serum AFP before and after first-trimester transabdominal chorionic villus sampling. *Prenat Diagn*, **15**, 699–703.

Bricarelli, F. D., Borrone, C., Mantero, M. M., Perfumo, C., Guelfi, M., Panucci, E. and Coviello, D. A. (1994). Maternal uniparental disomy for chromosome 14. In "International Symposium on Genomic Imprinting," University of Florence, p. 66.

Bridges, B. A. and Harnden, D. G. (eds.) (1982). Ataxia-telangiectasia. A cellular and molecular link between cancer, neuropathology, and immune deficiency. John Wiley & Sons, New York.

Brock, D. W. (1995). The non-identity problem and genetic harms—the case of wrongful handicaps. *Bioethics*, **9**, 269–275.

Brøndum-Nielsen, K. and Mikkelsen, M. (1995). A 10-year survey, 1980–1990, of prenatally diagnosed small supernumerary marker chromosomes, identified by FISH analysis. Outcome and follow-up of 14 cases diagnosed in a series of 12 699 prenatal samples. *Prenat Diagn*, **15**, 615–619.

Brøndum-Nielsen, K., Sand, A. and Tommerup, N. (1994). Investigation of Williams syndrome using dinucleotide repeat polymorphism in elastin gene. Deletions of maternal origin are equally frequent as paternal. In "International Symposium on Genomic Imprinting," University of Florence, p. 60.

Brook-Carter, P. T., Peral, B., Ward, C. J., Thompson, P., Hughes, J., Maheshwar, M. M., Nellist, M., Gamble, V., Harris, P. C. and Sampson, J. R. (1994). Deletion of the *TSC2* and *PKD1* genes associated with severe infantile polycystic kidney disease—a contiguous gene syndrome. *Nature Genet*, **8**, 328–332.

Brothman, A. R., Rehberg, K., Storto, P. D., Phillips, S. E. and Mosby, R. T. (1992).

Confirmation of true mosaic trisomy 20 in a phenotypically normal liveborn male. *Clin Genet*, **42**, 47–49.

Brown, C. J. and Willard, H. F. (1994). The human X-inactivation centre is not required for maintenance of X-chromosome inactivation. *Nature*, **368**, 154–156.

Brown, K. W., Gardner, A., Williams, J. C., Mott, M. G., McDermott, A. and Maitland, N. J. (1992). Paternal origin of 11p15 duplications in the Beckwith-Wiedemann syndrome. A new case and review of the literature. *Cancer Genet Cytogenet*, **58**, 55–70.

Brown, W. T., Houck, G. E., Jeziorowska, A., Levinson, F. N., Ding, X., Dobkin, C., Zhong, N., Henderson, J., Brooks, S. S. and Jenkins, E. C. (1993). Rapid fragile X carrier screening and prenatal diagnosis using a nonradioactive PCR test. *J Am Med Assoc*, **270**, 1569–1575.

Brueton, L. and Winter, R. (1993). Molecular aspects of morphogenesis. In "The new genetics" (I. Young, ed.). Ballière Tindall, London, pp. 345–373.

Bryndorf, T., Christensen, B., Xiang, Y., Philip, J., Yokobata, K., Bui, N. and Gaiser, C. (1994a). Fluorescence *in situ* hybridization with a chromosome 21-specific cosmid contig: 1-day detection of trisomy 21 in uncultured mesenchymal chorionic villus cells. *Prenat Diagn*, **14**, 87–96.

Bryndorf, T., Sundberg, K., Christensen, B., Philip, J., Yokobata, K. and Gaiser, C. (1994b). Early and rapid prenatal exclusion of Down's syndrome. *Lancet*, **343**, 802.

Buckton, K. E., Newton, M. S., Collyer, S., Lee, M., Spowart, G., Seabright, M. and Sanger, R. (1981). Phenotypically normal individuals with an inversion (X)(p22q13) and the recombinant (X), dup q. *Ann Hum Genet*, **45**, 159–168.

Budarf, M. L., Collins, J., Gong, W., Roe, B., Wang, Z., Bailey, L. C., Sellinger, B., Michaud, D., Driscoll, D. A. and Emanuel, B. S. (1995). Cloning a balanced translocation associated with DiGeorge syndrome and identification of a disrupted candidate gene. *Nature Genet*, **10**, 269–278.

Buiting, K., Saitoh, S., Gross, S., Dittrich, B., Schwartz, S., Nicholls, R. D. and Horsthemke, B. (1995). Inherited microdeletions in the Angelman and Prader-Willi syndromes define an imprinting centre on human chromosome 15. *Nature Genet*, **9**, 395–400.

Bunyan, D. J., Crolla, J. A., Collins, A. L. and Robinson, D. O. (1995). Fluorescence in situ hybridisation studies provide evidence for somatic mosaicism in de novo dystrophin gene deletions. *Hum Genet*, **95**, 43–45.

Burns, J. P., Koduru, P. R. K., Alonso, M. L. and Chaganti, R. S. K. (1986). Analysis of meiotic segregation in a man heterozygous for two reciprocal translocations using the hamster in vitro penetration system. *Am J Hum Genet*, **38**, 954–964.

Butler, M. G. (1994). Trisomy 18 mosaicism in a 24-year-old white woman with normal intelligence and skeletal abnormalities. *Am J Med Genet*, **53**, 92–93.

Buxton, J. L., Chan, C.-T. J., Gilbert, H., Clayton-Smith, J., Burn, J., Pembrey, M. and Malcolm, S. (1994). Angelman syndrome associated with a maternal 15q11-13 deletion of less than 200 kb. *Hum Molec Genet*, **3**, 1409-1413.

Byrne, E., Hallpike, J. F., Manson, J. I., Sutherland, G. R. and Thong, Y. H. (1984). Ataxia-without-telangiectasia: progressive multisystem degeneration with IgE deficiency and chromosomal instability. *J Neurol Sci*, **66**, 307–317.

Cacheux, V., Tachdjian, G., Druart, L., Oury, J. F., Sérero, S., Blot, P. and Nessmann, C. (1994). Evaluation of X, Y, 18, and 13/21 alpha satellite DNA probes for interphase cytogenetic analysis of uncultured amnioctyes by fluorescence *in situ* hybridization. *Prenat Diagn*, **14**, 79–86.

Callen, D. F., Eyre, H., Lane, S., Shen, Y., Hansmann, I., Spinner, N., Zackai, E.,

McDonald-McGinn, D., Schuffenhauer, S., Wauters, J., Van Thienen, M.-N., Van Roy, B., Sutherland, G. R. and Haan, E. A. (1993). High resolution mapping of interstitial long arm deletions of chromosome 16: relationship to phenotype. *J Med Genet*, **30**, 828–832.

Callen, D. F., Eyre, H. J. and Ringenbergs, M. L. (1990a). A dicentric variant of chromosome 6: characterization by use of *in situ* hybridisation with the biotinylated probe p308. *Clin Genet*, **37**, 81–83.

Callen, D. F., Freemantle, C. J., Ringenbergs, M. L., Baker, E., Eyre, H. J., Romain, D. and Haan, E. A. (1990b). The isochromosome 18p syndrome: confirmation of cytogenetic diagnosis in nine cases by in situ hybridization. *Am J Hum Genet*, **47**, 493–498.

Callen, D. F., Eyre, H., Yip, M.-Y., Freemantle, J. and Haan, E. A. (1992). Molecular cytogenetic and clinical studies of 42 patients with marker chromosomes. *Am J Med Genet*, **43**, 709–715.

Callen, D. F. and Sutherland, G. R. (1986). Normal female carrier and affected male half-sibs with t(X;5)(q13;p15). Location of a gene determining male genital development. *Clin Genet*, **30**, 59–62.

Callen, D. F., Sutherland, G. R. and Carter, R. F. (1987). A fertile man with tdic(Y;22): how a stable neo-X1X2Y sex determining mechanism could evolve in man. *Am J Med Genet*, **3** (Suppl.), 151–155.

Callen, D. F., Woollatt, E. and Sutherland, G. R. (1985). Paracentric inversions in man. *Clin Genet*, **28**, 87–92.

Campana, M., Serra, A. and Neri, G. (1986). Role of chromosome aberrations in recurrent abortion: a study of 269 balanced translocations. *Am J Med Genet*, **24**, 341–356.

Canki, N., Warburton, D. and Byrne, J. (1988). Morphological characteristics of monosomy X in spontaneous abortions. *Ann Génét*, **31**, 4–13.

Cans, C., Cohen, O., Lavergne, C., Mermet, M.-A., Demongeot, J. and Jalbert, P. (1993). Logistic regression model to estimate the risk of unbalanced offspring in reciprocal translocations. *Hum Genet*, **92**, 598–604.

Cantú, J. M. and Ruiz, C. (1986). On a prezygotic origin of normal/balanced translocation mosaicism. *Ann Génét*, **29**, 221–222.

Carakushansky, G., Teich, E., Ribeiro, M. G., Horowitz, D. D. G. and Pellegrini, S. (1994). Diploid/triploid mosaicism: further delineation of the phenotype. *Am J Med Genet*, **52**, 399–401.

Carothers, A. D., Buckton, K. E., Collyer, S., de Mey, R., Frackiewicz, A., Piper, J. and Smith, L. (1982). The effect of variant chromosomes on reproductive fitness in man. *Clin Genet*, **21**, 280–289.

Carpenter, N. J., Say, B. and Browning, D. (1980). Gonadal dysgenesis in a patient with an X;3 translocation: case report and review. *J Med Genet*, **17**, 216–221.

Cassidy, S. B., Lai, L.-W., Erickson, R. P., Magnuson, L., Thomas, E., Gendron, R. and Herrmann, J. (1992). Trisomy 15 with loss of the paternal 15 as a cause of Prader-Willi syndrome due to maternal disomy. *Am J Hum Genet*, **51**, 701–708.

Cassidy, S. B., Whitworth, T., Sanders, D., Lorber, C. A. and Engel, E. (1977). Five month extrauterine survival in a female triploid (69,XXX) child. *Ann Génét*, **20**, 277–279.

Castellví-bel, S., Milà, M., Soler, A., Carrió, A., Sánchez, A., Villa, M., Jiménez, M. D. and Estivill, X. (1995). Prenatal diagnosis of fragile X syndrome: (CGG)$_n$ expansion and methylation of chorionic villus samples. *Prenat Diagn*, **15**, 801–807.

Castle, D. and Bernstein, R. (1988). Cytogenetic analysis of 688 couples experiencing multiple spontaneous abortions. *Am J Med Genet*, **29**, 549–556.

Catalán, J., Autio, K., Wessman, M., Lindholm, C., Knuutila, S., Sorsa, M. and Norppa,

H. (1995). Age-associated micronuclei containing centromeres and the X chromosome in lymphocytes of women. *Cytogenet Cell Genet*, **68**, 11–16.

Chan, C.-T. J., Clayton-Smith, J., Cheng, X.-J., Buxton, J., Webb, T., Pembrey, M. E. and Malcolm, S. (1993). Molecular mechanisms in Angelman syndrome: a survey of 93 patients. *J Med Genet*, **30**, 895–902.

Chandley, A. C. (1988). Meiotic studies and fertility in human translocation carriers. In "The cytogenetics of mammalian autosomal rearrangements" (A. Daniel, ed.). A. R. Liss, New York, pp. 361–382.

Chandley, A. C. (1989). Asymmetry in chromosome pairing: a major factor in de novo mutation and the production of genetic disease in man. *J Med Genet*, **26**, 546–552.

Chandley, A. C. (1991). On the parental origin of de novo mutation in man. *J Med Genet*, **28**, 217–223.

Chandley, A. C. (1993). The relationship between meiotic chromosome pairing and chiasma formation. *Hum Genet*, **92**, 642–643.

Chandley, A. C. and Cooke, H. J. (1994). Human male fertility—Y-linked genes and spermatogenesis. *Hum Mol Genet*, **3**, 1449–1452.

Chandley, A. C., Fletcher, J. and Robinson, J. A. (1976). Normal meiosis in two 47,XYY men. *Hum Genet*, **33**, 231–240.

Chandley, A. C., McBeath, S., Speed, R. M., Yorston, L. and Hargreave, T. B. (1987). Pericentric inversion in human chromosome 1 and the risk for male sterility. *J Med Genet*, **24**, 325–334.

Chandley, A. C., Speed, R. M., McBeath, S. and Hargreave, T. B. (1986). A human 9; 20 reciprocal translocation associated with male infertility analyzed at prophase and metaphase I of meiosis. *Cytogenet Cell Genet*, **41**, 145–153.

Chang, H. J., Clark, R. D. and Bachman, H. (1990). The phenotype of 45,X/46,XY mosaicism: an analysis of 92 prenatally diagnosed cases. *Am J Hum Genet*, **46**, 156–167.

Chelly, J., Marlhens, F., Le Marec, B., Jeanpierre, M., Lambert, M., Hamard, G., Dutrillaux, B. and Kaplan, J.-C. (1986). De novo DNA microdeletion in a girl with Turner syndrome and Duchenne muscular dystrophy. *Hum Genet*, **74**, 193–196.

Chen, H., Chrast, R., Rossier, C., Gos, A., Antonarakis, S. E., Kudoh, J., Yamaki, A., Shindoh, N., Maeda, H., Minoshima, S. and Shimizu, N. (1995). *Single-minded* and Down syndrome? *Nature Genet*, **10**, 9–10.

Chen, K.-S., Gunaratne, P. H., Hoheisel, J. D., Young, I. G., Miklos, G. L. G., Greenberg, F., Shaffer, L. G., Campbell, H. D. and Lupski, J. R. (1995). The human homologue of the *Drosophila melanogaster* flightless-I gene (*fliI*) maps within the Smith-Magenis microdeletion critical region in 17p11.2. *Am J Hum Genet*, **56**, 175–182.

Cheng, E. Y., Chen, Y.-J. and Gartler, S. M. (1995). Chromosome painting analysis of early oogenesis in human trisomy 18. *Cytogenet Cell Genet*, **70**, 205–210.

Cheng, S.-D., Spinner, N. B., Zackai, E. H. and Knoll, J. H. M. (1994). Cytogenetic and molecular characterization of inverted duplicated chromosomes 15 from 11 patients. *Am J Hum Genet*, **55**, 753–759.

Chettouh, Z., Croquette, M.-F., Delobel, B., Gilgenkrants, S., Leonard, C., Maunoury, C., Prieur, M., Rethoré, M.-O., Sinet, P.-M., Chery, M. and Delabar, J.-M. (1995). Molecular mapping of 21 features associated with partial monosomy 21: involvement of the APP-SOD1 region. *Am J Hum Genet*, **57**, 62–71.

Chevillard, C., Paslier, D. L., Passage, E., Ougen, P., Billault, A., Boyer, S., Mazan, S., Bachellerie, J. P., Vignal, A., Cohen, D. and Fontes, M. (1993). Relationship between Charcot-Marie-Tooth 1A and Smith-Magenis regions: snU3 may be a candidate gene for the Smith-Magenis syndrome. *Hum Mol Genet*, **2**, 1235–1243.

Chevret, E., Rousseaux, S., Monteil, M., Pelletier, R., Cozzi, J. and Sèle, B. (1995). Meiotic segregation of the X and Y chromosomes and chromosome 1 analyzed by three-color FISH in human interphase spermatozoa. *Cytogenet Cell Genet*, **71**, 126–130.

Chia, N., Bousfield, L., James, S. and Nelson, J. (1992). Report of a severely retarded child with a duplication 18q derived from a paternal paracentric inversion (18q): a note of warning. *Bull Hum Genet Soc Australasia*, **6** (Suppl.), 48.

Chodirker, B. N., Greenberg, C. R., Pabello, P. D. and Chudley, A. E. (1992). Paracentric inversion 11q in Canadian Hutterites. *Hum Genet*, **89**, 450–452.

Choo, K. H., Vissel, B., Brown, R., Filby, R. G. and Earle, E. (1988). Homologous alpha satellite sequences on human acrocentric chromosomes with selectivity for chromosomes 13, 14, and 21: implications for recombination between homologues and Robertsonian translocations. *Nucleic Acids Res*, **16**, 1273–1284.

Christian, S. L., Robinson, W. P., Huang, B., Mutirangura, A., Line, M. R., Nakao, M., Surti, U., Chakravarti, A. and Ledbetter, D. H. (1995). Molecular characterization of two proximal deletion breakpoint regions in both Prader-Willi and Angelman syndrome patients. *Am J Hum Genet*, **57**, 40–48.

Chu, C. E., Donaldson, M. D. C., Kelnar, C. J. H., Smail, P. J., Greene, S. A., Paterson, W. F. and Connor, J. M. (1994). Possible role of imprinting in the Turner phenotype. *J Med Genet*, **31**, 840–842.

Chudley, A. E., Bauder, F., Ray, M., McAlpine, P. J., Pena, S. D. J. and Hamerton, J. L. (1974). Familial mental retardation in a family with an inherited chromosome rearrangement. *J Med Genet*, **11**, 353–366.

Chudley, A. E., Zheng, H.-Z., Pabello, P. D., Shia, G. and Wang, H.-C. (1983). Familial supernumerary microchromosome mosaicism: phenotypic effects and an attempt at characterization. *Am J Med Genet*, **16**, 89–97.

Clarke, A. (1995). The genetic testing of children. *J Med Genet*, **32**, 492.

Clarke, A., Fielding, D., Kerzin-Storrar, L., Middleton-Price, H., Montgomery, J., Payne, H., Simonoff, E. and Tyler, A. (1994). The genetic testing of children. Report of a working party of the Clinical Genetics Society (UK). *J Med Genet*, **31**, 785–797.

Claussen, U. (1980). The pipette method: a new rapid technique for chromosome analysis. *Hum Genet*, **54**, 277–278.

Claussen, U., Ulmer, R., Beinder, E. and Voigt, H.-J. (1994). Six years' experience with rapid karyotyping in prenatal diagnosis: correlations between phenotype detected by ultrasound and fetal karyotype. *Prenat Diagn*, **14**, 113–121.

Clayton, E. W. (1995). Removing the shadow of the law from the debate about genetic testing of children. *Am J Med Genet*, **57**, 630–634.

Clayton-Smith, J., Webb, T., Robb, S. A., Dijkstra, I., Willems, P., Lam, S., Cheng, X.-J., Pembrey, M. E. and Malcolm, S. (1992). Further evidence for dominant inheritance at the chromosome 15q11–13 locus in familial Angelman syndrome. *Am J Med Genet*, **44**, 256–260.

Clayton-Smith, J., Driscoll, D. J., Waters, M. F., Webb, T., Andrews, T., Malcolm, S., Pembrey, M. E. and Nicholls, R. D. (1993). Difference in methylation patterns within the D15S9 region of chromosome 15q11–13 in first cousins with Angelman syndrome and Prader-Willi syndrome. *Am J Med Genet*, **47**, 683–686.

Clayton-Smith, J., Webb, T., Cheng, X. J., Pembrey, M. E. and Malcolm, S. (1993). Duplication of chromosome 15 in the region 15q11–13 in a patient with developmental delay and ataxia with similarities to Angelman syndrome. *J Med Genet*, **30**, 529–531.

Clemens, M., Martsolf, J. T., Rogers, J. G., Mowery-Rushton, P., Surti, U. and McPherson, E. W. Pitt-Rogers-Danks syndrome: the result of a 4p microdeletion. Submitted, 1996.

Cobden, J. M., Verheij, J. B. G. M., Eisma, W. H., Robinson, P. H., Zwierstra, R. P., Leegte, B. and Castedo, S. (1995). Bilateral split hand/foot malformation and inv(7)(p22q21.3). *J Med Genet*, **32**, 375–378.

Cohen, A. J., Li, F. P., Berg, S., Marchetto, D. J., Tsai, S., Jacobs, S. C. and Brown, R. S. (1979). Hereditary renal-cell carcinoma associated with a chromosomal translocation. *N Engl J Med*, **301**, 592–595.

Cohen, M. M. (1994). Wiedemann-Beckwith syndrome, imprinting, IGF2, and H19: implications for hemihyperplasia, associated neoplasms, and overgrowth. *Am J Med Genet*, **52**, 233–234.

Cohen, M. M., Frederick, R. W., Balkin, N. E. and Simpson, N. J. (1981). The identification of Y chromosome translocations following distamycin A treatment. *Clin Genet*, **19**, 335–342.

Cohen, O., Cans, C., Mermet, M.-A., Demongeot, J. and Jalbert, P. (1994). Viability thresholds for partial trisomies and monosomies. A study of 1,159 viable unbalanced reciprocal translocations. *Hum Genet*, **93**, 188–194.

Cole, L. A. (1994). Multiple hCG-related molecules. In ''Screening for Down's syndrome'' (J. G. Grudzinskas, T. Chard, M. Chapman and H. Cuckle, eds.). Cambridge University Press, Cambridge, pp. 119–140.

Coles, K., Mackenzie, M., Crolla, J., Harvey, J., Starr, J., Howard, F. and Jacobs, P. (1992). A complex rearrangement associated with sex reversal and the Wolf-Hirschhorn syndrome: a cytogenetic and molecular study. *J Med Genet*, **29**, 400–406.

Colley, A. F., Leversha, M. A., Voullaire, L. E. and Rogers, J. G. (1990). Five cases demonstrating the distinctive behavioural features of chromosome deletion 17(p11.2p11.2) (Smith-Magenis syndrome). *J Paediatr Child Health*, **26**, 17–21.

Constantine, G., Fowlie, A. and Pearson, J. (1992). Placental biopsy in the third trimester of pregnancy. *Prenat Diagn*, **12**, 783–788.

Conte, R. A., Gupta, S., Brennan, J. P. and Verma, R. S. (1995). Rare variants of chromosome 9 with extra G positive band within the qh region are not alike. *J Med Genet*, **32**, 405–406.

Cooke, A., Tolmie, J. L., Colgan, J. M., Greig, C. M. and Connor, J. M. (1989). Detection of an unbalanced translocation (4;14) in a mildly retarded father and son by flow cytometry. *Hum Genet*, **83**, 83–87.

Costa, D., Borrell, A., Margarit, E., Carrió, A., Soler, A., Balmes, I., Estivill, X. and Fortuny, A. (1995). Rapid fetal karyotype from cystic hygroma and pleural effusions. *Prenat Diagn*, **15**, 141–148.

Coté, G. B., Katsantoni, A. and Deligeorgis, D. (1981). The cytogenetic and clinical implications of a ring chromosome 2. *Ann Génét*, **24**, 231–235.

Coto, E., Toral, J. F., Menéndez, M. J., Hernando, I., Plasencia, A., Benavides, A. and López-Larrea, C. (1995). PCR-based study of the presence of Y-chromosome sequences in patients with Ullrich-Turner syndrome. *Am J Med Genet*, **57**, 393–396.

Cotton, C., Cummins, M. and Smith, A. (1993). Alternate, adjacent 2 and 3:1 meiotic segregation products from a balanced t(13;18)(q12;q11) carrier. *Clin Genet*, **44**, 193–195.

Couillin, P., Zucman, J., Le Guern, E., Reguigne, I., Grisard, M.-C., Delattre, O., Novelli, G., Dallapiccola, B. and Boué, A. (1992). Molecular studies of a translocated (X; 22) DiGeorge patient using somatic cell hybridization. *Ann Génét*, **35**, 140–145.

Courtens, W., Petersen, M. B., Noël, J. C., Flament-Durand, J., Van Regemorter, N., Delneste, D., Cochaux, P., Verschraegen-Spae, M. R., Van Roy, N., Speleman, F., Koenig, U. and Vamos, E. (1994). Proximal deletion of chromosome 21 confirmed by in situ hybridization and molecular studies. *Am J Med Genet*, **51**, 260–265.

Court Brown, W. M., Law, P. and Smith, P. G. (1969). Sex chromosome aneuploidy and parental age. *Ann Hum Genet*, **33**, 1–14.

Couturier, J., Morichon-Delvallez, N. and Dutrillaux, B. (1985). Deletion of band 13q21 is compatible with a normal phenotype. *Hum Genet*, **70**, 87–91.

Couzin, D. A., Watt, J. L. and Stephen, G. S. (1986). Structural rearrangements in the parents of children with primary trisomy 21. *J Med Genet*, **23**, 470.

Cozzi, J., Chevret, E., Rousseau, S., Pelletier, R., Benitz, V., Jalbert, H. and Sèle, B. (1994). Achievement of meiosis in XXY germ cells: study of 543 sperm karyotypes from an XY/XXY mosaic patient. *Hum Genet*, **93**, 32–34.

Craft, I., Djahanbakhch, O., McLeod, F., Bernard, A., Green, S., Twigg, H., Smith, W., Lindsay, K. and Edmonds, K. (1982). Human pregnancy following oocyte and sperm transfer to the uterus. *Lancet*, **1**, 1031–1033.

Craig-Holmes, A. P. (1977). C-band polymorphism in human populations. In "Population cytogenetics. Studies in humans" (E. B. Hook and I. H. Porter, eds.). Academic Press, New York, pp. 161–177.

Creasy, M. R. (1989). Complex chromosomal rearrangements. *Am J Med Genet*, **32**, 560.

Croci, G., Camurri, L. and Franchi, F. (1991). A familial case of chromosome 16p variant. *J Med Genet*, **28**, 60.

Cross, I., Delhanty, J., Chapman, P., Bowles, L. V., Griffin, D., Wolstenholme, J., Bradburn, M., Brown, J., Wood, C., Gunn, A. and Burn, J. (1992). An intrachromosomal insertion causing 5q22 deletion and familial adenomatous polyposis coli in two generations. *J Med Genet*, **29**, 175–179.

Cuckle, H. S., Iles, R. K., Sehmi, I. K., Chard, T., Oakey, R. E., Davies, S. and Ind, T. (1995). Urinary multiple marker screening for Down's syndrome. *Prenat Diagn*, **15**, 745–751.

Cuckle, H., Nanchahal, K. and Wald, N. (1991). Birth prevalence of Down's syndrome in England and Wales. *Prenat Diagn*, **11**, 29–34.

Cunniff, C., Jones, K. L. and Benirschke, K. (1991). Ovarian dysgenesis in individuals with chromosomal abnormalities. *Hum Genet*, **86**, 552–556.

Curran, M. E., Atkinson, D. L., Ewart, A. K., Morris, C. A., Leppert, M. F. and Keating, M. T. (1993). The elastin gene is disrupted by a translocation associated with supravalvular aortic stenosis. *Cell*, **73**, 159–168.

Cussen, L. J. and MacMahon, R. A. (1979). Germ cells and ova in dysgenetic gonads of a 46-XY female dizygotic twin. *Am J Dis Child*, **133**, 373–375.

Dahoun, S. (1990). Un second cas d'inversion paracentrique *(de novo)* du bras court de l'X. *Ann Génét*, **33**, 52–55.

Dalby, S. (1995a). GIG response to the UK Clinical Genetics Society report "The genetic testing of children". *J Med Genet*, **32**, 490–494.

Dalby, S. (1995b). Reply to Michie and Marteau, 1995. *J Med Genet*, **32**, 838.

Dallapiccola, B., De Filippis, V., Notarangelo, A., Perla, G. and Zelante, L. (1986). Ring chromosome 21 in healthy persons: different consequences in females and in males. *Hum Genet*, **73**, 218–220.

Dallapiccola, B., Mastroiacovo, P. and Gandini, E. (1976). Centric fission of chromosome no. 4 in the mother of two patients with trisomy 4p. *Hum Genet*, **31**, 121–125.

Daniel, A. (1979). Structural differences in reciprocal translocations. Potential for a model of risk in rep. *Hum Genet*, **51**, 171–182.

Daniel, A., Hook, E. B. and Wulf, G. (1988). Collaborative U. S. A. data on prenatal diagnosis for parental carriers of chromosome rearrangements: risks of unbalanced progeny. In "The cytogenetics of mammalian autosomal rearrangements" (A. Daniel, ed.). A. R. Liss, New York, pp. 73–162.

Daniel, A., Hook, E. B. and Wulf, G. (1989). Risks of unbalanced progeny at amniocentesis to carriers of chromosome rearrangements: data from United States and Canadian laboratories. *Am J Med Genet*, **31**, 14–53.

Dar, H., Tal, J., Bar-el, H., Halpern, I. and Sharf, M. (1988). Paracentric inversion of Xq and ovarian dysfunction. *Am J Med Genet*, **29**, 167–170.

DeBrasi, D., Genuardi, M., D'Agostino, A., Calvieri, F., Tozzi, C., Varrone, S. and Neri, G. (1995). Double autosomal/gonosomal mosaic aneuploidy: study of nondisjunction in two cases with trisomy of chromosome 8. *Hum Genet*, **95**, 519–525.

Delabar, J.-M., Théophile, D., Rahmani, Z., Chettouh, Z., Blouin, J.-L., Prieur, M., Noel, B. and Sinet, P.-M. (1993). Molecular mapping of twenty-four features of Down syndrome on chromosome 21. *Eur J Hum Genet*, **1**, 114–124.

Delach, J. A., Rosengren, S. S., Kaplan, L., Greenstein, R. M., Cassidy, S. B. and Benn, P. A. (1994). Comparison of high resolution chromosome banding and fluorescence in situ hybridization (FISH) for the laboratory evaluation of Prader-Willi syndrome and Angelman syndrome. *Am J Med Genet*, **52**, 85–91.

Delhanty, J. D. A. (1994). Preimplantation diagnosis. *Prenat Diagn*, **14**,1217–1227.

Demczuk, S., Aledo, R., Zucman, J., Delattre, O., Desmaze, C., Dauphinot, L., Jalbert, P., Rouleau, G. A., Thomas, G. and Aurias, A. (1995). Cloning of a balanced translocation breakpoint in the DiGeorge syndrome critical region and isolation of a novel potential adhesion receptor gene in its vicinity. *Hum Mol Genet*, **4**, 551–558.

Demczuk, S., Lévy, A., Aubry, M., Croquette, M.-F., Philip, N., Prieur, M., Sauer, U., Bouvagnet, P., Rouleau, G. A., Thomas, G. and Aurias, A. (1995). Excess of deletions of maternal origin in the DiGeorge/velo-cardio-facial syndromes. A study of 22 new patients and review of the literature. *Hum Genet*, **96**, 9–13.

Deng, H.-X., Abe, K., Kondo, I., Tsukahara, M., Inagaki, H., Hamada, I., Fukushima, Y. and Niikawa, N. (1991). Parental origin and mechanism of formation of polysomy X: an XXXXX case and four XXXXY cases determined with RFLPs. *Hum Genet*, **86**, 541–544.

Desmaze, C., Prieur, M., Amblard, F., Aĭkem, M., LeDeist, F., Demczuk, S., Zucman, J., Plougastel, B., Delattre, O., Croquette, M.-F., Brevière, G.-M., Huon, C., Le Merrer, M., Mathieu, M., Sidi, D., Stephan, J.-L. and Aurias, A. (1993). Physical mapping by FISH of the DiGeorge critical region (DGCR): involvement of the region in familial cases. *Am J Hum Genet*, **53**, 1239–1249.

Dewhurst, J. (1978). Fertility in 47,XXX and 45,X patients. *J Med Genet*, **15**, 132–135.

De Arce, M. A., Costigan, C., Gosden, J. R., Lawler, M. and Humphries, P. (1992). Further evidence consistent with Yqh as an indicator of risk of gonadal blastoma in Y-bearing mosaic Turner syndrome. *Clin Genet*, **41**, 28–32.

De Boulle, K., Verkerk, A. J. M. H., Reyniers, E., Vits, L., Hendrickx, J., Van Roy, B., Van Den Bos, F., de Graff, E., Oostra, B. A. and Willems, P. J. (1993). A point mutation in the *FMR1* gene associated with fragile X mental retardation. *Nature Genet*, **3**, 31–35.

De Braekeleer, M. and Dao, T.-N. (1991). Cytogenetic studies in male infertility: a review. *Hum Reprod*, **6**, 245–250.

De Graaff, E., Willemsen, R., Zhong, N., de Die-Smulders, C. E. M., Brown, W. T.,

Freling, G. and Oostra, B. (1995). Instability of the CGG repeat and expression of the *FMR1* protein in a male fragile X patient with a lung tumor. *Am J Hum Genet*, **57**, 609–618.

De Grouchy, J., Bonnette, J. and Salmon, C. (1966). Deletion du bras court du chromosome 18. *Ann Génét*, **9**, 19–26.

De Grouchy, J., Royer, P., Salmon, C. and Lamy, M. (1964). Deletion partielle des bras longs du chromosome 18. *Pathol Biol*, **12**, 579–582.

De Grouchy, J. and Turleau, C. (1982). "Atlas des maladies chromosomiques" (2nd edn.). Expansion Scientifique Française, Paris.

De la Chapelle, A., Page, D. C., Brown, L., Kaski, U., Parvinen, T. and Tippett, P. A. (1986). The origin of 45,X males. *Am J Hum Genet*, **38**, 330–340.

De Perdigo, A., Gabriel-Robez, O., Ratomponirina, C. and Rumpler, Y. (1991). Synaptonemal complex analysis in a human male carrier of a 4;6 translocation: heterosynapsis without previous homosynapsis. *Hum Genet*, **86**, 279–282.

De Perdigo, A., Gabriel-Robez, O. and Rumpler, Y. (1989). Correlation between chromosomal breakpoint positions and synaptic behaviour in human males heterozygous for a pericentric inversion. *Hum Genet*, **83**, 274–276.

Del Porto, G., Di Fusco, C., Baldi, M., Grammatico, P. and D'Alessandro, E. (1984). Familial centric fission of chromosome 4. *J Med Genet*, **21**, 388–391.

Dhooge, C., Van Roy, N., Craen, M. and Speleman, F. (1994). Direct transmission of a tandem duplication in the short arm of chromosome 8. *Clin Genet*, **45**, 36–39.

Dietzsch, E., Ramsay, M., Christianson, A. L., Henderson, B. D. and de Ravel, T. J. L. (1995). Maternal origin of extra haploid set of chromosomes in third trimester triploid fetuses. *Am J Med Genet*, **58**, 360–364.

Disteche, C. M. (1995). Escape from X inactivation in human and mouse. *Trends Genet*, **11**, 17–22.

Dittrich, B., Robinson, W. P., Knoblauch, H., Buiting, K., Schmidt, K., Gillessen-Kaesbach, G. and Horsthemke, B. (1992). Molecular diagnosis of the Prader-Willi and Angelman syndromes by detection of parent-of-origin specific DNA methylation in 15q11–13. *Hum Genet*, **90**, 313–315.

Djalali, M., Barbi, G. and Grab, D. (1992). A further case of mosaic isochromosome 20q detected in amniotic fluid cells. *Prenat Diagn*, **12**, 71–72.

Djalali, M., Steinbach, P., Bullerdiek, J., Holmes-Siedle, M., Verschraegen-Spae, M. R. and Smith, A. (1986). The significance of pericentric inversions of chromosome 2. *Hum Genet*, **72**, 32–36.

Documenta Geigy (1982). "Scientific tables" (8th edn.) (C. Lentner, ed.), Vol. 2. Ciba-Geigy, Basle.

Donlan, M. A. and Dolan, C. R. (1986). Ring chromosome 18 in a mother and son. *Am J Med Genet*, **24**, 171–174.

Donnai, D. (1993). Robertsonian translocations: clues to imprinting. *Am J Med Genet*, **46**, 681–682.

Donnenfeld, A. E. and Kershner, M. A. (1993). Significance of mosaic isochromosome 20q on amniocentesis. *Am J Med Genet*, **47**, 1196–1197.

Dreesen, J. C. F. M., Geraedts, J. P. M., Dumoulin, J. C. M., Evers, J. L. H. and Pieters, M. H. E. C. (1995). RS46(DXS548) genotyping of reproductive cells: approaching preimplantation testing of the fragile-X syndrome. *Hum Genet*, **96**, 323–329.

Driscoll, D. J., Waters, M. F., Williams, C. A., Zori, R. T., Glenn, C. C., Avidano, K. M. and Nicholls, R. D. (1992). A DNA methylation imprint, determined by the sex of the parent, distinguishes the Angelman and Prader-Willi syndromes. *Genomics*, **13**, 917–924.

Driscoll, D. A., Salvin, J., Sellinger, B., Budarf, M. L., McDonald-McGinn, D. M., Zackai, E. H. and Emanuel, B. S. (1993). Prevalence of 22q11 microdeletions in DiGeorge and velocardiofacial syndromes: implications for genetic counselling and prenatal diagnosis. *J Med Genet*, **30**, 813–817.

Drugan, A., Greb, A., Johnson, M. P., Krivchenia, E. L., Uhlmann, W. R., Moghissi, K. S. and Evans, M. I. (1990a). Determinants of parental decisions to abort for chromosome abnormalities. *Prenat Diagn*, **10**, 483–490.

Drugan, A., Koppitch, F. C., Williams, J. C., Johnson, M. P., Moghissi, K. S. and Evans, M. I. (1990b). Prenatal genetic diagnosis following recurrent early pregnancy loss. *Obstet Gynecol*, **75**, 381–384.

Duckett, D. P. and Roberts, S. H. (1981). Adjacent 2 meiotic disjunction. Report of a case resulting from a familial 13q;15q balanced reciprocal translocation and review of the literature. *Hum Genet*, **58**, 377–386.

Duckett, D. P. and Young, I. D. (1988). A recombinant X chromosome in a short statured girl resulting from a maternal pericentric inversion. *Hum Genet*, **79**, 251–254.

Duff, G. B., Anderson, N. G. and Evans, L. J. (1994). Choroid plexus cysts in Christchurch. *Aust N Z J Obstet Gynaecol*, **34**, 543–545.

Dunger, D. B., Davies, K. E., Pembrey, M., Lake, B., Pearson, P., Williams, D., Whitfield, A. and Dillon, M. J. D. (1986). Deletion on the X chromosome detected by direct DNA analysis in one of two unrelated boys with glycerol kinase deficiency, adrenal hypoplasia, and Duchenne muscular dystrophy. *Lancet*, **1**, 585–587.

Duval, E., van den Enden, A., Vanhaesebrouck, P. and Speleman, F. (1994). Jumping translocation in a newborn boy with dup(4q) and severe hydrops fetalis. *Am J Med Genet*, **52**, 214–217.

Du Sart, D., Kalitsis, P. and Schmidt, M. (1992). Noninactivation of a portion of Xq28 in a balanced X-autosome translocation. *Am J Med Genet*, **42**, 156–160.

Earle, E., Shaffer, L. G., Kalitsis, P., McQuillan, C., Dale, S. and Choo, K. H. A. (1992a). Identification of DNA sequences flanking the breakpoint of human t(14q21q) Robertsonian translocations. *Am J Hum Genet*, **50**, 717–724.

Earle, E., Voullaire, L. E., Hills, L., Slater, H. and Choo, K. H. A. (1992b). Absence of satellite III DNA in the centromere and the proximal long-arm region of human chromosome 14: analysis of a 14p-variant. *Cytogenet Cell Genet*, **61**, 78–80.

Edwards, J. H. (1989). Familiarity, recessivity and germline mosaicism. *Ann Hum Genet*, **53**, 33–47.

Edwards, M. J., Park, J. P., Wurster-Hill, D. H. and Graham, J. M. (1994). Mixoploidy in humans: two surviving cases of diploid-tetraploid mixoploidy and comparison with diploid-triploid mixoploidy. *Am J Med Genet*, **52**, 324–330.

Edwards, R., Crow, J., Dale, S., Macnamee, M., Hartshorne, G. and Brinsden, P. (1990). Preimplantation diagnosis and recurrent hydatidiform mole. *Lancet*, **335**, 1030–1031.

Eklund, A., Simola, K. O. J. and Ryynänen, M. (1988). Translocation t(13;14) in nine generations with a case of translocation homozygosity. *Clin Genet*, **33**, 83–86.

Elakis, G., Moriarty, H., Saville, T., Purvis-Smith, S., Robertson, R. and Roach, T. (1993). Familial transmission of a rare centromeric fission of chromosome 10. *Bull Hum Genet Soc Australasia*, **6** (Suppl.), 40.

El-Fouly, M. H., Higgins, J. V., Kapur, S., Sankey, B. J., Matisoff, D. N. and Costa-Fox, M. (1991). DiGeorge anomaly in an infant with deletion of chromosome 22 and dup(9p) due to adjacent type II disjunction. *Am J Med Genet*, **38**, 569–573.

Elkins, T. E., Gafford, L. S., Wilks, C. S., Muram, D. and Golden, G. (1986a). A model clinic approach to the reproductive health concerns of the mentally handicapped. *Obstet Gynecol*, **68**, 185–188.

Elkins, T. E., Stovall, T. G., Wilroy, S. and Dacus, J. V. (1986b). Attitudes of mothers of children with Down syndrome concerning amniocentesis, abortion, and prenatal genetic counseling techniques. *Obstet Gynecol*, **68**, 181–184.

Elliott, M., Bayly, R., Cole, T., Temple, I. K. and Maher, E. R. (1994). Clinical features and natural history of Beckwith-Wiedemann syndrome: presentation of 74 new cases. *Clin Genet*, **46**, 168–174.

Elliott, M. and Maher, E. R. (1994). Beckwith-Wiedemann syndrome. *J Med Genet*, **31**, 560–564.

Elmslie, F. V., Vivian, A. J., Gardiner, H., Hall, C., Mowat, A. P. and Winter, R. M. (1995). Alagille syndrome: family studies. *J Med Genet,* **32**, 264–268.

Emery, A. E. H. (1986). ''Methodology in medical genetics. An introduction to statistical methods.'' Churchill Livingstone, Edinburgh.

Emery, A. E. H. and Pullen, I. M. (eds.) (1984). ''Psychological aspects of genetic counselling.'' Academic Press, London.

Engel, E. (1993). Uniparental disomy revisited: the first twelve years. *Am J Med Genet*, **46**, 670–674.

Engel, E., Crippa, L., Engel-de Montmollin, M., Tran, T. N. and Muhlethaler, M. (1981). Aneuploïdies sexuelles diagnostiquées par l'amniocentèse: implications pour le conseil génétique. *Ann Génét*, **24**, 107–109.

Epstein, C. J. (1986). ''The consequences of chromosome imbalance: principles, mechanisms, and models.'' Cambridge University Press, Cambridge.

Epstein, C. J. (1993a). Down syndrome. In ''The molecular and genetic basis of neurological disease'' (R. N. Rosenberg, S. B. Prusiner, S. DiMauro, R. L. Barchi and L. M. Kunkel, eds.). Butterworth-Heinemann, Boston, pp. 49–78.

Epstein, C. J. (ed.) (1993b). The phenotypic mapping of Down syndrome and other aneuploid conditions. Wiley-Liss, Inc., New York.

Epstein, C. J., Curry, C. J. R., Packman, S., Sherman, S. and Hall, B. D. (eds.) (1979). Risk, communication, and decision making in genetic counseling. *Birth Defects: Orig Art Series*, **15**(5C).

Erickson, R. P., Hudgins, L., Stone, J. F., Schmidt, S., Wilke, C. and Glover, T. W. (1995). A ''balanced'' Y;16 translocation associated with Turner-like neonatal lymphedema suggests the location of a potential anti-Turner gene on the Y chromosome. *Cytogenet Cell Genet*, **71**, 163–167.

Estabrooks, L. L., Lamb, A. N., Aylsworth, A. S., Callanan, N. P. and Rao, K. W. (1994). Molecular characterisation of chromosome 4p deletions resulting in Wolf-Hirschhorn syndrome. *J Med Genet*, **31**, 103–107.

Estabrooks, L. L., Rao, K. W., Driscoll, D. A., Crandall, B. F., Dean, J. C. S., Ikonen, E., Korf, B. and Aylsworth, A. S. (1995). Preliminary phenotypic map of chromosome 4p16 based on 4p deletions. *Am J Med Genet*, **57**, 581–586.

Estop, A. M., Bansal, V., Lin, A., Levinson, F., Karlin, S. M., Surti, U., Wenger, S. L. and Steele, M. W. (1994). Three unrelated cases of paracentric inversions of 1p in individuals with abnormal phenotypes. *Am J Med Genet*, **49**, 410–413.

Estop, A. M., Mowery-Rushton, P. A., Cieply, K. M., Kochmar, S. J., Sherer, C. R., Clemens, M., Surti, U. and McPherson, E. (1995). Identification of an unbalanced cryptic translocation t(9;17)(q34.3;p13.3) in a child with dysmorphic features. *J Med Genet*, **32**, 819–822.

Estop, A. M., Van Kirk, V. and Cieply, K. (1995). Segregation analysis of four translocations, t(2;18), t(3;15), t(5;7), and t(10;12), by sperm chromosome studies and a review of the literature. *Cytogenet Cell Genet*, **70**, 80–87.

Eunpu, D., McDonald, D. and Zackai, E. (1985). Down syndrome: rate in second degree relatives. *Am J Hum Genet*, **37**, A132.

European Polycystic Kidney Disease Consortium (1994). The polycystic kidney disease gene 1 encodes a 14kb transcript and lies within a duplicated region on chromosome 16. *Cell*, **77**, 1–20.

Evans, J. A., Hamerton, J. L. and Robinson, A. (1990a). Children and young adults with sex chromosome aneuploidy. Follow-up, clinical, and molecular studies. *Birth Defects: Orig Art Series*, **26**(4).

Evans, K. L., Brown, J., Shibasaki, Y., Devon, R. S., He, L., Arveiler, B., Christie, S., Maule, J. C., Baillie, D., Slorach, E. M., Anderson, S. M., Gosden, J. R., Petit, J., Weith, A., Gosden, C. M., Blackwood, D. H. R., St. Clair, D. M., Muir, W. J., Brookes, A. J. and Porteous, D. J. (1995). A contiguous clone map over 3 Mb on the long arm of chromosome 11 across a balanced translocation associated with schizophrenia. *Genomics*, **28**, 420–428.

Evans, M. I., Farrell, S. A., Greb, A., Ray, P., Johnson, M. P. and Hoffmann, E. P. (1993). In utero fetal muscle biopsy for the diagnosis of Duchenne muscular dystrophy in a female fetus "suddenly at risk". *Am J Med Genet*, **46**, 309–312.

Evans, M. I., White, B. J., Kent, S. G., Levine, M. A., Levin, S. W. and Larsen, J. W. (1984). Balanced rearrangement of chromosomes 2, 5 and 13 in a family with duplication 5q and fetal loss. *Am J Med Genet*, **19**, 783–790.

Ewart, A. K., Jin, W., Atkinson, D., Morris, C. A. and Keating, M. T. (1994). Supravalvular aortic stenosis associated with a deletion disrupting the elastin gene. *J Clin Invest*, **93**, 1071–1077.

Ewart, A. K., Morris, C. A., Atkinson, D., Jin, W., Sternes, K., Spallone, P., Stock, A. D., Leppert, M. and Keating, M. T. (1993). Hemizygosity at the elastin locus in a developmental disorder, Williams syndrome. *Nature Genet*, **5**, 11–16.

Eydoux, P., Kasprzak, L., Elliott, A. M., Shevell, M. and Der Kaloustian, V. M. (1995). De novo deletion of 22q11 in two male siblings with different phenotypes. *Am J Hum Genet (Suppl.)*, **57**, A113.

Falik-Borenstein, T. C., Korenberg, J. R. and Schreck, R. R. (1994). Confined placental chimerism: prenatal and postnatal cytogenetic and molecular analysis, and pregnancy outcome. *Am J Med Genet*, **50**, 51–56.

Fantes, J., Redeker, B., Breen, M., Boyle, S., Brown, J., Fletcher, J., Jones, S., Bickmore, W., Fukushima, Y., Mannens, M., Danes, S., van Heyningen, V. and Hanson, I. (1995). Aniridia-associated cytogenetic rearrangements suggest that a position effect may cause the mutant phenotype. *Hum Mol Genet*, **4**, 415–422.

Farag, T. I., Krishna Murthy, D. S., Al-Awadi, S. A., Sundareshan, T. S., Al-Othman, S. A., Mady, S. A. and Redha, M. A. (1987). Robertsonian translocation t dic (14p;22p) with regular trisomy 21: a possible interchromosomal effect? *Ann Génét*, **30**, 189–192.

Farah, L. M. S., Nazareth, H. R. de S., Dolnikoff, M. and Delascio, D. (1975). Balanced homologous translocation t(22q;22q) in a phenotypically normal woman with repeated spontaneous abortions. *Hum Genet*, **28**, 357–360.

Farah, S. B., Ramos, C. F., de Mello, M. P., Sartorato, E. L., Horelli-Kuitunen, N., Lopes, V. L. G. S., Cavalcanti, D. P. and Hackel, C. (1994). Two cases of Y; autosome translocations: a 45,X male and a clinically trisomy 18 patient. *Am J Med Genet*, **49**, 388–392.

Farrell, S. A. and Chow, G. (1992). Intrachromosomal insertion of chromosome 7. *Clin Genet*, **41**, 299–302.

Farrell, S. A. and Fan, Y.-S. (1995). Balanced nonacrocentric whole-arm reciprocal translocations: a de novo case and literature review. *Am J Med Genet*, **55**, 423–426.

Farrell, S. A., Summers, A. M., Gardner, H. A. and Uchida, I. A. (1994). Balanced complex chromosome rearrangement ascertained through prenatal diagnosis. *Am J Med Genet*, **52**, 360–361.

Faugeras, C. and Barthe, D. (1986). Transmission d'un chromosome 18 en anneau sur deux générations, chez des sujets Ö phénotype normal. *J Génét Hum*, **34**, 313–320.

Fechner, P. Y., Rosenberg, C., Stetten, G., Cargile, C. B., Pearson, P. L., Smith, K. D., Migeon, C. J. and Berkovitz, G. D. (1994). Nonrandom inactivation of the Y-bearing X chromosome in a 46,XX individual: evidence for the etiology of 46,XX true hermaphroditism. *Cytogenet Cell Genet*, **66**, 22–26.

Federman, D. D. (1987). Mapping the X-chromosome. Mining its p's and q's. *N Engl J Med*, **317**, 161–162.

Feldman, G. L., Weiss, L., Phelan, M. C., Schroer, R. J. and Van Dyke, D. L. (1993). Inverted duplication of 8p: ten new patients and review of the literature. *Am J Med Genet*, **47**, 482–486.

Feng, Y., Zhang, F., Lokey, L. K., Chastain, J. L., Lakkis, L., Eberhart, D. and Warren, S. T. (1995). Translational suppression by trinucleotide repeat expansion at FMR1. *Science*, **268**, 731–734.

Ferguson-Smith, M. A. (1983). Prenatal chromosome analysis and its impact on the birth incidence of chromosome disorders. *Br Med Bull*, **39**, 355–364.

Ferguson-Smith, M. A., Cooke, A., Affara, N. A., Boyd, E. and Tolmie, J. L. (1990). Genotype-phenotype correlations in XX males and their bearing on current theories of sex determination. *Hum Genet*, **84**, 198–202.

Fernández, J. L., Pereira, S., Campos, A., Gosálvez, J. and Goyanes, V. (1994). An extra band within the human 9qh+ region that behaves like the surrounding constitutive heterochromatin. *J Med Genet*, **31**, 632–634.

Ferrero, G. B., Franco, B., Roth, E. J., Firulli, B. A., Borsani, G., Delmas-Mata, J., Weissenbach, J., Halley, G., Schlessinger, D., Chinault, A. C., Zoghbi, H. Y., Nelson, D. L. and Ballabio, A. (1995). An integrated physical and genetic map of a 35 Mb region on chromosome Xp22.3-Xp21.3. *Hum Mol Genet*, **4**, 1821–1827.

Fewtrell, M. S., Tam, P. K. H., Thomson, A. H., Fitchett, M., Currie, J., Huson, S. M. and Mulligan, L. M. (1994). Hirschsprung's disease associated with a deletion of chromosome 10 (q11.2q21.2): a further link with the neurocristopathies? *J Med Genet*, **31**, 325–327.

Fineman, R. M., Issa, B. and Weinblatt, V. (1989). Prenatal diagnosis of a large heteromorphic region in a chromosome 5: implications for genetic counseling. *Am J Med Genet*, **32**, 498–499.

Fisch, G. S., Snow, K., Thibodeau, S. N., Chalifaux, M., Holden, J. J. A., Nelson, D. L., Howard-Peebles, P. N. and Maddalena, A. (1995). The fragile X premutation in carriers and its effect on mutation size in offspring. *Am J Hum Genet*, **56**, 1147–1155.

Fisher, E. and Scambler, P. (1994). Human haploinsufficiency—one for sorrow, two for joy. *Nature Genet*, **7**, 5–6.

Fisher, J. M., Harvey, J. F., Morton, N. E. and Jacobs, P. A. (1995). Trisomy 18: studies of the parent and cell division of origin and the effect of aberrant recombination on nondisjunction. *Am J Hum Genet*, **56**, 669–675.

Fitzgerald, P. H., Archer, S. A. and Morris, C. M. (1986). Evidence for the repeated primary non-disjunction of chromosome 21 as a result of premature centromere division (PCD). *Hum Genet*, **72**, 58–62.

Fitzgerald, P. H., Donald, R. A. and McCormick, P. (1984). Reduced fertility in women with X chromosome abnormality. *Clin Genet*, **25**, 301–309.

FitzPatrick, D. R. and Boyd, E. (1989). Recurrences of trisomy 18 and trisomy 13 after trisomy 21. *Hum Genet*, **82**, 301.

Flint, J., Wilkie, A. O. M., Buckle, V. J., Winter, R. M., Holland, A. J. and McDermid, H. E. (1995). The detection of subtelomeric chromosomal rearrangements in idiopathic mental retardation. *Nature Genet*, **9**, 132–139.

Fraccaro, M., Maraschio, P., Pasquali, F. and Scappaticci, S. (1977). Women heterozygous for deficiency of the (p21→pter) region of the X chromosome are fertile. *Hum Genet*, **39**, 283–292.

Franceschini, P., Martino, S., Ciocchini, M., Ciuti, E., Vardeu, M. P., Guala, A., Signorile, F., Camerano, P., Franceschini, D. and Tovo, P. A. (1995). Variability of clinical and immunological phenotype in immunodeficiency-centromeric instability-facial anomalies syndrome. Report of two new patients and review of the literature. *Eur J Pediatr*, **154**, 840–846.

Francke, U. (1984). Random X inactivation resulting in mosaic nullisomy of region Xp21.1→p21.3 associated with heterozygosity for ornithine transcarbamylase deficiency and for chronic granulomatous disease. *Cytogenet Cell Genet*, **38**, 298–307.

Francke, U. (1994). Digitized and differentially shaded human chromosome ideograms for genomic applications. *Cytogenet Cell Genet*, **65**, 206–219.

Francke, U., Harper, J. F., Darras, B. T., Cowan, J. M., McCabe, E. R. B., Kohlschütter, A., Seltzer, W. K., Saito, F., Goto, J., Harpey, J.-P. and Wise, J. E. (1987). Congenital adrenal hypoplasia, myopathy, and glycerol kinase deficiency: molecular genetic evidence for deletions. *Am J Hum Genet*, **40**, 212–227.

Franco, B., Guioli, S., Pragliola, A., Incerti, B., Bardoni, B., Tonlorenzi, R., Carrozzo, R., Maestrini, E., Pieretti, M., Taillon-Miller, P., Brown, C. J., Willard, H. F., Lawrence, C., Persico, M. G., Camerino, G. and Ballabio, A. (1991). A gene deleted in Kallmann's syndrome shares homology with neural cell adhesion and axonal path-finding molecules. *Nature*, **353**, 529–536.

Franke, U. C., Scambler, P. J., Löffler, C., Löns, P., Hanefeld, F., Zoll, B. and Hansmann, I. (1994). Interstitial deletion of 22q11 in DiGeorge syndrome detected by high resolution and molecular analysis. *Clin Genet*, **46**, 187–192.

Freeman, S. B., May, K. M., Pettay, D., Fernhoff, P. M. and Hassold, T. J. (1993). Paternal uniparental disomy in a child with a balanced 15;15 translocation and Angelman syndrome. *Am J Med Genet*, **45**, 625–630.

Freije, D., Helms, C., Watson, M. S. and Donis-Keller, H. (1992). Identification of a second pseudoautosomal region near the Xq and Yq telomeres. *Science*, **258**, 1784–1787.

Fried, K., Tieder, M., Beer, S., Rosenblatt, M. and Krespin, H. I. (1977). Mental retardation with 45 chromosomes 45,XX,−5,−14,+der(5)t(5;14)(p15;q13)mat due to familial balanced reciprocal translocation. *J Med Genet*, **14**, 68–72.

Friedrich, U. and Nielsen, J. (1972). Presumptive Y-15 and Y-22 translocation in two families. *Hereditas*, **71**, 339–342.

Fries, M. H., Lebo, R. V., Schonberg, S. A., Golabi, M., Seltzer, W. K., Gitelman, S. E. and Golbus, M. S. (1993). Mental retardation locus in Xp21 chromosome microdeletion. *Am J Med Genet*, **46**, 363–368.

Frohlich, G. S. and Falk, R. E. (1991). Trisomy 12 mosaicism. *Prenat Diagn*, **11**, 881.

Fryburg, J. S., Dimaio, M. S., Yang-Feng, T. L. and Mahoney, M. J. (1993). Follow-up of pregnancies complicated by placental mosaicism diagnosed by chorionic villus sampling. *Prenat Diagn*, **13**, 481–494.

Fryns, J.-P. (1995a). Syndrome of proximal interstitial deletion 4p15. *Am J Med Genet*, **58**, 295–296.

Fryns, J. P. (1995b). The concurrence of blepharophimosis, ptosis, epicanthus inversus syndrome (BPES) and Langer type of mesomelic dwarfism in the same patient. Evidence of the location of Langer type of mesomelic dwarfism at 3q22.3-q23? *Clin Genet*, **48**, 111–112.

Fryns, J. P., Bulcke, J., Hens, L. and Van den Berghe, H. (1980). Balanced transmission of centromeric fission products in man. *Hum Genet*, **54**, 127–128.

Fryns, J. P., Casaer, P. and Van den Berghe, H. (1979). Mosaic trisomy 13 due to de novo 13/13 translocation with subsequent fission. Karyotype: 46,XX,−13,+t(13; 13)(p11;q11)/46,XX,del(13)(p11). *Hum Genet*, **46**, 237–241.

Fryns, J. P. and Kleczkowska, A. (1986). Reciprocal translocation mosaicism in man. *Am J Med Genet*, **25**, 175–176.

Fryns, J. P. and Kleczkowska, A. (1987). Ring chromosome 21 in the mother and 21/ 21 translocation in the fetus: karyotype 45,XX,-21,-21,t(21;21)(p11;q11). *Ann Génét*, **30**, 109–110.

Fryns, J. P., Kleczkowska, A., Kubień, E. and Van den Berghe, H. (1992). On the excess of mental retardation and/or congenital malformations in apparently balanced reciprocal translocations. A critical review of the Leuven data 1966–1991. *Genet Counsel*, **2**, 185–194.

Fryns, J. P., Kleczkowska, A., Kubień, E. and Van den Berghe, H. (1986a). Excess of mental retardation and/or congenital malformation in reciprocal translocations in man. *Hum Genet*, **72**, 1–8.

Fryns, J. P., Kleczkowska, A., Moerman, P. and Van den Berghe, H. (1986b). Reciprocal translocations and full trisomy (trisomy 18 and trisomy 21) in the offspring. *Ann Génét*, **29**, 272–274.

Fryns, J. P., Kleczkowska, A. and Van den Berghe, H. (1986c). Paracentric inversions in man. *Hum Genet*, **73**, 205–213.

Fryns, J. P., Kleczkowska, A., Petit, P. and Van den Berghe, H. (1982). Fertility in patients with X chromosome deletions. *Clin Genet*, **22**, 76–79.

Fryns, J. P., Kleczkowska, A., Smeets, E. and Van den Berghe, H. (1988a). A new centromeric heteromorphism in the short arm of chromosome 20. *J Med Genet*, **25**, 636–637.

Fryns, J. P., Kleczkowska, A. and Van den Berghe, H. (1988b). Familial transmission of autosomal whole arm translocation. *J Med Genet*, **25**, 783–784.

Fryns, J. P. and Petit, P. (1987). Population cytogenetics of autosomal fragile sites. *Clin Genet*, **31**, 61–62.

Fryns, J.-P., Van den Berghe, H. and Schrander-Stumpel, C. (1994). Kabuki (Niikawa-Kuroki) syndrome and paracentric inversion of the short arm of chromosome 4. *Am J Med Genet*, **53**, 204–205.

Fu, Y.-H., Kuhl, D. P. A., Pizzuti, A., Pieretti, M., Sutcliffe, J. S., Richards, S., Verkerk, A. J. M. H., Holden, J. J. A., Fenwick, R. G., Warren, S. T., Oostra, B. A., Nelson, D. L. and Caskey, C. T. (1991). Variation of the CCG repeat at the fragile

X site results in genetic instability: resolution of the Sherman paradox. *Cell*, **67**, 1047–1058.

Fukushima, Y., Kuroki, Y., Ito, T., Kondo, I. and Nishigaki, I. (1987). Familial retinoblastoma (mother and son) with 13q14 deletion. *Hum Genet*, **77**, 104–107.

Gabriel-Robez, O., Ratomponirina, C., Dutrillaux, B., Carré-Pigeon, F. and Rumpler, Y. (1986). Meiotic association between the XY chromosomes and the autosomal quadrivalent of a reciprocal translocation in two infertile men, 46,XY,t(19;22) and 46,XY,t(17;21). *Cytogenet Cell Genet*, **43**, 154–160.

Gabriel-Robez, O. and Rumpler, Y. (1994). The meiotic pairing behaviour in human spermatocytes carrier of chromosome anomalies and their repercussions on reproductive fitness I: inversions and insertions. A European collaborative study. *Ann Génét*, **37**, 3–10.

Gabriel-Robez, O., Rumpler, Y., Ratomponirina, C., Petit, C., Levilliers, J., Croquette, M. F. and Couturier, J. (1990). Deletion of the pseudoautosomal region and lack of sex-chromosome pairing at pachytene in two infertile men carrying an X;Y translocation. *Cytogenet Cell Genet*, **54**, 38–42.

Gacy, A. M., Goeliner, G., Juranić, N., Macura, S. and McMurray, C. T. (1995). Trinucleotide repeats that expand in human disease form hairpin structures in vitro. *Cell*, **81**, 533–540.

Gadow, E. C., Lippold, S., Otano, L., Serafin, E., Scarpati, R. and Matayoshi, T. (1991). Chromosome rearrangements among couples with pregnancy losses and other adverse reproductive outcomes. *Am J Med Genet*, **41**, 279–281.

Gagnon, S., Fraser, W., Fouquette, B., Bastide, A., Bureau, M., Fontaine, J.-Y. and Huot, C. (1992). Nature and frequency of chromosomal abnormalities in pregnancies with abnormal ultrasound findings: an analysis of 117 cases with review of the literature. *Prenat Diagn*, **12**, 9–18.

Ganiats, T. G., Halverson, A. L. and Bogart, M. H. (1994). Incremental cost-effectiveness of incorporating oestriol evaluation in Down syndrome screening programmes. *Prenat Diagn*, **14**, 527–535.

Garber, A., Carlson, D., Schreck, R., Fischel-Ghodsian, N., Hsu, W.-T., Oeztas, S., Pepkowitz, S. and Graham, J. M. (1994). Prenatal diagnosis and dysmorphic findings in mosaic trisomy 16. *Prenat Diagn*, **14**, 257–266.

Gardner, R. J. M., Dockery, H. E., Fitzgerald, P. H., Parfitt, R. G., Romain, D. R., Scobie, N., Shaw, R. L., Tumewu, P. and Watt, A. J. (1994). Mosaicism with a normal cell line and an autosomal structural rearrangement. *J Med Genet*, **31**, 108–114.

Gardner, R. J. M., McCreanor, H. R., Parslow, M. I. and Veale, A. M. O. (1974). Are 1q+ chromosomes harmless? *Clin Genet*, **6**, 383–393.

Gardner, R. J. M., Monk, N. A., Allen, G. J. and Parslow, M. I. (1986a). A three way translocation in mother and daughter. *J Med Genet*, **23**, 90.

Gardner, R. J. M., Monk, N. A., Clarkson, J. E. and Allen, G. J. (1986b). Ring 21 chromosome: the mild end of the phenotypic spectrum. *Clin Genet*, **30**, 466–470.

Gardner, R. J. M., Rudd, N. L., Stevens, L. J. and Worton, R. G. (1978). Autosomal imbalance with a near-normal phenotype: the small effect of trisomy for the short arm of chromosome 18. *Birth Defects: Orig Art Series*, **14**(6C), pp. 359–363.

Gardner, R. J. M. and Veale, A. M. O. (1974). *De novo* translocation Down's syndrome: risk of recurrence of Down's syndrome. *Clin Genet*, **6**, 160–164.

Gardner, R. J. M., Veale, A. M. O., Parslow, M. I., Becroft, D. M. O., Shaw, R. L., Fitzgerald, P. H., Hutchings, H. E., McCreanor, H. R., Wong, J., Eiby, J. R., Howarth, D. A. and Whyte, S. E. (1973a). A survey of 972 cytogenetically examined cases of Down's syndrome. *N Z Med J*, **78**, 403–409.

Gardner, R. J. M., Veale, A. M. O., Sands, V. E. and Holdaway, M. D. H. (1973b). XXXX syndrome: case report, and a note on genetic counselling and fertility. *Hum Genet*, **17**, 323–330.

Gatti, R. A., Peterson, K. L., Novak, J., Chen, X., Yang-Chen, L., Liang, T., Lange, E. and Lange, K. (1993). Prenatal genotyping of ataxia-telangiectasia. *Lancet*, **342**, 376.

Gecz, J., Gedeon, A. K., Sutherland, G. R. and Mulley, J. C. (1996). Cloning of *FMR2*: a gene associated with FRAXE mental retardation. *Nature Genet*, in press.

Gedeon, A. K., Keinänen, M., Adès, L. C., Kääriäinen, H., Gécz, J., Baker, E., Sutherland, G. R. and Mulley, J. C. (1995). Overlapping submicroscopic deletions in Xq28 in two unrelated boys with developmental disorders: identification of a gene near FRAXE. *Am J Hum Genet*, **56**, 907–914.

Gelman-Kohan, Z., Rosensaft, J., Ben-Cohen, R. N. and Chemke, J. (1993). Homozygosity for inversion (2)(p12q14). *Hum Genet*, **92**, 427.

Genest, P. (1973). Transmission héréditaire depuis 300 ans d'un chromosome Y à satellites dans une lignée familiale. *Ann Génét*, **16**, 35–38.

German, J. (1993). Bloom syndrome: a Mendelian prototype of somatic mutational disease. *Medicine*, **72**, 393–406.

Gersh, M., Goodart, S. A., Pasztor, L. M., Harris, D. J., Weiss, L. and Overhauser, J. (1995). Evidence for a distinct region causing a cat-like cry in patients with 5p deletions. *Am J Hum Genet*, **56**, 1404–1410.

Giacalone, J. P. and Francke, U. (1992). Common sequence motifs at the rearrangement sites of a constitutional X/autosome translocation and associated deletion. *Am J Hum Genet*, **50**, 725–741.

Giampietro, P. F., Davis, J. G. and Auerbach, A. D. (1994). Fanconi's anemia. *N Engl J Med*, **330**, 720–721.

Gibson, R. A., Ford, D., Jansen, S., Savoia, A., Havenga, C., Milner, R. D., de Ravel, T. J., Cohn, R. J., Ball, S. E., Roberts, I., Llerena, J. C., Vorechovsky, I., Pearson, T., Birjandi, F., Hussein, S. S., Murer-Orlando, M., Easton, D. F. and Mathew, C. G. (1994). Genetic mapping of the FACC gene and linkage analysis in Fanconi anaemia families. *J Med Genet*, **31**, 868–871.

Gillessen-Kaesbach, G., Gross, S., Kaya-Westerloh, S., Passarge, E. and Horsthemke, B. (1995). DNA methylation based testing of 450 patients suspected of having Prader-Willi syndrome. *J Med Genet*, **32**, 88–92.

Gillon, R. (1987). On sterilising severely mentally handicapped people. *J Med Ethics*, **13**, 59–61.

Glenn, C. C., Saitoh, S., Jong, M. T. C., Filbrandt, M. M., Surti, U., Driscoll, D. J., Nicholls, R. D. (1996) Gene structure, DNA methylation and imprinted expression of the human *SNRPN* gene. *Am J Hum Genet*, **58**, 335–346.

Goldman, A. S. H. and Hultén, M. A. (1992). Chromosome in situ suppression hybridisation in human male meiosis. *J Med Genet*, **29**, 98–102.

Goldman, A. S. H., Martin, R. H., Johannisson, R., Gould, C. P., Davison, E. V., Emslie, J. E., Burn, J. and Hultén, M. A. (1992). Meiotic and sperm chromosome analysis in a male carrier of an inverted insertion (3;10)(q13.2;p14p13). *J Med Genet*, **29**, 460–464.

Goldstein, D. P. and Berkowitz, R. S. (1994). Current management of complete and partial molar pregnancy. *J Reprod Med*, **39**, 139–146.

Goodall, J. (1991). Helping a child to understand her own testicular feminisation. *Lancet*, **337**, 33–35.

Goodship, J., Cross, I., Scambler, P. and Burn, J. (1995). Monozygous twins with chromosome 22q11 deletion and discordant phenotype. *J Med Genet*, **32**, 746–748.

Gorski, J. L., Kistenmacher, M. L., Punnett, H. H., Zackai, E. H. and Emanuel, B. S. (1988). Reproductive risks for carriers of complex chromosome rearrangements: analysis of 25 families. *Am J Med Genet*, **29**, 247–261.

Gosden, C., Nicolaides, K. H. and Rodeck, C. H. (1988). Fetal blood sampling in investigation of chromosome mosaicism in amniotic fluid cell culture. *Lancet*, **1**, 613–617.

Gosden, J. R., Gosden, C., Lawrie, S. S. and Mitchell, A. R. (1978). The fate of DNA satellites I, II, III and ribosomal DNA in a familial dicentric chromosome 13;14. *Hum Genet*, **41**, 131–141.

Grass, F. S., Schwartz, R. P., Deal, J. O. and Parke, J. C. (1981). Gonadal dysgenesis, intra-X chromosome insertion, and possible position effect in an otherwise normal female. *Clin Genet*, **20**, 28–35.

Gravholt, C. H., Caprani, M. and Friedrich, U. (1994). Fluorescence in situ hybridization reveals a break in the α-satellite DNA of chromosome 1 in a family with a balanced whole-arm translocation. *Hum Genet*, **94**, 504–508.

Green, A. J., Barton, D. E., Jenks, P., Pearson, J. and Yates, J. R. W. (1994). Chimaerism shown by cytogenetics and DNA polymorphism analysis. *J Med Genet*, **31**, 816–817.

Greenberg, F., Guzzetta, V., de Oca-Luna, R. M., Magenis, R. E., Smith, A. C. M., Richter, S. F., Kondo, I., Dobyns, W. B., Patel, P. I. and Lupski, J. R. (1991). Molecular analysis of the Smith-Magenis syndrome: a possible contiguous-gene syndrome associated with del(17)(p11.2). *Am J Hum Genet*, **49**, 1207–1218.

Greenberg, F., Stratton, R. F., Lockhart, L. H., Elder, F. F. B., Dobyns, W. B. and Ledbetter, D. H. (1986). Familial Miller-Dieker syndrome associated with pericentric inversion of chromosome 17. *Am J Med Genet*, **23**, 853–859.

Groupe de Cytogénéticiens Français (1986a). Paracentric inversions in man. A French collaborative study. *Ann Génét*, **29**, 169–176.

Groupe de Cytogénéticiens français (1986b). Pericentric inversions in man. A French collaborative study. *Ann Génét*, **29**, 129–168.

Grudzinskas, J. G., Chard, T., Chapman, M. and Cuckle, H. (eds.) (1994). ''Screening for Down's syndrome.'' Cambridge University Press, Cambridge.

Guichaoua, M. R., Devictor, M., Hartung, M., Luciani, J. M. and Stahl, A. (1986). Random acrocentric bivalent associations in human pachytene spermatocytes. Molecular implications in the occurrence of Robertsonian translocations. *Cytogenet Cell Genet*, **42**, 191–197.

Guichaoua, M. R., de Lanversin, A., Cataldo, C., Delafontaine, D., Alasia, C., Fraterno, M., Terriou, P., Stahl, A. and Luciani, J. M. (1991). Three dimensional reconstruction of human pachytene spermatocyte nuclei of a 17;21 reciprocal translocation carrier: study of XY-autosome relationships. *Hum Genet*, **87**, 709–715.

Guichaoua, M. R., Quack, B., Speed, R. M., Noel, B., Chandley, A. C. and Luciani, J. M. (1990). Infertility in human males with autosomal translocations: meiotic study of a 14;22 Robertsonian translocation. *Hum Genet*, **86**, 162–166.

Guichaoua, M. R., Speed, R. M., Luciani, J. M., Delafontaine, D. and Chandley, A. C. (1992). Infertility in human males with autosomal translocations. II. Meiotic studies in three reciprocal rearrangements, one showing tertiary monosomy in a 45-chromosome individual and his father. *Cytogenet Cell Genet*, **60**, 96–101.

Guichet, A., Briault, S., Toutain, A., Paillet, C., Descamps, P., Pierre, F., Body, G. and Moraine, C. (1995). Prenatal diagnosis of trisomy 8 mosaicism in CVS after abnormal ultrasound findings at 12 weeks. *Prenat Diagn*, **15**, 769–772.

Guioli, S., Incerti, B., Zanaria, E., Bardoni, B., Franco, B., Taylor, K., Ballabio, A. and Camerino, G. (1992). Kallmann syndrome due to a translocation resulting in an X/Y fusion gene. *Nature Genet*, **1**, 337–340.

Guo, W.-J., Callif-Daley, F., Zapata, M. C. and Miller, M. E. (1995). Clinical and cytogenetic findings in seven cases of inverted duplication of 8p with evidence of a telomeric deletion using fluorescence in situ hybridization. *Am J Med Genet*, **58**, 230–236.

Gupta, J. K., Cave, M., Lilford, R. J., Farrell, T. A., Irving, H. C., Mason, G. and Hau, C. M. (1995). Clinical significance of fetal choroid plexus cysts. *Lancet*, **346**, 724–729.

Gustashaw, K. M., Zurcher, V., Dickerman, L. H., Stallard, R. and Willard, H. F. (1994). Partial X chromosome trisomy with functional disomy of Xp due to failure of X inactivation. *Am J Med Genet*, **53**, 39–45.

Guttenbach, M., Schakowski, R. and Schmid, M. (1994a). Aneuploidy and ageing: sex chromosome exclusion into micronuclei. *Hum Genet*, **94**, 295–298.

Guttenbach, M., Schakowski, R. and Schmid, M. (1994b). Incidence of chromosome 18 disomy in human sperm nuclei as detected by nonisotopic in situ hybridization. *Hum Genet*, **93**, 421–423.

Guttenbach, M., Schakowski, R. and Schmid, M. (1994c). Incidence of chromosome 3, 7, 10, 11, 17 and X disomy in mature human sperm nuclei as determined by nonradioactive in situ hybridization. *Hum Genet*, **93**, 7–12.

Haan, E. A., Hull, Y. J., White, S., Cockington, R., Charlton, P. and Callen, D. F. (1989). Tricho-rhino-phalangeal and branchio-oto syndromes in a family with an inherited rearrangement of chromosome 8q. *Am J Med Genet*, **32**, 490–494.

Haataja, R., Väisänen, M.-L., Li, M., Ryynänen, M. and Leisti, J. (1994). The fragile X syndrome in Finland: demonstration of a founder effect by analysis of microsatellite haplotypes. *Hum Genet*, **94**, 479–483.

Haddow, J. E., Palomaki, G. E., Knight, G. J., Cunningham, G. C., Lustig, L. S. and Boyd, P. A. (1994). Reducing the need for amniocentesis in women 35 years of age or older with serum markers for screening. *N Engl J Med*, **330**, 1114–1118.

Hagerman, R. J., Hull, C. E., Safanda, J. F., Carpenter, I., Staley, L. W., O'Connor, R. A., Seydel, C., Mazzocco, M. M. M., Snow, K., Thibodeau, S. N., Kuhl, D., Nelson, D. L., Caskey, C. T. and Taylor, A. K. (1994). High functioning fragile X males: demonstration of an unmethylated fully expanded FMR-1 mutation associated with protein expression. *Am J Med Genet*, **51**, 298–308.

Haig, D. (1993). Genomic imprinting, human chorionic gonadotropin, and triploidy. *Prenat Diagn*, **13**, 151.

Hajianpour, A., Murer-Orlando, M. and Docherty, Z. (1991). Germ line mosaicism for chromosome 5 "cri-du-chat" deletion? *Am J Hum Genet*, **49** (Suppl.), 217.

Hale, D. W. (1994). Is X-Y recombination necessary for spermatocyte survival during mammalian spermatogenesis? *Cytogenet Cell Genet*, **65**, 278–282.

Hales, H. A., Peterson, C. M., Carey, J., Hecht, B. K.-M. and Hecht, F. (1993). Prenatal detection of de novo paracentric inversion 46,XX inv(14)(q22q32.1) in a normal child: report and review of the literature. *Am J Med Genet*, **47**, 848–851.

Halliday, J., Lumley, J., Sheffield, L. J. and Lancaster, P. A. L. (1993). Limb deficiencies, chorion villus sampling, and advanced maternal age. *Am J Med Genet*, **47**, 1096–1098.

Halliday, J., Lumley, J. and Watson, L. (1995a). Comparison of women who do and do not have amniocentesis or chorionic villus sampling. *Lancet*, **345**,

704–709.

Halliday, J. L., Watson, L. F., Lumley, J., Danks, D. M. and Sheffield, L. J. (1995b). New estimates of Down syndrome risks at chorionic villus sampling, amniocentesis, and livebirth in women of advanced maternal age from a uniquely defined population. *Prenat Diagn*, **15**, 455–465.

Hamel, B. C. J., Smits, A. P. T., de Graaff, E., Smeets, D. F. C. M., Schoute, F., Eussen, B. H. J., Knight, S. J. L., Davies, K. E., Assman-Hulsmans, C. F. C. H. and Oostra, B. A. (1994). Segregation of FRAXE in a large family: clinical, psychometric, cytogenetic, and molecular data. *Am J Hum Genet*, **55**, 923–931.

Han, J.-Y., Choo, K. H. A. and Shaffer, L. G. (1994a). Molecular cytogenetic characterization of 17 rob(13q14q) Robertsonian translocations by FISH, narrowing the region containing the breakpoints. *Am J Hum Genet*, **55**, 960–967.

Han, T. L., Ford, J. H., Flaherty, S. P., Webb, G. C. and Matthews, C. D. (1994b). A fluorescent *in situ* hybridization analysis of the chromosome constitution of ejaculated sperm in a 47,XYY male. *Clin Genet*, **45**, 67–70.

Harper, P. S. (1993). "Practical genetic counselling" (4th edn.). Butterworth Heinemann, Oxford.

Harris, D. J., Hankins, L. and Begleiter, M. L. (1979). Reproductive risk of t(13q14q) carriers: case report and review. *Am J Med Genet*, **3**, 175–181.

Harrison, K., Eisenger, K., Anyane-Yeboa, K. and Brown, S. (1995). Maternal uniparental disomy of chromosome 2 in a baby with trisomy 2 mosaicism in amniotic fluid culture. *Am J Med Genet*, **58**, 147–151.

Harrison, K. J., Barrett, I. J., Lomax, B. L., Kuchinka, B. D. and Kalousek, D. K. (1993). Detection of confined placental mosaicism in trisomy 18 conceptions using interphase cytogenetic analysis. *Hum Genet*, **92**, 353–358.

Hasegawa, T., Asamura, S., Nagai, T. and Tsuchiya, Y. (1992). An unusual variant of chromosome 16 in three generations. *Acta Paediatr Jpn*, **34**, 166–168.

Hashish, A.F., Monk, N. A., Watt, A. J. and Gardner, R. J. M. (1992). A de novo insertion, detected prenatally, with normal phenotype. *J Med Genet*, **29**, 351.

Hassold, T., Arnovitz, K., Jacobs, P. A., May, K. and Robinson, D. (1991a). The parental origin of the missing or additional chromosome in 45,X and 47,XXX females. *Birth Defects: Original Article Series*, **26**(4), pp. 297–304.

Hassold, T. J., Pettay, D., Freeman, S. B., Grantham, M. and Takaesu, N. (1991b). Molecular studies of non-disjunction in trisomy 16. *J Med Genet*, **28**, 159–162.

Hassold, T., Hunt, P. A. and Sherman, S. (1993). Trisomy in humans: incidence, origin and etiology. *Curr Opin Genet Devel*, **3**, 398–403.

Hassold, T., Jacobs, P.A. and Pettay, D. (1987). Analysis of nucleolar organizing regions in parents of trisomic spontaneous abortions. *Hum Genet*, **76**, 381–384.

Hassold, T., Pettay, D., May, K. and Robinson, A. (1990). Analysis of non-disjunction in sex chromosome tetrasomy and pentasomy. *Hum Genet*, **85**, 648–650.

Hatch, M., Kline, J., Levin, B., Hutzler, M. and Warburton, D. (1990). Paternal age and trisomy among spontaneous abortions. *Hum Genet*, **85**, 355–361.

Hawkins, J. R. (1994). Sex determination. *Hum Mol Genet*, **3**, 1463–1467.

Healey, S., Powell, F., Battersby, M., Chenevix-Trench, G. and McGill, J. (1994). Distinct phenotype in maternal uniparental disomy of chromosome 14. *Am J Med Genet*, **51**, 147–149.

Healy, D. L., Trounson, A. O. and Andersen, A. N. (1994). Female infertility: causes and treatment. *Lancet*, **343**, 1539–1544.

Hecht, C. A. and Hook, E. B. (1994). The imprecision in rates of Down syndrome by 1-year maternal age intervals: a critical analysis of rates used in biochemical screening. *Prenat Diagn*, **14**, 729–738.

Hecht, F. and Hecht, B. K. (1984). Linkage of skeletal dysplasia gene to t(2;8)(q32;p13) chromosome translocation breakpoint. *Am J Med Genet*, **18**, 779–780.

Hecht, F., Hecht, B. K. and Berger, C. S. (1984). Aneuploidy in recurrent spontaneous aborters: the tendency to parental nondisjunction. *Clin Genet*, **26**, 43–45.

Hecht, F. and McCaw, B. K. (1977). Chromosome instability syndromes. In "Genetics of human cancer" (J. J. Mulvihill, R. W. Miller and J. F. Fraumeni, eds.). Raven Press, New York, pp. 105–123.

Hecht, F. and Sutherland, G.R. (1984). Fragile sites and cancer breakpoints. *Cancer Genet Cytogenet*, **12**, 179–181.

Heim, R. A., Lench, N. J. and Swift, M. (1992). Heterozygous manifestations in four autosomal recessive human cancer-prone syndromes: ataxia telangiectasia, xeroderma pigmentosum, Fanconi anemia, and Bloom syndrome. *Mutat Res*, **284**, 25–36.

Held, K. R., Kerber, S., Kaminsky, E., Singh, S., Goetz, P., Seemanova, E. and Goedde, H. W. (1992). Mosaicism in 45,X Turner syndrome: does survival in early pregnancy depend on the presence of two sex chromosomes? *Hum Genet*, **88**, 288–294.

Henderson, D. J., Sherman, L. S., Loughna, S. C., Bennett, P. R. and Moore, G. E. (1994). Early embryonic failure associated with uniparental disomy for human chromosome 21. *Hum Mol Genet*, **3**, 1373–1376.

Hendrich, B. D., Brown, C. J. and Willard, H. F. (1993). Evolutionary conservation of possible functional domains of the human and murine *XIST* genes. *Hum Mol Genet*, **2**, 663–672.

Henry, I., Bonaïti-Pellié, C., Chéhensse, V., Beldjord, C., Schwartz, C., Utermann, G. and Julien, C. (1993). Somatic mosaicism for partial paternal isodisomy in Wiedemann-Beckwith syndrome: a post-fertilization event. *Eur J Hum Genet*, **1**, 19–29.

Hersh, J. H., Yen, F. F., Peiper, S. C., Barch, M. J., Yacoub, O. A., Voss, D. H. and Roberts, J. L. (1995). De novo 1;10 balanced translocation in an infant with thanatophoric dysplasia: a clue to the locus of the candidate gene. *J Med Genet*, **32**, 293–295.

Hibbard, J. U., Loy, G. L. and Hibbard, M. C. (1994). Does chorionic villus sampling compromise fetal umbilical blood flow? *Prenat Diagn*, **14**, 1107–1112.

Hirsch, B. and Baldinger, S. (1993). Pericentric inversion of chromosome 4 giving rise to dup(4p) and dup(4q) recombinants within a single kindred. *Am J Med Genet*, **45**, 5–8.

Hirst, M., Grewal, P., Flannery, A., Slatter, R., Maher, E., Barton, D., Fryns, J.-P. and Davies, K. (1995). Two new cases of FMR1 deletion associated with mental impairment. *Am J Hum Genet*, **56**, 67–74.

Hirst, M. C., Barnicoat, A., Flynn, G., Wang, Q., Daker, M., Buckle, V. J., Davies, K. E. and Bobrow, M. (1993). The identification of a third fragile site FRAXF in Xq27-28 distal to both FRAXA and FRAXE. *Hum Mol Genet*, **2**, 197–200.

Hockey, K. A., Mulcahy, M. T., Montgomery, P. and Levitt, S. (1989). Deletion of chromosome 5q and familial adenomatous polyposis. *J Med Genet*, **26**, 61–68.

Hodge, S. E. (1989). Waiting for the amniocentesis. *N Engl J Med*, **320**, 63–64.

DAY SIX
SATURDAY, SEPTEMBER 15

TOPTICAL IPO LOOMS

By Lawrence F. Gooden
September 15

Next Wednesday, we'll experience the latest big IPO when San Francisco–based Toptical goes public. It is the hottest social networking company going and once again "experts" claim it will be the biggest in history. Millions of users are clearly standing in line to buy a piece of the site they use every day and have come to love. Investors, we're told, are salivating at the opportunity to get on board. Everyone's hoping to make out, but will they?

Consider first the state of social networking. With the possible exception of pornography, nothing has so taken the Internet by storm as have the various manifestations of such sites. Still, the decline for social networking companies appears to take place just when they go public. Facebook began experiencing bumps at that point as have others. There are many reasons for this, not the least of which is the heightened level of SEC scrutiny and the need to maintain stock value.

But there's another reason as well. Often these companies have run out of creative momentum just at that time. Their initial concepts have already seized the public's interest, but their shelf life fades rapidly after two or three years. Competitors come along focusing on key aspects more effectively and many users turn social networking sites into marketing vehicles. In fact, marketing through social media is turning the public off in general, as is the insatiable collection of personal data, which these companies then put to their own use. Privacy concerns are increasingly raising their ugly head.

Toptical CEO and cofounder Brian Cameron says his company is different. "We respect the privacy rights of our users," he said in a recent interview. Asked what guarantees the company was prepared to give he demurred. Toptical has yet to release the steps it takes to secure the private information of users.

There are more issues on the line next week. Toptical is just the latest social networking enterprise seeking to make its founders and initial investors mega rich. It's slicker than others, gives the appearance of greater control to users, and is ideally suited for business use, but in the end, it works because it asks you to tell it everything about you. The more forthcoming you are, the more effectively

Toptical works for you. And that's the rub. How long will users continue laying out the intimate details of their lives to a company's mainframes? They might call it the cloud but it is, in fact, just someone else's computer.

There are as well areas of concern surrounding next Wednesday's IPO, not the least of which is the new software the NYSE is going to employ. There are reports that two test runs encountered serious problems that have as yet to be resolved. Officially, all is well, but knowledgeable sources say that is not the case, in fact. The problem is that the NYSE has committed to its new program and can't back down now without admitting a mistake. Management, it seems, would rather take a chance instead.

Also in the mix is the initial asking price and the volume of stock being sold. There are experts who say the price is too high and that far too much stock is being offered. The result could be an almost immediate collapse in share value. No one will like that except the jackals who sell it short.

We'll know soon enough whether Toptical will be the next highly successful social networking company to go public, be a victim of IPO software gone amiss, or will be a financial debacle for those who climb on board.

32

You awake again?" Frank asked.

Jeff rolled onto his back, opened, then closed his mouth, feeling how dry it was. "Yes."

"Feeling any better?"

Jeff paused before answering. "A little. My head doesn't throb anymore, but I've sure got a headache."

"That's good, actually. Any double vision?"

"No, not since yesterday."

"I guess I can admit now I was a bit uneasy about taking you out of the hospital before the doc examined you. The MRI and X-ray looked good but there's nothing like an experienced doc seeing you eye to eye. But it seems like you're good to go. That's a relief. There's water beside you."

Jeff reached over, found an unopened bottle, twisted off the cap, finding his grip surprisingly weak, and drank it in a single pull. "That's good."

"You hungry?"

"I am. Very. But I feel really dirty. I need a shower."

"Even better. I've ordered pizza. It'll be here in a few minutes. You have time for a briefing and maybe a shower."

Jeff straightened up in the bed, moving the pillow so he could lean against it more comfortably. "So what have you learned?"

"Quite a bit," he said. "It turns out you're rich, to the tune of just over three million dollars. You've been a very naughty boy, and very greedy."

"What are you talking about?"

"When you were inside the Exchange's engines, you used some of your tools to plant a nasty piece of code that's been skimming trades. You've got a brokerage account in your name, opened after we started this job, and you funnel your ill-gotten gains directly to it."

"Brokerage account? I don't have a brokerage account."

"You do now."

Jeff's heart jumped. "How hard was this to find?"

"Not so hard. You've not only been naughty and greedy, you've been careless. Not like you at all. Your malware trades at a consistent rate. It makes no attempt to blend in with traffic so it was bound to attract attention. And, of course, you send the money directly into your account so it's easy to make the connection to you; almost like you put a flag on it. Then there's the really interesting part. This malware resembles the code you've been reverse engineering. I think that gives us a pretty good idea of what this case is really all about."

"Whoever did this used my tools?"

"Right. Some of those you distribute at conferences, none of the proprietary ones that have made you the success you are today." Frank grinned.

"So anyone could have planted it."

"In theory, yes, but think about it. Whoever did this has access to the system. Maybe they hacked it like we did or . . ." Frank's voice trailed away.

"They work there and already have access."

"I hate to think someone's been as clever as us and figured out how to hack into the New York Stock Exchange, but ego aside I must admit someone could. That said, it's unlikely. I'm persuaded that whoever is doing this has help on the inside. It's clear now that we stumbled on an ongoing operation. They needed to point the guilty finger at you before we figured out what they were up to, which suggests to my devious mind that it's an inside job."

"That sounds pretty shortsighted and desperate."

Frank swiveled all the way round in his chair. "I've been thinking about this. What it really says is they want to buy some time."

"How's that?"

"While our federal friends can be made to move quickly, as they did in this case, there is the risk that once they hear our side of the story they'll come to the same conclusion I have. Then they'll go after the real culprits."

"If they can find them."

"There's always that. But it would take us a few days, more likely a few weeks, to convince the SEC we're clean. I'm pretty sure that's their window."

"What window?"

"Well, they're going to try to erase all their tracks—that's a given—but why not take some more while they can, right? Makes sense. They'll have to close down soon, so make hay while the sun shines. This little scheme of theirs bought them some time."

"I guess we were close."

"I'd say so. I made some phone calls while you were out. This Alshon guy is every bit as tenacious as I was told he was. And he's not going to let go of us. He used to be FBI, we used to be Company. No love lost there. However, he's got an assistant named Susan Flores. She does the forensic work and is reputedly very good, and very fair. If she gets on this, how you were set up could become obvious."

"You really think so?"

"In time, yes, assuming she doesn't have ten other cases, assuming Alshon lets her and listens to her. But the longer you are the prime suspect, the less likely he is to admit he was ever wrong."

"Based on what you say, I can't believe I'm a suspect now. This is all pretty heavy-handed. Don't they realize I'd be smarter than that if I was crooked?"

"No. Crooks usually aren't that clever. They're driven by greed. Alshon will just figure you got in there, saw all that easy money, and couldn't resist."

"But using a brokerage account in my own name, come on, how dumb is that?"

"He'd reason you planned to erase your tracks, so why not? It was only for a few weeks. The risk was low."

Jeff eased back, his thoughts racing. "Frank, you don't have to do this. I'm the one they've set up. Just go in and tell them what's going on."

Frank smiled. "Don't be naïve. They're after both of us. They don't figure you did this alone. Anyway, I've got more. A fugitive warrant's being processed for our arrest. We'll be wanted men later today probably, definitely by Monday."

"That's just wonderful."

"Maybe there'll be wanted posters and we can pin them on the office wall later, when we have a laugh about all this."

"You have a sick sense of humor."

"So my wife says. I called an SEC defense attorney. I got a referral, so he gave me a phone consultation. He says Alshon's an SOB, and he'll already have hung a target around our necks." Just then, there was a knock on the door. "That'll be the pizza. Why don't you take a shower, then join me after?"

In the bathroom Jeff removed the bandages from his head, his thoughts afire at what he'd just learned. He undressed, then stepped into the bathtub and showered, taking special care with his scalp. Under the hot water he probed lightly. There was a tender spot toward the rear, a large goose egg that was very, very sensitive. His entire side ached and rubbing it did no good. His left forearm really hurt. When he peeled the wet bandages from it, it was skinned pretty badly. It hurt so much, he didn't want to use it. So don't use it for a while, he told himself.

After the shower, Jeff took several Advil, toweled off, confirmed the delivery man was gone, then dressed in fresh clothes. When he finished, he felt like a new man, an aching new man, but new nonetheless.

"So what did the lawyer say?" Jeff asked as he sat down, hefted a piece of warm pizza, and took his first bite.

"He said if we turn ourselves in, we'll get out on bond. The case will take about two years, not counting appeals."

"What? But we're innocent!"

"That's what they all say. He says the longer we wait to turn ourselves in, the tougher it will be to get out on bond, and the tougher the U.S. Attorney will be in dealing with us. Apparently they prefer criminals who make their job easy for them."

"I don't have a brokerage account. Someone else set that up."

"I know. But you'll have to show that and how do you prove a negative? The same goes for the malware. There's no proof you planted it, but there's no proof you didn't. It uses your code and you get the dirty money. Maybe you can get them to see reason, but it will take a long time."

"Jeez."

"The retainer is fifty thousand dollars. He estimates the defense would cost over two hundred dollars."

"Jeez." Jeff put down the pizza. "I'm not hungry anymore."

"I have the fifty thousand and about half of the rest. It would wipe out my savings though."

"How about a price break for two?"

Frank paused, then said, "He says he'll represent me only. You need to get your own lawyer." Jeff wrinkled his forehead. "It's so the feds can turn me, Jeff. Come on, you watch television. When the going gets tough, my lawyer will want me to flip on you. He's already thinking it. I could pick it up over the phone."

"Jeeze." Jeff rubbed his forehead. The headache was getting worse again.

"So here's what I say. Let's finish the pizza, then get cracking. Let's figure out what this hidden code does and see if the guys framing us have been careful. Maybe we can figure out who the inside guy is. At the least we'll know more and that can't hurt when the time comes to tell our story."

"That doesn't sound like much."

"It's better than nothing." Frank picked up a slice. "Anyway, we've got help coming." He grinned.

33

Sonia Lopes de Almeida disconnected her cell phone and grimaced. Her father. She was nearly twenty years old, and he still treated her like a child.

She glanced across the room. Victor was busy at his desk. She wondered what he did so diligently. He'd made it, he was rich, why work so hard? Once, when she'd told him as much, he'd only laughed. "Getting it," he'd said, "is the easy part. It's keeping it that's hard."

Keeping what? she'd thought. Just who was Victor Bandeira? Oh, she'd heard the stories—everyone had. Drugs, cartels, crooked businesses. You heard it all the time. The politicians were crooked, the businesses were crooked, the cops were on the take, it was the same everywhere. Who was she to draw some line? And how much of it was really true?

Once, just once, after he emerged from his helicopter, the wind had caught Bandeira's jacket and she'd seen the butt of a pistol at his waist. She'd never known a citizen to carry a gun before, and it caught her by surprise. Perhaps the stories were true. Why else would he carry a gun, especially since he was always surrounded by so much security?

She'd never told her father that she was seeing Victor Bandeira. The men were in business so normally she would have felt obligated to let him know but somehow, whenever she thought she might say something, she always hesitated.

Sonia lay back on the couch, lifted her magazine but watched him as she had in the past. He was a handsome man, a bit heavyset, but then, that always seemed to go with money and power. He could be generous with her, but she'd seen him be petty and parsimonious as well. There was, she'd observed, a slight cruelty in the occasional set of his mouth. Was it real? Or an act? They'd been together such a short time she still hadn't figured him out.

She had boyfriend, a real one. She'd never told Victor. At first, it didn't matter, but now he was turning her into his mistress. He hadn't discussed it with her. He just assumed that was their relationship. Still, there was no agreement between them, and she knew he'd been with other women since they were together. She even knew one of them. It wasn't as if she loved Victor. And Bruno was nothing like him. Slender, elegant in manner, quiet, soft spoken. But he could never give her what she really wanted. Only Victor could do that.

Her mother knew about her and Victor, and approved. "We are not as rich as you think, Sonia," she said. "It's time you knew. Our family has lost steadily since before you were born. If we hadn't, your father would never have allowed the bank to fall into Victor's hands. For now, it is important they do business together. Carlos doesn't like Victor, and Victor knows that. If you are—" She'd hesitated. "—if you are his lover, then he will not do anything against your father."

"You want me to be a prostitute?" Sonia retorted.

"Don't be silly. That's not what I said at all. You did this on your own. If you'd said something to me earlier, I'd have told you to stay away from him. You should have known better. But you're already there, aren't you? I'm telling you there is a lot at stake here so be careful. It's time you grew up, time you learned what a woman can do, and stopped being a spoiled child." She'd seized Sonia by the shoulders. "It's time you repaid your father for all he's done for you, for his years of sacrifice."

Sonia sighed. Victor had been fun at first, exciting since their affair was secret and forbidden. She'd even enjoyed cheating on Bruno, but she was growing weary of it. All she wanted, all she'd ever wanted, was to be Miss Brazil. Was that so much to ask for? Everything was corrupt, even the beauty pageant. She'd checked. Only the mistresses of the powerful ever won. When Victor first turned his attention to her, she'd seen her chance. She had a few years. If he wouldn't make it happen, then someone else would.

Sonia turned her attention to the magazine she'd been reading all morning. There was the current Miss Brazil, taking up half the pages. That's why she'd bought it. Sonia had seen her up close. She wasn't so much. Sonia knew she had a much better body.

"What are you staring at?" Bandeira asked.

"You," she said, quickly looking at him over the magazine. "I was wondering when you would stop working. I'm very lonely." She pouted.

Bandeira laughed, pushed himself away from the desk, stood up, and walked toward her. "What is it you want?"

Sonia turned the magazine toward him. "You know."

He laughed and sat down on the couch. "Miss Brazil? Is that it?"

She sat up, excited. "Think about it, Victor. Your lover would be Miss Brazil, the most beautiful woman in the country. Maybe, maybe even Miss World. Every man would envy you."

"They already do." He eyed her steadily. "I don't think you know what is involved to make this happen."

Sonia beamed as she sat up. "You checked? You found out?"

He nodded. "I made a few calls. There are many men, rich men with power, who would be doing the same thing for their woman. It can be very expensive and the outcome is not always guaranteed after you've spent all that money."

"But you have lots of money."

"Oh yes. And I'll have more if I didn't waste it on foolish chases like Miss Brazil."

"But . . ."

"My child, it would cost a great deal of money." Bandeira took her wrist, pulled her to her feet, then led her to the bedroom.

Though she knew she should be passionate, do the things he liked, she couldn't help being put off, a bit cold. Sometimes men were so taken with their own pleasure it didn't matter, but Victor wasn't like that. He was always attune to her. She didn't care. Her mother might want her to sleep with this man for the sake of the family, but she did it for her own reasons. When he rolled off her, he scowled and made a dismissive grunt. After his shower, she was still in a foul mood.

Bandeira made no attempt to cheer her up as he often did when she was down. He glanced at her from time to time, obviously enjoying the sight of her naked, as he took a call. She knew then he'd taken that little pill to boost him a bit. He'd want to do it again in an hour or so. He was so predictable.

"Tell me about yourself," she asked. "Are you who they say you are?"

He looked up from his phone. "Who do they say I am?"

"You know."

He made a face and lowered the phone. "People say all kinds of things. What have you heard?"

"That you are a *chefe*. The *chefe* of NL." Sonia was stunned at her audacity. She'd never even allowed herself to think the letters NL before now.

Bandeira smiled, and she saw a flash of the cruelty that always lurked in his face. "Why do you want to know?" She shrugged and pouted a little. "You are a child sometimes, Sonia. Men do not speak of such things."

She rolled off the bed and went into the bathroom. She spent a long time in the shower, not wanting to go back to the bedroom, not wanting him to mount her again. This time he might insist on her doing what he wanted. She hated that, hated being forced. If she was in the mood or been promised something nice, she was willing. But he was saying the opposite, that he'd do nothing to help her. She had to find another rich man, one easier to control. Her thoughts ticked off the possibilities. Finally, with no choice she climbed out of the shower, toweled herself slowly, then returned to the bedroom, sitting on a chair across from the bed.

Bandeira looked up at her. "So you want to know the kind of man I am. Suddenly that is important to you." He stood and walked toward her, naked. Sitting down like this, looking up at him, she realized he was twice her size.

"I just want to be Miss Brazil," she said, quietly realizing how badly she'd played her part.

"You will never be that, my dear. Never." Without warning he struck her on the side of her face with his open hand, the blow catching her by surprise, knocking her onto the floor. "Perhaps it could have been," he said, continuing. "I made the calls, laid out what was required. I was considering it to please you, and because it would have pleased me." He reached down and seized her bare feet, then pulled her toward the bed. "But then I learned about your little plaything. What did they call him? Bruno? Yes, Bruno, that is it."

Bandeira lifted her from the floor and tossed her bouncing onto the bed. She let out a cry, her hands clutched against the side of her face. "I have a video. Do you want to see it?"

Bandeira picked up the remote and punched a button. An enormous flat screen descended from the ceiling. Sometimes they watched pornography on it. There was a bright flash; then it came alive. She could see her boyfriend, Bruno. He was naked, his arms tied above his head. He'd been beaten.

"In the end," Bandeira said, "he wasn't so much a man." He looked at her, gauging her reaction. "You were cold to me earlier. Now you will be warm.

You will not say no, will you? All you have to do is watch the little show and see what is in store for my favorite *puta*. You will work hard, won't you?"

Bandeira turned her so she could see the screen more clearly. "Now," he said as he lowered himself to her, "now you will see who I really am." It was then that Bruno began to scream.

34

Daryl sat in the hotel lobby and watched for Frank. There was the usual foot traffic in and out. She could see the doorman, dressed like a college drum major, opening doors, putting guests into taxis, touching his cap to acknowledge a tip.

Since receiving Frank's telephone call, she'd been in a state of frenzy. It had taken no time to make her decision. She sent Clive an e-mail telling him she would be out of the office and city a few days on emergency personal business. Unable to catch the red-eye she'd booked an early-morning flight. She spent a restless night in her own bed, then packed and flew to New York. Once she'd settled into her room she'd called Frank to arrange a meeting.

So what was she really doing here? she asked herself as she waited. She'd already decided to help but wondered now if this wasn't really about trying to reconnect with Jeff. She wasn't married to the man, hadn't seen him or spoken to him in a year. What was he to her that she'd drop everything and fly across the country?

Frank and his wife, however, were college friends. Over the last few years, Frank had helped her more than once, at considerable career risk to himself. There was no question of her helping him. That's what she told herself as a man dropped onto the seat beside her. She ignored him, looked at her watch, then looked back toward the entrance. But part of her understood she was primarily here to help Jeff. He needed her.

"I took this class once," Frank said quietly. Daryl looked to her left in amazement. "The instructor said all this Hollywood stuff with false mustaches and makeup was a bunch of crap and useless in the field. He said there were simpler and more effective ways to disguise yourself. You're looking good, Daryl."

"I didn't recognize you." She stared at Frank again unable to put her finger on the transformation. Never an especially sharp dresser, he looked a bit shabby today, even though the clothes were typical for him. The man who'd sat beside her was older too, perhaps a bit sick.

"You weren't supposed to."

"You're fatter."

"Not really. Just some cotton between my cheek and gums. It gives me a sad sack look."

"There's more though."

"Not so much, mostly just my demeanor, my walk and stance, the way I look at things, interact with the world around me. I'm in loser mode right now. Like it?"

"Not especially, but it definitely worked."

"I picked up the jacket at a used clothing store, same with the shoes."

"You'll be standing outside asking for quarters later today."

"Hey, I'm just a bit down on my luck. All I need is a break to get on my feet." He paused, then said, "Thanks for coming."

"You've done the same for me." Daryl hesitated, then said, "How's Jeff?"

"He's good this morning. Hard at work on his laptop, trying to find a way to dig us out of this hole. He'll be all right, but it was close. Daryl, these are dangerous people. You're on-site now, so promise me you'll take this seriously and be careful."

"I promise."

"And you didn't have to fly across the country. I told you that. We're looking for hacker help with this."

"Better face-to-face. You know that. Now, tell me what's going on."

Frank filled her in, catching her up on what he'd learned that morning. She listened with growing disbelief at the audacity of it.

"This is no way to reward an American hero!" she snapped. "You of all people know what Jeff's done for this country, the risks he's taken. He's never asked for anything, not even a dime of the money he's spent chasing down terrorists. He's been shot, threatened, God knows what else."

"I couldn't agree more. But I don't think the people involved here know any of this. That was all so hush-hush."

Daryl composed herself before continuing. "So you've been set up."

"Right."

"Someone inside the Exchange or outside?"

"We think both. We're hoping you can help us pin that down. We need to point this Alshon guy at the right party to bring an end to this—and the sooner, the better. If we can identify someone working right here at the Exchange, that would be great."

"That will be the same somebody who's hacked the system."

"Absolutely."

Daryl thought about that for a bit. "How good a job did they do on you two?"

"Good enough to get the SEC in gear but frankly I think it's a bit over the top. In theory at least any fair-minded investigator should be willing to hear us out and realize we've been set up."

"But you don't want to take that chance?"

"Officially, we don't even know there's an SEC investigation, unless you count searching Jeff's place as a form of notice. Still, my source says warrants are coming out by Monday."

"That seems awfully fast for this type of crime. Is this connected to that bot Wall Street is upset about?"

Frank told her how they'd come to get the engagement. "The bot the *New York Times* is all upset about is harmless. Their source is exaggerating. Probably a disgruntled former employee."

"The market's reeling from the news."

Frank laughed. "If what we've found ever gets out, there will be a crash like no other in history. No one will have any faith in the stock market, no matter what they say about how secure it is."

"I guess we shouldn't be surprised after all we've seen elsewhere. So many institutions have gone out of business. Assets people thought were secure, like the value in their homes, vanished. Why should the New York Stock Exchange computers be immune?"

"I've made some calls," Frank continued. "Fortunately, I still have people I can trust on the inside. Alshon's pursuing this as an act of terrorism under the Patriot Act. That gives them a lot of authority."

Daryl grimaced. She hated to see laws meant for one purpose abused this way. She'd had this fight repeatedly within the National Security Agency. "Getting back to the hackers, being heavy-handed suggests they're only looking to get you two out of the way for a while."

"We agree but don't know where that takes us. The obvious conclusion is that they're just buying time to cover their tracks, maybe finish any looting they've got under way."

"All right, what do you want from me?"

"Like I told you over the telephone, we can use help in figuring out what exactly they are up to, but especially in backtracking to them. We have to hope they've left a clue somewhere. If they are inside the Exchange, that narrows the field of suspects considerably. If they are outsiders, that would tend to get us off the hook." He paused, then continued, "Since you're here, it occurs to me that it's useful to have a fresh face on the scene. You can go places we can't. We need to stay out of sight."

"Where are you two staying?"

"It's better if you don't know."

Daryl nodded. "Okay. I can see that." Neither spoke for a long minute. "Does he know you asked for me?"

"Yes, I told him."

"And?"

"He appreciates your help."

She looked Frank in the eye. "And?" she repeated.

"No 'and.' He appreciates your help. He knows how good you are."

"Okay, then. Tell him . . . tell him I'll do everything I can."

Frank touched her forearm. "He knows that."

Daryl blinked as she fought back tears.

35

ENFORCEMENT DIVISION
SECURITIES AND EXCHANGE COMMISSION
NEW YORK REGIONAL OFFICE
200 VESSEY STREET
NEW YORK CITY
2:51 P.M.

It was Saturday, but during a big case, weekends meant little in Robert Alshon's office. He had checked in with Flores and her team just after lunch. They were hard at the forensic examination of the computers seized from Red Zoya in D.C. When he'd caught her eye, she'd shrugged and shook her head.

He returned to his office. Maybe this guy was more clever than most, he thought. And he kept his dirt out of his office. If that was the case, Aiken would have a laptop with him from which he'd done everything. Alshon alerted his people and any federal officer who might arrest Aiken to acquire every computing device within reach.

Gene Livingston rapped lightly on his open office door. He was an understated man, both in size and demeanor, but Alshon had come to rely on him to perform the essential legwork outside Flores's province. He waved the man in and gestured at the chair.

"What do you have?" he asked pointedly.

"Just preliminaries at this point, boss, but there's some firm data here." Livingston lifted a legal tablet in front of him slightly. Approaching fifty years of age, with little hair remaining and out of date glasses, Livingston looked every bit the bookworm his job description made him out to be. He'd never married and had rented the same one-bedroom apartment for over twenty years. He brought his lunch to work and ate at his desk. Alshon once commented to a colleague that he wished he had ten more like him.

"I can find no connection between William Stenton and Jeffrey Aiken or Aiken's company. I've checked Stenton's finances, and there has been no significant movement in two years, nothing at all in the last three months. All indications are they'd never met before Stenton hired him and Frank Renkin. I've requested a digital and telephone screen and expect results back Monday or Tuesday, but I think we can expect it will confirm my preliminary analysis."

"I plan to meet with Stenton on Monday. I have a number of questions, and it will be better if I don't have to tell him he's a target. So do what you can to speed that along. What else?"

"Red Zoya is clean. Aiken owns it without partners. It pays its taxes, its corporation filings are up-to-date. It has a good credit rating. Basically, it's just an extension of Aiken for tax and liability purposes."

"And what about the man?"

Livingston smiled. "This is where it gets really interesting. He's a Ph.D., taught at Carnegie Mellon. You mentioned he once worked for the CIA." He looked up and Alshon nodded. "He was head of the Counter Cyberterrorism Unit, a four-man team in existence before 9/11. I can't find anything official but as I understand it he claimed to have uncovered the attack before it happened and later said no one listened."

"I've heard that story a few times."

"Anyway, he left after that and started his own company. It's got a good reputation, and he does too." He looked down. "There's more, but nothing official." Alshon raised his eyebrows. "Aiken also reportedly discovered a cyberterrorist attack against the West a few years ago. He flew to Moscow and Paris, engaged in a firefight, killed the brothers responsible."

Alshon looked at Livingston in disbelief. "Are you certain?"

"I am that it happened. It's pretty common knowledge in some circles. I just don't know the details. Two years ago, he's the one that found that virus that changes documents in a computer. He was involved in some incident in Turkey in which a plane crashed."

"Gene, this sounds like fantasy land."

"I understand your skepticism. I'll see if I can't nail down some facts."

"What about his finances?"

"He's done well, but he's not much of an investor. Basically, his money piles up in a savings account. Every few months, he transfers some into an indexed Schwab account. The rest he rolls into CDs. Of course, there's the recent activity. I'll get to that later."

"Not very imaginative."

"I guess not. He did pay off his town house in Georgetown last year. In general he works a lot and doesn't do much else."

"What about Renkin?"

"Renkin is former CIA as well. He left some months ago to go to work for Aiken. He was Deputy Director of Counter Cyber Research at the time. His finances are even more boring than Aiken's. Still has a mortgage, married, three children. Nothing stands out and no recent action."

Alshon grimaced. "You say there's nothing?" Livingston shook his head. "These guys are too clean. That's always a red flag. They're hiding something. What about recent weeks, since they came to New York?"

"Nothing on Renkin." Livingston consulted his tablet. "Aiken opened a brokerage account, and it's received just over three million dollars in the last few days."

"That's more like it." Livingston was pursing his lips. "What?"

"It doesn't smell right. He set the thing up in his own name. No attempt to hide anything. Then he's transferred market money straight into the account. It's almost like there's a spotlight on it."

"What was he supposed to do?"

"I don't know, something. Set up an LLC in Nevada and use it. That would have slowed a search down a couple of days to get back to him. Use any name but his own. Go offshore. Something. It's almost like he wanted to get caught."

Alshon swiveled in his chair and gazed out his window. "These are both Company men, Gene," he said after a bit. "They've been schooled in the craft. They think it through. My guess is he expected to erase his trail before anyone caught on to him. What we're seeing is a bitter man whose career was going nowhere, who has the chance of a lifetime to get back at everyone and set himself up for life. He figured he'd get away with it and laugh all the way to the bank. These guys like Aiken and Renkin, they think they're above the law." He turned back to his desk. "Keep digging. My guess is there's more."

"I do have more. Aiken was struck by a car Thursday night. He was hospitalized."

"What happened?"

"He was jogging near the reservoir and was attacked. He ran into a busy street to escape and was hit by a car. He was nearly killed."

"What do the police think?"

"They think a homeless guy went berserk."

"Nothing more?"

"Just that Aiken left the hospital without being released."

"I'd expect that. He's on the run now. All right, see what else you can find and keep digging. Send Susan in, please."

Flores arrived a few minutes later, looking very tired as she took a seat.

"What have you got?" Alshon asked.

"Not a thing. Zip. Nada."

"Details."

"It's all encrypted. I'd need the NSA to break it, and even then, it would take weeks, assuming it can be done."

Alshon thought about that, then asked, "How about his finances?" He often had Flores and Livingston cover the same ground just to be sure. They were aware of it and worked that much harder.

"That was actually pretty easy. Nothing out of the ordinary, just a Schwab account and some CDs. He pays his bills on time, owns his house." She looked up and in a rare moment of humor said, "In most regards he's a good catch."

Alshon snorted. "You'll be visiting him in prison."

"Not for me. For some women."

"Tell me what you found on the Exchange."

"It didn't take long to locate the tools Aiken used or his malware. He was employing it stupidly, though. Instead of blending in with traffic, he had it programmed to just keep working around the clock. The automated security scans would have picked it up but the way the malware was set up made getting caught even more certain. It was pretty carelessly done. And it leads straight to his brokerage account."

"So just as IT told us?"

"Pretty much." She tapped her teeth with her pen. "There's a rootkit in there. He'd been paying a lot of attention to it."

"Rootkit? That's some kind of cloaking device, right?"

"Right, it conceals a file's presence in a computer. He'd been working on this one."

"Maybe it's his."

"No. He's investigating it."

"What did you find out about it?"

"Nothing except that it's pretty sophisticated."

"It was just part of his job; good to go through the motions."

"I suppose, but a rootkit's got no business in the heart of the New York Stock Exchange's trading platform."

Just then, the telephone rang. "Yes?" Alshon listened intently, then hung up. "Take another look at his office data just to confirm we can't access it, then get back on the Exchange and see what else you can learn. Maybe he's one of those people who kept things separated, but not many do. Encrypting the files can only have one explanation."

"Maybe he works for sensitive clients and wants to protect his work product. That will be the explanation."

Alshon snorted. "He's hiding something. We need to find out what that is. I'm off to search his office over at the Exchange. The team will have more computers for you."

"Okay."

"With a great deal of luck they'll show up. I've got two arrest warrants." As he grabbed his jacket he gave her a very unpleasant grin.

36

Frank let himself into the small hotel room quietly, not sure if Jeff was sleeping. Instead, he found Jeff hunched over his laptop at the room's desk, deep in thought. Frank set his paper sack down and sat in the room's only chair.

"Any luck?" he asked.

"I've made some progress I think. What's in the bag?"

"Bourbon. I couldn't remember if you were a Scotch man or not, but I drink Bourbon so you can either share or get your own."

"Bourbon's fine."

Frank retrieved two glasses from the bathroom, unwrapped them from their plastic cover, then filled them halfway with amber liquid. "Here you go." They both took a sip. "So what have you got?"

"I think I've locked in what the malware does. It's pretty sophisticated. You're the expert on Wall Street, since unlike me, you've actually read a book so maybe it will make more sense to you. It looks like a trading algorithm programmed to hunt down certain traders and specific situations. When it finds them with a transaction matching the algo's parameters taking place, it rides it in, bypasses the Exchange's safeguards, and inserts itself at the head of the trading queue. It's a high-frequency trader that can always beat everyone to the front of the line."

"Like cutting in at the movies huh."

"Exactly. Only in this case, there are only so many tickets available at a preferred price. The algos suck that up. In effect, they drive up the price by taking the ready action, then dump, and repeat. They've held some of these trades hostage in the Exchange's computers for minutes while they pump and dump."

"How much?"

"Well, in terms of percentages, it's taking up to five percent of a trade, though usually less. Depending on the size it's a lot of money. I have found instances where it appears to have taken substantially more. I haven't figured out why those are treated differently."

"And the Exchange's IT department doesn't know about it?"

"Not from what I can see. They've done nothing to stop it."

"So the code is undetected and in operation."

"Yes, and hidden within the rootkit."

"That suggests to me someone with intimate knowledge of the Exchange's code." Jeff nodded agreement. Frank took a sip, then lowered his glass. "When did it start?"

"There's no way to tell so far. A few months, a year, perhaps more."

"Even if it's just a few months, that's a long time to operate in the heart of the New York Stock Exchange without being spotted."

"It is."

"Is it really that clever or are they just not very good at what they do?"

"It's clever, obviously. As for the rest . . . complacent is likely the word for it." He paused. "It's possible whoever is responsible for the type of security that would usually detect the malware is in on the action."

"Any clues?"

"No. Just something we should keep in mind."

"Any luck finding who planted it?"

"No, I've been working to figure it out. The code we've got in the engine has detected and copied the code out of our cloud server so whoever is doing this is active. We should be able to follow the files back to where they entered the Exchange and once we have a physical location we can get names."

"The other approach, I take it is—"

"—follow the money," the men said in unison.

"That will take a lot of time," Frank said. "Weeks, at the least."

"Yeah, and finding an end deposit is getting tougher every year. Do we have that much time?"

Frank shook his head. "In theory we do but like I've said already, the longer we're in the crosshairs, the harder it's going to be to get out. And this Alshon's going to think any perp we come up with is a fall guy. That's especially true since we'll be relying on computer records and trails. They can be made to point most anywhere."

Jeff nodded. "What we need is to catch one of the bad guys in the know and get him to talk."

"Good luck with that." Frank set his cup down and refilled it, gesturing to Jeff who held out his own. As he poured, Frank said, "Still, not bad for a guy who was just whacked on the head. We've got help in town now too."

Jeff took another sip. "How is she?"

"Daryl looks fantastic, what'd you expect? I can't believe you let her get away."

"I told you about it."

"You told me but you didn't convince me. She's here, Jeff. When you've got some time for your personal life, you should give that serious thought. If she didn't care, she wouldn't have flown across the country."

Jeff had already thought about that. "Does she believe us?"

Frank laughed. "What? You're having doubts? Of course she believes us. In fact, she's pretty pissed off. She's staying in midtown. I gave her access to the backdoors, and she's likely hard at work by now, trying to trace these guys."

"That's going to be the hardest part."

"Yep, they will stay as far from it as they can. Even if it turns out they're on the inside like we think, they'll have routed their work in such a way as to not point at them. As for the money, you can bet it's scattered far and wide. Maybe Daryl should work tracing the dough while you and I work on tracing its operation and finding a perp."

"Sounds good."

Frank opened his laptop and sent Daryl a message. "Want me to say anything from you?"

"Just thank her for helping."

"Okay, lover boy. That should melt her heart."

Jeff turned back to his computer but found he could no longer concentrate. He finished the bourbon, then poured more. Daryl. He was surprised to learn that she'd flown here, mildly irritated at the thought he might see her again. But when the reality set in, not just of his precarious situation, but that she'd cared enough to come, he found he was looking forward to seeing her.

The more he thought about their breakup, his reasons for it, the shallower they seemed. He wondered if the real problem had been that she wasn't conforming to what he wanted. She'd stayed the person he'd always known. If he really wanted a lasting relationship with her, he should have waited. Maybe he just had been looking for a reason to end it, to find one more reason to crawl back into his emotional shell. Because once she left, that's exactly what he did.

37

MACATUBA
SÃO PAULO, BRAZIL
4:41 P.M.

Victor Bandeira settled into his patio chair and laid the Cuban Robusto onto its slot on the ashtray. He took a sip of strong black coffee and looked across the expanse of his estate toward the virgin cluster of trees from which the stream emerged. The afternoon sun caught the clear water precisely and the effect was as if diamonds danced on the surface.

Sonia was still in the bedroom. When he'd finished with her, she lay there unmoving, softly weeping as he took his shower, humming to himself. Once his energy was recovered, he was considering having another go at her.

He'd found the entire experience depressing, though. She was such a child, and it had all been so easy. He'd known from the first time she'd been with another man, and now had made it clear to her that she was his and his alone. Women thought they were so clever about such things, but he'd always found it to be the opposite. He was sensitive to any change in their attentiveness or heightened passion, as both were signs. Women thought such compensation masked their infidelity, when in fact it only confirmed it.

Still, depressing as it had been, overall, the first moments of surprise and possession had been exhilarating. Unfortunately, he'd not be able to duplicate the experience—at least he could think of no way now. He had to be careful. If he crushed all life from her, he'd have a woman who was little better than a whore in his bed. He'd had enough of that when he was a young man.

Bandeira wondered if she'd tell her father. If she did, that could prove awkward. Carlos was at heart a weak man so there was that. But more significantly he was a man who needed Bandeira desperately. He'd managed the family bank too conservatively for too long and reduced it to a near state of bankruptcy. If Bandeira hadn't come along when he did, there'd be no more Banco do Novo Brasil. Perhaps it didn't matter if he knew. It would be amusing to see how he responded.

Bandeira sighed and picked up his cigar, suddenly angry with himself. When would he be man enough to give up such games? This was all nonsense. It was nonsense to let himself get distracted by that *puta* on his bed, nonsense to have bedded the daughter of a man important to his business, nonsense to have taken his pleasure with her as he had earlier. He mocked his predecessor, the *chefe* before him, both in his thoughts and in comments to his bosses, but he was no less indiscreet himself. These were all needless risks, and in the end, there was absolutely no way to predict the behavior of an outraged Brazilian father, especially one who had been made to look small at more than one board meeting.

Just then, Jorge César approached. Bandeira gestured for his head of security to come near, then left him standing as was his custom with underlings. "Jorge," Bandeira said, "we have a problem in New York. Two Americans have been making trouble for our financial enterprise. You know of this?"

"*Sim, Chefe. Casas de Férias.*"

"One of our men in New York took it on himself to attack the leader of these two and put him into a hospital. I did not want this as it might call attention to what we are doing, but he did it anyway."

"Should I contact someone in New York?"

"No, no. It's too late for that. We will take care of him later, after I no longer need him." Bandeira suppressed a fresh wave of anger. Matters should never have come to this. "No, I spoke to Abílio and have instructed that he leave a trail to lure the two men interfering with Casas de Férias to come to Brazil. You can take care of them here on our own turf."

César nodded. "When will the two men arrive?"

"I'm not sure but soon."

"Where will they go?"

"You remember the Mooca warehouse?" It had been a drug distribution center for a time. Lately it was unused. It was isolated, ideal for this purpose. "You have time to set up the ambush. Abílio has sent us their names and photographs."

César nodded. "And if they don't come?"

"That is possible, yes. If they stay in New York, you will have someone there take care of them, though I'd rather not. But I think they will come. The bait is nice and juicy."

"I will see to it at once and will use my best men. There will be no problems."

"I want them to vanish, you understand? It must appear they dropped off the face of the earth."

"As you wish."

Bandeira discussed other business with César, then sent him on his way. He was finishing his cigar and was considering a drink when he heard a voice calling for him from the bedroom. He rose and walked to the open sliding door. "What is it?" His voice was stern.

"I'm lonely," Sonia said.

Bandeira was momentarily startled. What was this? What game was she playing?

"Come to bed, my love. Please."

Bandeira moved closer, testing the situation. Then, satisfied at this unexpected turn he moved to the side of the bed and stood there. "What are you talking about?"

"Come to bed. I'm sorry, please forgive me. I was weak. It won't happen again." Sonia moved and the sheet slipped from her body. There was bruising there, but it only heightened his excitement. "Just don't be so rough this time." Then she smiled coyly. "Unless you think I need to be punished more."

38

Marc Campos exited the subway tunnel, stopped at the top of the stairs, and looked back as casually as he could manage. No one was following him from what he could see. He turned left and walked at a steady pace, stopping once two blocks later to tie his shoe, another time to pretend he was confused about where he was. Still no one.

And that was as it should be. There was no reason for the SEC to suspect him. He'd been careful, more careful than Richard Iyers. As he resumed his way, he put his thoughts to that particular problem. Just what was he to do? The man was out of control, gone rogue. He'd killed one man without permission, tried to kill another on his own. He was rash and he would be caught soon, for something. He knew too much, guessed too much, and had done too much. Iyers could tie Campos to one murder and another attempted murder. Never mind that Campos had nothing to do with either of them, the way American law worked, he'd learned, whatever Iyers did was the same as if Campos himself had done it. And when Iyers was arrested, as Campos was certain he would be at some point, he'd roll over in about five seconds.

I should have seen it coming, Campos thought bitterly. That night he'd pitched Casas de Férias to Iyers he'd seen the sudden light in the man's pale eyes. It had brightly flamed for several seconds and when it eased, Iyers had become animated, more aggressive than Campos had ever seen him.

Campos had already been criticized for hiring him in the first place.

Bandeira had chastised him directly when he'd learned about the use of a rootkit planted within the core code. What were the odds the one code writer with critical access he'd selected would turn out to be a psychopath? If anything else went wrong, Campos had to be concerned about just how much goodwill was left with his boss. That, he thought, will depend on just how badly things go. And with this rush to expand Casas de Férias and exploit Carnaval the chances of a disaster were more likely than they'd otherwise be. He had a sinking feeling about what lay ahead.

For one, NYSE Euronext was utilizing a new program for the Toptical IPO launch and there were always risks associated with that. For another, the high-frequency traders were going to be all over the IPO. They'd made a bundle on Facebook despite all the snafus, did very well indeed on Twitter, and were looking to score big again on this one. While this latest IPO was a golden opportunity for Carnaval it meant issues beyond their control could go wrong, disastrously so.

No, Campos thought, there is too much against us and we are being forced to do this too quickly, staking too much on a single operation. His every instinct told him that this was going to be a disaster and in more ways than one.

It was all so confusing. Campos was fully involved with Carnaval. In addition, he had his usual duties to perform at work; then he spent extra hours facilitating the updates and routes. It was complex, and he had to double-check and test everything. The Rio team was doing a good job, but he'd caught too many mistakes from them and couldn't help but wonder how much he was missing. Some errors meant nothing. The public would be shocked to learn how many bugs existed already in systems they relied on every day. But some of the mistakes could prove fatal to Carnaval. It would take a lot more time and more resources than Campos had to identify which ones.

And what to do about Iyers. Campos wanted nothing to happen to the man until after Carnaval so that gave him a bit of time. He needed him right now. But then what? He'd never killed a man, and from what he'd seen, Iyers's guard would be up. Even if Campos risked trying, the man's caution would make it more difficult. Now he understood why the Mafia kept its enemies close. He'd always wondered about that when he saw the movies.

Hire a killer? In that path were at least two risks. First, he'd be known to the man he paid. Second, the assassin might botch the job. Then he'd be in double trouble. Iyers would have no reason to remain loyal and the hired killer would have every reason to turn on him if he were caught.

No, hiring someone himself was out of the question. Anyway, he had no idea how to go about it. All he'd done since coming to New York was write code.

Did he dare suggest the killing to Bandeira? How long would it take for the *chefe* to set it up? Not long, Campos decided. His reach was extensive, but he'd be unhappy at being placed in that position. This was Campos's mess, and he'd expect Campos to clean it up.

Which meant he had to kill Iyers himself. Campos swallowed, his throat suddenly aching as he did.

He stopped and tied his other shoe. No one.

Satisfied but still uncomfortable walking the streets of Brooklyn at this hour, he stepped off more briskly. Brooklyn Heights was perhaps the most accessible area off Manhattan Island, which was why he'd chosen it initially. Originally the modest apartment had been nothing more than a bolt-hole in case things turned unexpectedly wrong, as well as a place to stash what he'd need in the event he had to run.

But over the years, he found he'd often come here, especially on pleasant Sundays. It was in many ways a different world from Manhattan and its skyscraper canyons. Even the people were different, more boisterous, more congenial behind their bravado, lacking the edge he dealt with every day across the river.

Montague Street was a delight. Trees lined much of it and the five-story redbrick buildings in their stately decline reminded him vaguely of home in Brazil. Mothers still pushed strollers along the sidewalks and children played in front of the apartment stoops. There were a few hotels built at the turn of the last century, some churches, thrift shops, and small restaurants. "Cozy" was not the word for it exactly, but he found it comfortable. If people didn't know one another, the lingering influence of Brooklyn's past dictated that they act as if they should.

Out of habit, Campos glanced back the way he'd come a final time, though if a tail had come this far, locating his destination would not be difficult. He saw nothing and mounted the steps. He entered the front door, then walked up the stairs to the second floor. On the back side of the building he let himself into a narrow one-room apartment. He closed the door behind him and stood silently, listening. The building had been settling, reacting to the changes in humidity, soil, and temperature for more than a century now, and he could still detect the slight creaks of its all but imperceptible movement. It was silly to listen for more he knew. He was alone. He turned on the high ceiling light, which cast a soft glow about the room; then he moved along the walls, turning on lamps one by one.

Campos opened the refrigerator and removed a small bottle of Coke. It was from Mexico, one of his Sunday finds here in Brooklyn. It was made with real sugar and tasted just like the Coke in São Paulo. He opened the bottle and drank half before setting it down on the Formica top of the two-chair kitchen table.

Beside the narrow bed was a small safe he'd bought and had delivered. A professional would have no trouble cracking it, a determined amateur would just carry it off, but it kept prying eyes away. Using his real birth date he opened the safe and removed its contents. He carried these in two hands to the kitchen table and sat.

When Abílio Ramos had first set himself up in America, he'd arranged for another identity. Two of them, in fact. He opened the Portuguese passport, examined the photograph again, then read the name. Rodrigo Emanual Braga. He could handle that. He set the maroon-colored passport down, then picked up the navy blue Brazilian passport. Jadir José Silva. Why not?

His real passport was in his apartment on Lower Manhattan just in case, for some desperate reason, he was forced to travel under his own name. Also there was the existing Portuguese passport in the name of the identity he would have to abandon—Marco Enfante Campo.

Now he fingered three stacks of cash. There was fifty thousand dollars in U.S. currency, mostly hundred-dollar bills, thirty thousand in euros with a fair number of five-hundred-euro bills, which kept the stack smaller, and five thousand in British pounds. Enough. There were also credit and debit cards for each identity.

Until this week, he'd never seriously considered that he'd have to run so soon. He'd always thought Casas de Férias would continue for several years and in time would be wound down into inactivity. Carnaval had been Pedro's idea initially but it was never intended to be the size Senhor Bandeira was now ordering.

The plan had always been that after a respectable period, Campos would just fade away. Now that was impossible. Either way, this was all coming to an end. He'd have to leave as soon as his involvement with Carnaval was not needed or if suspicion, even mild, was directed at him. Where to go? Portugal? It was part of the European Union and its security computer network.

He was wary of trusting his false identities in such a system. Still, as part of Europe, once he was in he'd be free to travel about with no questions asked. He could change his identity after arrival, then go . . . Where? Italy? Greece? They both appealed to him.

Or maybe his first stop should be Macau. That was tempting as it was in Asia and everything was for sale there, absolutely everything. But it was distant and he'd be trapped on a long flight with no idea who'd be meeting him when he arrived.

Madeira? With its heavy tourist presence, that might be ideal. It was Portuguese, and he'd blend in there but it was a small island and there'd be nowhere to easily run to. He could buy a boat he supposed, but he'd never sailed one on his own.

Brazil? Home? Yes, in time, but not right away.

Satisfied at his efforts and feeling better now that he'd confirmed everything was still here he debated what to do. Leave it and plan to come back if needed? Take it to his apartment? He smiled at that. Leave it, of course. That was the point of having it. Knowing it was here meant he could walk away at a moment's notice. In fact, now that he'd considered it, he'd move his real passport here as well. No one knew about this place. If there was trouble, it would focus on his official residence.

Campos placed everything back into the safe, closed the door, and spun the dial. He finished the Coke standing up, filled the bottle with water, rinsed, filled it again, and poured it out. His mother had taught him that. It kept ants away. He killed the kitchen light, kicked off his shoes, then stretched out on the narrow bed. He listened again to the quiet settling of the building, of the more distant nocturnal sounds without, and let his mind drift.

What to do about Richard Iyers. And when to do it.

39

Daryl curled her feet beneath her in the aspect of the Buddha as she studied the screen, her right hand resting on the mouse. She was tired but too keyed up to go to sleep. Anyway, her body clock told her the time was just approaching 9 P.M. Customarily a night owl, she was good for some time yet.

When she received Frank's message urging her to follow the money, she'd turned to the task with relish. She'd chased more than her share of money trails before, both for the government and while working with Jeff, as well as in her new job. It would be a lot more interesting than tracing the code back to its authors.

Daryl still didn't understand just how the malware worked—she'd leave that part to the boys—but once she'd focused on the cash her attention was drawn to the sequences of numbers she kept encountering. They were not all the same in length, nor did they appear in the same location in the code, but numbers were recurring throughout its functions.

Her first impression was that the numbers were encoded in such a way as to conceal the purpose they served. That was clever on someone's part. In the event the code was discovered it would still be difficult to decipher. As it was the numbers could be most anything. They could also be of either greater or lesser significance to the money trail. There was no way to know until she'd cracked exactly what they were.

Since this was a financial operation, Daryl's suspicion was that they were account numbers of some type, and that they'd be part of the routing path for funds once they were acquired. She suspected that the Exchange used internal identifiers for trading accounts, but hoped that the malware had a table of mappings between bank and Exchange accounts. If it didn't, this approach would be a quick dead end. With that in mind, she researched bank routing transit numbers. These were nine digit numbers appearing on all negotiable instruments including personal and business checks. They served to identify the financial institution on which the instrument was drawn. They were in essence an address. Originally, Federal Reserve Banks processed wire fund transfers by using them but now more people had money directly deposited into their accounts and paid their bills online.

But the numbers she was examining were longer than nine digits. Some were eleven, others as many as nineteen. She began slicing and dicing the numbers, searching for patterns. She recalled reading once that when spies sent messages, they did so in blocks of five numerical digits. Many of the numbers were not actually part of the message itself. They were intended to fill out messages to conceal those that were short or to establish authenticity. She doubted either was the case here, since the numbers were not of the same length, but seized on the idea that any sequence of numbers beyond nine was meant to conceal the fact these were bank routing numbers.

It consumed several hours, but finally she had it. Using a combination of code inspection and study of the numbers looking for patterns and correlations, she discovered recurring sequences of numbers. They were not always in the same order, but she was convinced they were meant to hide the actual number. At last she came up with sets of eight numbers. When she removed these numbers in specific patterns from the sequences, she was, in most cases, able to come up with a nine-digit number. She then ran the numbers through the fdic.gov Web site, and there they were—the names and locations of U.S. banks, one of them as close as Stamford, Connecticut.

So she'd been right. This part of the code was where the money trail began. If she could demonstrate that these numbers were part of a bigger, and longer lasting operation, one in which Jeff and Frank were not profiting, that would help enormously in getting them off the hook.

Daryl was impressed once she'd grasped the vast scope of the rogue code, as Frank had called it. There must be more than a hundred banks involved. If this routing system worked as others she'd cracked had, nearly all the financial institutions were bases the money scarcely touched before moving on. The money wouldn't come to rest until it had been carefully maneuvered and outpaced possible electronic surveillance.

Before 9/11 and the passage of the Patriot Act, such efforts had not been all that complicated. Money would leave a company, or in this case the Exchange, go offshore and vanish. As long as the country with the offshore bank refused to cooperate with American law enforcement, drugs lords, organized crime kingpins, and tax evaders were free to conceal their assets from the Internal Revenue Service and other government agencies. And most other countries did not cooperate unless a great deal of pressure was brought to bear on them.

If the launderers wanted to be doubly safe, once the money was offshore, they'd move it two or three times, say to Latvia, then to Belgium, then Switzerland, then back to an offshore bank. There a lawyer would set up a perfectly legal company and invest the money back into the U.S. stock market.

But the Patriot Act changed all that. In the guise of chasing terrorists the U.S. government now had the power to strip many foreign bank accounts of their protective shield. If a bank—or, more important, the country—where it was located wanted to have any dealings with the United States, then they cooperated with requests for data. Not every country played ball but most did and it took someone very knowledgeable to keep moving money from bank to bank, country to country, always staying with those prepared to stonewall Uncle Sam.

That was the trail Daryl had to follow, and her first efforts suggested it was going to be too much, at least too much in the time she had. There had to be a faster way.

Seeing Frank had been sobering. His effective disguise and the seriousness with which he presented their problem struck home. She'd understood that their situation was critical; otherwise, she'd never have climbed on an airplane, but she'd not really appreciated just how serious this was. Though Frank had been his usual self, she couldn't help but notice how he kept an inconspicuous eye on the lobby. And though he'd seemed casual in his manner, she knew him well enough to know he'd been tightly coiled.

Daryl wondered how Carol, his wife, was taking this. Then she realized he likely hadn't told her. What was the point? If things turned really ugly, there'd be time enough to let her know; otherwise, it was just so much needless worry.

What impressed her was Frank's tradecraft. She was pretty sure that was the word. She'd heard it from her CIA colleagues when she was still with the NSA. She'd always considered him another computer expert, better at handling the ins and outs of bureaucratic politics than most, but she'd never thought of him as a spy.

She knew he'd been an operative, though. On occasion when he had a bit too much to drink, he'd tell stories of that time, but they were always more travelogues than espionage stories. Listening to them, you'd have thought he'd been working for IBM, and he never related an incident that even hinted at danger. But watching Carol during those moments Daryl had noticed some reserve when she joined in the laughter, her hand placed protectively on her husband, a subtle tightness around her mouth.

Carol knew Daryl realized. She knew just how close to death Frank had come in the years before they met.

Now he was employing all that experience and skill to keep himself and Jeff out of harm's way. Daryl appreciated that he had such abilities, but wished it wasn't necessary. But his tradecraft had given her an idea.

40

Frank stood and stretched, feeling the tension ease from his muscles as his joints yielded a slight popping sensation. He looked over at Jeff who'd fallen asleep atop the bedspread in an exaggerated X. Frank was worried about him. Jeff should still be in the hospital under monitoring, not hiding out in a dump like this.

Not for the first time, Frank suppressed the emotions that welled up inside him. He'd never been in precisely this position before, though he'd seen it happen to a colleague in his field days. That hadn't turned out so well, which was just one more reason he'd elected to fix the problem himself rather than hire a lawyer and fight it out in the system.

He went into the bathroom and scrubbed his face. He'd thought days like this, nights in nameless hotels in the rougher part of town, were behind him. He'd turned in his 007 card and taken to the office and was surprised at how easily he'd made the transition. His bachelor cowboy days were behind him, and he'd transitioned into a suburbanite with remarkable ease. Carol had helped, actually made it possible. She'd intuitively understood what he was giving up and made his reason for giving it up a good trade every day. Then the children had come and there'd been no turning back.

Now this.

Frank wondered just how rusty he was. It was one thing to remember the moves, to still have the contacts, yet another to get into the action. Until now, he'd primarily spent his time on the computer and kept to ground but that was about to change.

He looked at himself in the mirror in the harsh light. He was old, slow. He'd worked at staying fit but only someone who'd worked the field as many years as he had knew how much more finely honed his reflexes needed to be than they were. He'd talked to one of the older agents about it years before. They'd been holed up in Venezuela on a surveillance operation and there was nothing to do but talk, swap stories, and tell lies. He'd asked how the man did it now that he was middle-aged.

"Experience and judgment make up the difference," he'd said. "There's no point in fooling yourself that you're the man you were but you know a lot more, have picked up a trick or two. Actually, what you learn is that most of the action was never necessary, that there'd been another way to do it all along, but you hadn't known enough to use it." Then he'd smiled. "Bringing along a young stud like you, of course, always helps."

Frank wondered if that spy made it to retirement. They'd lost touch after that operation. He hoped so. He wanted to think he had, that he was on a sunny beach where his only concern was drinking too much.

Frank went back into the room and sat before the laptop. He ran through the code again, then began tracing it step by step.

Jeff stirred from his sleep, slid off the bed, and sat on its edge for a long time, muttering something about going back to work, finally rose, used the bathroom, then sat in front of his laptop. As he accessed it an e-mail came in. A message was written across a photograph of two bodies lying in a field, their heads placed beside them like a pair of jack-o'-lanterns.

STOP! DO NOTHING OR YOU WILL DIE!
WE KNOW WHO YOU ARE!
YOU CANNOT RUN FROM US!
THIS IS YOUR ONLY WARNING!

"Look at this," he said, suddenly wide awake.

Frank glanced up from his computer, then moved over. "They're running scared."

"That's one way to look at it. Aren't you troubled that they know enough to send me an e-mail?"

"Jeff, they knew enough to frame us. This just confirms what we already know: There's someone on the inside in this." He studied the screen. "This is almost reassuring."

"You're a sick man."

"Not so much. I've just been around. Take a hard look at the photo. It might have some useful data." He flashed a knowing smile. "I'm betting it does."

DAY SEVEN
SUNDAY, SEPTEMBER 16

SECURITIES EXCHANGE COMMISSION MOVING MORE AGGRESSIVELY

By Gordon Field
September 16

New York—After years of complaints over alleged inaction, the SEC reports it is now acting more aggressively when wrongdoing on Wall Street is detected. "The days of moving at a gentlemanly pace are over," Carl Levitt, Director of the Manhattan Enforcement Division, said in a recent interview. Changes in federal law have given SEC investigators more powerful tools and the New York Regional Office is not reluctant to use them when faced with the facts.

"We have broader subpoena power than in the past and can, in specific situations, cause an arrest warrant to be immediately issued," Levitt said. "Such measures in and of themselves will, we believe, have a sobering effect on malfeasance in the securities industry."

With the advent of computer trading the SEC has often found itself under attack for moving too late and too slowly. Given the speed with which trades now take place, often within a single second, enormous sums change hands free from direct scrutiny. "We are increasingly concerned about actual abuse and the potential abuses of high-frequency trading," Levitt admitted. "We now have the means to effectively investigate them."

Critics disagree however. In a recently published article Tamara Greene, a former SEC investigator, wrote, "The relationship between the NYSE and the major high-frequency traders is more than cozy, it's incestuous. The Exchange simply makes too much money from these players to want to rein them in. That's a reality the SEC cannot get around." No matter how aggressive the SEC is, she asserts, the NYSE consistently runs interference for them.

Levitt disagrees. "I respect Tammy very much, but she's speaking of a different time." He then cited several recent examples of the new laws in action. "We issue subpoenas and arrest warrants early in key investigations. Our Enforcement Division now emphasizes its law enforcement capabilities. This alone will have a sobering impact on wrongdoers."

Greene viewed the changes with dismay. "Turning the SEC into the secret police isn't the answer. Until the unethical bond between the NYSE and high-frequency traders is broken abuses will continue."

Others discount her criticism, claiming that the Exchange is not in bed with high-frequency traders. They argue that they are just another player in securities trading who should be regulated for the common good rather than singled out.

Another source, formerly with the SEC and who asked not to be named, stated, "The Enforcement Division of the SEC has turned into a modern Gestapo. They are quick to judge guilt and often move before the facts are adequately known. Their primary concern is intimidation through aggression. In the end, they don't really care if their targets were actually guilty, just so traders see the havoc they wreak on their lives. It's hard to believe we still live in America."

Levitt dismissed the accusation with a laugh, then asked for the source's identity.

Digital Wall Street

41

ENFORCEMENT DIVISION
SECURITIES AND EXCHANGE COMMISSION
NEW YORK REGIONAL OFFICE
200 VESSEY STREET
NEW YORK CITY
9:07 A.M.

Robert Alshon reviewed the search report from the office used by Jeff Aiken and Frank Renkin with disapproval. His team had done an outstanding job but the forensic examination of the physical evidence had turned up nothing of use to him. The preliminary examination of the computers was negative as well. The pair had been too crafty to be caught red-handed, leaving no obvious trail.

The search of their hotel rooms had been no more productive. The frustrating part was that his people had arrived too late. Their personal effects, specifically their computers, were gone. They'd been alerted by the security system in D.C. and moved one step faster than he had. Not for the first time, he regretted that he could not make the arrests at the same time he'd conducted the search.

Alshon's supervisor had already expressed concern with the investigation. He wasn't focused on this case as yet but the message was clear to him. He needed to close the circle ASAP.

His stomach burned. He reached into the right desk drawer for an antacid. He chewed two large pink tablets, then downed them with tepid black coffee. It was Sunday, he reminded himself again. He'd like to be doing something else. He spent too many weekend days in this office.

The good news was that the arrest warrants were out. He'd sent an alert to the NYPD and called his contact at the FBI Manhattan Field Office. With their cooperation he had local assets on the ground and was confident they'd flush his targets. New York was a big city but these two were from out of town, with no contacts. They'd need to use a debit or credit card soon enough, and then he'd have them. Plastic was always the Achilles' heel for such criminals.

Though Alshon wasn't all that certain in this case. He'd already tried tracing their cell phones. Both of them were inoperative. Aiken and Renkin had been smart enough to remove the batteries and were no doubt using burners. They'd also have ways to obtain false identities. They might even have access to cash to keep themselves off the electronic grid. He hated chasing spooks. They knew too much.

Alshon's initial thought had been that this pair were computer geeks and would be easily snared. He'd done it often enough since coming to the SEC. Computer experts could write code and engage in all kinds of chicanery, but when it came to fleeing, they were amateurs. But not in this case, apparently.

Alshon's immediate concern was how expert they were, what contacts they possessed he could not know about. Had they both or either of them been operatives at one time? He made a note to find out, grimacing as he wrote. The Company would drag its heels, it always did. The supposed post–9/11 camaraderie was a façade. No agency cooperated with another, not unless there was something in it for them or you had a personal contact inside. Not for the first time, he regretted not having cultivated one at the CIA.

But he just couldn't stand spooks. The CIA was simply sleazy from his experience. They worked in the shadows, never told the truth, and never the entire truth even when forced to come clean. They routinely engaged in misdirection, were never straightforward. In Alshon's view they were downright un-American in their conduct, and since their creation had caused far more harm than good.

In his experience, they also had an excess of money, power, and resources, and too many agents went into business for themselves taking advantage of what they learned and the contacts they'd made. It was disgusting, and it was a nasty business.

Alshon was forming the opinion that was the case here. He wondered just how far the web spread. Could just two men have done what the IT report claimed? There could very easily be more to this than met the eye. Whose nest were they feathering? How much help would others give them?

Alshon ran his right hand across his scalp. He was sweating. He closed his eyes. God, he wanted to nail these guys, nail them good. But what resources did they have access to? He fought off the sinking feeling that the pair had already slipped from beyond his grasp.

Just then, Susan Flores rapped lightly at his open door. He nodded for her to come in and sit.

"What do you have?" he asked sharply.

"We're still at it but I know more than when we spoke last time."

Alshon knew she'd been up most of the last two nights. She looked it. He'd have to back off on pressing her; otherwise, her efficiency would plummet. But time was critical right now, and he had no regrets about his manner. Everyone needed to know this case was urgent. They'd slip into the long-haul mode soon enough if he didn't catch a break.

Flores referred to her notes. "It's a big operation, bigger than it initially appeared. Like we thought, it's been going on for about a year from what we can tell. The software uses a special high-frequency trading algo and exploits its preferred position within the Exchange's trading platform. We haven't traced any of the money yet but know that it's scattered. The algo targets many companies, taking a bite everywhere; it doesn't steal from within the Exchange itself. Candidly—" She hesitated just a millisecond before finishing. "—we're wondering if this can possibly be a two-person operation."

Alshon opened his desk drawer and shook out two more pink pills.

"We think they've been at this for several years, moving very carefully as they set it up. We were able to do a 'before' and 'after' of one of their updates and, frankly, it looks to us like more work than two men can accomplish within a reasonable time frame. It also has all the hallmarks of an inside job. Do these two have connections within the Exchange?" Flores stopped and looked up.

"I don't know." Alshon made a note. "I'll have a background done on every key employee who could work this from the inside. Can you give me those names?" Flores nodded. "We'll find the link if there is one."

"The other part of this, sir, is that the operation is ongoing."

Alshon was shocked. "You mean they're still at it?"

"Absolutely. If anything, it looks like its accelerating in frequency."

Alshon wrinkled his forehead. "They're on the run. How can they do that? Are you positive this isn't automated?"

"Yes. What's happening is being human directed. My thinking was the same as yours initially, that they'd have to shut down in the circumstances, that if they did anything, it would be to delete code and cover their tracks. I think we really need to consider that a number of others are involved. Or—" She hesitated. "—whether these two are even involved at all."

"What do you mean?"

"Unless we can connect them with someone on the inside going back several years I think we need to consider that they've been set up."

"Set up?"

"Right. Assume for a minute, they are fall guys. They were brought in to conduct a penetration test. We know they succeeded. In doing so they encountered the code for this illegal operation. Whoever is doing it could have made it look like they were the culprits to discredit them and divert attention."

"That seems a stretch."

"Yes, but I don't find it any more implausible than Aiken opening a brokerage account in his own name and carelessly dropping malware the IT security trolls were sure to spot."

"I'll keep it in mind, but innocent men come forward. They don't run and these two are running like rabbits."

"Yes, sir. That's your area. I just wanted to point out the possibility. Just keep in mind that if they are guilty, they're doubtless part of a much bigger team. This is very sophisticated. And I really don't see how they can be doing what is currently taking place from a hotel room with laptops."

"I've been at this a lot of years, Susan. I know crooks when I see them. These two are bent. I can smell it. I've alerted NYPD and local FBI. They'll flush them out, and when they do, they'll roll over like all the rest."

"Yes, sir," Susan answered, her eyes steadfastly planted on her notes.

42

The office was as busy as on any workweek. Bill Stenton scanned the cubicles. Everyone was here. He'd not given orders, but somehow word had spread that this wasn't a weekend to spend time at home.

He sat back in his chair, swiveled away from his door, closed his eyes, and wondered how things could ever had gone this far. Yesterday had been a disaster. Alshon from the SEC had stormed in with a search warrant and a team of investigators, ostensibly to search the office where the Red Zoya men had worked. In fact, Alshon's team had been everywhere, eyeing trusted employees suspiciously, looking across desks distrustfully, obstructing the hallways, intruding in the normal flow of work. It had been terrible.

Alshon had made it worse by speaking to Stenton in such a way as to indicate that he wasn't entirely trusted. Maybe that was an over interpretation, Stenton thought, but the investigator had answered questions with questions and had not taken him into his confidence.

When the SEC was finished, "for now" Alshon said, his team had stripped bare the office Aiken and Renkin had used, leaving nothing but fixtures and the desks behind. What was the point of that other than as a show of power? All the equipment they'd taken belonged to this office but Stenton was in no position to complain, nor did he want to. It was the turmoil and suspicion that troubled him.

Afterwards, he'd gone with his senior staff to a quiet watering hole. The discussion had inevitably turned to what had taken place earlier. From what they'd witnessed and what investigators said, it was apparent that Aiken and Renkin were suspects in a major crime. His colleagues kicked around what they'd heard, talked about it, and decided that this time the SEC was barking up the wrong tree. More than one on his team knew Aiken by reputation and refused to believe he was a criminal. "They don't always get it right," one said.

"Yeah, but they always make it look like they do," another answered.

And that bothered Stenton because he was now having serious reservations about what was taking place. He'd called the colleague who'd recommended Aiken so forcefully and quizzed him at length.

"Jeff's the best there is," the man had repeated. "I've known him for years. It was a shame he left the CIA, but he's proved his worth time and again." The man related two incidents when Aiken had uncovered malware that was steadily looting companies. "You recall that Anonymous hack of RegSec? It was Jeff who figured that out, plus he came up with a way to identify the hacker at the conference he was attending."

When Stenton continued to express reservations his colleague had told him stories he'd heard, how Aiken had hunted down two cyberterrorists in person, how his girlfriend had been kidnapped by a gang and he rescued her. "He's as straight as they come," he'd said. "Check around, Bill. You'll see I'm right."

Stenton had declined to say why he'd called but had taken the man up on his suggestion and called two more contacts in the industry, people he'd not talked with before. Both knew Aiken by reputation and both spoke very highly of him.

Now Alshon was telling him that Aiken was dishonest. How could that possibly be true given what Stenton was being told? People don't just change their nature. Aiken had had plenty of chances to steal before, and in places with far less security. Here, he was all but sure to be caught.

Alshon had let drop that something was amiss in their system and had been for some time. Stenton found that impossible to believe, the harmless bot notwithstanding. The system had performed as expected, and their security measures, the finest in the industry, had detected nothing. Absolutely nothing.

And if Aiken were the guilty party, how could he have managed to steal for a year and then arranged for Stenton to hire him?

It was impossible. There was simply no way he could have hacked their system before he was hired, but that was what Alshon was suggesting. And if it was a coincidence, that was too improbable to even consider. Stenton had conducted a nationwide search for just the right man and ended up hiring the hacker who'd already penetrated his system?

Impossible was the word for it.

Stenton's head throbbed. He'd kept his drinking under control with his staff but later, at the bar near his apartment, he kept at it until after midnight. He turned slightly toward his desk, picked up the Red Zoya summary, and flipped through it again. The papers quivered ever so slightly in his shaking hand.

Frank Renkin had left this summary of their findings. It was all there. How they'd successfully penetrated the impregnable system. How they'd discovered rogue code in it, code that had been there a year or more, just like Alshon had said. Renkin and Aiken had asked for a face-to-face to go over their findings in detail.

Stenton lifted the last page. The pair had recommended that Stenton get the IT people on the rogue code at once to get it neutralized, then reverse engineer it to determine what it did and how it managed to penetrate their system.

Was that something criminals would do? Hardly.

Then there was the attack on Aiken to consider. One of his employees had speculated that it could be related to his work somehow.

Could it? Stenton hadn't even considered the possibility until then. But when he finally examined Red Zoya's summary, he could see plenty of motive for someone to want to put Aiken out of action, though it looked as if they'd moved too late. What if Aiken was on to something and someone decided to stop him? It was far-fetched though not impossible. Assuming that to be true, where did it lead? Who would want to stop him? The hackers obviously, assuming the report was correct.

The first question to consider was who would know Aiken was working here. Stenton had kept the hire discreet and no one knew what he'd been hired to do. His staff had seen the men at work, but Aiken and Renkin were low key, not attracting attention to themselves. Next, and most troubling, was who would know they claimed to have discovered this rogue code? The obvious answer was the one he disliked the most—someone working in this office. Because that meant the hacker was a trusted employee.

Stenton knew all these people; he'd personally hired many of them. He rubbed shoulders with them every day. He'd never experienced the slightest doubt about their integrity. But from long experience, he knew that anyone can violate a trust. He'd seen it before. One of his employees at Wells Fargo had been caught in a pretty basic computer theft. It turned out she had a biker boyfriend who'd given her no choice. So it could happen.

Then there was the media and the frenzy the *Times* article about that bot was causing. The market had taken a real fall on Friday, and the international markets were suggesting it was in for more of the same on Monday. He'd been forced to meet with his boss and assure him that the accusations of the disgruntled former employee who leaked the story were unfounded, that the bot was simply harmless. Stenton's response, he told him, had been to bring on board the finest team he could locate to conduct a pentest to locate and plug any holes.

He'd felt sick to his stomach defending himself that way, realizing too late that his superior might have already heard about the SEC investigation. Fortunately, the raid hadn't happened until the next day, but Stenton knew he'd be back before his boss on Monday, trying to talk his way out of all this. His story was losing credibility even to himself. There'd been a harmless bot, he'd hired a company, the men were suspected by the Exchange's IT department of looting accounts, and the SEC had launched an investigation, searching their office, questioning his staff. He'd heard warrants were outstanding for the pair.

This was his area, he was responsible. It almost didn't matter what the truth was any longer because events were discrediting him with every passing hour. When it came time for heads, or a head, to roll, he hadn't the slightest doubt his would be on the chopping block.

Stenton turned away from the door. He didn't need this, not on top of his usual responsibilities and the endless meetings he was attending about the pending Toptical IPO. He'd never expressed his reservations about the new algo the Exchange was going to use as it had not been his decision and no one had asked. But the test runs had all experienced glitches and there was a pervasive sense of unease he could detect among those responsible for it. The IPO had to come off without a serious problem. With the stock market reeling the credibility of the Exchange was at stake. Too much depended on its success for there to be a failure like that experienced by BATS or even a snafu like the Facebook IPO.

What a disaster that would be, Stenton thought.

On Friday, he was asked specifically about the integrity of the Exchange's trading platform, and he'd answered there were no problems, despite what

The New York Times was reporting. Looking back at the Red Zoya summary, though, then recalling the earlier report from the Chicago office, he realized something very likely was amiss. Could it have anything to do with the IPO? There was without question enough money at stake to make it a ready target. And the fact that the Exchange was employing a new algo was common knowledge. The *Wall Street Journal* had dedicated a long article to it. New algos were always a place for shenanigans as the unexpected often occurred, even without interference.

Stenton found himself taking shallow breaths and forced himself to fill his lungs deeply. His uncontrolled eyelid tic was back. His wife had complained about the weekends he was working, among other things. He promised her that wouldn't happen when he'd taken this job, and now it turned out he'd promised something he couldn't deliver. And she didn't even like living in Manhattan.

But Stenton had a more pressing issue, one that had gnawed at him ever since he'd first learned of Alshon's investigation. Stenton had hired Jeff Aiken. What if, despite everything he'd been told, Aiken was guilty? What if he'd planted this rogue code the previous year?

God, Stenton thought, no one will believe my hiring him was a coincidence. No one. He'd be finished, not just here, but anywhere significant. And he'd deserve it, because it was him who'd let the fox into the hen house.

He glanced at his watch. Too much time. His first drink was at least three hours away.

43

A ROCHA
EDIFÍCIO REPÚBLICA
RUA SÃO BENTO
SÃO PAULO, BRAZIL
12:33 P.M.

A Rocha restaurant occupied the entire tenth floor of the Edifício República. To dine here meant Victor Bandeira did not have to leave the building, and his bodyguards could position themselves inconspicuously near the elevator.

The restaurant was busy as usual on a Sunday. Many of those who dined here regularly brought their wives and families directly from Mass. Bandeira sat at his usual corner table with the commanding view of the floor, acknowledging nods in his direction. He ordered a drink as he waited, wondering why he should be waiting.

He'd been drinking too much lately, he decided. He'd confided his concerns to no one. That was one of the prices he paid for being on the top. There was no one with whom he could share everything. Information was power and the more information he gave away the weaker he became. Such had been his experience.

Carnaval was the most ambitious operation of his career and must succeed. He'd spoken directly with Ramos about it and the man had expressed his unease. "I'm concerned that it's too much, too fast," he'd said respectfully.

Bandeira understood, but the allure of $10 billion in a single stroke had been more than he could resist. Now he was committed, and there was no turning back. He was satisfied that Grupo Técnico in Rio was doing what had to be done. Ramos had assured him the same was taking place in New

York. Still, it was asking a lot, and though Bandeira gave the orders, he understood he was pressing his skilled staff to the breaking point.

But that's what they were paid to do. If this work were easy, anyone could do it. They were bright, no question about it. But could they pull it off?

Any troubles they had, Bandeira believed, were connected to the fact that Pedro didn't like taking direction from Abílio. He wanted to be his own man. He occasionally resisted instructions, which was bad enough but primarily he squabbled with his New York counterpart, clashing with him over ultimate authority. As if anyone but Bandeira was in charge. The situation was improved but it was still a source of concern to him.

He thought about his son and wondered if other fathers had the same troubles. He'd coddled the boy, he belatedly realized. An only son is a burden as everything rested on him. Perhaps it had been a mistake to put Pedro in charge of Casas de Férias. Of course, at the time he'd had no idea the operation would by now be poised to take $10 billion from the New York Stock Exchange, to make him and those with whom he did business richer than any of them had ever dreamed. Now, with everything depending on success, he was stuck with Pedro playing a key role. Everyone was expecting the big payoff. Bandeira had to deliver. He wondered if his son understood that.

Failure would be a disaster from which he could never recover. Bandeira was unconcerned about the operation being traced to him. That was of no consequence. The problem would be in disappointing those in power he depended on. So far, his career had been free of major missteps, but he'd studied previous *chefes* and had taken from them one important lesson: The perception of success is the mother of power. When those who can hurt you see you fail, then the power seeps from you like water from a cracked pot.

Bandeira's fresh Scotch arrived and he lifted it to his lips. The first danger with Carnaval was that something might go wrong and would point to the ongoing Casas de Férias operation and possibly to the men working at the Exchange before they had a chance to get away. It wasn't anything Bandeira thought couldn't be handled, but it would be an unnecessary complication. He was satisfied that NL was sufficiently removed from the operation even in that eventuality.

What ate at him was the consequence of success. Ramos had expressed his concern that taking so much from the IPO could have a catastrophic cascading effect on the market. "Lesser amounts have caused serious disruptions," he cautioned.

Bandeira found that hard to accept. The NYSE transacted billions of dollars every day. Ten billion would scarcely be missed but Ramos had explained that even a few billion when linked to the algos of the high-frequency traders had caused temporary chaos in the market previously. "Everyone is looking for the next event," he said, "and when it happens, we can't predict with total confidence how they will react. We could have a stock market crash unlike anything in history. Everything is set up for it to happen at some point. No one has faith in the Exchange to have in place the necessary controls."

And there it was, the real source of Bandeira's concern. He could not be seen as responsible for an international collapse of the financial markets. He required a functioning stock market. He needed a financial system with all the flaws the current one had to milk it. A restructured, rebuilt system would make what he'd been doing, and what he planned to do in the future, impossible. A catastrophe would also wipe out the fortunes of many powerful men. Guilt would need to be placed, a scapegoat found. Bandeira wondered if he could escape the blame of a concerted worldwide effort to find the culprit.

Was his ambition at last too much? Bandeira thought as he finished his drink and gestured for another. Had his ego finally become too much? Esmeralda had cautioned him once about that. She'd been the last person able to speak to him with such candor. He'd dismissed it at the time. Great men did great things. It was the way of the world. Still, it was peculiar that her words came back to him at this moment.

Ego had been the final undoing of his predecessor, Joaquim de Sousa Andrade. Known simply as Bibo, he'd been *chefe* for just a single year. He'd been satisfied with the status quo, content with the wealth and power that flowed his way and made no changes except the ill-advised one of moving Bandeira to the number two position. Andrade had thought the car accident that made his final elevation an act of God. Everything, it seemed to Bandeira, went to the man's head and in the end it was vanity that did him in. He'd wanted a hair transplant, the bags under his eyes removed, his jowls reduced or eliminated, and opted to do it all in a single secret procedure. He trusted Bandeira with the news as he'd be out of commission for a week or so. He didn't survive the procedure, nor did the doctor and his team. Bandeira had passed off their brutal elimination as revenge for their carelessness in allowing the great Bibo to die.

Just then, Carlos Lopes de Almeida, president of the Banco do Novo

Brasil, entered the restaurant. Bandeira watched him smile and wave, then weave his way across the crowded room, shaking a few hands, gesturing to others along the way.

He was of slightly below average height compared to the new generation. His scalp shined in the bright light, the wreath of gray hair about it trimmed short. He wore heavy framed glasses in the Latin style. He smiled broadly as he reached the table. Bandeira rose and the two men embraced.

"I am so sorry to be late, my friend," Almeida said. "I was detained at home and the traffic is just terrible."

"Of course. I understand. I only just got here myself."

Bandeira didn't like depending on men like Almeida, men of privilege. They came from the highest ranks of Brazilian society, were intermarried with each other's families, and were traditionally those who controlled the nation. That had changed in recent decades but such men were still important to someone like Bandeira who needed connections in such circles.

That was what irritated him. For all his wealth and power Bandeira would never be invited within that group. That was just one reason why he needed Almeida, why his involvement with Sonia was so reckless. Yes, he controlled the bank, but he still needed the father.

And just what game was she playing? He'd known women who enjoyed it rough. Typically they started fights knowing they would end in only one way. Over the years, he realized that these were not just women who came from violent childhoods but also women of social standing, women who had been pampered all their lives. Was he to believe that Sonia was one of them? You never knew with young women, not until it happened. He wondered sometimes if they knew. Had Sonia discovered this about herself only now? It would seem so, and if he was right, it opened up new opportunities for him with her, opportunities so much more reckless than what had gone before.

Almeida gestured for drinks; then the men ordered their meal. It had been Almeida who wanted to meet, so Bandeira waited, indicating by his silence that he intended to get to business. He had plans for later.

Almeida hesitated, then said, "I am concerned about the cash flow into the bank."

Bandeira raised an eyebrow. "I thought banks liked money."

Almeida smiled. "Oh we do, but lately it has been too much. It is getting difficult to manage without attracting attention. The Banco do Novo Brasil might be old and respected, but it is no longer a major bank in our nation."

"It soon will be, Carlos. We've discussed my plans."

"Oh yes, yes, I quite agree," Almeida said eagerly. "But . . . too much, too fast is a problem, you understand?"

Bandeira pursed his lips. "I can see that." The waiter set their drinks down, then drifted away. "How are the special accounts doing?"

The "special accounts" were those established for key politicians and government officials, all the corrupt elite who had to be taken care of. One of the reasons for acquiring control of the bank had been to give Bandeira a legitimate way of paying them off. Almeida's principal service to him was to arrange this as routine business.

"There are no problems. It all goes smoothly."

"Carlos, over the next week to ten days you will receive perhaps a billion U.S. dollars." Almeida blanched. Bandeira held up his hand to stop him commenting. "I will be meeting with our friends before then, arranging special payments. I will give you the figures in a week. Move the money on to their outside accounts, you understand? Do not keep it in the bank."

"I understand." Almeida lifted his drink gulping down half before lowering the glass.

Bandeira smiled. "In this case the bank records are important to us so don't work too hard at concealing them."

"I . . . I thought . . ."

"Yes, usually. But this time I want my friends tied very closely to me. Don't be concerned, Carlos, the secretary of the Ministry of Finance will receive a significant sum. All is well."

"As you say." Almeida ran his bare hand across the top of his head. He removed a handkerchief and wiped it unconsciously.

This was insurance. Almeida would bind the powerful in Brazil to Bandeira so completely, implicate them in Carnaval so thoroughly, if the necessity came they would save him in saving themselves. It was going to cost a great deal but it was worth it.

Business done, Bandeira turned to chat. "And how is your family?"

"Oh, that. It is why I was delayed coming. My daughter, Sonia—you've met her—she is having boyfriend trouble."

"Young women always have trouble with their romantic life."

"You are lucky to have a son. You have no idea what a curse it is to have so beautiful and willful a daughter. It is not like the old days when a father simply told his daughter what to do."

"She told you about this trouble?"

"Nothing like that. You know women. I think she told my wife who became very upset." Almeida leaned closer and lowered his voice. "I think he was physical with her. She is wearing too much makeup on her left cheek."

"Ahh. He has no right. They are not married."

"Exactly!" Almeida blinked quickly several times. "But since I'm not sure what happened, I don't know what to do." He clenched his jaw. "But if he really hurt her, that *filho da puta* will pay, I promise you!"

Bandeira suppressed a smile. He could not imagine Almeida doing anything in such a situation. "These young people, they are always having troubles like this. We spoil them."

"Yes, I know. I know." Almeida picked up his glass.

"Who is she seeing? Do you know?"

"I've never met him. I asked once, just showing interest, and she glared at me. I asked my wife and she said nothing."

"Difficult."

"Yes, it is very hard." The man uncharacteristically finished his drink. "I've been thinking," Almeida said, "and want to make a suggestion. An idea I have to bring us closer together, bind our relationship and solve this problem I have."

"Yes?"

"You find my daughter attractive. I'm sure you do. She is lovely. Perhaps you could spend some time with her. It would be a great favor to me as it would get her away from this vile man who abuses her. Perhaps, if you think it would be an agreeable match, you would do me the honor of considering marrying her."

Bandeira was stunned.

"Ah, there they are." Almeida rose to attract the attention of his wife and Sonia as they entered the dining room. His wife wore a fixed smile on her face, as plastic as that on a mannequin. Sonia, dressed in something light and sunny, kept her eyes down, looking up just once, her eyes passing across Bandeira's face without expression. For all anyone watching could know, this was the first time they'd ever seen each other.

Bandeira carefully watched as she sat. Then, for the briefest of moments, she caught his eye with a sly, hungry gaze.

44

Daryl grimaced at the sight of the hotel where Frank and Jeff were staying. She looked carefully about the lobby as she entered and decided it was safe enough. The unshaven desk clerk eyed her as she went straight to the elevator but said nothing. She punched the button for the fifth floor, then stepped through the opening doors. The elevator swayed slightly as it rose, strange metallic sounds coming from above and below, echoing in the shaft.

The car stopped and the doors slowly parted. Daryl found the door and rapped lightly. A moment later Frank opened it half an inch, then pulled the door wide and greeted her with a smile.

"Good to see you," he said, hugging her. "Come on in. Come on in."

A bachelor's effort had been made to clean the place, but it was obvious two men had been sharing the cramped room. The trash basket was filled to overflow with a pizza box and take-out containers. Papers on the dresser had been neatly stacked, sort of. Jeff was seated beside his laptop in the room's only chair. There were white bandages on his head. He stood and smiled lightly.

"Hello, Daryl." He didn't approach her. She nodded in reply.

Frank closed the door behind her. Daryl moved to the first bed and sat. "Little short of sitting space, I see."

"Yes," Frank answered. "It's turn-of-the-last-century modern. Hope you didn't have any trouble getting here."

She shook her head. "No. I took three cabs, traveled back and forth on the subway for an hour, then had a coffee for a bit before coming. That's as good as I can do it. The area's not as bad as its reputation, though a bit dodgy." She took in the faded wallpaper. "This place is kind of a dump."

"Manhattan. Gotta love it. They take cash, gladly." Frank looked at Jeff as if giving him a prompt.

"Thanks for coming, Daryl," Jeff said. "We both appreciate it very much."

"How's the head?" Frank had assured her it was nothing serious, though it certainly *looked* serious to her untrained eye. Jeff was pale, seemed weak to her, appearing as if he'd been sick for a long time. The change was remarkable from when she'd last seen him. He'd lost at least ten pounds.

"It's been better. Still aches a bit but nothing I can't handle. The swelling's gone down, but I've still got a pretty good knot. I'll ditch the bandage before we go out. It'll be fine."

"You've not seen a doctor?"

"Not since the hospital, no. Frank's been my primary care physician." He said the last with a small smile.

Frank shrugged. "What can I say? Emergency field medical management, EFM as we called it for short. The training came back." He sat on the other bed, creating a conversation triangle for them.

Daryl reached into her purse and withdrew a white packet she handed to Frank. "Fifteen thousand dollars. You didn't say anything but if you're going to be fugitives, it's better not to do it on a credit card. You can pay me back when this mess is over."

"Thank you. This is very kind. You can never have too much in a situation like this." Frank placed the packet on the dresser. "What have you found?"

"I have an answer for those numbers. A lot of them track to banks. I think they're part of the routing protocol for moving the captured money."

"What banks?" Jeff asked.

"They're everywhere. Cayman Islands, Latvia, Costa Rica, Belgium, Switzerland. There are a lot more. Many of them right here in the U.S."

"The U.S.?" Jeff said.

"Just touching points I'd guess," Frank answered. "And the other numbers?"

"I'm still working on that. At least one of them is in Connecticut. I think it's all part of the same money distribution and vanishing operation. I don't know if I can run any of the money trails down to a final source, and if I do, if I'll be able penetrate the shell corporations that will be set up. My guess is I can't, not anytime soon, and not without a lot of help." She paused. "What have you got?"

Frank looked to Jeff who cleared his throat. "As you know, the code is designed to exploit its favored position within the Exchange's trading platform. It loots money from specifically defined trades from carefully defined entities. You've confirmed what we suspected, which is that the money then goes offshore as soon as it's generated." Daryl nodded. "We've reached the conclusion that there is at least one inside player. There is definitely someone responsible for the core trading system involved."

"Maybe there is more than one employee involved," Daryl suggested.

"We don't rule out the possibility, but the more there are, the greater the security risk," Frank said. "It seems more likely there is just a single conduit within the Exchange, someone well placed. We aren't ruling out the existence of an extra hand or two, just think it unlikely."

Daryl nodded. "Maybe someone penetrated from outside, and there is no insider."

"We've considered that," Frank said. "But with the single exception of the rootkit the rogue code is too smoothly integrated to the trading functions to be accomplished by outsiders. Someone in the know is doing it. Now, it's possible it's a former employee, or perhaps someone who worked on the system as a contractor. We've not dismissed the possibility they set up a backdoor they're accessing. The stock exchange has undergone many changes these last few years with the creation of the super hubs and the merging of various international trading networks. A lot of people have worked on these projects during that time and one, or some of them, could be responsible. That would be a job for the SEC or the Exchange's security team to undertake. But we think it's someone still there.

"Now the kernel of the trading platform is very sophisticated, very smooth. The code is altered periodically and the rogue code has to be modified with every update of the trading platform's operating system. They do that almost seamlessly. It's difficult to plant anything without attracting the attention of the automatic security audit monitoring. We think that's what the rootkit was about. Someone got a little sloppy and didn't want to put in the time to properly integrate the malware within the system. He took the easy way. It's worked so far with the automated system but it was always vulnerable to being discovered by people like us who'd look for something like that."

"So there is definitely an outside group involved," Daryl said.

"Exactly," Frank agreed. "Someone, somewhere else, is writing the code and keeping it on point."

"Any hints?" she asked.

"More than a hint. We've got a location. The company is called Companhia Cero. It's located in São Paulo."

"Brazil? The bank data has two or three Brazilian banks in it."

"That's to be expected," Frank said. "Any international laundering operation is bound to touch Brazil at some point, even land there eventually. It's tolerant of white-collar criminals so it's a likely end point for people doing something like this."

"So you two think that it's being run out of Brazil?" Daryl asked.

"We don't know," Jeff said. "We just know that's where the New York code is originating. Whether or not it's the origin point we can't say, but someone in São Paulo probably knows the answer. The indicators point there."

"All right. Look, you two have been working with the IT team. You must have met most, even all, of those with the kind of in-house access you suspect is necessary for this operation. Anybody come to mind?"

Frank made a face. "We've kicked it around a bit but to be honest we had our noses to the grindstone when we were there. No one was to know about the penetration test, so we made a point not to mingle much. If we're right, and one or more of them is involved, maybe we spoke to them but it's more likely we just passed them in the hallway."

"Any hints? Brazilians?" She grinned at how obvious that would be.

"No," Jeff said. "You, Frank?"

"No. Not that I know of. There were some Asians, a guy from Italy or Portugal if I got that right, an Aussie. The rest were all native-born Americans from what I could see."

"Anybody can be a crook."

"You got that right," Frank agreed.

"As Frank mentioned," Jeff said, "they've been regularly modifying and updating their code. There's been a sharp increase since we went on the run. That suggests to us they're in a hurry to do something, definitely something big."

"Like what?"

"We don't know. Perhaps you can figure that out."

Daryl paused, then said, "Maybe it's time to go to the SEC with what we have."

"There's a warrant out for our arrest," Frank said. "They'll be eager to lock us up. It'll take days to even get access to someone who'll listen and there's no guarantee it will do any good."

Daryl blanched at the news. "You can try the NYPD, FBI, some other agency." Her voice faltered just a bit.

"We've talked about that but it works out the same way unfortunately."

"How about sending what we've detected to the SEC through back channels, maybe find a source who'll listen."

"Yeah, that's a possibility," Frank said, "but in the end, it comes down to the same thing: two suspects pointing the guilty finger at someone else. It's the same ol' same ol' as far as the SEC's concerned."

"This is absurd!" Daryl blurted. "Hasn't anyone done a background check on you two? If you were crooked, it would have shown up years ago. Frank, you've been an operative, for God's sake. Jeff, just look at all you've done for this country these last years. I just can't believe someone can so easily frame you. It's just not right!"

"We both appreciate that," Frank said. "But I really think we need to pin this down ourselves."

Daryl wiped a wet eye carefully so her mascara wouldn't run. "What's that mean?"

"We need to find the source," Jeff said, "get access to the computers and original code. If we're lucky, we'll locate a body and get him to squeal. Is that still the word?" He looked at each of them in turn.

"You mean tell what he or she knows," Frank said.

"Okay, I can see that," Daryl said. "But how does that work?"

"We think whoever is doing this in São Paulo is a good starting point," Jeff said.

"They might be the origin or they might be a conduit," Frank explained. "We can't tell, but if someone working there doesn't know anything, which we think is highly unlikely, they should lead us to someone who does. We find that someone and suddenly we've got credibility, then all the rest we've come up with falls into place. With a bit of luck we can grab some computers as well. That would ice it."

"What if this magic person doesn't want to talk?"

"Daryl, Daryl," Frank said. "There are ways."

"What are you talking about?"

"I promise, no marks of any kind, but by the time I'm finished they'll squeal like a greased pig." He looked at Jeff. "Squeal I think is the right word."

"This sounds dangerous," Daryl said.

"Staying here is dangerous," Frank said. "The local cops dropped off a flier downstairs earlier today with our photos on it. I was concerned it was them when you knocked. The clerk made a point to show me one. I slipped him a hundred, but that won't hold him long. We've got to move now."

"How hard was identifying São Paulo?" she asked suspiciously.

"Hard, but not impossible," Frank said.

"Tell me," she insisted.

Jeff looked at Frank, who answered. "We received a photograph. They hadn't stripped the metadata and the GPS coordinates map to a warehouse district in São Paulo. Companhia Cero is the only company listed with offices at that location."

"What photograph? Who would send you a photo? Of what? What are you talking about?"

"It was just a . . . gentle warning," Jeff said.

"A warning? In a photograph? Let me see it."

"Daryl, really, that's not necessary," Frank said quietly.

She was stunned. "You two, you're going to get killed, you know that?" She reached into her purse, removed tissue, and blew her nose. As she put it away she said, "They go to the trouble of sending you a photograph and just accidentally leave the GPS in it. Someone is baiting you. They just put out the hook and you're going to bite. You've thought of that, right?"

"First idea we had," Frank said. "But we can't stay here and São Paulo is the only physical lead we've got, tainted or not. And Brazil is perhaps the best place in the world for us to go right now."

"And how does that work, exactly?" she asked.

Frank looked offended. He pulled open one of the top drawers in the dresser. "Here." He handed over two Canadian passports.

Daryl fingered them both, then leafed through the pages, scrutinizing the visa stamps. "Are these any good?" she asked. "They look all right to me but will they pass?"

"They're as good as originals. In fact, they are originals except for the fact the final product wasn't officially created, though the Canadian computers say they were. And there's a credit card or two to go with each of them, but we'll only use them where cash will raise suspicions."

Daryl looked distraught as she handed the passports back. "So when are you going?"

Frank checked his watch. "We're leaving here in about an hour. We're booked out of Newark, changing planes in Miami, then on to São Paulo. We'll be there midday tomorrow; then we'll work on finding the location."

"Frank, please. Do you really know what you're doing? You could end up in a Brazilian prison the way you're talking."

"It'll be fine. You'll see. Trust me." Frank's smile was dazzling.

45

ENFORCEMENT DIVISION
SECURITIES AND EXCHANGE COMMISSION
NEW YORK REGIONAL OFFICE
200 VESSEY STREET
NEW YORK CITY
2:41 P.M.

Susan Flores rose from her desk, stretched her body with exaggeration as her yoga instructor had once taught her, repeated the movement three times, then slowly drew several deep breaths. She held each, then released them slowly.

She acknowledged the others working on her way to the ladies' room. A computer forensics expert, she'd worked for Robert Alshon for nearly two years. Her specialty was the NYSE Euronext software architecture and specifically the trading system security mechanisms. This particular examination had proved problematic, since she didn't know that much about malware, which was beyond the scope of her usual tasks. The NYSE IT computer security team did great work in her estimation, and she had always been careful not to step on their toes in the past. She'd made several requests for their resources, asking for data and access to log files and trading records. Though she had a court order, it was better if this was all done cooperatively. There'd be other investigations after all.

She'd been flattered when Alshon selected her as his go-to contact for such work. It was a big step up so early in her career. But the man was more than a little intimidating to work for and not very forgiving of failure. He'd made more than a few enemies even since she'd joined his team, and she didn't want to go down that path. He demanded nothing less than excellence, and she wasn't surprised he'd been divorced twice. She didn't want to think what he must be like to live with.

Susan Flores had been raised in Tucson, Arizona, the oldest child of Mexican immigrants. She'd attended the University of Arizona, majoring in economics and computer science. She'd gone to work at the IT department of Nabisco after graduation and it was there she'd become interested in computer security. Though she'd been uneasy about moving to Manhattan, she loved her job with the SEC. It was a great place to apply her education, training, and experience. The only real downside was Alshon being so difficult to work with. As a result she lived in constant fear of perceived failure and worked under stress she'd not had before her move.

After stopping by the restroom, Flores went for coffee and considered why she felt so uneasy on this assignment. She had it. Alshon was behaving with an excess of passion. She was reluctant to admit it, but it seemed to her the fact that he'd once been with the FBI and that the targets in this case had formerly been CIA had a lot to do with it. She recalled previous disparaging comments he'd made about the CIA. Up to then, his attitude hadn't seemed to influence his work but now she wasn't so sure.

Red Zoya wasn't the only examination on her desk. She'd been doing other important work, but he had her drop everything to work on this. And it wasn't going as expected.

She poured some kind of artificial creamer into her black coffee and considered again how unhealthy her job was. Proper exercise was challenging. She enjoyed Central Park but so did most of the city on beautiful days. Sure, she could get off on a subway stop farther from the office, but finding time was difficult. She'd given up yoga and saw how quickly she was slipping away from what she'd been taught. It was so easy to turn into one more fat computer nerd. Maintaining fitness had been easier in Tucson, a bit challenging in New Jersey, but in Manhattan it was proving almost impossible.

Flores closed her eyes for a moment. When had she last slept more than an hour? She couldn't remember. Two nights, at least.

She was to meet with Alshon later and mentally reviewed what she would tell him. Aiken and Renkin, her targets, had to be part of a much larger operation. She estimated as many as half a dozen software writers were involved, though she understood that such estimates were inexact. What she was sure of was that no two men were doing this.

The success and expanse of the penetration had come as a shock to her.

She realized it had been a bit naïve on her part, but she'd honestly believed that it was impossible for someone to hack the Exchange's trading platform. She found the reality more than a little unsettling.

Her most recent forensics data drop from the trading engines contained an updated version of the malware, confirming that the operation was ongoing. NYSE IT remained unaware of the malware's existence and as a result they had yet to shut this operation down. She wanted to take her findings to her contacts there, but Alshon had explicitly instructed her not to. He didn't want to act before he had a clear view of the extent of the infiltration, especially if there was an insider involved. Tipping their hand prematurely could result in the destruction of evidence or, worse, a rash act by the culprits or even the NYSE IT department that could take a bad situation and make it a disaster.

This was a complex and widespread operation, delicately interwoven within the kernel of the trading platform. Even after they were alerted NYSE IT would move cautiously and it would take more than a few days to act as they'd be concerned about disrupting normal operations by committing an error in negating the malware. The law of unintended consequences flourished in just such situations, especially when things were rushed.

The speed and size of the updates was just one reason she was certain so many people were involved. And it was ridiculous to think that two men on the run were making the recent changes from a hotel room somewhere. The scope and frequency of the additions and changes suggested to her an urgency by the hackers, and she increasingly felt a sense of unease that something very bad was about to happen, as if she and her colleagues at NYSE IT were the lookouts on the *Titanic*, who'd just spotted the iceberg dead ahead.

Which only heightened her suspicion. As she'd told Alshon, it wasn't her place to analyze motives and character but the casual way Aiken had set up his brokerage account shocked her. He was surely cleverer than that. She'd researched his company and saw the rave reviews it received. Renkin was more difficult to research, as his computer career had been in the CIA, but she'd found no hint of concern about him or his work.

Not for the first time did she wonder if Alshon had this wrong. Her suggestion that the two had been set up was slowly turning into an opinion, one she knew would be unwelcome. She reminded herself to stay focused on what the code was doing. That was troubling enough.

Flores returned to her desk, sipped the hot coffee, set the cup down, then placed her face into her hands, her eyes burning slightly. Should she risk a nap? She feared she'd be down for the count if she did.

This high-frequency trading algo malware deeply concerned her. It was manipulating trades across the spectrum, and she suspected it was stealing money from them. She could see how the funds were routed out of the system, scattered about into what she believed were various banks and trusts. It had all the hallmarks of a classic financial fraud operation. The difference was its level of sophistication, its presence within the NYSE trading engines, and the implementation of a HFT algo. It was like multiple bank robberies occurring simultaneously on fast forward and the implications were staggering.

Flores sighed and went back to work. Her job was to tie these two to the operation. Failing that, she was to see where it led and who else was involved, if possible. It was up to Alshon to make the command decisions. She just hoped he knew what he was doing.

46

Pedro Bandeira couldn't recall the last time he'd put in so many hours. Now, with blinding speed, everything was coming to an end. When this was over, he'd decided, he'd start his own computer company, providing legitimate services. Much of what they did was in fact not illegal and would be of use to companies. He'd even take his staff with him.

This idea of assuming the leadership of the Nosso Lugar after his father, something his mother frequently brought up, was absurd. He'd never be a criminal, at least not like his father was. What Pedro wanted was a quiet way out of what he was doing, a way to lead a normal life in the years to come.

Pedro turned his mind to business. What was nagging at him was his concern as to whether or not they could really pull this off. Right now it didn't look to him as if it were possible. They were being asked to do the impossible.

In his last conversation with Abílio in New York he'd been sure he detected some doubt in his counterpart as well. Pedro might not have liked the subordinate role he'd held for most of the last five years, but he'd never doubted his boss's expertise. Abílio was on-site. He saw everything firsthand. If *he* was worried, Pedro knew he had every reason to be as well.

Grupo Técnico had the Universal Trading Platform code for the NYSE engines. Obtaining it had been time consuming, and one of Abílio's jobs was to ensure their version was always current. This gave them an engine core behaving exactly as it did at the New Jersey hub. They ran new and modified code within a simulated framework where they placed bids and offers and observed how their code worked in the complex environment. This allowed them to confirm it worked as predicted before insertion into the live trading engines.

They'd made several revisions to their code in recent days without difficulty but now they'd received a copy of the latest NYSE code drop the Exchange was uploading in preparation for the major IPO on Wednesday. And that had thrown a monkey wrench into their plans because the revised code was now incompatible with their simulation framework. The parameters of the various internal subroutine calls had been changed significantly, and his team was having a hard time understanding their purpose. Their limited goal was to get their own software functioning properly and every few hours, they thought they had it, but each time they ran a test with the latest code the simulator either hung up or crashed. They seemed no closer to a resolution now than they'd been when they'd run their first test.

Renata had given him a progress report earlier that afternoon. Five billion dollars of the Wednesday take was to come from several Casas de Férias operations against specifically targeted companies. They still hadn't identified enough of them but most troubling was that, in her view, they had too few holding accounts and an insufficient number of exit channels for the money.

"I'm worried that it can be traced," she'd said. "We haven't generated enough targets to properly conceal it. There's another concern as well."

"What?"

"Ten billion is dangerous, Pedro. I know this is going to be a big IPO and there will be a lot of action surrounding it but that is a great deal of money. There's the potential of something beyond our control going very wrong and we'll get swept up in it."

"I pointed that out and was told to go ahead anyway."

"All right. But what if we cause a crash in the market? Something really serious? It could be very bad for us."

He'd told her that he understood and sent her back to work. She'd raised the very question that most troubled him. An IPO of this size was drawing players who controlled unimaginable sums of money. These HFTs would be using their sophisticated algos to break the IPO their way. He simply couldn't predict how that would affect Carnaval. He hoped those wouldn't influence Carnaval at all, but the more he read about the Toptical buzz, the more concerned he became.

Should he talk to his father again? He looked at his staff. He'd have to give them a break. The botched update was a warning. If he continued to demand they work like this, there'd be more mistakes, and he didn't dare risk that, not with what was on the line.

His Skype program rang. Pedro opened it, then accepted the call. "My son," Bandeira said, "how are things going?"

"We're working on the last update. I don't know if we can get it ready before Wednesday morning."

"It must be done," Bandeira snapped, then smiled. "You can do it, Pedro. I know you can."

"It's like I told you before, I have too few people for all the work we have to do. If you scaled back how much you plan to take, things would be much easier."

"That's not possible."

"As you wish. The good news is that our IPO algo looks good. We just have to get it working properly with the new code. We're also having a problem with the other targets. They are scattered and it is more complicated."

"Pedro, I have made commitments. The figure I've given is the one you must reach."

"I'm doing my best, Father, but you are asking a great deal."

"Just do it! We'll talk Tuesday night, and I expect everything to be in place. Now, enough of your complaining. Be a man for once!" Bandeira ended the call.

Pedro sat back in his chair. This was the ugly side of his father, the one he despised. How many times had he been treated like this over the years? Too many. He considered what would happen if he missed the target, or if there was a disaster beyond his control. What would his father do?

Nothing significant to him, he realized. Humiliate him, shut down the operation, force him into a lowly job, but he couldn't help feeling concern for his staff. He'd heard stories about what his father did to those who disappointed him. Until recently he'd not believed them. He could see the top of Renata's head from where he sat. Would his father really kill her, a single mother?

There was a gnawing in the pit of his stomach. He knew the answer.

As for the $10 billion, Pedro knew what that was all about. Ego, greed, the pleasure his father took in setting an impossible demand and then insisting it be met. It was to be $10 billion because his father said so. There was no other reason.

47

Jeff examined his Canadian passport, wondering exactly how Frank had managed to get one for each of them so quickly. Not only had he accomplished it on short notice, but he also expressed absolute confidence in them.

Jeff wasn't so sure. He ran his thumb across its surface. It definitely *felt* official. It looked it as well, on the cover and inside. But passports were now linked into vast computer networks. You didn't just have to fool an individual when boarding the plane or when clearing immigration on arrival; you had to fool a sophisticated database.

He looked again at his new name: Douglas Bennett.

Was he even real? Or was the name simply a creation?

He'd asked Frank for specifics, but his friend had simply smiled, then patted his arm. "Let me worry about details. You just get well and take it easy."

Easy to say but Jeff couldn't help but be concerned. And if they were caught leaving the country, he didn't want to think how badly that would reflect on them. Not one official would believe they were on their way to prove their innocence. They'd interpret this as two fugitives fleeing to avoid getting caught.

What a mess. Jeff slipped the passport back into the inside pocket of his jacket and closed his eyes. Frank was off buying water, snacks, and pain pills. Jeff was feeling better all the time, but right now couldn't remember the last time he'd felt so run-down. And he still had a ten-hour flight ahead of him.

He placed his hands on his head, inadvertently touching the tender spot. He'd removed the bandages before sneaking out of the hotel in Manhattan. He'd not said anything to Frank, but he wondered if he had internal bleeding on his brain, some slow seepage that would send him into a coma and kill him. He'd done an Internet search on the subject. There would be no symptoms until it was almost too late. That's why patients with head injuries were kept in hospitals until the doctor was certain.

The airport was busy. Planes landed and took off every few minutes. Hordes of travelers moved about, usually in waves going one direction or another, pulling luggage behind them, wearing backpacks, texting and talking on their phones as they went. Not for the first time, he stared in amazement at the clothes people chose to wear on airplanes. The businessmen and women were obvious enough and there were a large number in cargo pants, comfortable walking shoes, and polo shirts. But the others . . . He had vague memories from his childhood when people dressed up to take a flight because such occasions were special and everyone wanted to look their best. Now the clothes looked pulled from a charity bin.

Seeing Daryl again had been both wonderful and awkward. He'd been relieved to see her looking good. He realized that he'd been worried about her but saw she'd flourished away from him. San Francisco apparently suited her. He'd considered embracing her as a longtime friend, but he'd hesitated, not sure the gesture would be welcome, and by then the moment had passed. From there on the personal aspect of seeing each other went downhill.

Daryl had talked mostly to Frank, only occasionally looking at him. Her departure had been as awkward for him as her arrival. So in the end, he was left with the work she'd done and with that he was very satisfied.

"Jeff! Jeff Aiken!" someone called.

Jeff looked up and spotted a woman in her fifties smiling as she walked up to him. Agnes Capps was wearing her distinctive purple glasses and was dressed in flamboyant Gypsy style, a mauve scarf wrapped about her neck with a flourish. She was a writer who late in life had carved out a niche for herself reporting and speaking on cybersecurity issues. Though not generally well regarded by computer security experts, as she tended to gloss over details and occasionally got things wrong, she was popular with various news shows. She produced a weekly article and a book nearly every year.

"My word," Agnes said, "imagine running into you here of all places." She sat beside him, a bit winded from her rush over. "Where are you off to? Or are you just coming back?"

Jeff had last seen Agnes the year before at CyberCon in San Diego. She'd been on one of the discussion panels. It had been unique in that the hacktivist group Anonymous had joined remotely.

Jeff didn't want to lie, but then, he was traveling under a false identity. "Where are you off to?" he asked, answering her with a question of his own.

"Back home to beautiful Oklahoma City, if a tornado hasn't flattened the homestead. I've been doing some research here. You would be shocked at what the U.S. government is secretly doing with all this social networking information people put out there so casually. It's like *Brave New World* or *1984*, one of those books. They know everything about us—*absolutely* everything—and they don't even have to listen in to our telephone calls."

"I doubt much would surprise me," he said. "They have the ability to collect it and from their perspective, why not? They've got a country to keep safe."

She snorted. "That's what they say but it's not true, believe me. You know," she whispered, "I think that kind of information was used to influence that last presidential election. That's why the polls were so far off." She looked around to check that no one was listening. "I can prove the government used mass fake social networking accounts in the campaign, coordinated across Facebook, Toptical, and Twitter, and that they planted online articles to influence public opinion. They softened public outrage against the IRS, NSA, and other scandals with those same tactics." She moved even closer, her body touching Jeff's, and with her lips nearly touching his ear said, "If the truth were known, it would come out that the NSA is engaging in wholesale securities fraud to fund government black budget projects. They've been at it for years."

What to say? "It wouldn't surprise me a bit."

"So . . . where are you off to?"

"Just coming back. Going home."

"Ah, well, that's always nice, isn't it? And how is the lovely Daryl? I've not seen her in ages."

"Good." He hesitated. "But we're not together anymore."

Agnes raised her eyebrows. "She's a keeper, young man. You can take it from me. Don't let her get away." She glanced at her watch. "I must be off." She stood. "See you soon."

Jeff watched her walk away with a wave of relief.

"Agnes is looking good," Frank said as he joined him. "I thought I'd wait until she left. Did you mention me?"

"No. I told her I was on my way to D.C."

"Good. Keep it simple, logical. What say we check into international departures and get that out of the way?"

They took their carry-ons with them and entered the security checkpoint. Jeff held his breath as the heavyset woman accepted his passport, scanned it, looked at the screen for several seconds, then handed it back. He moved on, placed his laptop into a container, shoes and belt, wallet, keys and change into another. The alarm sounded when he went through the machine, and a stoic man had him pass through again, this time without incident. Jeff recovered his items and sat down to put his shoes back on.

"So far, so good," he said as Frank sat beside him.

"Don't think about it."

The pair walked down the long hallway to their departure lounge. Two hours later, they boarded. Another woman looked at his passport, matched it to his boarding pass, then let him on. Jeff didn't breathe easy until they were in the air.

Now all he had to worry about was clearing immigration in São Paulo.

48

Though her part of the operation was to follow the money, Daryl instead turned her attention to the code itself. She reasoned that Jeff and Frank had been in motion since the previous day, and she knew they'd had little if any time to work on the rogue code.

Frank had sent her a summary of their findings and suspicions before the pair left. She'd spent late Saturday night reviewing the code and tinkering with the malware. Now all day Sunday, she'd devoted herself again to the task.

She'd reached some conclusions, which to her seemed self-evident. She'd traced the stolen money to the bank accounts through which it was routed. According to Frank's report, they'd decided that the money originated from outside traders, not from accounts within the Exchange itself.

This made a great deal of sense to her. If they were taking money from within the trading software of the Exchange, then security would easily discover it. But if they took the money from someone making a trade, then routed it through the Exchange, they could diffuse suspicion to any number of targets. And since none of the thieves were part of the NYSE, it would not be of concern to its ongoing security efforts.

So just as the money was dispersed into hundreds of bank accounts so too was it likely taken from a vast array of traders and brokers. As she worked the heavily obfuscated code in the malware she eventually located a store of

IDs and what appeared to be trade amounts. She looked through the documents Jeff and Frank had gathered, remembering that one was a spreadsheet that listed the IDs the Exchange assigned to stocks. Sure enough, the IDs in the malware matched the ones in the spreadsheet. Attached to them as well were other symbols but a bit of research revealed them to be prefix designations to identify the type of trading vehicle.

One of the symbols was that for Toptical, TPTC. That was no surprise. Now that it was about to be publicly traded, it needed one—and starting Wednesday, it was going to be a heavily traded stock, at least initially. Its presence within the malware told her that the IPO was going to be a target.

As she knew little about them, Daryl researched IPOs to see what prior experience said on the subject. Major IPOs, she learned, created enormous volatility in the market during the first few hours. This occurred because there was pent-up demand by those who used the product, which in cases like this one represented millions of people. Toptical was enormously popular and a great number of the faithful users were going to want to own a piece of the action.

Another reason was that the public generally had a positive opinion of IPOs. There was the undeserved belief that they were always successful and that those who got on board early did very well. There were plenty of public offerings to testify against that opinion, but for some reason, that reality didn't capture the public consciousness.

Then there was the host of brokers representing hundreds of thousands if not millions of clients. Public offerings were always a part of their portfolios and in this case they'd be under pressure to take part. There were as well hedge and retirement funds, enormous piles of cash looking to diversify under favorable conditions.

There were also speculators, individuals and traders who believed they understood the market better than most and were persuaded they saw an opportunity. Some of them would buy early and if a specific price point was reached late Wednesday, they'd sell, looking to make their money quick and easy. Others would gamble that the stock was overpriced. They would sell short and make their money during the price collapse.

Finally, there were the high-frequency traders, some of which fronted those big piles of cash. The difference with them was their ability to incrementally manipulate the price, then exploit the conditions they'd created. They were seen as major factors in previous IPOs, and they relentlessly expanded their algos, tweaking their systems for each new opportunity. They could make money on the rise, on the fall, and on the thousands of variations in price in the meanwhile. They would have enormous influence on the IPO, especially in establishing a perceived level of trade volume.

What concerned her was that Jeff and Frank had already concluded that the rogue code was itself a high-frequency trader and whoever was behind it had gone to a lot of trouble to get the two of them out of the way. The only conclusion she could take from that was that they'd been too close. The malware wasn't just any high-frequency trader; it was a trader without a monetary reserve. In other words, it had no backing. In the real world it could be said that in many, if not most, cases it made its play by some form of cheating.

Looking at the data dumps that Jeff and Frank's code had funneled out of the engine to her C2 servers via the backdoor, Daryl observed the code had been updated twice since the Exchange had loaded its new IPO software and updated its trading platform code. Now TPTC seemed to be interlaced everywhere within it. A third update that afternoon disclosed it as the rogue code's primary target, the numbers controlling the size and frequency of the trading skims representing as much as half of all the projected rogue code action.

How much would that be? she wondered. What she saw convinced her it was more than a billion dollars.

She turned her attention to the malware's trading logic, carefully stepping through it and following the numbers flow across it and into functions that were obviously its connections with the actual NYSE trading engine. After several hours, she decided that she could make an estimate of how much money it had siphoned out of legitimate trades in the last year, $50 to $100 million.

Employing this information as a baseline, she now tried to determine how much action the latest code and configuration were designed for when it came to Toptical. She knew her best estimate would be inexact, that it had to be inexact because even those who wrote the algo didn't know with precision how many opportunities it would encounter on IPO day. But even an imprecise estimate was better than a guess.

Seven to fifteen billion dollars. That was the potential spread.

Daryl was staggered. She double-, then triple-checked her analysis, but the results didn't change. Hadn't one of the significant problems with the market been caused by a much smaller trade? After a few minutes, she found it. On a day in which total volume was $200 billion, the Flash Crash had been caused by a trade of just $4 billion.

She wrote up a report of her findings to the "boys," as she thought of them, concluding, "I'm no expert, but if these guys are looking to take seven to fifteen billion Wednesday, that is going to cause a great deal of economic trouble. And if there is a problem with the rogue code, or with HFTs or with the NYSE's new trading software, we could be looking at a disaster worse than 1929. These exchanges worldwide are so interlinked that a multibillion-dollar scam of this sort could be the catalyst for truly terrible events. Look at what that harmless bot has done to the market. There's another editorial in the NYT today attacking security at the Exchange. The market is expected to fall even more tomorrow because of lost confidence. If Wednesday is a disaster, I don't even want to think what the consequences will be. We need to stop this!"

Daryl stepped away from her laptop and prepared for bed, scrubbing her face, combing out her hair, brushing her teeth. She was tired but knew she could still put in several hours yet. Back at the desk she connected to one of the C2 servers and looked for a new data dump from the engine, but found none. She checked and saw that the jump server backdoor was not in the logs. They had either been discovered and shut down, or some change in the Exchange's security configuration was blocking their outbound access.

Her shoulders sank as the reality set in. They were cut off from access into the Exchange beyond the jump server, with no access to the rogue code or chance to trace it back to whoever was planting it. She tried again. No luck. After sitting for several long minutes in shock and dismay, she composed herself and sent another message to Jeff and Frank. "Beacon is down on the backside."

Daryl stood up. What to do? How much more could she learn on a computer? How much could she expect to accomplish from her hotel room? Where could she best spend the next day?

She undressed, then climbed into the shower, soaping head to foot, scrubbing herself clean as she emptied her mind. Outside the shower as she toweled off it came to her.

Plan B. Boots on the ground and all that. There wasn't much time. Still . . .

She was humming as she set her alarm and crawled between the sheets.

DAY EIGHT
MONDAY, SEPTEMBER 17

HIGH-FREQUENCY TRADERS POISED TO EXPLOIT TOPTICAL IPO

By Arnie Willoughby
September 17

As the next major IPO approaches, high-frequency traders are gearing up for what promises to be an eventful and highly profitable day. "HFTs make real money on big trading days with plenty of volatility," Shannon Woodruff, publisher of the highly regarded *Woodruff Report,* said in remarks earlier this week. "The Toptical IPO promises to provide both."

High-frequency traders, or HFTs as they are more commonly known, earn enormous profits by exploiting small changes in stock valuation. They identify these changes before anyone else, then complete their trades at lightning speed. Backed by billions of dollars they are the 800-pound gorilla in the stock market and Woodruff says they are able to bully their way through traditional traders.

"With enough capital, the latest algos, and proximity hosting, HFTs have a disproportionate advantage over everyone else," Woodruff said. "The NYSE regulators are moving too slowly and too ineffectually to rein them in." The price investors pay because of their dominate place in trading is a higher cost for the securities they buy, or reduced earnings for those they sell. "The HFTs scoop up the difference even though they serve no meaningful role in public trading," Woodruff observed. "They are the three-card monte game of the stock market."

High-frequency traders have been with us since the beginning of programmed computer trading. The advantages computers brought with their incredible speed and the ability to handle enormous volumes of data were recognized from the start. HFTs are always one step ahead of regulators in their latest exploits. "Despite recent changes in law the SEC essentially cleans up after them," Woodruff said. "They give the illusion the HFTs are under control, but they are not. It's the Wild West out there, and IPOs are the major shootouts."

Though HFTs prefer to remain under the radar, it is becoming increasingly difficult for them to remain out of sight as they now account for the overwhelming majority of all security trades. While the Toptical IPO is officially being downplayed as just one more major public offering, unofficially key investors believe it has the potential of being the largest IPO in world history. "Investors are eager for the next big thing, and their desire may well be a self-fulfilling prophecy," Woodruff said. "If that is true, we could be headed for disaster. The HFTs have never been greedier. They know heavier regulation is inevitable at some point. This may be their last shot at a big killing."

He cautions that increasingly HFTs behave in unison and that could spell trouble in the wrong circumstances. We'll find out Wednesday.

READ MORE: HIGH-FREQUENCY TRADING, NYSE, TOPTICAL IPO

US Computer News, Inc.

49

CHARLES STREET
GREENWICH VILLAGE
NEW YORK CITY
9:13 A.M.

Richard Iyers leaned back in his chair and considered the weekend with distaste. Bored Saturday night, he'd gone to the Union Jack where he'd been pleased to spot the blonde he'd had his eye on for several weeks. She was even mildly intoxicated and in a playful mood, which made everything he had in mind that much easier. She'd seen him there before, and he had no trouble striking up a conversation. She was with a brunette girlfriend who was playing darts.

Iyers was his engaging best, and shortly after midnight, the pair had stumbled out of the bar and taken a taxi to his apartment. The rest had been by the numbers, and while in his view there was no such thing as bad sex, this had been a near thing. First and inexplicably, she'd wanted to be coy. After that, she'd wanted to be coaxed. He'd played her game, more than a little disgusted by it and with himself. Then it turned out that she had no imagination and was easily put off by almost everything he wanted. Worse, she didn't like it rough, getting angry at one point, and the last thing he wanted right now was trouble, so he'd reined it in and settled for the ride. Disappointing was the word for it, especially when he realized—too late—that she wasn't a natural blonde.

He'd wanted her to leave, but she passed out almost as soon as he was finished, and he'd been kept awake by her snoring. The only real fun had been Sunday morning, when he'd made her pay the price. He'd taken her without preamble, hard and fast, not given her any time to warm up to the experience. That had pissed her off, and she'd slammed the door on the way out.

Iyers smiled at the memory.

He peered idly out the opening of his cubicle. So what to do about Marc? The guy had him working like a maniac. The trading platform had been updated, and Marc alerted him that the Carnaval program was itself both updated and expanded at the same time. The changes had proved problematic and Iyers labored to fix the mess. He still wasn't sure it was functioning properly. And he understood Rio was still laboring over yet more changes.

Iyers was irritated with Marc for leaning on him so hard. He'd done little but give Iyers hell about his use of the rootkit, describing it as sloppy. What Campos refused to admit was that he'd placed Iyers under undue pressure, had imposed an arbitrary deadline that had left Iyers with little choice except to take a shortcut. He'd intended to fix it later but it worked so well and was so unlikely to be detected that, in the end, he'd left it alone. The code was clever and would give them an extra layer of protection from snooping eyes. Now Marc had seen to an upgrade that was worse than anything Iyers had ever done.

And Marc still claimed he was getting no outside help. What a joke.

Iyers was glad the end for Vacation Homes was in sight even if his future plans weren't yet set. The sooner he was rid of Marc, the better, in his view. The guy was a wimp. Iyers was seriously considering demanding he be paid what he was owed before doing anything more. Marc needed him right now, and there'd never be a better time. But with so much more money on the table he cautioned himself not to risk it.

The only thing he really felt good about now was how effectively Marc had run Red Zoya out of the building. That had been sweet. At first, he was worried when he'd not killed Aiken, but in the end, it didn't matter. That ham-handed frame job Marc planted had done the trick. The SEC had stormed the place like the Gestapo. They'd all but stripped the office the pair used and spread suspicion around the office.

It was perfect. Rumors were flying everywhere about the looting of accounts, and not just by Aiken and Renkin. The story was they were all going to be served with subpoenas. People were talking about hiring lawyers. Now he heard that Aiken had left the hospital without permission and that the two men were on the run. It couldn't have worked out any better.

Then there was the media hype about that bot they'd had weeks earlier.

Newspapers were questioning the ability of the Exchange to maintain the security of their trading system. Stenton was more than his usual nervous wreck. Iyers's only concern was the stumbling stock market. He couldn't anticipate how that would influence the Toptical IPO. Traders might stay away, reducing the volume, which would give Carnaval a greater possibility of exposure, or they might jump in with both feet, looking to make up losses incurred these last few days. There was just no way to know.

Iyers turned to what he'd been doing. With its acceleration and the dominance of Carnaval, the end time for Vacation Homes was in sight. He checked his watch. It was important to his future that Carnaval go off like clockwork. There were less than forty-eight hours to go. And the code still looked like crap.

50

Samantha Mason watched the blanket of heavy fog from her office window, feeling as depressed as she ever had in her life. In the distance came the moan of the warning foghorn. She wondered why she'd ever thought she liked San Francisco.

It was an utterly artificial city, smug in its conceit and political correctness. Families were being systematically driven out and the upwardly mobile singles who remained were consumed with themselves. And it was cold, and wet. She longed for the sunny Valley. Even the burning heat of a Valley summer was preferable to this.

She glanced at the final prospectus. She'd consulted with her attorney the previous Friday to hear her options again and learned there were no new ones. Her attorney was a pro at this, having specialized in dot-coms from the first. He'd been down this road with other clients. "Take the money," he'd said, "bide your time under the terms of the IPO, then sell as much stock as you like and leave. You have your whole life ahead of you. You can do whatever you like, including starting another company if that's what you want."

Sound advice, Sam knew. Her own preference, to facilitate a takeover by an established company that would have given them the terms they wanted, had been rejected. Everyone, except for Molly Riskin, had their eye set on maximizing the money. Nothing was getting done, not a bit of work. All the talk was about Wednesday's IPO and how much they'd all soon be worth.

Gordon Chan was wandering the hallways with that smirk on his face, as if he were the master magician who'd pulled this off. Even Adam Stallings had lapsed into uncharacteristic cynicism.

Poor Molly. She looked as if she was having a breakdown. She'd developed an uncontrollable facial tic and was now wearing so much makeup, her face looked painted on. She was like a wound-up toy as she wandered the hallways. Sam had told her to go home, as much because she couldn't stand to see her in this state, as for concern about her.

For three days Sam had studied the prospectus, and she found it no more reassuring than she had when she'd first read it. There were red flags woven throughout it. The IPO was oversubscribed. Worse, much worse, she'd asked Adam to call his contact at the Exchange's IT department for an update on their new IPO software. "It stinks," he'd told her Sunday, when he'd agreed to meet at a Starbucks. "My contact says it's so buggy, managers are starting to distance themselves from it. A senior executive even argued it not be implemented as the potential for disaster is so great."

"Then why are they going forward? They don't need another black eye. Just look at all the heat they're taking about security because of some bot that crept into their system."

"You know bureaucracy. They publicly committed. They aren't going to back away from it. It's up to the software engineers to make it happen. And if it fails, they'll be forced to take the blame."

"It won't be that easy."

"No, it won't." Adam had grimaced. "You're right about this, Sam. I just wish Brian had listened."

Brian. Mr. Cool.

She knew better. How many nights when they'd still been lovers did he confide to her how out of his depth he felt, how overwhelming the sudden growth of Toptical was? Since they'd come to an end, the situation had only become more intense, the company even larger. He had a new girlfriend now, some model he'd met a few months earlier. Sam saw her just once, but it had been obvious she was a gold digger. She hoped Brian knew how to write a prenup because he was going to need it.

The foghorn moaned again. Enough, Sam thought. Enough.

She stood up and went to Brian's office, walking right past his secretary. Inside, she found him talking on his cell phone, the look on his face making it clear to her it was a personal call, and she had no doubt who was on the other end, sharpening her fangs.

"We need to talk," Sam said, then sat down.

"I'll get back to you," Brian said, looking up at Sam. Pause. "Same too huh." She knew the phrase. It was the one he'd used with her. "What's up?"

"Brian, you know I'm very unhappy with how our IPO has been handled. I understand the decision to not seek a takeover was made by the group and don't blame you alone. That's not why I'm talking to you."

"So why are you talking to me? This is a very busy time."

Sam smiled unpleasantly. "Yes, 'same too huh.' Must be busy indeed." She couldn't help herself.

Brian glared at her. "Why don't you get to the point?"

"The point is that I'm out of here. I'm taking everything I'm legally able to, selling as quickly as the terms of the IPO allow, then I'm exiting. No comment to the media, nice going away party, then I'm outta here. Okay?"

Sam had expected that Brian would have been relieved to see her gone. New management was coming on board shortly. He'd have his hands full with them. Not having to deal with her would only make his life simpler.

Instead, squirming in his seat, he said, "Samantha, please, don't do this."

"Excuse me?"

Brian cleared his throat, then continued, "We started this. It was the two of us." He paused. "We're a team."

"Team? Brian, we haven't been a team ever since the IPO date was set. There isn't a single idea I've proposed you adopted. You've shot them all down."

"I don't think it's been that drastic."

"It has. I can give it to you point by point if need be."

"If that's true, then I'm sorry you think it's been personal. I've been making decisions for the good of the company. I've turned away ideas from everyone." He smiled wanly. "You're not the only one who's mad at me."

"I'm not mad, Brian. I'm just tired and more than a bit disgusted."

"Disgusted?" He gestured expansively. "Toptical is what we set out to make it. If anything, it's more than we imagined. And neither of us dreamed it would become a reality so fast, mean so much to so many."

"You sound like Molly."

"I guess I do. But it's true."

"I'm disgusted by the greed. Have you walked the hallways lately? Seen the groups standing around speculating about how much money they're going to make in two days?"

"I've seen it. I've even tried to get people back on track but for everyone here this is the biggest event of their life."

"I guess. I just hope it doesn't turn out to be the biggest in my life. That's why I'm leaving."

"Samantha." He hadn't called her that in two years. "Sam, don't make this final. Stick with me . . . us. We need you. It'll get better once we have this thing behind us. All the distraction, the money guys, that'll be over."

Sam shook her head slowly. Brian sounded sincere, but she knew he was fooling himself. "No, it won't. Starting Thursday, every day before you come to the office, you'll have checked our stock price. Every day. And when you sit in this office, every single decision you make will be driven to some degree or another by the need to keep that price up. What you've been through this last year? It's the new norm for Toptical. And I want no part of it. I can see that now. When I do something like this again, I won't repeat the mistake of going public. I'll keep it small, closely held and private. It'll be my thing, not some public monstrosity."

"I had no idea that's what you think of Toptical. A monstrosity."

Sam hesitated. "It just came out, Brian, but now that I think about it, yes, 'monstrosity' is the right word for it. And what's this about needing me? You haven't needed me, personally or professionally, in nearly two years."

"That's not true. That's not true at all. Is that what this is about? You're the one who ended us, not me." His voice dropped to a whisper. "I begged you, Samantha. I begged you not to leave me."

Sam didn't know how to respond. She said nothing for a long moment. "You left me, Brian. You shut me out. It was over but you couldn't see it. You were too full of—" She looked around the room, taking in the entire building. "—all this to even know it." There was a very long pause. Her throat ached. She said, "You broke my heart."

Brian rose, turned to the window behind him, and stared into the fog. Neither spoke for a long time. "You know I'll do whatever I can to make this easy for you, Samantha. I hope . . . I sincerely hope you'll change your mind." Just then, his cell phone rang. He picked it up. "I have to take this."

"Of course you do," Sam said, then left the room.

51

PACIFIC EASTERN BANK
BELL STREET BRANCH
STAMFORD, CONNECTICUT
11:39 A.M.

Dressed in a navy blue business suit and carrying an oversize matching purse, Daryl stepped from the train platform and walked the short distance to the bank branch. She paused, reached into her purse, removed a mirror, and checked her appearance. She slipped on a pair of glasses that didn't distort too much, which she'd picked up at a secondhand store and gazed at her image. With her hair pulled back, she decided she looked like a porn star pretending to be a schoolteacher. She closed her eyes. The things I do, she thought.

Daryl had intended to tell Jeff and Frank about this when they met, but after they'd said they were leaving for Brazil, she decided not to. She knew they'd have just tried to talk her out of it. The reality was that she'd never develop the information they needed working from her hotel room. She was fairly confident this would work. Every woman, certainly every reasonably attractive one, had used her femininity to her advantage at one time or another in life, though she'd always disdained such tactics.

This bank was one of the landing spots for the money streaming out of the country from the rogue code and was within easy reach of Manhattan. She placed a smile on her face, walked through the doors, and went directly to the sign-in sheet.

"Welcome to Pacific Eastern Bank. May I help you?" the receptionist asked.

"You may. I just need a few minutes."

"Mr. Scofield is with a customer right now, but can be with you in a few minutes. Just have a seat. Can I get you coffee?"

"No, I'm fine. Thanks." Daryl took a seat from where she could watch the cubicles. There was only one man working with a couple. A few minutes later, he finished with them and escorted them out the door. He went back to the receptionist counter, glanced at the name, then looked to Daryl and came over. "Naomi Townsend. I'm Pat Scofield. How can I help you?"

Scofield was young, like every bank employee seemed to be these days, not yet thirty. He was a handsome young man with widely set pale eyes and a prematurely receding hairline. He wore a bright gold wedding band.

"I'd like to make a deposit into a trust you hold."

"Why, certainly. Come on back to my desk."

As they sat down, she presented him with one of the business cards she'd had printed that morning. She had made several with various identities and positions. He looked it over. NAOMI SWENSON-TOWNSEND, it read. ASSISTANT CFO FOR APPRECIATION TRUST, with an address in Hartford.

"I've got the account number if you need it. I'm afraid I don't have a deposit slip with me."

"Let me see what I have first," he said. "You could have made this deposit in Hartford." She didn't know if he was testing her or making conversation.

"I forgot. I'm on my way into the city and realized at the last second I promised to do this Friday. What a mess."

"I understand. Here it is. I've got the account. Let me fill out a deposit slip for you. How much?"

"Two hundred fifty thousand dollars. You can see why I didn't want to forget."

"Yes, that would take some explaining. I see you usually do wire transfers."

"That's right."

Scofield took out a blank deposit slip and then, comparing the information on the screen, looking back and forth, filled it out. Daryl opened her purse to find the check and fumbled around a bit. "Oh dear."

"Problem?"

"I'm not sure it's here. Can you imagine?" She dug in the purse again, then sighed. "Could I call my office, please? I want to ask my assistant if I left it on my desk." He looked at her as if wanting to say something. "I left my cell phone too." She smiled brightly. "I'm afraid it's been one of those days."

"Help yourself," he said, gesturing to his phone. "Dial nine and that will get you an outside number."

When he made no move to give her privacy, she stared at him without touching the phone. "I've got to check in with the cashiers," he said after a moment, "so take your time."

Without punching nine, Daryl dialed a number in Los Angeles she'd memorized. The phone was answered on the second ring. "Hi," she said, "this is Pat Scofield in Connecticut." She was calling on their internal phone system so the call was taken as authentic. She'd been ready to leave and to find another branch if the manager was male, but as luck had it the manager had an androgynous name. She was gambling that a bank employee in California had no idea that Pat Scofield in Connecticut was a man. "Our system is down and I need information on an account: Appreciation Trust. Here's the number. Thanks."

Daryl stepped into a Starbucks, ordered a latte, then sat at a small table, opening her laptop. Scofield had been very understanding when she told him she had in fact forgotten the check and apologized for taking up his time. He said he'd be happy to help her anytime and walked her to the door.

Now she went online with the application information she'd obtained with the two telephone calls she'd managed to make from the bank's phone system. The Appreciation Trust accounts with Pacific Eastern Bank had been opened in the name of Dick Iver. The business address, it turned out, was a UPS store in Hartford. She did a search for the company and found absolutely nothing, which didn't surprise her. Next she accessed Data Retriever Solutions using the CyberSys account and ran the number. It was for a man who died in 2005. Again, no surprise.

A dead end—for now. But with this information she could follow the money to the next stage. Still, her heart sank at the prospect. How many stages would there be? Too many she feared.

She drank her coffee and considered the odds. She had tonight and tomorrow for computer time. Maybe she could turn up something, but didn't think it likely. What she needed was to link what was taking place to the rogue code's real authors. The ease with which she'd fooled the bank manager had set her mind to considering another option. But first, there was something else she could do now. She picked up her cell phone to call her boss, Clive Lifton, in San Francisco. He answered at once.

"Daryl, when are you coming back? I need you."

"I'm not sure, Clive. Things are complicated. Listen, I need your help." For the next ten minutes, she filled him in on what was taking place. His company, CyberSys, Inc., was small but highly regarded in the cybersecurity community. His annual CyberCon was one of the most respected of its kind and was attended by both private contractors and government agents. His contacts throughout the cybersecurity world were extensive.

"That's quite a story," he said when she'd finished. "So the SEC is convinced that Jeff and Frank are thieves. But from what you tell me the setup isn't all that clever."

"Robert Alshon is the senior investigator. I'm hoping you know him."

"Alshon. Alshon. I have a vague memory of a large man with a shaven head and mustache. If that's him, we met once, briefly, but I should know people who know him. It's the same everywhere. What do you want me to do?"

"Talk to him. At the least slow him down, get him to dig deeper before he lands on Jeff and Frank with both feet."

"You say that warrants have already been issued?"

"That's what Frank said. Alshon was able to get the NYPD involved. That's why they left the city."

"Where are they?"

"The less you know, the better, Clive. Will you do it?"

"Of course I'll do it. I just don't know if it will do any good."

52

POUSADA VERDE NOVA
RUA MANUEL DE PAIVA
SÃO PAULO, BRAZIL
2:34 P.M.

The hotel's Web site had been true to the nature of the Pousada Verde Nova. Frank had selected it during their layover in Miami primarily because of its location. Tropical in design with a cobblestone parking area, the small hotel had a restaurant and featured both inside and outside dining. Quiet, with Wi-Fi throughout, it was situated three blocks from the nearest busy street. It was the kind of hotel that appealed to out of country travelers. It made you want to lounge about, drink too much beer, and do absolutely nothing. It was ideal for their purposes as it was easy to blend in.

Jeff had found the long flight south both physically and mentally exhausting. The passports cleared Newark and Miami without difficulty and there'd been no trouble at the Guarulhos International Airport. Frank had assured them that traveling as two Canadian businessmen would be easy.

Once they'd left Miami, Frank had offered him an Ambien, but Jeff had refused. He'd taken the drug once before, and it had left him dazed for the next twenty-four hours. He couldn't afford such a luxury right now.

When Frank first announced his intention of flying south to collect information at the likely source or to find someone in the know, Jeff had objected, arguing that it was too dangerous. If anything went wrong, they'd end up in a Brazilian jail.

And just how reliable was the information on São Paulo anyway? They found nothing when they'd first cracked the code, and they'd looked hard for such a connection. Now, out of the blue, came this picture. Daryl was right. They'd been lured here.

He didn't share Frank's optimism, if that's what it was. There seemed to Jeff virtually no chance they could run this thing down here or find someone who could confirm their suspicions and be made to talk. They had no idea if São Paulo was even the end of the trail. For all they knew it was just another stopping point for the money. And as for the hackers, the operation could very easily have been outsourced to them from most anywhere in the world. In Jeff's view this was the longest of shots. He'd told Frank this as forcefully as he could before they'd left New York.

"If we stay here in New York, we'll be arrested, with all that means," Frank had argued. "We've already discussed it at length. Even with Daryl's help we can't do this working only with computers. You need to come with me."

"To Brazil?"

"Absolutely. We can't stay here. If we do, it's just a question of time. A moving target is a lot harder to find. We've got cash and in Brazil cash is king. If this lead comes to nothing, we'll hole up there and work this for the long run. There are few better places in the world in which to be a fugitive. The Brazilian authorities won't cooperate with the SEC or FBI. They don't view so-called white-collar crime the same way as the U.S. And we don't have to show identity cards to function there so we can assume whatever name we want. There's also a larger expat community in Brazil than you realize and in the south there's a large number of Brazilians who originated largely from Germany. We'll be invisible or close to."

"I don't know."

"I speak the language."

"You speak Spanish, Frank. The language in Brazil is Portuguese."

"Close enough. Jeff," Frank said with a winning smile, "trust me."

After checking in to the Pousada Verde Nova, they showered and changed, then had a light snack with bottles of Brahma, a local beer. Frank had unspecified business and left, saying he'd be back in a bit.

Jeff lay on his bed and tried to sleep, but his restless mind refused to shut down. Running into Agnes had been upsetting. His mind had been filled with fear, fear that she knew there was a warrant out for his arrest, that she'd been playing him and had run off to tell the police where to find him. It was ridiculous he knew, but he'd had to fight to suppress the surge of terror that threatened to engulf him.

When Frank returned, Jeff said, "Frank, I appreciate your commitment to secrecy, I really do, and understand the culture. But in this case, I think it's misplaced. You want me to trust you and I do, but put yourself in my place. I need to know more. Tell me about this." He held up the passport.

Frank sat in a chair, a fresh bottle of beer clutched in his hand. "You've got a point. Old habits. I'll just give you the highlights, since there are necks on the line here." He took a pull, then continued, "The Company does a lot of its business off the books."

"You mean it outsources."

"Yes, but not just that. A contract operator has less of a trail back to the Company if anything goes wrong. Deniability. For one, he's got a life insurance policy on him so the U.S. government isn't paying his widow death benefits. It's a 'no questions asked' situation, and they've used it a lot, especially since the start of the war on terror, as it's known. The problem is that outsourced agents can't get what they need directly from the Company. This is not a new issue. When the CIA was created, it set up companies in the U.S., Europe, and around the world, run by agents at first, later by patriots. With Company resources and good business management you'd be surprised at how successful some of them have become. You'd even know a name or two. So when an operator needs cash, a job title, things like that, these companies step up.

"So . . . passports. Not every such operation is legal. That's how independent operators get weapons, communications gear, and the such. At least one of them specializes in identities. They have a stash of perfectly legitimate blank passports from a number of countries, including Canada. They prepare them just the way the Canadian government does. Now, here's the tricky part; they've got a source inside Passport Canada. That's a quasi-independent government agency that reports to the Citizenship and Immigration office there. It's been a disaster from the first. Passport Canada hires people without proper clearance, issues felons passports; it's a mess. So this guy working there inserts all the information directly into the official government database. I'm telling you, Jeff, these passports are in effect the real deal. Now, I need you to trust me. I'm as exposed as you are."

"All right, then. Thank you."

Frank removed a cell phone from his pocket and slid it over. "Here's a throwaway. Keep it charged and with you. There's a strip of masking tape across the back with your number and mine."

Jeff glanced at the phone, then slid it into a pocket. "Should we be worried about Agnes?" He hadn't expressed his concern or fears in transit not being entirely sure their conversations were secure.

"Naw. I was once in . . . now, where was it? Oh, yeah, Rome. Anyway, I was in Rome, eating dinner with someone I was running, when this guy comes up all smiles. We'd gone to high school together, wanted to know how my wife was, shook my hand until I thought it would fall off, gave me his business card, hinted he wanted to join us, then seeing I wasn't going to invite him he moved on."

"Awkward. What did you tell the man you were with?"

"Mistaken identity."

"Did he believe you?"

"No. The funny thing about it was I'd never seen the other guy before. I'd never gone to school with him, and he didn't know me. He had my name wrong and that of my wife. It really was mistaken identity. So there you are. Agnes won't be a problem. If we become a national story or the cyber community spreads word around, then she'll try to put two and two together. If she likes you, she's not likely to call the authorities because she'll have her doubts, especially Agnes. Federal law enforcement has lost a lot of credibility since the Patriot Act and PRISM. And even if she tells someone about seeing you, the Miami airport feeds lots of places in the world."

"It's the gateway to South America."

Frank nodded. "There's that. But, Jeff, you give them too much credit. You're not traveling under your own name. They'd have to use facial recognition to spot either of us and take it from me, since my group developed that software to its current state, it is nowhere near as fast or simple as the movies make it seem. I know their capability, and it's limited. Mostly they catch people because people do stupid things, or act guilty. That's why you need to put this out of your mind. For the next little while, you are Doug Bennett. Think about your cover story, don't flash too much cash and ogle the babes. That's the national pastime down here."

"What about Carol?" Jeff asked. He had no one who needed to know he was on the run but Frank had a wife and family.

"Carol is fine."

"I don't understand. How can she be fine with all this going on?"

Frank took a pull of his beer. "She knew what I was when we met, or at least not long after we met. She's the reason I made the career change but that didn't happen overnight. She's lived with this before. We have a code, just in case."

"What kind of code? What's it for?"

"It's for emergencies when I might have to go to ground. I was still in the field for over a year after we started living together, so I gave her a code expression. Whenever she heard or read it from me it meant I was fine but had to vanish for a while and couldn't be in touch with her. She was to do nothing. Not call anyone, not talk about it."

"Couldn't someone from the Company keep her posted, so she wouldn't worry?"

Frank smiled. "Jeff, you are an American original. The Company might very well be why I was pulling my vanishing act."

"You're not serious."

"After all you've been through since 9/11, and especially these last few days, you still don't get it. The field is no different than Langley was. Remember those days? Management has its own agenda, the best and brightest are few and far between, motives are muddled. As often as not out there my adversary was the home office. Dealing with the official enemy was pretty straightforward and with most of the enemy operators there were rules we followed."

"Rules? In espionage?"

"Of course. We all had families. One rule was that they were off limits. There were others."

"So how many times did you have to hide from the Company?"

"That was just an example of why I needed a private code. I actually only kept my head down from the home office once and that was just for a few days until the situation corrected itself."

Jeff started to ask, then stopped. What Frank might very well mean was that he'd corrected the situation personally. "Okay."

"You never know when your past might catch up with you, so I kept the code alive. I called Carol when we went to ground so she knows I'll be out of touch for a while."

"Still, she must be worried."

"Oh yeah. No matter how hard you try you always worry."

53

Jonathan Russo looked up from the code and nodded to Alex Baker with approval. "We're getting there," he said.

"How much are we committing?"

"Everything. Opportunities like this don't come along that often. We have no idea how many high-frequency traders will be in on the action, skimming the cream, and we have losses to make up for."

"I'm concerned no matter how good our algo looks. The new IPO software the Exchange is using is still buggy. I called a contact there, and she's not sure it'll be fixed by Wednesday."

"Are they going with it anyway?"

"She says they are, though there's a revolt going on with the staff. But the Exchange committed to it publicly, and they are being told it has to fly."

"That's a hell of a way to run a railroad."

Baker shrugged. "You know what they're like."

"I'm afraid so. I like what I see here," Russo said, indicating his screen, "but I want you to triple-check our exit code. We've established parameters in which we'll do well. If the trades migrate out of the parameters, we have to be sure we're no longer participating. I think we're secure in that regard."

"I'll be working on that all day tomorrow." Baker stopped but seemed poised to say more.

"What?"

"I'm concerned the algos are getting too complicated."

"They are sophisticated, no doubt about it."

"They are time consuming to trace and too much of the code has been generated by other code. I have to use tools to understand some of it."

"Nothing new there."

"In this case, though, it is. I frankly don't understand some aspects of our algos. I know that the tools say they're fine and that they test out on our machines but . . ."

"So what's the problem?"

"I don't understand them except in the most general way. I could write a short paper describing how they function but I can't explain the details of the functionality."

"Yes, it's not like the old days, but we're going to see more and more of this, Alex. The day will come when code will write all code. We'll just tell it what we want it to do."

"Not soon, I hope. I don't trust it."

Russo leaned back. "Don't tell me that you want to hold off? If the algo really isn't ready, we shouldn't use it. But you don't know that, do you?"

"No. I'm just uneasy is all."

"It's always that way with something new. We've never been this aggressive before, this committed."

"That's it I guess, plus we had that problem last week, when the test had run just fine. Okay, late tomorrow, I'm shutting it down to changes, then we'll run a number of scenarios in-house. If all goes as expected, we'll be good to go. We'll deploy the update two hours before trading begins Wednesday morning."

"I'm depending on you. I'm exhausted. I'm going home for some rest and I'll be in late tomorrow. We've a long day ahead of us once I get here."

Russo watched Baker leave his office. He understood what the man was saying. When he started out, he'd written code from scratch. Later, he basically copied and pasted, then adapted code he had crafted already. Only when he went to work for Jump Trading, had he returned to writing code from scratch, at least in the beginning. Now every high-frequency trading company copied where it could, duplicated functions, producing nearly identical algos. They made money even then, but every edge you could encode meant a lot.

In Russo's view this code was conservative compared to what he'd really like to do. He was already thinking of how it would be rewritten for the next major IPO. He'd squeeze the other HFTs out, that's what he'd do. They'd never know what hit them. He was expecting to do well on Tuesday, and was prepared to bail out at signs of trouble, even overriding the program if he didn't like what he saw. Despite his desire to plunge after the algo problems and losses of the previous week, there was too much on the line to be taking needless risks.

54

Back in Manhattan, Daryl had found an image of a NYSE employee ID online, printed a copy at Kinkos, affixed a passport photo she had taken there, laminated it, and attached it to a lanyard. While it looked authentic, it didn't have the RFID chip on it that would open secured doors when swiped past a reader.

The name on the card was that of a woman from the Server Systems Group at the Exchange taken from the employee information Jeff and Frank had compiled during their reconnaissance. Besides being on vacation and from a department that would give Daryl latitude to move around, she bore a vague resemblance to Daryl, at least based on the small photo in the company directory.

Daryl now stood outside the Wall Street building housing the offices for Trading Platforms IT Security and waited for a crush of employees, preferably one with several young women. It didn't take long. She blended in with a stream, hanging close to three laughing and chatting women. Each swiped her card as she passed through a waist-level security gate. Daryl hurried behind the woman in front of her, sliding through before the gate closed while swiping her card. The security guard's attention was elsewhere and the chattering group hadn't noticed her tailgating behind them.

She stayed tight with the three women, then rode the elevator with them, wanting to get off the ground floor and away from the security guards at once. They exited on the fourth floor. Daryl looked around. It didn't seem right. At the closest cubicle, Daryl asked, "Where is IT Security? I'm afraid I left my directions at the office."

The young man scarcely looked up from his screen, "Fifteenth floor, if you're looking for admin. It's also housed on the sixteenth and seventeenth floors."

"Thanks."

Daryl returned to the elevator, then stepped off on the seventeenth floor, glanced about, then walked along the hallway, which encircled the primary work area. Perhaps a third of the cubicles she saw were unoccupied, employees in meetings, taking breaks, sick, unfilled vacancies.

When she'd first considered this infiltration in the euphoria following her success earlier with the bank manager, it had seemed easy. Now she wasn't so sure. She knew she couldn't just stand around looking confused. Someone would ask if she needed help. In an empty cubicle she spotted a number of loose sheets of paper. She stepped in, picked one up, then walked steadily along the hallway as if she knew where she was going. She'd read somewhere that people carrying a piece of paper looked purposeful.

It was a busy office and for that she was grateful. Anyone she encountered was obviously busy while those in their cubicles were intent on their work. She drew a look from every man she passed but there was nothing new in that. The best news was that once at their station employees rarely displayed their identity cards. She'd noticed the women with whom she'd entered had taken theirs from purses and put them back as they walked to the elevators.

She went by a copy room, an empty manager's office, then realized she was about to lap the floor, so she slipped into the unoccupied ladies' restroom, entering the first stall. She stood there taking several deep breaths. So far, so good.

Women entered and went straight to the mirrors. ". . . our fault. I can't believe we've had two meetings in three days over this nonsense. It's not like we did it." Her voice sounded very young.

"If the *Times* writes about it, if it's in the news, we have to pay the price. You know that." The second voice seemed a bit older.

"It was harmless. It happens to every company one time or another. Now he wants to change everything. You watch. We'll spend the next three months focused on the wrong things just to cover his ass. In the meanwhile our real work will get ignored."

Faucets were turned on and off, water splashed, there was more chit-chat, then the women left. Daryl waited before stepping back into the hall-way and resumed her walk, looking for an open workstation.

Richard Iyers spotted the blonde as he was on his way to the men's room. "Well, hi," he said when she was close. "I haven't seen you before."

Daryl stopped and smiled. "I'm from SSG." The Server Systems Group was big and housed in a separate building. She was gambling not everyone working there was known by sight here.

"That explains it. My name's Richard. I work over there." Iyers gestured across the top of the cubicles. "If I can do anything for you, just let me know. I'm an infrastructure specialist. We should have a lot to talk about."

"Thanks. I'll keep that in mind." Daryl looked for his badge to get his last name and saw he had it tucked into his pocket. She moved around him.

"I didn't catch your name," Iyers said as she walked past him.

"Kelly," Daryl replied over her shoulder.

This second time through, she thought she had a sense of the place. She selected a cubicle not directly seen from the hallway and sat. She couldn't put her finger on it but as she examined the work area it gave her the impression that no one had worked at it recently. She slid into place and turned on the computer.

The backdoors into the system that Jeff and Frank had constructed were of necessity composed of several pieces. One bit was code they had planted in the trading engine. This connected to more code on the jump server, which in turn connected to still more code on other computers they'd compromised, including the essential Payment Dynamo servers. These connected out of the Exchange to the C2 servers they'd rented in public cloud providers such as Amazon EC2 or Microsoft Windows Azure. This was the tunnel Jeff and Frank employed and from which they could accomplish anything they wanted, from spying on employees on the IT side to injecting more code into the trading engine if that proved necessary.

A serious problem Daryl now faced was that the link from their C2 servers to the Exchange and possibly the jump server and their code in the trading engine had been disrupted. Her first order of business was to check to see if she could reestablish a path.

From her purse Daryl removed a USB key to boot one of Jeff's tools. This enabled her to change the local administrator password on the operating system. Once done she rebooted the computer normally and logged on. Now that she was in, she ran a tool to leverage the passwords Jeff had collected to give her access as if she were the users to whom they belonged. Using that access, she connected to one of the Payment Dynamo backdoor servers via the IT side of the Exchange network. Holding her breath, she scanned the list of processes running for their backdoor. There it was, still active. She exhaled. She could connect to the backdoor from the system she was using and regain access to the jump server. This allowed her to monitor the software uploads through the jump server and if she positioned herself correctly, she hoped she could prevent them from passing through.

With her ability to monitor and interfere with the rogue code restored, Daryl turned to following up on the Brazilian connection. Jeff and Frank needed all the help they could get and while Frank suspected the lure was intentional she was sure of it. She was convinced that things would go very badly for them no matter how confident Frank seemed.

She navigated to the internal employee directory Web site and set about scanning it slowly searching for Portuguese names or variations in the event they'd been Anglicized. As a prodigy Daryl had discovered a natural aptitude for languages very early in her life. Before she was a teenager she already spoke Spanish, Portuguese, and Italian fluently. In her teens, she'd added both Latin and French. Her parents thought she'd become a linguist, but Daryl had also been drawn to mathematics and computers. At age fifteen, she was spending most of her time with pimple-faced geeks. It had been the combination of languages and computing skills that had led to her recruitment by the National Security Agency.

The problem in searching for a Portuguese surname was that they were Latin and so many were identical to Italian and Spanish family names, and immigrants often dropped the specific distinctions to simplify assimilation. After an hour, she had a working list of thirteen possible names: Alvaro, Braga, Camacho, Campos, D'Souza, Esteves, Fernandes, Gonsalez, Mateos, Nunes, Parra, Rodriguez, Silva.

Braga, D'Souza, and Nunes were almost certainly Portuguese in origin. The others might or might not be. She next went through the thirteen names in turn to determine what access to the trading engines each had and from that produced three who were in an easier position to insert malware. Braga, Campos, and Esteves. Of course, she knew any on the list could have used their position of privileged access to hack into the system but these three were in the best position, and she had to start somewhere.

Daryl memorized the names, titles, and office numbers. She recalled that she'd seen the name Esteves on one of the manager offices on this floor. She drew a deep breath, stood up, and went back into the hallway. Esteves's office was unoccupied. The two others were on the fifteenth floor.

She stepped off the elevator and resumed her movement around the next floor. It seemed identical to the other. Employees walked by her, intent on their own concerns. As she'd noticed on the other floor, there was a sense of restlessness in the air, not exactly one of urgency but rather of unfocused frenzy. The cubicles had no names for occupants. Apparently you were expected to know who worked at the station. Braga and Campos were not managers. What to do?

"Excuse me," she said to a chubby young woman standing in the hallway talking to someone in a cubicle. "I'm looking for Marc Campos. I don't know him by sight."

"Marc?" The woman repeated the name as if she'd never heard it before. "Marc," she said again, looking down. "This lady wants to talk to you." With that she said good-bye, glancing at Daryl from the side as she moved away.

"Marc Campos?" Daryl asked as she moved to the cubicle opening.

"Yes." Though he was sitting down, she could tell Campos was tall. He was in his early thirties, with olive skin, an average face, though with slightly bulging eyes. She knew that he was on the core trading platform team at the heart of the trade matching engines. He looked very tired. "What can I do for you?"

There was just the slightest trace of an accent and for reasons Daryl could not explain she knew this was her man. "I'm Kelly," she said. "I'm with SSG. Do you have a minute to talk?"

"Sure," Campos said, gesturing to a chair in the corner. "You have a card?"

Daryl smiled, then dipped her hand into her purse and extracted one of the cards she'd printed earlier. She handed it to him. Campos read it, then set the card down, looking back at her expectantly.

"I'm following up on the bot that's been in the news."

Campos laughed. "It's amazing how those things can get blown out of proportion. I know the former employee who is the source. He's just disgruntled. Almost everything being reported isn't true. And the market is rebounding today. It always does."

"Have there been any others since you came to work here?"

Campos shook his head. "I don't recall any but then, unless it was in the trading software, it's not likely I'd have heard about it. And I can't imagine anything like that getting through the jump server."

"How long have you been here?"

"Five years," Campos answered before looking at her card again.

"Campos," she said. "Is that Spanish?"

"Portuguese," he said warily.

"*Eu falo Português. Onde é que sua família vem?*"

"Porto," Campos said.

"*Porto é muito bonito.*"

"Yes, it is."

"*Você deve falar Português?*"

"Of course." Campos began to sweat. Daryl arched her eyebrows in expectation. Then he said, "*Sim, é claro que eu falo Português.*"

And there it was. It was all Daryl could do not to yell "gotcha." He'd tried, even in his short admission that he spoke Portuguese to disguise his accent but there was no hiding it. The region about Porto spoke some of the most traditional Portuguese in existence, while those from Brazil spoke a variation tempered by the climate, the distance from the source of the native language, peppered with African words and idioms unique to their region. Porto Portuguese was like Castilian to Mexican Spanish, Prussian to Bavarian German.

Campos was Brazilian.

Daryl continued speaking to him a bit, almost enjoying his efforts to conceal his accent. Finally, uncomfortable with the exchange, Campos said in English, "If there's nothing else, I need to get back to work."

I'll bet you do, Daryl thought. The Toptical IPO is less than two days away. "Of course. Nice meeting you. It was good to practice my Portuguese. It's been too long." She extended her hand.

When she was gone, Campos lifted up her card. Kelly Vogle. He punched the listed SSG number into his phone. It rang three times before an electronic voice said, "You have reached the voice mail of Kelly Vogle. Please leave a message."

Shit!

What did SSG want with him? They'd found the trail he'd planted leading to Aiken and reported it to the SEC just as he'd wanted. Why would they come snooping around here? Why ask about the bot? The publicity it was causing?

And why talk to him? Why send someone who spoke Portuguese? What were the odds it was a coincidence?

Campos stood up and went into the hallway, his legs unsteady. She was gone. He sat back down and stared ahead, realizing that his hands were trembling.

Merda!

55

ENFORCEMENT DIVISION
SECURITIES AND EXCHANGE COMMISSION
NEW YORK REGIONAL OFFICE
200 VESSEY STREET
NEW YORK CITY
5:11 P.M.

Robert Alshon pulled the drawer out and removed two more pink tablets, chewed, then washed them down with coffee. He looked at his watch. Time was racing away.

He fingered the report he'd received earlier. Uniformed NYPD officers had located a fleabag hotel uptown the previous day where two men matching the descriptions of his target had holed up. The clerk said he had no doubt they were the pair on the flyer but by the time a SWAT team arrived and stormed their room the birds had flown.

Alshon had been furious on receiving word. Whatever happened to cops just doing their job? Why wait on a special tactics team? Just go in and make the arrest. It seemed to him every routine law enforcement procedure was morphing into a big deal. It was, in his view, just one more way to avoid responsibility.

So Aiken and Renkin were gone. Where?

Nowhere close, that much he was sure of. Alshon couldn't shake off the thought they were long gone. He'd missed his best chance to snag them. By now they could be anywhere. Most likely they'd gone to Canada as it was so close. As Company men they'd know how to go to ground. If they didn't already have new identities, they could get them there. A Canadian passport was as good as an American one, and they were a lot easier to obtain. You didn't even have to get a false one. And that assumed they didn't have one already lined up.

They could have gone south, Mexico. Simple enough by bus or by buying a used car and making the drive. Once below the border, they'd simply vanish and even if they were traveling without new identities those were easily obtained in Mexico City, where false documents were a booming business.

There was a knock at his open door. "Come in, Gene," Alshon said. "Give me some good news. I could use it."

Gene Livingston entered holding his customary legal tablet and took a seat. He pushed his glasses back onto his nose, then said, "I won't get the telephone and e-mail information on Stenton, Aiken, and Renkin until tomorrow, so I have nothing new to report there. I did retrace my steps a bit and widened the search, but I still can't find a connection to Stenton before he hired Red Zoya." He looked up. "Sorry I couldn't get this done as soon as I'd expected."

"It's good news, though. I prefer to have Stenton on my side in this. So what's new?"

"I've been working on Stenton's staff since this was an inside job. It occurred to me that these two might have another ally there."

"Good thinking."

"What I came up with is Marco Enfante Campos. He works on the trading platform team on one of the modules at the heart of the trade matching engines. That's as sensitive as it gets. He's been there for five years. According to his application, he's from Porto, Portugal. He attended college in the U.S. and worked for New York Life before joining the Exchange. He's a trusted, reliable employee. He's moved up steadily in responsibility. He's single and lives a quiet life from what I can see."

"What else?"

"He's working here on a green card. Okay, I got into the New York Life records—don't ask, you don't want to know—and while there is a cursory record of his employment, it isn't fleshed out like that for the other employees."

"I don't understand."

"It looks to me like it was inserted."

"Inserted?"

"Let's say you want to establish a work history. You hack a company computer and insert your personal data. When the prospective employer checks, some clerk goes into the records and says 'Sure, he worked here from such-and-such a date until such-and-such.' No one gives out any real information anymore because of lawsuits. And that's all the prospective employer is looking for—confirmation the applicant actually worked there."

"You're saying his record looks funny."

"Right. I checked out the data for employees with similar responsibilities and it is far more extensive. His is really stark."

"That's pretty thin."

"There's more. I checked with Tufts University, and there's no record of him ever attending."

"Maybe the records have it wrong. Maybe he used a different name or took them as special classes."

"That's possible. But it was enough for me to really focus on him."

"And?"

"He's a creation. I can't tell you who this Marco Campos is but I'm prepared to guarantee that his real name isn't Campos, and my bet is he's not even Portuguese."

"He looks like their inside man, then?"

"That could be. But when I looked, I couldn't find any link between Campos, Aiken, and Renkin. Actually, Mr. Alshon, if I were looking at the data fresh, I'd say Campos is your man, not Aiken and Renkin. He's been there five years, he's the one who has been in position to set this operation up."

"We've got Aiken red-handed!"

"Maybe," Livingston said evenly. "But think about it. You've been running a long con for five years, you've been making money for the last year, then these hotshots from outside come in and stumble on what you're up to. What would you do? Run?"

Alshon eased back in his chair. Livingston was solid as they come. He needed to listen. "Run makes sense. Why set them up? That in itself is a great risk."

"Yes, it is. But you'd do it if you wanted to buy time because maybe you've got something big coming up."

After Livingston left, Alshon summoned Flores and assigned her to personally check out Campos without telling her what he'd already been told. When she left, he gnawed at his lower lip until his cell phone rang.

"Alshon."

"Mr. Alshon, my names Clive Lifton. I run CyberSys, Inc., out here in San Francisco. We met two years ago in Atlanta. Perhaps you recall. I'm sorry to bother you, but a matter has just come to my attention I need to discuss with you urgently."

Alshon's mind raced. Lifton? He had no recollection of meeting the man but that was no surprise. He met a lot of new people in a typical year. CyberSys, Inc. was familiar to him. When he'd been with the Bureau, they adopted one of its security systems.

"What can I do for you, Mr. Lifton."

"I've known Jeff Aiken for a number of years. I've tried to recruit him for most of them. I understand you think he's committed a crime of some kind."

"Where did you hear that?"

"A colleague notified me. It's not important who. I was able to confirm that a warrant has been issued for his arrest so we aren't dealing in confidences here."

"I'd still like to know who told you."

"Let me tell you about Jeff, including information you won't find in official records, or at least not those you can access. I think when you learn just who he is, you'll rethink the direction of your inquiry."

"I'm listening."

After Alshon disconnected, he was furious. He'd had targets pull weight before. It was inevitable in any significant investigation and all of his were significant. He'd anticipated a call such as this at some point, though, this was a bit early from his experience; but he'd never had one claim his target was innocent on national security grounds before, and he didn't like it one bit.

Just who did these people think they were? When he'd been with the Bureau, he encountered this from time to time. Someone who'd provided information to another government agency would pull a string and the boss would get a call. Snitches were devious people in his opinion, and those who sold information to the Company, or the Defense Intelligence Agency or any of the alphabet soup agencies involved in national security were weasels. They were only on the side of the angels by accident. They'd learned what they learned by working with the bad guys, by doing bad things. They had no commitment to anything beyond their own survival. Calls like this had never succeeded at the Bureau, at least not in his experience.

This Lifton had told Alshon quite a story. You'd think Aiken was James Bond to hear him tell it. He saved the world at least twice. Well, it wasn't going to work. Alshon knew bad apples when he found them, and these two were rotten.

But as the workday drew to its exhausting close, as he prepared to go home for a few hours' sleep, Alshon's thoughts turned back to what Livingston had told him about Campos. It made sense that Aiken had an inside man. It made no sense to him that this was a Campos operation. No, it was the Company men; of that, he was certain.

56

The warehouses were laid out in the shape of a square-cornered U. The open end through which deliveries and shipments were made faced the rear away from the street. The entry opening was a secured expanse of steel grating topped with spear points and electric wiring. In the middle were large sliding automatic doors controlled from a guard post there. This was the only way in or out. The exterior of the warehouses was a solid wall fifteen feet high, lacking a single window or doorway. This outside wall was also topped with spear points and electrical wiring.

All of this was standard in Brazil. What was new, and unseen, were the motion detectors and sophisticated surveillance cameras Jorge César had installed in anticipation of his two visitors. The warehouse had not been used for some months, and the contained loading area showed the evidence of disuse, dirt blown into corners, bits of paper gathered here and there, the entire expanse looking abandoned. Only the offices of Companhia Cero had remained operational, and César had sent that small staff home as soon as he'd received his orders.

The warehouse had been owned or controlled by Nosso Lugar for more than two decades. It was located in a commercial district, and though there were city efforts to revitalize the Mooca District with some success, they'd not yet extended to this area. When they did, Bandeira would sell the facility for a nice profit. For now, its advantage to the organization lay in its relative isolation as it was surrounded by similar structures and because it lent itself to a wide range of activities. In just the last decade it had been a transfer point for human trafficking, a processing facility for soft drugs, a storage and transfer point for hard drugs, and a weapons cache. Now, with César's practiced eye at work it had been turned into a killing zone.

The security chief had placed his three best men, Didi, Zico, and Cafu, on the roof to establish triangulated fire. He occupied the office in which he kept on lights after dark. With him was Paulinho, a former special operator with the army. These two gringos, Aiken and Renkin, had no chance.

The plan was simple enough: Ramos in New York had made it possible for the men to know that what they wanted was in São Paulo. He'd sent them a threat in the form of a digital photograph, careful to leave in place the GPS coordinates to this location. He'd told César that these men would discover it, and with the heat on them in the United States it was highly likely they'd take the bait, if for no other reason than to get away.

The *chefe* was confident, and even Ramos said he thought it would work. Still, César thought the likelihood the pair would show up to be quite low. In César's experience only trained agents of some kind would travel so far with the intention of taking proactive measures. It was far more likely the two would just go to ground. That was the human reaction for most smart men. Those not so smart went home and waited for the police.

It was possible they'd come and if not, he knew whom he'd contact in New York to take care of them. In the meantime, he had his orders. The only hard part of the operation was all the waiting, which was why he'd selected his best men. He had a score who knew how to shoot, only a handful who knew how to wait.

Bored with scanning the security screens on the computer, César stood back from one of the office windows overlooking the loading area so he could not be seen and examined the loading area again. He'd looked at it from outside, both by day and night, to see the impression it formed. At either time it was apparent that the Companhia Cero offices was the only occupied point in the facility. They'd be drawn to it, under the guns of his snipers.

And they would come at night, which was why the lights were on. They'd want to find the offices unoccupied so they could access or steal the computers. That was what they were after. And if it was going to happen, it would be tonight, or the following at the latest, though it was possible they could come anytime in the next week. If they hadn't arrived by Friday, he planned to inform the *chefe* there was no reason to maintain the operation beyond keeping a single gunman in the office.

Scrutinizing the scene, he was satisfied. He'd had the men damage the security gate to make it consistent with the current condition of the warehouse. There was no guard at the post and it was possible to simply push either of the gates back by hand far enough to slip in. He'd done it himself.

César lit a cigarette and returned to his seat. Paulinho sat in the corner, his IMBEL MD97 resting on his lap. César offered him a smoke, and he shook his head.

Let's hope it's tonight, César thought.

57

After seeing Campos, Daryl rode the elevator up a floor and headed directly to the ladies' room. It was the one secure place for her in the building. In the farthest stall she gathered her thoughts. She had her man, she felt sure. What to do next?

Daryl wondered if she'd aroused his suspicion. She'd pressed the issue with him, and he'd clearly been uncomfortable. But what was he going to do about it if she had? What *could* he do? Call security and have them check her out? Hardly. No, he'd be confused about how to react. Most of all, the man had his own secrets, and the last thing he'd want would be to draw attention to himself, which was what would happen.

She decided to return to the unoccupied cubicle and see if she could uncover incriminating information about this Campos. Perhaps from his e-mail she could find an accomplice within the building, or even better, confirm the link to Brazil and the Companhia Cero office in São Paulo. With that she'd have enough to go to the SEC and this nightmare would be finished.

Back at the computer she tried to backtrack accesses to the jump servers. After copying them off to her laptop, she scanned them visually. The logs were voluminous and recorded tens of thousands of standard connections and attempted connections over the past several days that constituted the usual background noise of a computer network. The logs included regular backup account connections, policy management software, and security scanning software accounts. From the logs, she hoped to identify unusual behavior, then by tracing it to its senders connect Campos and any allies he had to the malware. This would constitute hard evidence the SEC would not be able to ignore and even if it failed to lead immediately to vindication for Jeff and Frank it would begin the process of revealing the truth.

Not spotting anything visually, she ran one of Jeff's log analysis tools. Given the size of the logs it would take an hour to get results, so she turned to researching Campos by entering his name into DRS to see what she could learn about him. It took twenty minutes for her to eliminate names before identifying the right Campos out of the one hundred or so that matched.

His full name was Marco Enfante Campos. He'd attended university in the United States and worked for New York Life for a time before joining the New York Stock Exchange. He wasn't on Facebook, LinkedIn, Toptical, Twitter, or any other social network she checked. She was able to locate an address and telephone number for him. She ran a credit check, and he came back above average but not with a top score as he didn't have enough debt. She could follow up, but it would take more time than she had. And what was the point? She was checking out a cover identity because Marc Campos from Porto, Portugal, was clearly not who he really was.

She turned back to Jeff's program, which had just finished. He had logged the accesses he and Frank had used so she wouldn't confuse their activities with those of the rogue code authors. She soon listed the other connections that stood out because of their infrequency or irregularity. It noted several that corresponded to the record of the history Jeff and Frank had given her of the connection times. It also called out several others over the past week that were unusual because they were sporadic and came from a single system, employing the account of the user who managed the server.

It was highly unlikely these were legitimate. Someone had hijacked the account and was using it to upload software in order to conceal his true identity. Daryl worked to trace the trail back to the actual originator by analyzing the logs from the source system, but had no luck. He'd hidden his path well. The only conclusion she reached was that he had to be working within the system, which meant he was on one of these three floors. She considered trying this from Marc Campos's end, but knew how secure his system would be. He'd probably have installed alerts to notify him when unexpected connections were made to his computer. Instead, she kept at it from the other end, trying different parameters on Jeff's program that might highlight something it hadn't caught the first time.

After another hour, she decided it wasn't going to work, not today at least. Every time someone passed in the hallway she tensed. She knew it was hurting her concentration. But she didn't want to just walk away with what little she had. She needed more. And she needed a different approach.

Back in the hallway she saw the number of workers was reduced by about half. She wondered when the rest would finally leave. She felt conflicted because she needed bodies for cover, though the more employees there were, the greater the likelihood she'd be discovered.

Daryl took the elevator back to the fifteenth floor. She'd decided on two or three follow-up questions in the event Campos was still working. In addition to his usual work he was managing a major fraud and the clock was running.

She braced herself as she reached his workstation. Empty. She looked about her, then stepped in. His jacket was on a coat hanger. She patted his pockets, found something hard, reached in, and drew out a cell phone. She stepped outside and went directly to her auxiliary office, the last stall of the ladies' restroom.

If necessary, she was prepared to steal the phone even though that would alert Campos beyond whatever suspicion he already had. She'd rather just copy its data, but it was locked with a PIN. It was running Android, and that was good. Two years earlier, when she'd been working with Jeff, the two had been hired by the U.S. government to discover vulnerabilities in the Android operating system. They'd found several. Eventually, the government had notified Google, and they were fixed, but cell phone companies were in the business of selling phones and services, not updating software, and it was too common for even known vulnerabilities to never be patched. The logic was that the owner would buy another phone before anything bad happened. With luck he'd have a vulnerable one.

She ran her exploit code app on her phone. It listed the Bluetooth devices nearby, the only one of which was Campos's phone. The very first vulnerability she had found was a bug in the Bluetooth driver. She selected it, and the app successfully exploited the vulnerability, dropping code into the phone, which unlocked it. This gave her access to the phone's apps, including e-mail, photos, call history, and voice mail. She copied all of these into her laptop. Though the download proceeded quickly, it seemed to take forever. She found herself sweating and drew several deep breaths to calm down.

Finished, she put her laptop away, left the stall, and pressing her lips together, hurried back to the cubicle. No sign of Campos. She returned the cell phone to the same pocket and went directly to the elevator, as excited as she'd ever been. Surely, surely, there was something useful in what she'd taken. There had to be.

58

Frank pulled the São Paulo city map from his inside pocket. He'd been studying it earlier. "Companhia Cero is about eight blocks from here. The Internet tells me it's in an industrial area, so this time of night, it should be quiet. I'd like to observe it for a while before doing anything." He looked over at Jeff. "I can do this alone if you aren't up to it."

"No, I'll come."

"Good. That's better, since I'll need you later."

Both of them had made efforts that afternoon to access the Exchange's software but the backdoor was down. "We're locked out," Jeff said. "Looks like coming down here was our only option after all. I hope Daryl can find something in the samples we pulled out before the connection went down."

They'd agreed to a late lunch. Afterwards, Frank said he had more things to buy and suggested Jeff get some rest. He lay on his bed and tried to sleep, but his mind was racing at the pace of events. He wondered how all this could happen, how it could so quickly have reached this state. He tried to devise alternative options, measures that wouldn't involve possibly going into an ambush but didn't see any that led to a resolution.

He thought Frank's intentions here a long shot, always had, but he'd agreed at the time that leaving the United States was a good idea. He didn't like the thought of staying in Brazil long term if it came to that, but compared with a three-year legal battle that might very well end with a prison term, it was the better choice. He didn't know how they were going to prove they were innocent, but he was determined they find a way. So long shot or not, he'd decided to trust Frank.

He wondered what Daryl was doing. The loss of the backdoor had to be frustrating her efforts, as it had theirs. Frank had sent her his new cell phone number in the event of an emergency but told her not to contact them otherwise. Even this was a risk as they had no way of knowing how far the investigation had progressed or what level of cybersecurity measures were in place. But they had to keep a channel open.

Her last message to them expressing her concern about the Toptical IPO on Wednesday was disconcerting. The rogue code updates were focusing increasingly on it. With the recent turmoil he really had to question how much more the stock market could withstand. It seemed to have rebounded, once again, from a perceived cyberthreat but with the increased attention on high-frequency traders and their role in the market Jeff questioned if the next flash crash wouldn't be catastrophic.

For all his concerns Jeff was still recovering from his injuries and was exhausted. At some point he nodded off, his dreams consisted of unsettling flashing images, someone in the distance calling for help, remote accusing voices.

Frank shook his shoulder to awaken him. "Rise and shine, Sleeping Beauty."

Jeff stirred slowly, sat on the edge of the bed, then went into the bathroom to wash up. When he returned, Frank said, "Seriously now, Jeff, how do you feel? You haven't been out of the hospital long."

"All right. I've still got some pain where you'd expect especially in my forearm but I'm feeling a lot better. I've recovered some of my energy."

"You don't have to do this."

"I'm fine."

"Okay. Wear dark clothing," Frank told him. "No reason to make us too easy to spot. And put your new phone on vibrate. We don't want it going off at the wrong time."

When Jeff came out, Frank was seated on his bed, carefully inserting items into a black canvas shoulder backpack he'd bought at a store down the street: nylon line with attached large hooks like something you'd use to catch a whale, a pry bar, binoculars, a large hunting knife, various items Jeff couldn't identify, a revolver, and a heavy semiautomatic handgun. Jeff didn't ask questions as he put on the darkest clothing he had, a pair of newish jeans, a long-sleeve plaid shirt, and running shoes.

"Ready?" Frank asked. Jeff nodded, feeling anything but.

Outside, the temperature was pleasant, nearly eighty degrees. They left the cobblestone hotel parking area and turned right at the street. The sidewalks were constructed of small flat stones. The pressure of bodies over time gave them a curious undulating effect and made for cautious walking, but they were otherwise in good repair. There were mature trees and shrubbery masking houses, usually well trimmed, but not always. It was not a poor section of the city, but it wasn't especially affluent either.

They passed along narrow streets, then wide boulevards, moving up and down gentle hills. There were tracks laid on some streets they crossed, overhead wires for trolleys not operating at this time of night. Aging single-story buildings and houses were interspersed with five-story office buildings, graffiti marking walls everywhere. Though it was a worknight and in Jeff's mind getting late, there were couples, young and elderly, strolling, chatting, holding hands. Not for the first time did Jeff realize how much his own country had changed in his lifetime.

Traffic remained busy and aggressive, though a bit lighter than earlier. Auto pollution controls were lax, and when trucks roared by, Jeff and Frank were engulfed in the blue-tinged acrid smoke of diesel.

Frank had memorized the route. The landscape slowly turned more commercial; then after they crossed one street, it became entirely industrial, so much so they were now conspicuous on foot. Frank continued walking at a steady pace for several minutes, until he finally slowed before ducking into the shadows created by the nearly constant walls that abutted the sidewalk. There was just a single distant streetlight. "That's it there," he said.

Jeff looked. All he could make out was one more solid wall. "You're sure?"

"That's it. Though this part of the warehouse faces the street, this is actually the rear. See the driveways on both sides? Those go to the back, which we'll find open, covered by a security wall. That will be the entrance."

"Google Earth, right?"

"That and images. I'm always amazed what's available on the Internet. If only I'd had these resources back in the day. My main concern right now is finding an observation place."

"You've not forgotten this is very likely a setup," Jeff reminded him.

"I remember. We're going to be very careful. This way." He led them across the street, then up an access drive to an irregular paved expanse. Jeff concluded that it was an area for large trucks to maneuver in and to facilitate their movement between the various businesses away from the public street. It was lit only by ambient light.

Frank walked with measured steps, keeping to the shadows. He slowed and then came to a stop when they could see into the facility. He reached into the bag, searched for something, then extracted the binoculars. Vague illumination glowed behind two windows at the far end of the buildings. Otherwise, the facility looked abandoned.

There was movement in a shadow against the warehouse wall. Jeff searched for it, moved his line of sight slightly to the side, and saw what appeared to be a small animal, a cat most likely, perhaps a small dog.

There was a restless wind, occasionally enough to move the gathered street trash a few inches. The area about them smelled of used oil, diesel, and gasoline. But every few minutes, the wind carried the pungent smells away briefly bringing a floral fragrance, sweet like jasmine.

"What do you think?" Jeff asked a bit uneasily.

Frank lowered the binoculars. "It's not a fortress, but like everything here it was built with security in mind. We're going to hang out for a while. Relax if you can. It could be a long night."

"Do you think it's a setup?"

"It's sure got the look. We're out here away from any interference. The beckoning light in the window appeals to a primeval instinct in us. Even those automatic gates look slightly ajar, inviting as hell."

"Maybe someone's working late or it's a night-light."

"There are no vehicles, so we're supposed to assume no one's working. I'd say it's supposed to be a night-light."

"So you think it's a trap."

"I don't know. That's the beauty of these things. You promise someone what they want, keep it plausible, make it alluring, and even against their better judgment people fall for it. And for all our suspicion this could be exactly what it appears to be. The bad guys could very well be working out of here; it's sure as hell a good spot for it. The threat to us was just that, a threat, and whoever sent it didn't know about the embedded GPS code. That's all entirely likely. So either way, we'll settle in and watch."

"I think this is broken glass I'm standing on."

"I never said we'd be comfortable."

59

Back in her hotel room, Daryl took a shower and then ordered room service. After toweling herself dry, she wrapped herself into the soft hotel robe. She ate half of a club sandwich, then sat at her laptop and examined what she'd downloaded from the cell phone.

Daryl vividly recalled identifying this vulnerability. She and Jeff had made it a game, each seeing if he or she could find more of them, faster. Hers had been the first coup, and she'd made a point to be a poor winner, reminding him repeatedly over the following days of the job that she was not only first, but also remained ahead of him in count.

It had been fun, more a game than work. When they were together, she recalled almost everything had been fun. The problem was that they weren't together often enough, or long enough.

So now she had Campos's digital world. She first checked his photos and found almost nothing, just three street scene shots: a juggler, a tree-lined lane that didn't look like anywhere in Manhattan she knew about, a plate of food at a restaurant.

Next his call history. It came as no surprise that he'd placed no calls to Portugal. There were calls to the same local number but far more to one in Brazil, often more than one a day. She noted that the frequency had dramatically increased recently.

She called the number herself, using his phone. After several rings, a recorded man's voice came on the line in Portuguese. "You have reached the offices of Grupo Técnico. We are not available. Please leave a message, and we'll get back to you as soon as possible."

Grupo Técnico. That was not the name Frank had used in São Paulo. She opened her browser and typed in the name along with the word "Brazil." There were a number of hits as the name was so generic, but nothing that looked right. There was no Web site for the company.

Next she checked voice mail and found one pending, also in Portuguese. "Abílio," a young man said, "I need you to get back to me. I know you are busy but so are we. Call as soon as you get this, regardless of the time."

Abílio. Could that be Marc Campos's real name? Probably.

So . . . just where was Grupo Técnico? Was it part of the company Jeff and Frank were going to in São Paulo, Companhia Cero? Or was it somewhere else altogether? The thought brought her up cold, because if it was somewhere else, then São Paulo was a trap.

60

COMPANHIA CERO
MOOCA DISTRICT
SÃO PAULO, BRAZIL
11:14 P.M.

Jorge César shifted in his seat and fought off boredom. He scanned the security screens again. Nothing.

From time to time, he said something to Paulinho to confirm he was alert, but they both knew from long experience that real conversation was a distraction. The rooftop snipers—Didi, Zico, and Cafu—checked in every ten minutes, their familiar voices coming into César's earpiece. He was out of cigarettes and Paulinho didn't smoke. "I'm making coffee," César said. Paulinho nodded, the fingers of his right hand caressing the IMBEL MD97, the Brazilian Army semiautomatic assault rifle.

A few minutes later, with two cups of black coffee, César returned from the small kitchen and handed one to Paulinho. He sat and scanned the screens again. Still nothing. Too late he'd realized he should have placed two cameras with infrared capability to cover the public street. He had considered the idea but dismissed it as risky, since they could be spotted. Now, though, he'd rather have taken the chance. He was blind out there.

Anxious, the hot cup grasped in his hand, he stood where he knew he couldn't be seen from outside. The loading and parking area was empty. He sighed and returned to his seat, bored as ever.

Frank lowered the binoculars. "Someone's inside."

"You're sure?"

"Reasonably. He didn't go to the window, but there was a slight change in the light."

"Maybe they've got a watchdog."

Frank turned to face him. "Now, there's a thought." He resumed scanning the structure. "But I don't think so. The change was from higher up in the room. The roof appears clear, or if someone's up there they are very, very good."

"How long do you want to wait?"

"I'm not sure. I'm going to keep an eye on that window for a while. I'm pretty sure you're wrong about a security dog, but better a dog than a guard, especially one making such an effort not to be seen."

61

HOLIDAY INN
LAFAYETTE STREET
NEW YORK CITY
11:22 P.M.

Next were the e-mails, since it was possible Daryl would find a physical address in one of them.

Nearly all she saw were from or were sent to P.Bandeira@grupotecnico. com.br. She quickly read through the messages with a growing sense of excitement. This was it. There was no doubt at all. This P. Bandeira was sending code to Campos in New York. Most of the messages were tied to a previous message and lacked a signature. She searched for an original message from P. Bandeira. Finally, taking longer than she'd thought, she finally found one with the company signature located just below the telephone number and e-mail address:

Pedro Bandeira
Presidente
Grupo Técnico
Rua Adolfo Mota, 108
Tijuca – Rio de Janeiro – RJ

Next she entered "Grupo Técnico" and "Companhia Cero" into her search engine, looking for a connection. She found none.

Biting her lower lip she sent a message to Frank's phone.

62

COMPANHIA CERO
MOOCA DISTRICT
SÃO PAULO, BRAZIL
11:54 P.M.

Okay," Frank said lightly. "The roof still looks clear, and there's been no more change in the light. Maybe a window is open and the wind moved a curtain. Or, as you suggest, they've got a dog in there. We're going to take this very carefully, though, Jeff. I just want you to cover me." He reached into the bag and pulled out the revolver Jeff had seen earlier. "Take this." He removed the automatic and slipped it into his waist.

Jeff took the weapon. It was heavier than he expected, used but well oiled and maintained. He was not a novice with a handgun, having taken target practice with his grandfather growing up. In fact, one summer as a teenager, he'd become quite accurate. But he'd never hunted, he'd never killed anything in his life. He thought for an instant about asking if this was really necessary, but realized how foolish that would sound. Of course it was.

"You know how to use it?" Jeff nodded. "Okay, then. We're ignoring those inviting doors. If I'm wrong about this, that open area is a kill zone. Just stick with me but I want you to hold back ten to twenty feet, depending on how much distance you need. Now, here's the hard part: Force yourself not to watch what I'm doing. It's going to be much harder than it sounds. Your job is to be the lookout, to watch all the things I can't because I'm busy. Keep an eye out around us but primarily scan the roofline. I haven't spotted anyone up there but that could just mean they are good. If there's a roof lookout, at some point I'll make enough noise to attract him. He should quietly check me out, and when he does you should see him. If he's really good, he won't move. He'll wait for when I'm on the rope or just coming over the wall on top. Either way, if he exists, he's not alone. You understand?"

Jeff's mouth was suddenly dry. "You really think we need to do this?"

"If this isn't a setup, then what we need is inside that office. In ten minutes, we can be there, with unlimited access. Even if this just proves to be a transfer point, we could very well take away enough data to clear us, or at least to get the Feds to focus somewhere else. And if Daryl's right, we'll have the data to prevent a potential Wall Street meltdown. It's worth the risk. You ready for this?"

"Yes."

"Okay, then. Let's go."

Frank moved out back the way they'd come until they were midpoint along the extended wall of the warehouse. He hesitated, listening and watching, then quietly moved across the access drive until he was at the base of the wall. There he set his black bag on the ground and reached in for the nylon rope with attached hooks.

César's ear came alive. It was Zico.

"*Movimento abaixo,*" he said quietly. "*Olhê embaixo.*" Movement below. Look down there.

César scanned the cameras. Nothing. Whoever Zico heard was in a blind spot. "*Alguém,*" he told Paulinho quietly. Someone. The man nodded but didn't move. His job was to cover the office. Zico could take care of his roof section by himself.

César waited, no longer bored, that familiar excitement suddenly coursing through him. He notified the other two snipers, Didi and Cafu, to be vigilant.

Jeff scanned the area about them. A motorcycle sped by on the outside road. He glanced back where they'd been standing and saw nothing out of the ordinary. He looked to the skyline just visible against the ambient light of the city and sky. Nothing.

Frank had the rope out and was skillfully looping it so when he tossed the grappling end onto the roof it would feed out cleanly.

Above them, Zico was intent on the slight motion he was sensing below. Not sure this was the moment he'd been on watch for, he moved his assault weapon to the ready. There was no need to work the slide. A bullet was already chambered. He slipped the safety off and placed his finger on the trigger, long experience telling him not to put pressure on it—yet. The weapon was on full automatic. At this range it would slice his target in half in under a second.

Below, Frank was poised for the toss. He looked back at Jeff, who was standing perhaps ten feet behind him, scanning the roofline. Jeff shook his head, certain he could make out the motion. Frank stepped back from the wall and started to twirl the rope. It moved slowly at first, almost touching the ground; then Frank increased the speed, creating a slight whirring sound. Just as it seemed to Jeff he was going to let fly, he slowed the motion, then without letting the metal hooks touch the ground and make a noise he stopped. He reached into his pocket and removed his cell phone. He placed it away, carefully put the rope and grappling hooks back into the bag, and approached Jeff.

"We're leaving. Now."

On the roof, Zico waited. Then he detected a slight sound, almost like a wire vibrating in the wind, but very faint. Try as he might he couldn't tell where it came from and it was so soft he wondered if he was imagining it. It faded. He listened intently. He thought he heard steps, but he had heard similar noises from time to time in the two nights he'd stood vigil. Cats, dogs probably, even the wind moving something.

"*Alarme falso,*" he whispered into the mouthpiece as he moved his finger and reset the safety.

In the office César looked to Paulinho and shook his head slightly. He relaxed back in his chair and scanned the security screens, utterly bored again.

Frank and Jeff moved cautiously along the black shadows painting the wall, Frank leading the way. After covering a careful twenty feet, Frank flushed a cat that screeched at being disturbed, then shot across the access alley.

On top Zico heard and spotted the cat as it raced out of darkness. Something else was moving below. He repositioned himself against the low roof wall and peered below. His eyes long accustomed to the dark, he spotted two men, crouched, moving cautiously away from the warehouse toward the street.

"Eles estão aqui." They are here, he whispered into his mouthpiece. He rose and fired in a single motion.

The shot was not ideal, as Zico was right-handed, and though he leaned well out, it was difficult from this angle to get a direct line on his targets. He knew at once he'd missed and leaned even farther as he instinctively adjusted his aim.

Below, the blast of the fully automatic assault rifle was like a cannon going off or lightning striking a few feet away. A line of bullets laced inches away just beside Jeff and Frank.

"Run!" Frank shouted as he shot forward, pulling out his automatic as he did. Instinct took over, and he understood the shooter would quickly adjust his aim. Frank turned as they ran, slowing just an instant as he looked to the rooftop. He saw the flash and fired into it three times as trained, the shots coming so rapidly they sounded like one.

Zico felt the IMBEL MD97 reel in his hands. At the same instant, a heavy blow struck his left arm and another his shoulder. The weapon fell away as he jerked back, pain suddenly spreading across his body. *"Fui atingido!"* he grunted. I'm hit. He slid to the rooftop, groaning.

"Todo mundo atrás deles!" Everyone! After them! César shouted into his mic.

Paulinho shot from his chair and raced out the door. On the roof Didi and Cafu ran to the street side of the structure. Didi was first and spotted two figures just crossing the street below, fleeing into the shadows. He fired.

Frank dived behind a broken block wall. "Get down!" he snapped. Jeff sank beside him. When Didi opened fire the second time, Frank again fired three times. On the roof Didi took one shot through his right eye, the back of his head popping open as the bullet passed through. He collapsed across the low wall of the roof, half of his body hanging over the side.

Just then, Cafu arrived. He looked at Didi an instant, then, cautiously, into the street. He could see nothing.

At almost the same instant Paulinho reached the street from below and, careless of his safety, ran out so he could clearly see. In the distance he made out running figures beneath the dim yellow streetlights. He raised the weapon to his shoulder and fired, knowing he'd need luck.

Frank, hearing the fire, spun, letting Jeff race past him, crouched, then fired in two bursts of three at the flash points he saw.

Paulinho saw the discharge, heard two shots whip by him so closely, he thought his hair was trimmed. He pitched off the road, then from greater safety peeked back down the street. The men were gone.

DAY NINE
TUESDAY, SEPTEMBER 18

NYSE IPO SOFTWARE CRITICIZED

Toptical IPO May Be at Risk, Critics Charge

By Dietrich Helm
September 18

The New York Stock Exchange is aggressively seeking to manage tomorrow's Toptical initial public offering. It has promised a seamless trading day in what some experts believe will be the most expensive IPO in history. Toptical management was vigorously courted by other exchanges but in the end went with the granddaddy of them all, in large part because they want to avoid the troubles that have plagued recent offerings.

Now some critics claim the NYSE is risking its reputation by employing a new program expressly designed for tomorrow's big day. Insiders report they have as yet to run a single test without significant problems. "They're not ready," one knowledgeable insider reported. "They've had nearly a year to get this right, and it still doesn't work as intended."

The new program is expressly designed to handle new issues related to high-frequency trading. HFTs are expected to dominate the first hours of the IPO, accounting for as much as 80 percent of the action. Highly sophisticated and very aggressive algos will be unleashed on the Exchange in a focused effort that experts say it has never previously experienced. Amid allegations that HFTs are able to manipulate the price of stock to their advantage the program is intended to prevent such efforts and safeguard the trading for the public at large.

"There is tremendous interest in Toptical stock and we want everyone to have an equal opportunity to take part," Paul Feldman, NYSE trading spokesman, said in a statement released Friday. He describes the new program as "the most sophisticated ever employed in a public offering."

Last week's revelations that malware was discovered within the trading software of the Exchange has shaken confidence. Though the market has largely rebounded from its 1,156 drop on Friday, questions linger. "The NYSE cannot afford to bungle this," Jason Lim, a respected stock market analyst, said yesterday. "I'm extremely concerned if they do. If the Toptical IPO turns into a disaster, major players are this time prepared to abandon the field and that includes the stock market altogether. They'll migrate into alternative trading vehicles for future trading. We could potentially see a collapse of confidence that will have worldwide and lasting consequences. No one can anticipate how destructive it could be but I've moved out of the market altogether until I see how this plays out. I'm not alone."

Feldman makes light of such criticism, commenting that doomsayers can always be found.

The competition to handle IPOs has never been keener and by delivering a seamless day Wednesday, the NYSE expects to solidify its position as the most reliable exchange for major players.

The market opens at 9:30 tomorrow as usual with the Toptical IPO scheduled for half an hour later. By midmorning tomorrow, we'll know if their gamble on a new software program was a wise move, or the disaster some critics fear.

TAGS: TOPTICAL, NYSE EURONEXT, IPO, TRADING PLATFORM

Cyber Security News

63

Daryl had wanted to get back into the building earlier, but most workers arrived at this hour, and she needed a crush for her makeshift card to work. She had no idea what would happen to her if she was caught, but she knew that without her help, Jeff and Frank were in very serious trouble. When a cluster of young women went to the open doors, she joined them, swiping her sterile card as she passed the distracted guard. Then she was in the elevator and on her way to the seventeenth floor.

She was a familiar face to some now and received a reassuring nod from several workers as she returned to the out-of-the-way workstation she'd selected. She hoped no one was assigned to it today. She'd brought a few things with her and placed them about: a pad of pastel-colored sticky notes, two pencils, a black pen, and a picture frame she'd picked up in a drugstore, the photograph of two smiling boys looking back at her. The space was hers now, until someone showed up and demanded to know what the hell she was doing.

Once settled, she returned to analyzing the logs, since they remained the key to what she needed to discover. With tweaks to the anomaly filters, what she uncovered over the next two hours were clear patterns, which she was confident were the work of those uploading malware but none of it constituted the kind of proof she needed and none led directly back to Campos. She also saw how busy the Exchange had been executing multiple uploads through the jump servers, which she believed were related to the next day's IPO. This activity, she concluded, was the new software being deployed and updated.

But there were also clusters of uploads she was just as certain were modifications or expansions of the rogue code. They came from some of the suspect sources she'd identified from examining the logs. Campos, she was convinced, was behind them. If she'd had any doubts something big was coming related to Toptical, she set them aside. There was a storm brewing and it would strike when the stock market opened the next morning.

She decided to risk coffee while she gathered her thoughts. Taking a break was natural and the recognition she received gave her confidence. As she stepped into the break room she saw the light-haired man Richard holding a cup of coffee as he fingered creamer into it. He looked up at her, and his pale eyes were suddenly alive. "Well, hi, Miss SSG. How are you this fine morning?"

"Very good. How's the coffee?"

"Average, I'd say, but around here that's pretty good."

She extended her hand. "I'm Kelly Vogle. You're Richard, right?"

He eyed her evenly for a second, then said, "Good memory. I am indeed Richard. Nice to meet you, Kelly. How long are you going to be with us?"

"I'm not sure. A few hours now and then, I think. It's really more a media cover-your-ass thing, you know?"

"Oh yeah. Not the first time. If you're still around later, let's have lunch."

Daryl paused, then said, "Let's do that." She poured coffee as Iyers left the room. Now, why did I do that? she thought. He'd told her that he was an infrastructure specialist. She could learn a lot from him over lunch. Working on this only from logs could take more time than she had.

Anyway, she thought, he's cute.

64

Jeff had been surprised he could sleep at all. When they'd arrived back at the hotel, it was nearly two in the morning. Frank had taken them the long way, ducking into alleys, hiding in darkened yards behind walls, watching, doubling back, making absolutely certain they'd not been followed. At first, there'd been sirens as police responded to the gunshots, but they'd never seen a police car, nor any suspicious vehicle on the prowl for them.

When they'd entered the room, Jeff said, "Why'd you call it off just before all the shooting happened?" There'd been no chance to ask sooner, and he knew it could wait.

"I got a message telling us we were in the wrong place."

"Daryl?"

"Who else? Let's talk about it tomorrow. I'm bushed and still have work to do."

Frank had made two phone calls, taken a shower, then gone to bed. Jeff followed him with a shower, finding Frank already fast asleep as he stepped out of the bathroom. In bed he had trouble sleeping, the night scenes of the firefight running through his mind again and again. He'd never fired his weapon, never even thought about it, nor had he been frightened. There'd been no time.

But now, in bed, alone in the dark quiet, he realized how close a call it had been. Those had been automatic weapons fired at them. The shooters had been near enough for him to hear the bullets ricochet off the cobblestone and block walls, to see the sparks when a bullet struck something metallic. A gnawing anxiety replaced the adrenaline of the firefight and their flight, and it was this that Jeff struggled to suppress. As he thought about it, grateful neither of them had been struck, he slid into a restless slumber of flashing gunfire and distorted images.

Frank let him sleep, but when Jeff awoke, he said, "Join me on the patio for a late breakfast, okay?"

It was a lovely late morning outside. The hotel was just far enough removed from busy streets to be relatively quiet. Birds sang in the overgrown courtyard trees. Two couples sat at other tables, tourists most likely, Jeff decided.

The breakfast was a buffet, and he loaded up his plate, emphasizing the ripe fruit and fresh bread. The coffee was strong and bracing, just what he needed. He sat and ate while Frank chatted as if nothing had happened the night before.

"What about that message?" Jeff finally asked, when it was clear he needed to bring the subject up.

"Daryl said it was a trap. Get out. So that's what we did. If it hadn't been for that damn cat, they'd never have known we were there."

"How'd she know?"

"She sent a message later. She's identified the inside man as a guy named Marc Campos. She got access to his cell phone and traced his calls and e-mails to a company in Rio named Grupo Técnico. That's our target."

"Rio? How far away is that?"

"About a five-hour drive. Don't worry about it. I've got it covered. Just eat up."

As Jeff was finishing they were joined by two nondescript men. Frank stood up with a broad grin. It was like old times for the three of them, lots of hugging and back pounding. The trimmer man of the pair turned to Jeff and introduced himself. "Hi, I'm Jeff," the man said.

Frank laughed. "No, he's Jeff."

"Oh. Hi," the trim man repeated, "I'm Carl. This is Oscar."

Oscar shook his hand; then the two men joined them, passing on breakfast. "We had a bite earlier."

From what Jeff had seen on the streets he would have taken the pair to be natives. Neither was over six feet tall. Carl was a spare man, looking very much like an accountant to Jeff, or a librarian. He wore glasses and had a retreating hairline. Oscar was only slightly bigger and, though he seemed in decent shape, had the same look—that of a man who spent a lot of time indoors. He had a thick head of dark hair just turning gray at the temples. Neither man was young any longer but neither looked especially old. There was a vagueness about them that made it difficult to pin them down in his mind.

"So how do you three know each other?" Jeff said. "Or can't I ask?"

"Oh, you can ask," Oscar said. "You'll even get an answer, but why go there?"

"We know each other from the old days, Jeff," Frank said. "I'm lucky they're here."

"It seems . . ."

"What?" Frank asked.

"I don't know, too much of a coincidence."

"See?" Frank said to the others. "I told you."

The men laughed, then lapsed into small talk that only they understood. They rarely finished a sentence, yet the other two knew what was being said. It was clearly a reunion.

"Listen," Frank said a bit later. "I need to talk with Jeff here. Why don't you bring the car around and we'll load up in, say, fifteen minutes. We've got a long drive ahead of us."

"No problem," Carl said as the pair stood up and left.

Back in the room, Jeff said, "Frank, I need to know who your two friends are."

"Actually, Jeff, you don't. The less you know, the better for all concerned. I know them, I trust them. Each of them has gone to considerable trouble to help us."

"I'm serious. You're going to have to tell me."

"You can stay here."

"I wish I could, but if we get access to Grupo Técnico's computers, it'll take both of us. I can't stay out of it so this concerns me as much as you. Anyway, I've already been shot at. And I take it Carl and Oscar aren't computer geeks?"

"No-o. Their specialties lie in other areas."

Jeff sat on a chair, leaned forward with his elbows on his knees, and said, "Tell me."

Frank was seated on the bed. "Jeff . . ."

"I'm serious. I won't go into this blind. You wouldn't in my place. Now, who are they?"

Frank sighed. "You've got a point there. I just wish you'd let this stay 'need to know.' That way if things go wrong, you aren't in a position to hurt anyone." Jeff said nothing. Frank continued, "You don't need their real names. I've worked with each of them singly more than once. Very dicey situations each time, none of that *Mission: Impossible* crap they put in movies but dicey enough for the real world. They're steady professionals, absolutely reliable. We worked as a three-man team on my last assignment before I gave up field-work. It lasted for six weeks, and when it was over, each of us spent some time in a hospital."

"They're Company?"

"Were, are. We didn't discuss it. In their field, it's not important as you never really leave. Anyway, Oscar's working out of Rio now. Officially, he's doing security with an oil company. I'm sure he's doing Company work as well. It's none of my business. He was in Curitiba when I called."

"Why's he here?"

Frank looked at Jeff in surprise. "He's here because I told him I needed him here. I contacted him last night. He just got in. Jeff, I've been out of this line for a long time. I'm soft and I'm slow. You saw how things are. We need help."

"You had me fooled last night."

"That? That was nothing. Instinct. And we were very lucky."

Jeff considered that, then said, "And Carl?"

"Carl's from São Paulo. He's definitely still with the Company; he runs some kind of front business here. I don't know what he's doing exactly but knowing him, it's interesting."

"They seem pretty nondescript."

"They're supposed to. They've spent decades getting that look down. Jeff, you need to trust me in this. I've already told you too much. But understand this: forget their looks. These guys are the best at what they do."

"You think we need them?"

"Oh yes. I absolutely think we do."

65

R ichard Iyers sat down and smiled across the table at Daryl. She was, without question, the loveliest woman he'd ever seen in person. He couldn't believe his luck.

The restaurant was crowded but the manager knew Iyers as a regular and had shown him to a corner spot, as quiet as was possible this time of day in Manhattan. They ordered, then Iyers made small talk, mentioning a bit of his origins in Upstate New York, bouncing the conversation back to Daryl from time to time. She found him an attractive man with his ready smile and dancing eyes, hinting a bit at a mischievous nature that held a certain appeal. Since Jeff he was the first man she'd so much as given a second look, but she intended to do nothing about it. This was work, and she was operating under a false name. She turned the conversation away from their personal stories.

"Are you involved in this new IPO program?" she asked to get it started.

Iyers drew back a bit, giving a cockeyed smile that said he knew she'd just changed the subject. "Not directly. I monitored it when it was initially uploaded and have followed up on each update but my only concern is to confirm it doesn't affect the trading platform in general. Not worried are you?"

Daryl shrugged. "All I know is what I read. There seems to be some skeptics."

Iyers nodded. "I understand. The Exchange is an enormous operation. You know that. But we have so many checks, it's amazing we're able to respond to changing needs at all. I'm giving it the benefit of the doubt."

"*The New York Times* thinks otherwise."

"Those guys. What do they know? I knew the snitch who told them that stupid bot story. He's an ass. He's just trying to get even."

"Still, it was malware that found its way in."

"It was a harmless bot and never went past the public-facing servers. I wouldn't be surprised if the snake didn't insert it himself when he suspected he was getting laid off. That's really the only way anything can get past our security. In my experience, it's always the human factor. Our digital security is all but impenetrable."

Their food arrived, and for a few minutes they said little. Daryl enjoyed good New York deli and wished she could focus more on her pastrami on rye. She looked around the noisy room. Why was it that nowhere else she'd ever been captured this mood? It was uniquely New York. It made San Francisco seem almost quaint. She looked back at Richard. How to go about this?

But before she could speak, Iyers said, "Kelly, I've really enjoyed this and I'm quite serious when I say I'd like to see more of you. But you should know that about six months ago I was one of two from the infrastructure team to attend a joint meeting with SSG. You'll never guess who I sat next to. Yes, Kelly Vogle." He smiled. "So who are you? FBI? SEC? Private?" His smile spread into a grin that said he didn't care which.

Stunned, the only thought Daryl could summon was gratitude this wasn't happening back in the IT offices with all the security. "Private," she said at last with no attempt at evasion. What was the point? He had her. "I'm a colleague of Jeff Aiken and Frank Renkin. You know them?"

"Sure. I was always trying to get them to use my gym. So what's your real name?" She shook her head lightly. "Okay. What's this about? You think they were set up?"

"They were framed without question."

"I liked them. And I researched Jeff. He's all right. I thought this whole thing was funny, you know? And the SEC have been assholes about it, accusing everyone. Some very hardworking, dedicated people are now under suspicion." He smiled. "I'm probably one of them."

"They were too close. I think they were set up by someone working at the Exchange, someone who wanted to get them out of the way."

"Too close to what?"

Daryl drew a breath. Here goes. She told Iyers what Jeff and Frank had discovered, malware concealed by a rootkit within the trading platform code. "There's an ongoing operation," she continued. "It's taking money out of the system. That's what they uncovered."

"You're telling me they penetrated to the trading engines?"

"Yes, absolutely. They had the run of the place."

"I find that very hard to accept. We've seen no sign at all. Not of any attempt, definitely not of anyone mucking around in there."

"They are very good."

"And they say they found a rootkit there? It can't be done," Iyers said. "There are too many safeguards."

"Well, take my word for it, it's there. I've seen it."

"You've seen it? You've been in the trading software?" She just gave him a look in reply. "Okay, I'll take your word for it. But you can't take money out of the Exchange without getting caught. It just isn't possible. Everything is tracked, and the automated systems call any anomaly to our attention."

"That may be but the looting takes place with a high-frequency algo that watches for bids and offers on a set of stocks at specific prices and puts itself at the front of the queue, taking a percentage of those trades. The accounts the trades go into route the money offshore. Except for working out of the Exchange trading platform it doesn't touch what is going on there. The theft takes place at the moment of the trade and is detectable only by the trading partners who are watching bids and orders at nanosecond granularity. If the amounts are small enough, I doubt they can even notice. If they do, it just looks like the buy came in lower than it first looked when the deal was approved."

"Clever but I don't see how software like that can get into our system without our knowing."

"Someone on the inside is doing it. That someone realized Jeff and Frank were getting close and set them up. Framing them was done very crudely. They opened a brokerage account in Jeff's name, put trading malware into the engine that was sure to attract interest, then sent the money straight to his account. You know the rest."

"Interesting. You have any idea who?"

Daryl hesitated. He might be cute, but she had no idea who he really was. "No. That's what I'm doing on-site. I'm looking for the mole. Are you going to let me work on this? Or turn me in?"

Iyers said nothing for several long moments. "What you say makes a lot more sense than what the SEC was insinuating. From how you describe it this frame job was pretty sloppy. We should be able to trace it back to your mole."

"'We'?"

"Sure. After you finish your coffee, let's go back to the office. You can show me what you've got. No one knows the system better than I do. I can help."

"Why would you do that?"

"Well, besides the fact that your explanation makes a lot more sense to me than the one the SEC is putting out there, I'd like to see this alleged rootkit for myself. I really can't believe it exists. And anyway, I'd like to get the bastard just as badly as you do. It'll be a feather in my cap." He smiled again. "Ready to go?"

On their way back to Wall Street, Daryl quickly ran through her mind the wisdom of this. The smart thing might be to just keep going, to say good-bye now and return to her hotel. Richard didn't know her real name.

Part of her was telling her to be cautious, not to trust this stranger, while another reminded her of just how effective she could be with a key infrastructure specialist working with her. She couldn't be the only one who thought how Jeff and Frank had been framed was too obvious. Richard would see it for himself soon enough. And if that didn't convince him, surely the rootkit would.

But what if this was a trap? What if he was just luring her back so she could be arrested?

That made no sense at all. He'd known from the first moment he'd heard her name that she was lying and had done nothing. Maybe he was working with the SEC, but that made even less sense. For the time being everyone at the Trading Platforms IT was to one degree or another under suspicion.

No, she'd take her chance.

A plum didn't fall into Iyers's hands very often, and he was still dazed by events. As he was going home the previous night, his thoughts returned repeatedly to the dazzling beauty he'd spoken to briefly. This morning, he'd made an effort to hunt her down. When she'd told him her name, it was all

Once the slender security chief was star
me about last night."

"Shortly before midnight, Zico repo
beside the warehouse. When it didn't rep
Then a cat attracted his attention. He s
return fire he was wounded in the arm
Didi was shot dead on the roof. Paulinho
nor Cafu were wounded."

"How many did they get?"

César cleared his throat. "I could find
that doesn't mean we didn't."

"How many were involved?"

"Based on what I heard and what my r
and seven."

"And where were you during this gur

"In the office, of course. The engage
signed to lure us away."

"There was nothing there to steal."

"No, but they didn't know that, and
out whoever tried the office. I had good r
They didn't need me."

Bandeira gathered his thoughts bef
this. We lure two computer nerds here a
no sign we even touched whoever came
any sense."

"We don't know it was them. I'm incl

"Then what was it?"

César shrugged. "A burglary gone wr
they thought we were storing somethin;
likely than it was the two we are waiting

Bandeira opened his mouth to dismi
sponsible, then stopped. Was that poss
from the first? "I don't see how," he said
If these were local men, we'll hear abou
been responsible for last night, he neede
consider the implications. And there was
his attention.

he could do to quell his excitement. She didn't know it yet, but he owned her, lock, stock, and barrel.

In his view, he'd had no alternative but to pretend he believed her, to offer to help. He needed to know what she knew, whom she suspected, and just as important, whom she'd told. They were down to the final twenty-four hours—less, actually. Tomorrow was going to be the biggest day of Iyers's life, and he planned to stick to whoever this woman was as if they were joined at the hip.

"Perhaps we should increase security at Grupo Técnico," César suggested. "Just to be on the safe side."

"It's not necessary. Keep good men at the warehouse. But I need you and Paulinho with me."

"As you say."

EDIFÍCIO REPÚBLICA
RUA SÃO BENTO
SÃO PAULO, BRAZIL
12:49 A.M.

Victor Bandeira replaced the telephone i
window without pleasure. Carlos Almeida
His anxiety over his coming windfall was b
to bear. He'd been complaining for months
to be the modest income stream of Casas de
ing online the task of handling the increase
for him. Bandeira was tired of holding the
ished, it was time to kick him upstairs and
into power. He shuddered to think that ther
ally confided in the man.

Bandeira had been amused at the sugge
then intrigued. The Almeidas were one of
Brazil. It would introduce Bandeira into a
tolerated him. To be married to such a wil
problem. He would do as he wished, just as
husband there would be no question of his
intrigued but not convinced. The child cou
was worth to him.

But Bandeira had no time for such tho
Carnaval. He told his assistant to send in (

67

Returning from lunch and her presumed alliance with Richard, Daryl decided to take a different, more direct, approach with her investigation. He went to his workstation while she settled in at her purloined cubicle. Time was running out, and she still didn't have the evidence she needed to clear Jeff and Frank. First, though, she needed to know who this Richard was. She accessed the administrator account Jeff and Frank set up previously when they compromised the Payment Dynamo server, since that account had access to most of the infrastructure. The account allowed her into the employee account database and human resource systems.

All she had was his given name, Richard, but she needed to know who he was. She was grateful for his offer of help but suspicious as well. It struck her as too easy, too opportune. Still, she'd overheard enough to know that the SEC was not popular here. Their execution of the search warrant and treatment of staff was still a popular topic. Richard could very well be telling her the truth.

She navigated in search of the infrastructure team but found them spread out in several subcategories. On a slip of scratch paper she wrote out, "Richard, Rick, Rich, Dick," then, looking down from time to time to remind her, she slowly worked through the employee lists. After ten minutes, she had five names, two of them using Richard, only one of which was an infrastructure specialist. Richard Iyers. That must be her man.

Something tickled in the back of her mind. Richard Iyers. Hadn't she seen that name before? She thought, but nothing came to her. It would in time, she was certain. For now, just to be on the safe side, she connected to Iyers's computer, which was identified in the network directory, and installed Jeff's monitoring software. This would allow her to read Richard Iyers's e-mail and log his keystrokes. She configured it to alert her whenever he sent or received e-mails. Next she copied off his access logs and scanned them visually and with Jeff's tool, but they showed no accesses to the jump server.

The logs were the key, though. As she continued to work on them she was identifying patterns of suspicious behavior, mapping it all out, dating it. This information established correlations with logs from other systems, fanning out into a complex map of interconnections, the majority of which would be red herrings. These patterns came from a number of different staff, but she was convinced they originated with Campos and whoever else was involved. Eventually she'd have enough of the map to find her way behind those cutouts, following the trail back to the originator. Knowing Campos was a target helped narrow the data, but it was still tedious work.

Then there was the IPO. She had access to the jump server and one advantage for her was that every update had to go through it. What she needed was a way to block any more updates, but most important, to ride into the system and turn off the rogue code.

From time to time her thoughts drifted to Brazil, to the danger Jeff and Frank were in. For security reasons contact was at an absolute minimum. She'd only received a text message after her two messages, thanking her and saying all was well.

But she'd given them the right address, the one in Rio, and she knew they'd be going there. One hard drive from the right computer, one person involved in the operation willing to talk, would bring this all to an end. She'd rather have worked out the answer entirely from computers but understood the logic of what they were up to. She just couldn't get over the sinking feeling she experienced every time she thought of them.

Marc Campos was both furious and scared. His fear came from the fact that the code he'd been receiving from Rio was not ready to be implemented. He was exhausted from rewriting and editing, from demanding that Pedro get his team on the ball. The clock was running down.

He was angry because Iyers wasn't doing his job. Even when Campos had code ready to upload, Iyers often wasn't available or was slow to respond. Campos had even gone to see him, something he almost never did in the office, only to find him away from his workstation. He searched and been stunned to see him standing in the hallway, leaning into a cubicle, talking to Kelly from SSG of all people.

Campos still didn't know what to make of her and her questions. At the time, the entire experience had been odd in the extreme, and he'd been sure he was uncovered. Seeing her at a workstation was reassuring to some extent as it suggested she was who she said she was. It was peculiar for someone from SSG to be working on-site, but not without precedent. He'd been afraid to check her out in detail as it would only call attention to himself.

Seeing Iyers talking to her led to only one conclusion, that once again he was distracted by a pretty blonde. It had happened before, though never at such a critical moment. As Campos had turned away he was suddenly seized by an overwhelming anxiety. What if the two were up to something? Here she was asking odd questions, and there was Iyers, the crucial cog in his operation, looking very friendly indeed.

Back in his office Campos called Iyers on his cell phone. When he answered, Campos said, "Meet me at the coffee shop, right now! Don't say a word, just do it!"

Ten minutes later, Iyers entered the narrow shop, glancing about as he always did, searching for women. He spotted Campos in the rear booth and joined him. Iyers told the waitress he'd take coffee, then turned to face Campos. "You look like shit," he said.

"What the hell are you doing with that woman?"

"Who? You mean Kelly?"

"Yes, Kelly. She questioned me yesterday."

"Questioned? How does she even know about you?"

"She's from SSG. She said she's here following up on that bot because of all the heat it's generated."

"Yes, but why talk to you?"

"I don't know. She didn't tell me. What are you doing talking to her?"

Iyers's coffee arrived. He sat back as he stirred sugar into it, then poured cream. He took a sip. "She's not SSG and she's not Kelly Vogle."

Campos found he couldn't breathe. His eyes widened in alarm. His tongue licked across his lips. "What are you saying?"

"I've met Kelly Vogle and this isn't her. I had lunch with this woman earlier and confronted her to try to find out what she's up to. I thought she might be official, working undercover or something."

"My God," Campos said, lowering his face into his hands. "It's over."

"Relax, amigo," Iyers said with a cocky grin planted on his face. "Everything's fine. We'll pull through."

"What . . . what are you talking about?"

"She's with Aiken and Renkin. She's here to try to clear them."

Bewildered, Campos said, "What do you mean?"

"What I said."

Campos processed what he'd heard, struggling to compose himself. Finally, he said, "Why did she talk to me? Did she tell you?"

"No. I don't know why. Aiken and Renkin aren't just running, they're trying to figure out who put the finger on them. This woman's working with them on that. They've come up with something that pointed to you."

"Jesus! That can't be. I've been so careful."

Iyers hunched down, moving closer to Campos, and lowered his voice. "She's not certain, Marc. Sure, she can try and blame you, and you and I know how bad that would be, but she needs to be positive before she takes that step. We don't need a lot of time here, and she doesn't know that. Toptical goes off tomorrow, in less than twenty-four hours. We'll have made our haul by this time tomorrow. She's working from Ann's old station. I'm sticking close to her, to see what she's up to, figure out how much she knows."

"Why would she let you do that?"

"Because I told her I think Aiken and Renkin are innocent and I want to help. She believes me."

"Why should she trust you?"

"Having someone on the inside will make what she's doing a lot easier." Iyers grinned. "And I've got a way with women. You know that."

Campos looked at Iyers and wondered how he could ever have recruited this man. This was supposed to be a cyberjob, computers only. Now because of Iyers, he had a murder and attempted murder on his hands. Only God knew what else.

"I need you to do our job. Carnaval is backed up."

"This is important too, to keep us out of jail, Marc. I'll take care of the rest. Don't worry about it. But don't you see? This makes it all easier."

"And how is that?"

"We're about to be blown. That means tomorrow night we take off. We don't risk sticking around. I just have to keep her on the string until then, and that won't be hard. I know what she's looking for."

Campos closed his eyes and thought. He swallowed several times, trying to work some moisture back into his mouth. Finally, he said, "Maybe—" He stopped. "Maybe, she needs your special attention." He couldn't believe he'd said it, but it was the only way.

"What's that?"

"We can't run tomorrow. We need to stay here and cover tracks as the money is funneled. It's part of the job."

"I don't get you."

"She's the only one who suspects, right?"

"There's Aiken and Renkin."

"They're being taken care of."

"Is that right? You never said anything to me about that."

"We just need to see to this woman."

"Oh, I get it. You're giving me the green light."

"Just don't be sloppy like you were in the park."

"No problem, amigo. It's about time you came around." Iyers picked up his coffee.

Campos glared at him. "Don't call me amigo."

68

Carl and Oscar rapped lightly on the door, then let themselves in. Frank had been asleep on the couch. He roused himself, went into the bathroom, then came out just as the other two retrieved bottles of water and made themselves comfortable in overstuffed, worn chairs. They looked as if they'd been out for a stroll, and perhaps in their world they had. Carl was in tan chinos with a light blue polo shirt while Oscar wore light green cotton pants with an untucked embroidered white shirt, Latin style. He had a cigar tucked in one of the pockets.

Jeff had watched them from over his laptop. He'd been in the safe house for some three hours now. When they'd arrived, Jeff asked if the CIA knew they were using it and been answered with laughter all around, then told not to worry about it. He closed the laptop and moved to the couch.

"What'd you find?" Frank asked.

"It's a two-story mansion converted into office space," Carl said. "The street is a mixed neighborhood with businesses and residences. It's surrounded by a ten-foot wall with the usual stuff on top. There's a car entrance with an electronic gate, a door for foot traffic, and a guard post. There were four vehicles parked inside. The grounds are neat, grass with no trees or significant shrubbery. In the rear is a helicopter landing pad with what looks like a storage building to the far side. We think the bottom floor is dedicated to security, and the offices we're after are on the second floor. All in all, not a bad setup if privacy and security are what you want while still looking legitimate."

"How many?" Frank asked.

Carl shrugged as he pushed his glasses up onto the bridge of his nose. "I made three. How about you?"

"Same," Oscar said. "Just one at the guard station, another on the grounds, a third inside watching the monitors. They all looked bored. It's possible there's a fourth on the second floor. We stayed as long as we could but weren't able to tell how many others are inside. They've got security cameras covering the grounds and two along the wall facing the street, which also takes in the entrance. We'll scope the setup tonight and do another count."

"When's the equipment coming?" Frank asked.

Oscar glanced at his wristwatch. "In about half an hour."

"Good. What about the second floor?"

"It looked busy," Oscar said. "Lights were on. We saw movement. Two guys, office types who came out for a smoke break looking pretty haggard. They stood away from the guards. There was no interaction with them. I'd say no more than six work upstairs, maybe less."

"It looked pretty busy," Carl agreed.

"I'm thinking around midnight," Frank said.

"Should be less security at night. We'll need time to observe before we move."

"They're on deadline," Jeff said. "It could be very busy tonight."

"So security may stick around, you think?" Oscar asked.

"It's a thought," Jeff answered.

"Maybe, maybe not," Frank said. "Guards are creatures of habit. Unless they've got some reason to think tonight is special, they'll leave the standard night shift."

"Probably one, then," Carl said. "Definitely no more than two."

"Your fracas in SP might have alerted them," Oscar suggested.

"Maybe they've made no connection," Jeff said. "They have no way of knowing we've learned about the Rio operation. Their lure sent us to the other site."

"Good point, but still, they might increase security," Frank said. Oscar and Carl looked at each other. "What?"

"I ran a check on the warehouse where you had the trouble and on this location," Carl said. "You aren't going to like it. Both places are buried in paperwork, but in some databases, they are identified as belonging to Nosso Lugar. It means 'Our Place.' It's commonly identified as simply NL."

"And what is NL?" Jeff asked.

"It's one of the major gangs out of SP," Carl said. "Slicker than most, well established. The *chefe* is Victor Bandeira. A thug but more enlightened. Big in banking and cybercrime."

"NL is big locally in banking and a major world operator in Internet gambling," Oscar said. "It fits what you've uncovered in New York to a tee. Apparently Bandeira has branched out."

"Bandeira, you say?" Frank repeated. "Daryl followed up last night's text warning with a copy of this address. The e-mail she used to locate it has a Pedro Bandeira listed as president. He seems to be running the operation in New York."

"A relative," Carl said. "A key position like that would only be trusted to someone close."

"What difference does this make?" Jeff asked. "We've suspected all along there was a criminal organization behind this."

"It only makes a difference in that these are very tough people," Frank said. "If security is increased we'll have our hands full. Ideally, we need to get in and get out without attracting attention. I'm thinking we go for the computers and skip taking a body."

"It won't matter," Oscar said. "Either way, once we make our move they'll be after us with a vengeance." Jeff moved uneasily. Oscar looked at him, the only outsider to their black ops world. "We've got this covered, Jeff. Don't be concerned. We just want Frank here to know what we're up against."

"From what you say they've made no connection between what happened last night and us. Otherwise, this place would be flooded with security." Frank stretched. "I'm going on an equipment run for me and Jeff in a few minutes. You two should get some sleep. We'll bring food in about eight, then do a gear check. Let's move out at ten thirty, be in place by eleven. Sound right?"

Carl and Oscar nodded. "Sounds good."

69

From inside his office, Pedro heard the helicopter drawing close, but gave it no thought. Helicopters were common in Rio, though this one was lower than usual. But when the volume increased, he looked out the window, wondering what was going on. Seeing nothing, but with the noise even louder he went through the offices to the downstairs.

The guard from the monitor was standing at French doors watching the back corner of the lot. "What's going on?" Pedro asked.

"*El Chefe* is landing," he said.

Papai? Pedro thought. Now what the hell is he doing here?

The Colibri midrange helicopter was in clear view now. The craft was slowing, the engine noise causing the shades to vibrate, the wind storm created by its rotors kicking up leaves from the grass lawn, the craft lowering itself slowly until at last it settled within the walls, some thirty feet from where Pedro stood.

As the rotors slowed César climbed out of the craft, holding his suit jacket close to his body, looking out of place with his dark sunglasses. Paulinho came out next. He was followed by Victor Bandeira who stepped from the craft clutching a briefcase. He lowered his head and came directly to the door. The guard all but snapped to attention. Seeing his son, Bandeira embraced him with a wide grin. "Caught you by surprise, I can see." He laughed.

"Show me what you are doing." He stepped off for the stairs leaving Pedro to catch up.

In his office Bandeira took Pedro's seat. The young man closed the door and sat in front. "What's going on?" his father asked. "We don't have a lot of time."

For other men of Bandeira's age and in other companies his presence would have been ludicrous, an aging manager pretending he understood the complexity of the sophisticated code Pedro's team produced. But Bandeira had worked with computers from the start and understood the basics of software, the demands of good code, and the creation of stable architecture. He'd required at least weekly briefings from Pedro during the development of Casas de Férias.

"Abílio stopped automatically forwarding our drops into the trading engines late yesterday. With our increased output, it was the only way to get the job done. Now we've been denied direct access."

"He told me. He said your code wasn't ready to upload and he needed to clear everything first."

Pedro wanted to take offense but what his father said was correct. "We've been under enormous strain, as I've told you. Increasing the take to so much in such a short time period has been more than we could handle with the same safeguards we've had. Not to mention the frequent trading engine code updates as the Exchange readies for the IPO." His father shot him a look but didn't interrupt. "I've got the team reworking code. Then it comes to me for review. When I think it's ready, I send it along to Abílio. The quality is better, but we're going too slowly. I'm concerned."

"What's the main problem?"

"The IPO module looks good. Even Abílio seems happy with it. Our test runs were largely glitch free, with just a few bugs. He's working on cleaning those up and plans a final upload later tonight."

"It's not already in place?"

"No, we held off as we didn't want to risk attracting attention in New York. If we'd uploaded earlier, we'd have to have done several updates and with the controversy over the bot their security level is heightened. We also have only so many opportunities to piggyback on the normal software updates. Abílio says there's a final Exchange IPO software update scheduled at three tomorrow morning. The Exchange, even with its vast resources, has been having many of the same problems we've got. We're riding in on it."

"Abílio says it will be ready?"

"As ready as we can make it. Our primary problem is in setting up the targets for the Casas de Férias aspect of Carnaval, the account module. Half the money will come from it. We've managed to identify a sufficient number of targets, companies and funds we know will take part in the Toptical IPO. Our difficulty has been in writing the configuration for each one and in securing enough routes to get the money out of the United States quickly. I've had to make some compromises."

"What compromises?"

"This past year, as you know, we've limited our take to around five percent. In some cases, when the trade was small-time enough that the players didn't have enough clout to have their complaints acted on, we've increased the take significantly. I am using those increased parameters now with essentially the same account module."

"Good. It's proven software. This is the final operation. How much is the increase?"

"Depending on the action and our ability to hide within it we are programmed to take as much as half of any trade."

Bandeira's eyebrows shot up. "You think we've got cover?"

"We think this will be the most confused IPO in history. Abílio says the new IPO code is simply not ready. He expects all kinds of problems including interruptions, signficantly increased latency, and volatile volume as the high-frequency algos kick in. God knows what they've got up their sleeves. We think our action, big as it is, will be well concealed. In time, of course, months from now, after the inevitable SEC investigation into the IPO, our take will stand out, but by that time the money will be long gone and the electronic trail erased or so obfuscated, they'll never be able to follow it to a meaningful end."

"You've done well. You look tired. Well, in a few hours, you can rest."

"Why are you here, *Papai?*"

"I told you. This is important. I'll be here through the IPO. I've got an important meeting tonight but will be back later." He smiled. "We can watch the operation unfold together. This is a great moment for NL and for us." He rose, came around the desk, and placed his arm across the young man's shoulders.

"I will enjoy that," Pedro said, realizing as he did that he really meant it.

70

Richard Iyers grimaced as he sat at his workstation. When he'd met with Campos and assured him that he'd stay on the woman he'd completely forgotten the meeting he had to attend. The new IPO software was scheduled for the daily upload in a few hours, and the presence of all the senior infrastructure specialists was mandatory. There would be a final triage of the outstanding bugs, and there were more than a few. Not that there was anything much they could do at this point. The decision was made, the timing was set. They would have to hope the bugs wouldn't impact the IPO or surrounding trade activity. The market would open at nine thirty the next morning, as usual—with the Toptical IPO scheduled for ten o'clock.

Iyers checked and saw three sets of code modifications Campos wanted him to review, bundle, and insert with the next Exchange update. Iyers sighed. It would take hours, and he'd probably get more yet. It was going to be a long night.

But his real concern was the woman. He had no idea what she'd been up to all afternoon. In his experience women were no better than average when it came to this kind of work, so he wasn't unduly concerned. Aiken and Renkin had impressed him with their calm assurance but this hot chick was something else. Such women liked to talk a good game but lacked the intuition that understanding complex code and network systems like the Exchange required. The only disturbing aspect of their conversation was that she knew he'd used a rootkit. He assumed either Aiken or Renkin had found it.

Still, for now, the Rio code would have to wait.

Since returning from lunch, Daryl had continued to analyze the logs with the aim of finding the digital trail to Campos. No employees interrupted her at her appropriated workstation. Alerts from Iyers's e-mail had distracted her throughout the afternoon, but they were all routine Exchange business. But what she did note was the high number of them between Iyers and Campos.

Daryl paused. Something was nagging at her. Something she knew she'd missed. Then it came to her. She hurriedly pulled out her laptop and quickly went to her notes from the previous day. There it was. The Appreciation Trust accounts with Pacific Eastern Bank had been opened in the name of Dick Iver.

Richard Iyers. This was no coincidence. For a chilling moment she recalled the assault on Jeff. These were desperate men. She needed to stop thinking about this as a purely computer problem.

"Kelly," Iyers said, "hard at it, I see."

Daryl glanced up from her screen. Her throat caught for an instant. She switched to another screen. "Hello, Richard. Still here, I see."

"Busy night. We've got the big IPO tomorrow, and there's a much larger update than usual scheduled at three A.M. Lots to go over. Sorry I haven't been able to come by sooner to help out. I've been in a meeting. What have you been doing?"

"I've not accomplished much so far. This is all very sophisticated, much more demanding than the code I usually work with." She gave him her "I'm only a girl" smile.

"Don't feel bad about it. We hire the best, and it takes months before anyone can navigate the system with confidence, let alone rework code. Have you tried the logs?" The only real worry Iyers had was if she turned to the logs, found the right ones, and proved good at reading them. He and Campos had discussed them many times over the years because they were the Achilles' heel of their operation. They'd hidden their trails within the work of others and believed they were covered but if they could create them, someone with enough determination, time, and expertise could trace them back.

"Not really. They're pretty complicated. I was thinking maybe you could spend some time with them, since you know the system better than I do. It's hard for me to know what's legitimate activity."

"Sure. It'll have to be tomorrow, though. I'm packed with work before then, probably not surprisingly."

Daryl looked disappointed. "If you have to. I can't hang around here much longer though. Someone's going to ask questions at some point." She brightened. "What did you think of the rootkit?"

Iyers was startled. He'd not bothered to look at it. After all, he'd planted it and knew it was there. "Really something. I didn't think it was possible. It's going to be quite a coup for me when I officially report it."

"Don't act too fast," Daryl cautioned. "Wait until I'm out of here."

"I will. Don't worry." Iyers stared at her a moment. Was it possible he'd overestimated her even with his reservations? Right now, she didn't sound bright enough to be a threat. "Well, I've got to get back. You know where I'll be." He stopped, then added, "At some point tonight, we both need to stop. Let me buy you a late dinner or early breakfast, depending, okay?"

"That would be nice," Daryl said, as no other answer was acceptable.

Once she was satisfied he'd left she returned to the logs.

71

The streets were largely calm as the four men drove to the Grupo Técnico offices in Carl's Camry. Still, people were out, though not that many and the traffic was light, mostly small commercial trucks.

No one spoke. There was a slight mood of tension in the air but nothing extreme or uncomfortable, much like a college classroom just before the big exam. Carl drove by the stadium, then turned down a narrow residential street two blocks from the office, pulled into an open parking space, then killed the lights and engine.

The men climbed out of the car and shut the doors quietly. In the near distance a dog yapped. Oscar opened the trunk and handed a dark sports bag to Frank. He gave a smaller one to Carl, who swung it from his shoulder while Oscar did the same with a matching one. Then Oscar lifted a small black plastic suitcase from inside the trunk and closed the lid.

The case held heat sensor equipment that had been mysteriously delivered to the hotel. Jeff hadn't seen the man, if it had been a man, but been shown the suitcase contents. Frank had explained that with this they'd be able to know exactly how many people were within the mansion and their locations.

Frank, Oscar, and Carl took three cell phones from their pockets Frank had acquired earlier. They turned them on, secured them on their belts, put their earpieces in, and clipped mics to their collars. Without a word, they set out toward the office building, Jeff following closely. A few minutes later, Frank stopped in the shadows on the opposite side of the street. Oscar and Carl separated from them and, it seemed to Jeff, vanished.

A small motorcycle buzzed by. Jeff caught a glimpse as it passed. Pizza delivery.

They were still well down the street from the entrance, out of range of the security cameras. Inside his pocket, Jeff grasped the revolver Frank had given him. It felt heavy, and lethal. Several minutes passed. Frank murmured quietly into his mic, then said, "The boys are in place."

"How are they going to use that equipment with the wall blocking them?"

"They've got an elevated location."

A short time later, Frank mumbled again into the mic. Then he looked to Jeff. "There's a helicopter in back of the main building."

"Reinforcements?"

"We're getting the count now."

After ten minutes, he spoke. "There are five guards, four inside the building. We make three on the second floor. One on the ground floor, seated at a table or desk. The fifth is on foot, staying generally near the guard post at the gate."

"What do you think?"

"Let's move. It's as thinly manned as we can hope."

There were more lights here than along some streets Jeff had seen but it was still very dimly lit. It was a narrow street and traffic was sparse. Frank and Jeff went closer to the entrance.

"What now?" Jeff asked quietly.

"Just watch," Frank whispered.

Oscar approached the front entrance by himself. With his slight build, glasses, and accountant demeanor he looked utterly innocent and a bit confused. He said something through the metal gate. A stout man in a tan uniform and peaked cap stepped toward him. He was wearing a thick black bulletproof vest, had an automatic pistol on his hip, and carried a military-style rifle across his chest, a common look for Brazilian security guards from what Jeff had seen. He moved closer to the entrance, stopping a few feet back. He said something in Portuguese.

"Oscar's asking directions," Frank whispered. "When you follow me in, close the gate behind you."

There was an exchange of words; then the guard noticeably relaxed, came right up to the gate, and gestured down the street as if giving instructions. Oscar shot a hand through the gate and almost instantaneously the guard crumbled.

"Now!" Frank said as he ran to the entrance, Carl sprinting to meet them from the other direction. By the time they arrived Oscar had the gate slid open. The three men squeezed through and shot across the driveway toward the front door to the mansion. Jeff hesitated over the fallen guard but saw no blood. By the time he entered the building the single guard there had his hands in the air. He'd been seated at a desk in front of a computer monitor.

"Upstairs," Frank ordered. Oscar joined them and the three went up leaving the guard with Carl.

Pedro was scowling at the screen. Everyone was so exhausted no one was functioning efficiently, even him. Well, it wouldn't be much longer. Abílio would need the final Carnaval code in the next three hours so that he could plant it with the Exchange update. Abílio said it was a big one as there were still changes being made to the new IPO software. After that, Pedro planned to sleep a bit to be ready for when the Toptical IPO started seven hours later. He'd be watching that with his father.

He heard loud steps pounding on the stairs and wondered what that was about. Had his father come back? Then he heard orders barked in the outer office and felt a chill. Before he could react, a strange man entered his office, holding a gun in his hand.

"Push away from the computer," Frank ordered in English, sure the boss would speak it.

"American? What are you doing here?" Pedro said. "Get out!"

"Move from the computer," Frank repeated.

Pedro looked into his eyes, then at the weapon, then stood and backed up, pushing his chair from the desk. Frank came around, turned him to face the wall, then secured his wrists with the type of plastic strip that served police as temporary handcuffs. "Sit," he ordered, directing Pedro back into the chair.

Jeff, still near the door to Pedro's office, looked into the outer office and saw the three coworkers uncomfortably seated on the coach, their hands behind their backs. Renata's eyes were wide with terror. Oscar was hovering over them, looking ominous.

Frank shut the door and turned to Pedro. The color had drained from the young man's face. His eyes bulged and he blinked spasmodically. Still, he managed to speak. "Who are you?

"Who we are isn't important."

"What have you done with Gustafo and Luís?"

"They're fine, for now."

If Jeff hadn't known how much of this was a bluff, he'd have bought Frank's threatening manner.

Pedro stared at the two gringos. They were grim-faced, serious men. He gathered his courage. "What do you want?" he said.

"Let me tell you what we know already so we can save a bit of time here. You and the others outside have written malware and infiltrated the New York Stock Exchange with it. You've been stealing money for about a year now. How am I doing?"

Pedro's wide eyes grew wider. "I don't know what you're talking about."

"If you expect to get out of this, you're going to have to get a lot smarter than you're acting right now." Frank crossed his arms. "Put your thinking cap on. Just who do you think we are?"

That, Pedro thought, was an excellent question. Possibilities came to him in a wave. "I don't know."

"Let me give you a hint. The Exchange hired someone to run a test of their trading platform. The people doing that encountered your malware, crudely hidden I might add in a rather quaint rootkit. Any ideas forming about who we are?"

Pedro looked at Frank with fresh interest, then at the tall man standing to his side and slightly behind him. "No."

"This is where it gets interesting." Frank squatted down. "One of the two guys doing the penetration test went for a run in Central Park. He was attacked and nearly killed. Now he's really pissed off, so is his friend. How are the brain cells working now?"

"Attacked?" Could it be? He stared at the men, at one, then the other, back and forth, as if he could decipher their thoughts.

"Whoever did it didn't care if he lived or died. At the same time one of

your helpers in New York planted code making it look as if they were stealing the money, instead of you."

My God! Pedro thought. This can't be! "You?"

"Yes," Jeff said. "Us. We're the men you framed and tried to murder."

"No, no, not me, I . . ." Pedro stopped.

"Now, listen, we have a deal for you. It's important. If it works out, you
get to live." Frank waited for that to sink in.

Pedro licked his lips. "What deal?"

"You stop what you're doing. Turn it off, take it down, whatever you
have to do, but you stop it. Then you tell us all about your operation, most
importantly, the name of your helper in New York."

"I don't know what you're talking about."

"Too late, Pedro. We know you do."

"You're wrong."

"Now, listen, kid," said Frank. "We can have a talk like adults, you can
get back on your computer and stop this operation, or I can hurt you, hurt
you in ways you've never considered, and when I've finished, we'll still have
that talk and you'll still bring this operation to an end. The only difference
is how much and for how long you suffer, and how hard you make me work
because when this is over, I have to decide if it's worth letting you live."

It was a bluff, Jeff knew. The objective was to make the young man believe it. Then he wondered. Frank might very well be serious. Not for the
first time, Jeff considered just how far things had gone.

Frank let the threat linger in the silence. Pedro looked at him, then to
Jeff, then back again. He licked his dry lips, suddenly thirsty. "I can't stop
it," he said finally. "It doesn't matter what you do to me. I can't."

"It's the only way you're getting out of this in one piece," Frank said.

"You don't understand. I'm blocked out. If I tried to shut the operation
down, the man in New York would see it, even if I found a way to do it.
He'd just report the effort, and undo what I did."

"Who would stop you from shutting down this operation?" Jeff asked.

"I . . . I can't say."

Frank reached down and gently touched Pedro's knee. The young man
recoiled as if he'd received an electric shock.

"Abílio. His name is Abílio Ramos," he said, forgetting in his fear Abílio's assumed name.

"Where does he work?" Frank asked.

"At the Exchange. I told you." Pedro was sweating. The acrid smell coming from him was pungent.

"Where? It's a big operation."

"I don't know. I never asked. I wasn't supposed to ask. Please."

Frank lifted his hand.

"Who would he report the effort to?" Jeff asked.

Pedro's tongue darted across his lips. He said nothing.

"You're going to tell us, Pedro. Trust me in this," Frank said.

"My . . . my father."

"And who is your father?" Frank asked.

"Victorio Bandeira." Pedro hesitated, then with a rush of pride said, "He is *chefe* of the Nosso Lugar!"

72

COPACABANA PALACE
AVENIDA ATLANTICA
COPACABANA
RIO DE JANEIRO, BRAZIL
11:37 P.M.

Victor Bandeira looked at Carlos Almeida and made sure to disguise his disgust. The banker sweated profusely, had even used his dinner napkin to wipe the gleam from his bald pate. The third man at their table was Ernesto Dayan, president of the Banco Central do Brasil. Dinner was over, and they were smoking Cubanos and drinking brandy.

Dayan was one of the new breed of technocrats who dominated Brazil's economic policy. New to the job, he came from a long line of bankers. Bandeira understood there was a family connection with the Almeidas. Dayan's hairline was in significant retreat, and he compensated with a trimmed beard. He wore rimless glasses on his bland, pasty face and was not amused by the evening. They'd dined well on the finest North Italian cuisine, a hotel specialty, and Bandeira had ordered only the most expensive wines, but he was certain he'd made no dent in the man's concerns.

The entire purpose of this meeting had been to reassure Dayan. To that end, Almeida had been his backup, and he'd played his part badly. If anything, his nervousness had only disturbed Dayan even more. But the harm was done, business was finished. When Bandeira had assured him that the operation was on track, Dayan had only looked at him with dead eyes. He'd then dismissed Bandeira's mention of a woman with a noticeable curl of his upper lip, as if he'd just been insulted.

Other meetings had not gone smoothly, either. In the end, it came down to the money. When Dayan's Swiss account bulged with the Carnaval take, all his concerns would be set aside. It was always that way.

They made their goodbyes, and after Dayan was gone, Almeida remained. "I think it went well."

"Yes," Bandeira said, "quite well. Give my regards to your lovely wife and daughter."

"Perhaps . . . perhaps you'd care for another drink at the bar?"

"I wish I could, but I have yet another business meeting," Bandeira said.

"So late?"

"With my son. Tomorrow is a big day for us, Carlos. Remember?"

"Oh, yes, of course."

They parted in the lobby. César had already summoned the car. Sergio, who'd also flown the helicopter, was driving. Paulinho, one of Bandeira's oldest and most trusted men, sat beside him. The four drove through the streets back to Grupo Técnico.

73

R ichard Iyers finished editing a portion of the Carnaval code Campos had sent earlier and moved it into the deployment for later. There was still more to come. He glanced at his watch. Three hours.

He went to the break room and poured a cup of black coffee. Standing at the sink drinking it, he noticed that his hand trembled slightly. Back at his computer he opened the logs for the jump and deployment servers and for those of his own system. Once or twice he'd seen something that caught his attention in his earlier scans, but nothing that in the long run proved a worry. Tonight, though, he saw that the deployment server was being accessed by another infrastructure specialist who he know for a fact had left work earlier that night for a break, planning to return after midnight. This was one of the systems he and Campos used to access the server, which meant someone out there was being clever.

Someone, like a gorgeous blonde who wasn't nearly as dumb as she acted. Iyers had hoped to enjoy his time with the woman but there was too much at stake for such an indulgence. And events were moving quickly. He had the green light from Campos and strong evidence she was too close. The only danger was in waiting.

With a growing sense of anticipation Iyers made his way to Daryl's workstation. Though it was positioned to be largely hidden, he knew this floor intimately. He positioned himself so he could watch her unobserved while he thought about how to do this. He eyed the back of her head and admired her blond hair. There was no doubt it was real. If he ever learned her real name, he was certain he'd discover she was of Scandinavian origin, perhaps German. She moved once to the side and he caught sight of a breast. He felt a stir. He stepped toward her.

Daryl was making progress. As the number of staff diminished, she'd been able to work with greater concentration. Just then, she sensed someone behind her. She closed the log analysis, which snapped up another window with irrelevant logs, then turned.

"Hello, Richard," she said. "You still here?"

"No rest for the wicked." He lowered his voice. "We need to talk."

"Okay." She waited.

"Not here. Somewhere private." When he saw her hesitate, he added, "I've found something you need to know about. There's an all-night coffee shop right next door. We won't be gone twenty minutes. Trust me. It's worth your while."

"If it's that important, let's go." Daryl stood, slipping her purse strap onto her shoulder.

74

On the ground floor, Carl had tied up and gagged both guards. He'd next gone outside to the gates and confirmed they were in their usual closed position. Oscar had taken the three staffers downstairs, binding their wrists and seating them on a couch, while Frank moved Pedro into the outer office to give Jeff free rein at the computer.

For several minutes, the pair questioned the trio with no luck. It was obvious they were far too frightened of something worse than them to talk. Renata simply lowered her head, shut her eyes, and gently moved her head back and forth. The other two repeatedly exchanged looks at each other but neither spoke a word.

"What do we do with them?" Oscar finally asked. "We haven't got all night."

Carl considered their next move. "We can come back to them if necessary. Let's move them outside for now. There's a storage building of some kind. Looks like it might have been a horse stable back in the day."

The men took the five prisoners outside, across the darkened yard to the structure. The door was unlocked. They moved everyone inside and ordered them to sit against the wall. They bound their ankles with plastic straps.

Back in the office building Oscar checked the security system and found it deficient. There were too many blind spots. He went to Carl and took him aside. "I'm setting up visual security. We should assume we don't have much time."

Upstairs, Frank told Jeff, "Don't forget to collect paper and find something to stash it in. Assuming it's in Portuguese, I should be able to read it with a little help from a translator." He eyed Pedro who was pretending not to listen.

"Right," Jeff said. "We'll also take hard drives. No reason to hang around here longer than we need to." He went to the office, located a trash basket, emptied it, and then started examining the papers he found neatly piled on the credenza. After a minute spent examining them, he just piled every-thing into the basket. Then he went on his knees and began unscrewing the hard disks of Pedro's system. He'd have them out in two minutes; then he'd take the disks from the three computers he'd seen outside.

In the outer office Frank called to Oscar below. "Any luck with the geeks?"

"None. They won't talk. They're much too scared of what will happen to them. We put them outside with the guards. Given a bit of time they could be persuaded but we've got the big guy's son, right? Let's take him. It's sim-pler and he's running the show. Why waste time on the little guys?"

"My thought exactly." Frank looked to Pedro and grinned.

On the street outside, Sergio slowed before the gates and waited. After a moment, Paulinho said, "Where's Luís?"

"What's that?" Bandeira asked, looking up from his iPhone.

"Luís, Chefe," César said. "He's supposed to be at the gates or very nearby at night. Should I honk?"

Bandeira looked toward the mansion. Nothing seemed out of place but . . . "What do you think, Jorge?"

Jorge's keen eye swept the yard and building. He'd seen it many times at this time of night, and it didn't look the same. "Maybe last night wasn't what we thought. We should be cautious."

"Yes, I agree," Bandeira said. "Pull up here on the street. We'll go in on foot."

Once they'd parked, the men exited the vehicle, closing the doors qui-etly. "The trunk," Bandeira said. Sergio opened it and removed two IMBEL MD97s, Bandeira taking one, Paulinho the other. The others pulled heavy automatic pistols from their waists as they all went through the pedestrian doorway, then made their way silently across the driveway toward the man-sion entrance.

FINAL DAY
WEDNESDAY, SEPTEMBER 19

TOPTICAL IPO LOOMS

By Lawrence F. Gooden
September 19

"Unease" is the best word to describe today's Toptical initial public offering. Touted as the biggest public offering of all time in some quarters with figures in excess of $100 billion being bandied about, insiders have sought to downplay expectations for weeks, asserting the IPO will not exceed $30 billion. The reality is that there is no way to know where the valuation will land as expectations often dictate outcome.

For nearly two years, Toptical has been the hottest social networking platform on the Internet, attracting users because of its seamless interface and perception of control. Businesses like the clever way marketing has been designed into the system. This has addressed the most serious problem social networking sites face upon going public—they have to make money or at the least demonstrate the path to it. Now payday has arrived for the company's founders and early investors. And that's just one of the problems.

The Toptical IPO is heavily skewed in favor of insiders, that is, those who have been invested with the company from early days. As many as half of the shares being offered come from them. This is far more than is common and suggests to some observers that those in the best position to know have no long-term faith in the company. Others argue that there are just a lot of players looking to profit and that the big percentage of total stock coming from them is not all that out of line when applied in each case.

The sheer volume of stock being made available raises serious questions as to whether or not the stock is oversubscribed. If it is, and it may very well be, too much stock will dilute share value. This will put the price into a nosedive initially and no one will be able to accurately predict at what price it will settle. This uncertainty is causing many principal clients of Morgan Stanley to reconsider their position.

The tip-off came a few days ago, when Morgan Stanley issued a last-minute revised prospectus. Readable between the lines of what was ostensibly an upbeat report was the suggestion that institutional investors exercise caution today. It is unlikely such caution will be demonstrated by the average investor for whom Toptical is often considered a close digital companion.

Looming over today's IPO are two issues not commonly appreciated by the investing public. The first of these is the fact that the NYSE is employing new software to handle this IPO. Reports indicate it is still buggy. Given the track record of special software for IPOs there is legitimate concern. You need look no further than the disastrous BATS offering, and it was in the business of IPOs. A major meltdown by the software isn't even required. A single glitch at the wrong moment can send a tremor through the marketplace that could become a self-fulfilling prophecy. We're told there are no problems but that's what they always say.

The second major issue is the role the high-frequency traders will play today. It is estimated that as many as 80 percent of the trades will be their creation. HFTs have come in for a lot of criticism of late, and deservedly so. The problem for the public and for Toptical is that most of the abuses HFTs engage in have not been eliminated. We can be certain that at least some stock price manipulation and false volume will be solely their creation. This alone will cause uneasiness and hesitation on the part of big players.

The primary problem associated with HFTs is that they make money if the stock goes up, or if it goes down. The consequence is that they have no vested interest in maintaining value. The algos HFTs use tend to act in unison with slight variations as each seeks an advantage. If the HFT algos decide Toptical is going up, they'll join in the ride and from their participation we may witness the largest public offering in world history. But if the algos decide the stock is tanking the HFTs will pile on and drive the stock into oblivion. Either, or neither, could happen today.

What experts recall is that a trade of just over $4 billion when the average volume was $200 billion on a single day created the infamous Flash Crash. They claim that the measures taken since then will not prevent a repeat of it. We can expect more than one trade today to exceed $4 billion dollars. The consequence is that what is at stake isn't whether or not people make money. It is if Wall Street can sustain the shock of another Flash Crash incident. And if it cannot, then the world financial system could very well totter on the brink of collapse. All it will take is a single push to shove it into the abyss.

75

Daryl noted how clean the air was outside on the street after the stuffy, closed space of the Exchange with all its electrical devices. There was a light, cool breeze, heavy with the smell of the Atlantic sweeping the Wall Street canyon, and she drew her suit jacket close in front of her.

"The coffee shop is just there," Iyers said with his usual smile. "It's not bad. The best part is that it's open 24/7."

Daryl had noticed it before. Iyers took the outside position as they walked toward it.

This was a situation she was uncomfortable with, but she didn't know how else to deal with it. Iyers was part of the operation, though she had no reason to think he knew that she knew. Still, she couldn't help but be on edge. She'd made good progress with the logs and copied the suspect ones to a thumb drive. With the two in-house names and the incriminating information she'd collected leading to Brazil she was satisfied she had enough to get the SEC to back off Jeff and Frank and take another look at what was really going on.

What she needed to do now was block the rogue code so it wouldn't be operational when the IPO launched. The more she'd seen of the operation, the more it frightened her, and the speed with which changes had been made to the code in recent days suggested to her a lack of proper care. High-frequency traders, even the Exchange itself, took months to carefully craft every bit of code they inserted into the trading engines, yet glitches still happened. How much damage would a group of freebooters, their common sense dulled by greed, cause with sloppy code?

Iyers was chatting, and she feigned attention, glancing up at him from time to time, as if this were a first date. He was an attractive man, no doubt about it, but she'd seen enough of him to realize there was a forced congeniality in his interactions. There had been moments when it struck her that he was acting.

How different Jeff was. If anything, when they'd been together she found his lack of spontaneity almost too much. Looking back on it, she realized how refreshingly honest he was. Even when he was ending their intimate relationship, he'd been unable to be anything but candid. She'd taken offense at that, had nursed her anger for a wasted year. Now she understood how rare it was. If she ever got a second chance, she told herself, she'd embrace his candor, not see it as something to deal with.

As they passed an alleyway just short of the coffee shop, Iyers looked up the street, then down. Without warning, he bodychecked her off the sidewalk into the gaping blackness. Stunned, Daryl staggered, recovered her balance, then opened her mouth to scream. Iyers struck her on the side of her face with his fist, like a prizefighter delivering a knockout blow. Daryl fell, her head swimming as she struggled to remain conscious.

Iyers looked quickly back toward the sidewalk for any sign of alarm. Seeing none he seized Daryl's feet and dragged her deeper into the dark, pulling her beyond two overloaded Dumpsters. Satisfied they could no longer be seen, he stopped and stood astride the prostate woman like a conqueror, breathing heavily.

From the ambient light and dim glimmers from windows facing the alley he could see her prostrate form. Her skirt had been pulled up above her waist revealing her panties and legs, looking pale and vulnerable. He was suddenly aroused to a fever pitch.

He reached down and jerked her out of her jacket, her body twisting side to side as he pulled it off with force. Next he tore at her white blouse, angry when it refused to give at once, tearing at it harder, finally ripping it apart to reveal her bra.

Iyers had never raped anyone before, though it was one of his recurring fantasies. Until now, he'd always taken his victims drunk or drugged, sometimes dazed from his rough handling. They were always unwilling, or at the least in no position to be willing. Still, he'd had to be careful they'd not report him and that caution had always limited what he could do.

But not tonight, not now. He could do what he wanted before killing her. It was that realization that excited him. He'd be gone in a few days after all. There was no reason he'd be suspected, no reason to hold back.

Daryl moaned and Iyers slapped her. Then he knelt beside her and began clawing at her panties.

76

As they approached the parking area in front of the wide stairs leading to the French doors, César gestured for the men to stop. He stood examining what he saw. After a moment, he turned and whispered to Bandeira. "*Chefe,* wait here while we approach. It doesn't look right. There's no guard on the grounds and I can see no one at the desk."

"My son is in there," Bandeira said in a nearly normal voice so all could hear. "Nothing must happen to him."

César gestured for the other two to follow, then moved cautiously toward the building. Bandeira held back, then, unwilling to wait, moved with them, his weapon at the ready.

Carl was watching the outside approach. "Trouble," he said. "We've got visitors, and they're moving like a combat patrol, weapons ready."

"Shit," Oscar said as he took out his automatic pistol and moved to position.

"Four armed men approaching cautiously, Frank," Carl said into his mic. "They aren't sure about us yet, but they soon will be."

"I'll be right down." Frank gave Pedro a "stay right there" look, then moved to the door as he pulled out his weapon. "We've got company. I'm going down. You need to get in here and keep an eye on this one. He's our ace in the hole. And keep your head down."

Jeff had just pocketed Pedro's hard drive and was about to move into the outer office to start on the computers there. He came into the office as Frank was running down the stairs. He looked at Pedro. "Don't move."

Pedro nodded. His father was back and with him was César and two bodyguards, hard men he'd often seen over the years. These Americans were in serious trouble. This whole raid had struck him as lunacy. What did they expect to gain from it? No one here was going to talk. He certainly wasn't. And the way things were going, they'd be dead in a few minutes.

In the short time he'd been seated, Pedro had steadily worked at the plastic strip binding his wrists. It still held him fast, and he doubted he could free his hands, but he had to try.

César halted the men once again. He still could not see either of the guards who should have been in plain sight.

"Spread out. I think we have trouble. Be careful of your targets," he ordered.

"Anyone who harms my son dies, along with his family," Bandeira hissed.

Frank, Oscar, and Carl spread themselves about the ground floor, taking up firing positions they'd instinctively selected when entering the building. Each had cover and together they provided a lethal triangulated firing zone anyone foolish enough to use the front entrance would find unforgiving.

Frank spoke into his mic. "Think we can bargain using the son?"

"Maybe but I wouldn't bet on it right now," Oscar answered. "They don't look in the talking mood."

"One of you know where the light switches are?" Frank asked.

"Behind Oscar," Carl said.

"All right. Once we know they mean to fight kill the lights. Until then, let's see if they want to talk."

They didn't have long to wait and no chance to communicate.

Sergio came through the entrance first, kicking the doors open, moving fast and low, followed immediately by Paulinho with his heavier weapon, one darting left, the other right. Oscar reached for the switches. Paulinho fired from his position against the front wall, striking Oscar in the stomach just as he slapped the lights off. He fell to the floor, clutched at himself, an excruciating pain rendering him all but immobile.

Carl returned fire, aiming at the flash point of the assault rifle. But Paulinho had already moved to the side. Sergio fired back at Carl and was struck in the chest by three bullets from Frank's handgun.

"Sergio!" Paulinho called out. "Sergio! Are you all right?"

César was now inside, moving to his right toward Paulinho. Behind him he realized Bandeira had come in as well. "Over here, *Chefe!*" he shouted. If something happened to him, César knew his days were numbered.

Paulinho opened up with a full auto blast, bullets striking the wall behind Frank, pictures shattering and falling, plaster flying from the walls.

"Pare! Você está louco? Meu filho!" Stop! Are you crazy? My son! Bandeira shouted.

"Paulinho, single fire. And careful!" César ordered. Sergio and Paulinho had been close friends for years.

César saw flickering light behind him. A fire had started on a curtain, lit by a sparking wire exposed by the bullet holes in the wall behind it. César turned to see if he could risk putting it out but decided against it. The flames would make him a target.

"Oscar," Frank said into the mic. "Are you all right?"

"It's bad," Oscar groaned.

"Carl?"

"I'm clear," came the answer.

A lull had come to the firefight. The only sound was the snapping flames of the growing fire.

Upstairs Jeff clutched the revolver. He'd been startled when the lights went out below, but the reason had come at once when the gunshots began. He went to the doorway at the top of the stairs and turned out the lights upstairs as well. Should he go and help?

Behind him, Pedro had given up on his hands, but he had to do something. He was certain that his father was down there, risking his life to save him. In the darkness he could just make out the tall American standing in the doorway, not far from the top of the stairs. Impulsively, he shot to his feet and charged him.

Jeff felt the blow from behind and was shoved through the doorway toward the top of the stairs. He twisted around fumbling to grab the young man who was grunting as he struggled and pushed him. Jeff clung to the revolver in desperation, trying to use both hands against the young man but

Pedro was strong, stronger than he'd looked. Before Jeff had control, the two of them were on the landing, then tumbling down the stairs.

The fire had spread across the front wall. It licked at the office furniture, inching along the carpet and casting the room in a fiery glow. Paulinho had moved to his left, checked Sergio, and found him dead. Filled with rage he lay prone and searched for someone to kill.

"Pick your targets, Carl," Frank said into his mic. "Oscar's hurt. We need to make short work of this."

Carl used an old dodge. He felt around on the floor, found an object that felt like a heavy ashtray that had fallen, then tossed it away from him. Paulinho fired at the sound, Carl instantly returning fire. Paulinho grunted from the impact of the bullets, slumped flat onto the floor, and was dead within a minute.

César replied to Carl's shots with controlled semiautomatic fire but Carl had already moved. Frank fired on César, who twisted away as a bullet burned its way through his left bicep. "*Merda*," he cursed under his breath as he rolled onto his back.

Looking behind him as he tried to determine how bad the wound was, César saw that the room behind him was now engulfed in flames, smoke beginning to spread everywhere. There was no turning back, but then, that had never been an option.

77

Consciousness came to Daryl like a bad dream. Something weighty had struck her. She had a vague memory of being pulled across rough ground, worried as her dress rode up to her waist. Then something was hitting her, grabbing at her. The sensations were remote, though, almost as if they were happening to someone else. She felt no pain, no discomfort of any kind. It was as if she'd lost all sense of feeling, as if her body had turned numb.

Then suddenly she was awake, the cocoon of silence that had engulfed her filled with sound. The rough asphalt of the alley, the debris under her, was harsh against her exposed skin. And her face hurt as if she had a terrible toothache. Above was more sound, moaning, and she felt her body being pushed back and forth.

Daryl opened her eyes and saw at first just darkness interspersed with faint light, foggy and undistinguished. A form hovered above her, near, weaving back and forth, muttering to itself, the words slurred, impossible to make out.

Richard. The name shot into her memory. *I'm being murdered.*

The realization came as a shock. Then, feeling her panties pulled from off her feet came the other realization. *I'm being raped!*

Without thinking her self-defense training took over. She'd been taught to simply act if this ever happened to her. An attacker, she'd been told, is stronger than you, may have a weapon, but he is vulnerable.

Iyers had surrendered utterly to the drives within him. Desires long suppressed were now raging out of control. He was no longer, strictly speaking, human. He wanted to possess, to destroy, to kill.

On his knees, sound coming from his mouth that made no sense, he unbuckled his belt and lowered his trousers. Daryl, no longer feeling his hands on her, forced her eyes to focus. He was standing right there, his legs slightly parted. With all her strength, following her training, she raised her right leg, and before Iyers could react, shot her foot into his groin like a bolt.

The pain coursed through Iyers's lower body, sickening in its intensity, the nausea almost overwhelming as he doubled up. Daryl pulled her leg up again, then kicked him a second time, now in the face, with everything she had.

Iyers cried out, then rolled away, writhing on the ground, one hand on his broken nose, the other clutching himself. Blood was streaming, clogging his throat, and he thought for an instant that he was choking to death.

Daryl also rolled, then with a sense of urgency, she pushed herself up and onto her feet. Run! Run! That's what she'd been taught. She looked and could just make out the street beyond the Dumpsters. She could be there in seconds, long before Iyers had any chance of recovery.

She took a step, then another, finding it very hard to move her feet. She was walking like a zombie. She felt naked and held her arms across her body. She took another step, then another. It wasn't far. She could see cars driving by.

She reached the first Dumpster. Exhausted, she braced her hand on it to draw a deep breath, to gather her strength. Just then, Iyers leaped on her from behind. They fell to the dirty pavement, Daryl trying to push him off, Iyers's hands clutching at her throat.

He was too heavy, too strong, she knew. This wouldn't work. She tried rolling right, then left, but the man used his legs to pin her down. In desperation Daryl spread her arms and searched the ground about her, looking for something, anything, to help.

Nothing.

She could no longer breathe, and for just an instant, the thought formed that this was the end, that her life would extinguish in this filthy alley, at the hands of a rapist. She felt a sense of loss, of regret.

Then her right hand had it. She didn't know what "it" was but it was heavy, with sharp corners. She slammed it against Iyers's head, glancing off it. His hands relaxed on her throat, and she drew a lungful of welcome air. She struck again, and this time he fell from her.

Daryl struggled to her knees but stayed where she was. He'd come after her again if she ran. He'd come. She knew it. She lifted the object and struck his head again, then again, then again, until finally she knew he wouldn't chase her, that he'd never chase anyone again.

78

Sergio and Paulinho were dead. César could see their bodies in the light of the raging flames. The fire was to the ceiling now and had begun to spread along the walls. Wooden furniture here and there was spontaneously combusting under the intense heat, making sounds like popcorn in a kettle. How many men was he facing? Four, five? He couldn't tell but surely his team had hit someone. Sergio and Paulinho were too good to have missed entirely.

Bandeira crawled from where he'd been hidden to César, his weapon at the ready. "We have to get out of here before we are burned alive. Have you seen Pedro?"

"No. He's probably upstairs."

"I hope you're right. Rush them," he ordered. "I'll cover you."

Rush? César thought. Yes, stand up, run forward, draw fire, and *chefe* will kill them. And I'll be dead. He didn't move.

"I said 'rush them'!"

Just then, a voice called from across the room. "We've got Pedro! Leave us while there's still time. We'll be in touch. We'll release him unharmed afterwards."

It was Bandeira who answered. *"Filhos de putas!* Release my son now, and you'll live! Otherwise, you and your families are all dead!"

Bandeira aimed at the direction of Carl's voice and opened fire. The bullets churned up the woodwork around Carl, rising in an irregular line along the wall, then bore down toward him. Carl rolled away from the lethal spray.

Frank fired three times at the muzzle flash, then an instant later felt a blow to his side followed a moment later by pain. He too rolled away, grabbing at his side.

"*Agora!*" Now! Bandeira ordered and this time César leaped forward, firing as he did.

Across the room Carl saw the figure rise, then rush forward in a crouch. He fired and the man stumbled, then fell. Bandeira opened up on his gun's flash but Carl had already moved, one bullet stinging as it struck his boot.

On the stairs, Jeff and Pedro were struggling, but one-sidedly as the young man's hands were behind his back. Still, the young man kept at it, pushing at the American, instinctively trying to shove him the rest of the way down the stairs, into the open, where someone would surely see and kill him.

Though still limited primarily to the walls and ceiling, the fire crawled into the living area. The flames now reached the lower steps of the stairs, blocking them intermittently. The air was filled with heat and smoke, and it was becoming increasingly difficult to breathe.

Carl moved to Oscar and found him still alive but unconscious. He looked near death. "Come on," he said, hoping Oscar could hear him. "Time to go." He took Oscar by his arms and dragged him along, crawling away from the inferno toward the rear door and escape.

Jeff and Pedro continued to struggle. More than once Jeff had Pedro against the railing but each time the young man had found a way off. Finally, Jeff pinned him and shoved with all his strength. The railing gave and Pedro screamed as he was pitched off the stairs, Jeff teetering but managing to keep from falling after him. Pedro plunged backwards fifteen feet, falling headfirst to the floor, where he lay unmoving. His body wasn't far from Frank who saw at once that the man was dead. So much for the ace in the hole.

"Jeff!" he shouted into his mic, no longer sure the cell phones even worked. "Jeff! Get out of here. I'll cover."

Jeff could see Frank below and heard him over the roaring flames.

"Get the others and go!" Frank shouted. "I'll go out the second floor and meet you outside."

Lying on the floor, Bandeira watched César die and was stunned. What had he done? His three best men, all dead within minutes. Then he looked up and there were two men struggling on the stairs. Suddenly, one of them, his son, had plummeted to the floor.

He saw another figure bolt across his line of fire but was too shocked to shoot. His son. His only son. He began moving toward him, hardly registering the man in front of him, to his left, pulling someone from the flames. The heat was intense. The acrid smoke bit his nostrils. When he finally reached Pedro, he could no longer see the man.

The salon was becoming an inferno of yellow and red flame. Smoke made it almost impossible to breathe. Bandeira knew if he remained here much longer, he'd be dead. He reached out and touched Pedro's still face, felt his hair. An image of him as a toddler learning to walk flashed in his mind.

Bandeira forced his mind back to the now. He looked up to the second floor and saw his son's killer crawling up the stairs, away from the flames and smoke toward the upper office. In a rage, Bandeira aimed and fired, bullets piercing the stairs. He fired his IMBEL MD97 empty, and he dropped it, pulled out the automatic pistol he often carried, and ran to the foot of the stairs, which were nearly engulfed in the fire. He paused, judged the dancing flames, then plunged across, scrambling up the steps, only one thought on his mind. To kill the man who'd murdered his son.

Jeff had seen the bullets lacing through the staircases and thrown himself against the wall. When the firing stopped, he rushed to the second-floor landing as Frank ordered, still clinging to the pistol. The smoke was now so thick, he could scarcely breathe and his throat ached. He turned, instinctively searching for his friends below but could see nothing beyond the bright flames and heavy smoke. He went into the offices, then to the back room and straight to one of the windows.

It was barred against burglary, and he could see no way in the dark of opening it. He stepped back and kicked, then kicked again. Behind him he could hear the fire. All around him the smoke filled the room. He coughed, then gagged. He knew that he'd pass out soon.

At the top of the landing Bandeira suddenly emerged, his clothes smoldering from the flames, his hair singed, his eyebrows nearly burned off. He spotted the figure at the window and fired.

The glass shattered in front of Jeff. He turned and there was Bandeira.

Jeff dived to the side, Bandeira snapping off a round as he did. Bandeira reached the doorway, low against the floor, and risked a quick look. Spotting Jeff, he fired again, missing him, then ducked back from the doorway.

Jeff fired in return, then moved his aim and fired twice into the wall next to the door, as if it weren't there, recalling from his childhood how often bullets easily penetrated seemingly solid objects. But he could see from the holes left in the paint that the interior walls of the mansion were made of brick and plaster and were all but impervious to bullets.

Bandeira rushed through the doorway, firing a snap shot toward Jeff as he did to keep him down, and came to a stop concealed on the other side of the desk.

For a long minute, the only sound was the raging fire. The heat through the floor was intense, and Jeff expected flames to burst into existence any second. Smoke had filled the room like a dense fog.

Out of time, Jeff lowered his face to the floor, could just see his adversary under the desk, his foot, knee, and lower leg. He fired.

Bandeira screamed, rolled in pain, then lay on his back, his head and arm just beyond the desk, he raised his pistol to shoot again. Before he could, Jeff had him in view and fired twice into his chest.

Bandeira let out a low groan. The weapon fell from his hand. He looked out of the office toward the stairs and his dead son. He felt nothing. No pain, no desire. Nothing. And he thought nothing as his life ended.

79

Daryl lay with her head against the Dumpster, utterly exhausted, sucking air, grateful just to be alive. The sweet sensation of existence swept through her, nearly matched by enormous relief. She wasn't going to die. She would live.

She stayed like that for some minutes, unable to move, unable to think clearly, simply being.

Finally, she stirred and as she did the pain returned. It took her a good minute to get to her feet. When she was standing, she saw the dark form not far away. Iyers hadn't moved. She had no intention of checking on him. He was dead. She knew it.

She spotted her jacket. She'd need it. Not far away was her purse, which had been dragged with her by the shoulder strap. She took them both, clutching them to her breast.

She swooned momentarily. When her balance returned, she reached into Iyers's pocket and took his badge. That would get her back in the Exchange, and hopefully the night guard wouldn't notice that she wasn't a Richard. Then she began walking along the alley toward Wall Street, taking baby steps, stopping whenever the effort was more than she could manage. As she neared the exit there was more light, and for the first time, she considered her appearance.

She couldn't leave the alley looking like this. Someone would call the police. By the time she explained what happened, the urgency of her work in the Exchange, 3:00 A.M. would have come and gone. By then, it would be too late to stop the operation.

But could she just leave a dead body in the alley in the heart of Manhattan? She laughed, then kept laughing. It happened all the time, why not now?

She got control of herself and began the process of fixing her appearance. She straightened her skirt, brushing off the worst of what clung to it. Her blouse had been ripped apart. She brushed the sleeves of her jacket, then slowly buttoned it in front of her, fixing the white blouse collar so it showed above the jacket. She reached for her hair, realizing at once there was nothing much she could do with it here. She rubbed her hands all over her face.

She removed her mirror from her purse but could scarcely make herself out in the darkness. She put the mirror away and removed her makeup compact. She ran the pad across her cheeks, sure it would be an improvement.

The street was quiet. The life and death struggle in the alley had gone completely unnoticed. She turned right and walked as deliberately as she could to the coffee shop, the bright lights like a welcoming beacon. She pushed open the door and walked into a wave of warm air, humid from the kitchen and bodies, the ripe smell of fast food and coffee almost overwhelming her.

She kept walking toward the rear, where she knew the bathrooms would be. A young waitress carrying paper-wrapped silverware said, "Miss, are you all right?"

"I'm fine."

One of the men eating in a booth stared at her as she passed but said nothing; then she was at the restrooms and inside. She went into the stall and sat, holding her head in her hands for a long time, her mind numb. Get yourself together, she said silently. You've got work to do yet. You can collapse tomorrow.

She looked in the mirror with alarm. The left side of her face was already bruising and her eye was turning dark. There were livid scratches on both sides of her face. One of her earrings was gone. She removed the other. Her hair was a mess. She let it out entirely, then removed a comb and brush from her purse. When she had it as good as it could look, she removed her makeup compact. She gingerly applied a coat to the bruising, covered the scratches, which stung like hell, then used her pinkie to lessen the darkening around her eye. She finished with lipstick.

After she'd put everything away, she raised her eyes and took a hard look in the mirror. She looked like a hooker who'd just been beaten by her pimp, but it would do. She'd had a hard night, maybe a fight with a boyfriend, but there was nothing she could see that she couldn't explain away if need be.

She removed her soiled jacket. She dampened several paper towels and worked over it. The worst was the back, where she could do only so much. When she finished, it was dark from moisture but would look better when it dried. She removed her skirt and repeated the process. It wasn't as bad because it got turned inside out when she'd been dragged, leaving most of the damage on the inside.

With fresh damp towels she cleaned her legs. She took out her compact again and applied makeup to the worst spots. She slipped on her skirt, struggled into her jacket, buttoned it in front, fluffed the blouse collar, then looked again.

You'll do, she said to yourself. You'll do.

Outside, she took a seat in an empty booth far from the other customers. The same waitress came up with a menu. "You're looking a lot better," she said. "Rough night?"

"You have no idea."

80

Jeff kicked at the window bars again but they refused to give. He kicked, then kicked again. It wouldn't go.

His lungs were burning and every breath was an effort. He turned away from the window, stepped over the dead man, then went to the landing. The room below was a raging inferno, the heat unbearable.

He was trapped.

But unable to get out from the second floor, Jeff had no choice but to race down the stairs. He dived through the fire at the bottom, hoping he was not diving into a blaze. He rolled, then came to a hard stop, balanced uneasily on his feet and hands. Just ahead, in the dancing flames, he spotted three prone forms. He crawled toward them, gagging and coughing as he did.

Carl and Oscar were overcome by the smoke. Carl had collapsed atop Oscar, shielding him from the fire. A few feet away lay Frank, bleeding and moving ever so slow.

"Frank! Frank!" Jeff shouted. "Get out of here! I'll get the others."

Frank looked blankly at Jeff as if seeing an apparition. Then comprehension came to his eyes. He nodded and began to crawl toward the rear door.

Jeff moved over to Carl and Oscar. "Oscar!" he shouted over the roar and snapping of wood. There was no answer. Jeff looked around. Frank was nearly to the door, which was not far away. They'd almost made it.

Jeff took the unconscious, bleeding Oscar by the arms and began dragging him. He knew he had little time but could move only so fast. He'd drag him, stop, then drag. All the while the fire raged, the smoke stinging his eyes and filling his lungs. He coughed until he thought his guts would come out; then he'd coughed some more.

Finally, he was at the door. Frank lay there unmoving. Jeff raised an arm, felt the white-hot handle, disregarded the shooting pain, and turned it. He tried to push it open with no success. He moved, leaned against the door with his back, and pushed.

A draft of cold night air was sucked into the inferno, creating a strong breeze that momentarily drove the flames and smoke back. Jeff drew a lungful of fresh air, staggered to his feet, and with all his effort pulled Oscar out of the building into the night. He kept dragging him until he was satisfied he was clear.

He could hear sirens now. The sound of emergency vehicles. Help was coming.

Then he turned and ran back in for Frank, pulling him to Oscar.

He looked up and could see flashing lights. He looked back at the mansion. The infusion of air had whipped the fire into a frenzy. The doorway was a wall of flames. Jeff turned, and for the last time, plunged into the inferno.

81

Back at her workstation, Daryl was beginning to feel something close to normal. It was as if what had happened in the alley was a bad dream, not an actual event. She'd had three cups of black coffee and forced herself to eat half a breakfast at the coffee shop. When she finally left to return to the office, she'd passed the entrance to the alley, not looking into it, sensing and seeing nothing that told her Iyers's body had been discovered.

She'd scanned Iyers's badge, the sleepy security guard paid her no attention, then ridden the elevator up. She found perhaps a third of the day shift was still at it. Everyone looked exhausted. She'd thought to check on Campos, but there was no reason. The man was busy. With his helpmate out of the way, he would be busier than ever.

Now she turned to the rogue code. She'd had time to think about it and believed she could stop its functionality, but she still had a lot to learn about the deployment system first. Also, she'd have to sabotage it at the last minute, as it landed on the jump server; otherwise, Campos might discover what she'd done and override it.

Her plan was simple enough. Once she understood the key functions of the code she planned to obfuscate them by corrupting the files. She'd didn't want to delete them, since there might be automated checks for missing files.

But first, she had to find these key files, and she had to do it in just over one hour.

Marc Campos couldn't understand what was going on in Rio. There'd been no updates for hours. He'd sent work to Pedro earlier and heard nothing back. He'd tried calling with no luck. The call simply went to voice mail. He'd tried Skype and again there'd been no answer.

It was possible the system in Rio was down but that was highly unlikely. He had expressly selected the location for Grupo Técnico with that in mind. The company had the services of two Internet companies. It also had a backup electric generator system. It was important it never be offline or unable to function.

Something was wrong.

He tried calling Jorge César. He'd rather not but it had to be done. No answer.

Did he dare call *el chefe*? It was the middle of the night in Brazil as well. And what could Bandeira do in the short amount of time left? No, he'd make do.

His other problem was that Iyers had vanished. He'd done nothing on Carnaval for nearly two hours. The time for the upload was rapidly approaching and Campos needed him for that. Campos could do it himself in a pinch but it was a job Iyers had always done in the past because it fit his job function. Campos would be running a risk of getting noticed.

He had tried calling Iyers with no luck. He'd sent him secure e-mail and text messages. Again, nothing. He'd finally risked going to Iyers's workstation. Empty.

Where could he be?

Campos returned to his work. If Iyers didn't show soon, he'd have to go with what he had. The code was 90 percent there. Carnaval would function as it was. He'd have to do without the other 10 percent. He checked his watch. He'd spend the next hour fixing what he could; then he'd follow up with Iyers. If he still couldn't find the man, he'd handle the insert himself.

Then a thought came to him: What about the woman? Had Iyers seen to her? That would explain his absence. Maybe he was being too hard on him. He couldn't be in two places at once. Maybe he'd decided he couldn't risk having her in the building. That would explain everything except his failure to answer his cell phone.

Campos resisted the impulse to check on the woman. Unless she was already dead—the thought startled him with the ease with which it came to him—she'd be at that workstation. He could drop by later. Right now, he had more important work. Iyers would show. Too much was on the line for him not to.

Daryl was now satisfied she'd identified the files that were key to the function of the rogue code. It was only twenty minutes until the scheduled 3:00 A.M. deployment, so she assumed the final version was already on the jump server waiting to be copied into the trading engine. She doubted the last update would change the structure in any significant way, so she corrupted two of the files. When she merged her changes with the final deployment, she would in effect render the malware inoperable.

She looked at her watch. Less than ten minutes to go. How long could she wait before pressing the Enter button? If Campos was working on or watching the code, he'd see the change. It would take him only a few seconds to replace it with an untainted version.

On the other hand, she didn't dare wait too long. If the update took place early, she'd miss her chance. Still, she was certain the malware was going to ride in with the IPO and standard nightly updates. She had to have a target opportunity, and that was it.

Her work was nearly done. She ached from head to foot. She wondered if she should go to a hospital. At the least she needed to see a doctor.

And what about Jeff? And Frank? What were they doing in Brazil? Had they acted on the new address she'd given them? She knew Frank had once been a man of action, a super-secret special agent as she'd once called him after too much wine. Everyone at the table had laughed, though Daryl knew it was largely true.

But Jeff was no secret agent. He wrote code. He understood computers. Sure, he was in good shape, and she knew from previous experience that when everything was on the line, he rose to the occasion, but still . . . how much could reasonably be expected of him? He was barely out of the hospital.

She wished she had a message from Jeff and Frank telling her everything was fine. In a few minutes, she planned to send one telling them that she had the evidence to clear them and that the rogue code had been stopped in its tracks.

She leaned back in her chair and closed her eyes.

———————

Campos had still heard nothing from Iyers or from Pedro, so proceeded on his own. He would check on the woman when he was done.

He completed his work fifteen minutes before 3:00 A.M. He went through the steps to make the insert, steps designed in part to conceal the fact that he was doing it. Then he copied the rogue code onto the jump server. The master stroke was in position, all that was needed for Carnaval to be in place when the market opened was the last Exchange update.

The hallways were largely empty as Campos made his way to Daryl's workstation. She'd picked it carefully as he recalled.

There she was. Her arms were crossed and she looked asleep. He was amazed at her audacity, simply insinuating herself into the offices of Trading Platforms IT. In theory this should have been impossible, but he'd long noted how lax security had become. He and Iyers had obviously taken advantage of it many times over the years.

He looked at her monitor and was shocked at what he saw. It was a core part of Carnaval, files essential to its operation. She'd done something to them, he knew. That's why she was here. He stepped toward her.

Daryl jolted awake, experiencing an instant of vertigo as she did. It took a moment for her to realize where she was. She immediately checked her watch. 2:57 A.M. Time to go to work.

Just then, she sensed movement behind her. She turned and there was Campos, looking wild-eyed and angry. "What are you doing?" he demanded as he barged into the small work space.

"I don't know what you mean. Just a second and I'll be right with you." She reached for the Enter button.

"Stop! Stop!" Campos shouted as he lunged at her.

The two toppled off the chair onto the floor, Daryl experiencing a sense of déjà vu. But Campos wasn't the psychopath Iyers had been, nor was he as strong. The two wrestled on the floor, grunting in effort. Daryl struggled to get to her feet, Campos pulled and tugged at her to keep her away from the keyboard.

Finally, Daryl rolled on top, briefly pinning Campos. She struck him in the face with her fist. An image of Iyers flashed in her mind, and she struck the man again and again, no blow enough to knock him unconscious but the flurry momentarily dazing him.

Still, Campos was both bigger and stronger than Daryl, and her superior position didn't last long. He heaved her up and off him, then moved to place himself between her and the computer. "I'm calling security," he said breathlessly. "You should leave."

Daryl reached onto the desk beside her and grabbed her purse. Fumbling inside she removed the pepper spray and before Campos could react, she sprayed him, right to left across the eyes just as she'd practiced. He screamed, grabbed his eyes, and all but fell to the floor.

She leaned around him, reached for the keyboard, and pressed Enter.

She stood back as Campos danced in a circle screaming for help and looked at her watch. 2:59 A.M.

82

Jonathan Russo stood with most his employees, watching the giant monitors arrayed across the wall of the office. Everyone was tired, but they'd made it. The new algo was in place. Over the next two or three hours, all the recent losses would be recovered and Mitri Growth would earn upward of $100 million. It was the most exciting day in Russo's life.

He looked around. Everyone was sitting at their desks or standing and watching the screens. In fact, they'd not know the outcome for at least an hour, but they would be able to confirm the algo was functioning properly. It had worked in the tests, but the sting of their failure the previous week was still with them. Nothing was certain.

"Here we go," someone said as the IPO trading began. No one said a word for some minutes.

Colored graphs arrayed across the displays grew in height as trading volume surged. The Toptical stock best bid and offer prices, known as National Best Bid and Offer, or NBBO, which were displayed in a large font on the primary wall screen began to change. The initial Toptical price had been set at thirty dollars. Speculation was that too much stock was being made available and that the price might very well fall at first. And that's what happened. But not for long. The Mitri algo was designed to take a large position at the start of trading. It responded at once to the drop by executing thousands of small sales, a process called quote stuffing.

This move was part of Russo's secret sauce. Mitri's sophisticated statistical algo was based on past market behavior to determine optimal sale sizes and price drops, the small trades incrementally squeezing money out of the system and slowing the reaction of other algos with their sheer magnitude. Only collocated algos like theirs would be immune to the delays in getting an accurate view of the NBBO.

The pent-up demand of regular investors now kicked in as the price looked like a bargain below thirty dollars, joining Mitri and no telling how many other high-frequency traders following the same course of action. The impact of the HFTs was greater than they'd calculated but they'd allowed even for that possibility. The price began to rise. A small cheer went up.

Mitri Growth's special Toptical IPO algo assumed that it possessed an advantage in latency over everyone else, that is, it acted based on the programmed belief that it knew the true price just slightly ahead of everyone else. The increase in HFT trading was pushing the limits of that advantage but Russo and Baker were convinced they still possessed it.

Next the combination of regular investors, both institutional and personal, taken with the high-frequency activity, caused the quotes even to the collocated algos to start to lag behind actual prices, just as in 1929 with the ticker tape. Unknown to anyone until days later, the lag was initially just a second, but it was soon five seconds, then fifteen, then a minute, then three to four minutes.

Nearly all of the HFTs algos immediately moved into a rhythm with the other high-frequency trading algos that were seeing different prices and as was the case in the infamous Flash Crash the price was quickly driven down. In usual trading the New York Stock Exchange applies artificial "brakes" in such a situation, to allow latency to catch up, to permit traders a few moments for reflection or to override their computers, but such safeguards don't apply to IPOs. This was a free for all and the stock, for now, would be allowed to go where the trading took it.

Toptical rose to $32.43, then at 10:21 A.M. began to fall steadily: $31.19, $30.44, $29.56, $28.23, $28.02, $27.06, $25.37, $24.01.

"My God," someone said, "look at that."

$23.46, $22.43, $20.09, $18.33, $12.56, $9.07.

The free fall continued until 10:33 A.M., when the New York Stock Exchange suspended trading. Toptical's price was frozen at $2.22. Those watching were stunned by what they'd witnessed.

A pall of gloom spread across all trading on Wall Street. The market recorded a loss of 11.2 percent, one of the largest in history. But there was no collapse, no worldwide panic, no end to the international financial market as it was known.

Later that morning, Baker brought Russo the figures. "We made a hundred thirty-seven million dollars," he said with a grin. "A lot more if you include Toptical, but we have to wait to see what the Exchange does with it."

"What a collapse," Russo said. "I never imagined."

"No, but the code we wrote did. Congratulations."

83

Samantha Mason was in her office. She'd seen the writing on the wall much earlier, and left what was supposed to be a celebratory party. She was sitting at her desk, playing around with a game she'd been designing in her free time when Brian came into her office, shut the door, and took a seat.

"How bad?" she asked as she looked up.

"Two twenty-two," he mumbled.

She could barely hear him. "I'm sorry, Brian. I know how much this meant to you."

"What happened?" he asked. "I just don't understand it."

"I'm not exactly sure. Morgan Stanley did us no favors. They were serving at least two masters, and I think we were the less important one. We may find out it was the Exchange's new IPO algo. It was buggy. But my guess right now is that it was the high-frequency trading algos. Their greed, and recklessness, finally caught up with them. We just paid the price."

"Two dollars. How do I go out in public?" Brian said.

"How's Heather taking it?" Heather was Brian's former model live-in girlfriend, Sam's replacement in his life. It was nasty to ask she knew. She didn't care.

"Heather?" Brian looked at her as if hearing the name for the first time.

"I don't know. We haven't talked. I think . . ." He paused. "I just don't know."

"We've both still made a lot of money, Brian. We're rich, just not mega rich."

"I don't think so. Gordon talked to his people at Morgan Stanley. They think the whole trade's going to be voided, like it never happened."

"Wow. That's something. I didn't think of that."

Brian said nothing for some time and Sam left him alone, waiting. "I've been thinking," he said finally. "I hope you'll reconsider your decision to leave. I need you. We all need you. This IPO thing was a mistake. You were right. I should have listened. We're back to square one now. We've got to make Toptical a sustainable business model. I think together we can do it."

"I'm leaving, Brian. I've had enough."

"Sam . . ."

"Listen to me. I don't want to spend any more of my life on this. I don't even understand what's been going on this last year. It simply isn't what I want to do. I've got other plans. I'm sorry not to get the money but I've got other dreams, and I'm going to go after them. This—" She gestured grandly.

"—is in my past, even if I'll still be here for a few weeks or a month or so to help in the aftermath. I still owe some of our people."

"Sam—"

Just then, Gordon stuck his head in without knocking. "Brian, you're needed on a conference call right now."

"What's going on?"

"Morgan Stanley needs our consent to announce the IPO is canceled. We need to work on the language of the press release."

"Okay. I'm coming." Brian looked back at Sam. "I need you."

"Yes, you do," she answered. "But I'm still leaving."

Brian stood motionless for a moment, then quietly left.

Sam sat at her desk without moving until there was a knock at the open door. It was Molly. "Isn't it wonderful?" she said as she came in and flopped in a chair. "The whole thing just collapsed! Now we get rid of all those finance assholes and get back to building Toptical. I know I shouldn't show anyone how happy I am—everyone's so depressed—but I know you understand. This really is the best thing that could happen to us."

"I guess."

"You don't think so?" Molly looked crestfallen.

"I don't know what I think," Sam said. "Come on, Molly. I'll buy you a drink. You've been putting in too much time here."

"Really? At this hour?" Then Molly looked over her shoulder to see if anyone was watching, like a schoolgirl about to play hooky. "Okay!"

84

Jeff awoke lying on a bed. He ached across his entire body. The CIA doctor, if that's what he was, had told him he'd be fine. He'd bandaged three or four places on Jeff's forearms and neck where flames had touched him, then applied a greasy cream to other spots that gave off an angry glow. The hand Jeff had grabbed the doorknob with was wrapped in thick gauze. The doctor told Jeff to keep the cream applied and watch carefully for infection.

Frank was seated in front of the television in a worn armchair. He wasn't wearing a shirt and his upper torso was also bandaged, especially around the right side. The television was off, and he was just ending a phone call with his wife.

"How's Carol?" Jeff asked when Frank disconnected.

"Okay. She knew something was up but not what. She and the kids were glad to finally hear from me."

"Did you tell her you got shot?"

Frank smiled wickedly. "I'm saving the best for last."

"I thought the doc wanted you in a hospital," Jeff said.

"He said something like that, but I told him I didn't want to risk it even under an assumed name, so it was better to be here. He says I'll be all right. He just doesn't want any bleeding to start. I'm supposed to take it easy for a few days."

"Any word on Oscar?"

"It was a near thing. He was in surgery for four hours, but they think he's going to pull through."

"I'm glad to hear that. I guess he's in trouble, along with Carl."

Frank stared at Jeff, then said, "You still amaze me at times, Jeff—you really do."

"What do you mean?"

"We're using a Company safe house, they got sophisticated surveillance equipment from the Company, a Company doctor is tending us—doesn't any of that tell you something?"

"What are you saying?"

"Once Oscar and Carl knew the NL was involved, they called it in and got approval."

"You're telling me this was a CIA operation?"

"In the end, after a fashion. And the station chief is a very happy man right now. NL had been on the radar for a long time. Victor Bandeira, a really bad guy, is dead. So are his top enforcers, from what they hear. This was a good day for the good guys."

Jeff absorbed the news. "I'm just glad everyone's going to be okay."

"That's the bottom line. You should know that there's also been some heat brought to bear on this SEC thing." Frank had told him about his earlier conversation with Daryl and the evidence she'd uncovered. "We're no longer suspects. The warrants have been quashed." Just then, Frank's phone rang. It was a Skype video call. Jeff heard Daryl's voice when Frank answered. Frank held the phone out to him. "Someone wants to talk to you."

Jeff took the phone and saw Daryl's face on the screen. "Hi," he said. She was wearing more makeup than usual, and he was sure he could detect scratches. He decided not to ask, not now.

"Hi to you. I see you're still with us," she said.

"Absolutely."

"You'll have to tell me all about it when you get back."

"Sure thing. How are you?"

Daryl had not told Frank about Iyers or Campos. She'd save the explanation for when they were together. "Just fine. Tired. Did Frank tell you we stopped the rogue code?"

"He did earlier. But don't you mean that you stopped it?"

"It was a team effort."

"Thanks for helping. And it sounds like we can come home soon."

"Good." Daryl hesitated, then said, "Jeff, I've had some time to think about what happened with us. I want . . . I want to come back. Let's do this right this time, okay?"

For a moment Jeff couldn't speak. "Yes, let's do it right." He was almost choking when he said, "I'll see you soon."

Daryl smiled. "Can't wait."

MEMORANDUM

DATE: October 15

FROM: Seth Kaufman
Special U.S. Attorney
United States Attorney's Office
Southern District of New York
Securities and Commodities Fraud Division

TO: Eleanor Kaschnitz
National Security Advisor

RE: Summary of Related Events to NYSE Malware Episode

Last week, you asked me to follow up, informally, on some matters resulting from the events surrounding the discovery of the ongoing malware operation in the Exchange's trading engines and the Toptical IPO. Here's what I've come up with. If you need more detail, just let me know.

I'll begin with Toptical. As I'm sure you know, it's been acquired by Tencent, a major Chinese media company.

As I'm sure you've also heard, the SEC and NYSE are, once again, considering serious regulation of high-frequency traders. They haven't got it right in the past, and I doubt they will this time.

The major credit for stopping this unprecedented criminal penetration of the Exchange software goes to Robert Alshon, Senior SEC Investigator in NYC. He'd been on this case for a week. When he saw the IPO going askew, he strongly urged trading be suspended. He's scheduled to take over the SEC New York Regional Office. We need more like him.

Yes, you were correct. The operation was being run by an organized crime family in Brazil. Our sister agency that handles such matters has been vague on details, but I'm assured we can confidently expect the operation to be shut down for good.

As for Jeff Aiken and Frank Renkin, they had no involvement in the rogue code. They were set up by those responsible. It is regrettable they were ever suspects, but these things happen. I'm assured they just want it all laid to rest.

The actual perpetrator was Abílio Ramos, aka Marc Campos, a longtime and trusted employee of the Exchange IT security department. After learning of the death of the leader of the criminal cartel for which he worked, he elected to cooperate in exchange for a reduced sentence. He managed the fraud with the assistance of just one other in-house employee, Richard Iyers. Iyers was found murdered in the alley not far from the Exchange. Police don't know if this is a coincidence or related. There are no suspects.

All in all, what we have is a satisfactory ending to what could have been a very messy outcome. I'll be in D.C. next week. Let's get together if you have time.

Bibliography: Additional Information on High-Frequency Trading

BOOKS

Arnuk, Sal. *Broken Markets: How High Frequency Trading and Predatory Practices on Wall Street are Destroying Investor Confidence and Your Portfolio*, FT Press, 2012.

Bodek, Haim. *The Problem of HFT: Collected Writings on High Frequency Trading & Stock Market Structure Reform*, Decimus Capital Markets, LLC, 2013.

Connaughton, Jeff. *The Payoff: Why Wall Street Always Wins*, Prospecta Press, 2012.

Durbin, Michael. *All About High-Frequency Trading*, McGraw-Hill, 2010.

Harris, Larry. *Trading and Exchanges: Market Microstructure for Practitioners*, Oxford University Press, 2002.

Narang, Rishi. *Inside the Black Box*, Wiley, 2013.

Patterson, Scott. *The Quants: How a New Breed of Math Whizzes Conquered Wall Street and Nearly Destroyed It*, Crown Business, 2010.

———. *Dark Pools: The Rise of the Machine Traders and the Rigging of the U.S. Stock*, Crown Business, 2012.

WEB SITES

"The Professional Page of Haim Bodek," accessed March 2014, http://haimbodek.com/.

"Scott Patterson Reports," accessed March 2014, http://www.scottpatterson reports.com/.

"NYSE Euronext Markets," accessed March 2014, http://usequities.nyx.com/markets.

"TabbFORUM," accessed March 2014, http://tabbforum.com/.

"Nanex," accessed March 2014, http://www.nanex.net/.

"Themis Trading," accessed March 2014, http://blog.themistrading.com/.

"Modern Markets Initiative," accessed March 2014, http://modernmarket sinitiative.org/.

"U.S. Securities and Exchange Commission Market Structure," accessed March 2014, http://www.sec.gov/marketstructure/.

PAPERS

Senator Kaufman's nine-point plan for market structure reform, August 5, 2010. Accessed March 2014. http://www.sec.gov/comments/s7-27-09/72709-96.pdf.

Dolgopolov, Stanislav, "The Maker-Taker Pricing Model and Its Impact on the Securities Market Structure: A Can of Worms for Securities Fraud?," February 23, 2014. Posted February 24, 2014. http://papers.ssrn.com/sol3/papers.cfm?abstract_id=2399821.

Dolgopolov, Stanislav, "High-Frequency Trading, Order Types, and the Evolution of the Securities Market Structure: One Whistleblower's Consequences for Securities Regulation," Last revised January 23, 2014. Posted August 22, 2014. http://papers.ssrn.com/sol3/papers.cfm?abstract_id=2314574.

Joint CFTC-SEC Advisory Committee, "Recommendations Regarding Regulatory Responses to the Market Events of May 6, 2010," February 18, 2011. Accessed March 2014. http://www.sec.gov/spotlight/sec-cftcjoint committee/021811-report.pdf.

U.S. Securities and Exchange Commission, "Concept Release on Equity Market Structure," 2010. Accessed March 2014. http://www.sec.gov/rules /concept/2010/34-61358.pdf.

"NASDAQ OMX Order Type Guide," April 2013. Accessed March 2014. http://www.brainshark.com/nasdaqomx/vu?pi=zF7zJ6aUZzoG0z0.

"Direct Edge Order Type Guide," Accessed March 2014. http://www .brainshark.com/DCS/vu?pi=zGwzPWcfUz3QRKz0.

VIDEOS AND PODCASTS
"Haim Bodek—HFT is an Artificial Industry," YouTube video, 43:40, from a presentation by Haim Bodek to TradeTech USA 2013 on February 27, 2013, posted by Trade TechTV, Apr 26, 2013, https://www.youtube.com /watch?v=ItfAKguEdAE.

"Discussing HFT with Haim Bodek," The LoopCast recording, posted March 3, 2014, http://www.theloopcast.com/2014/03/03/discussing-hft -with-haim-bodek/.

"The Wall Street Code," YouTube video, 50:31, posted by VPRO Blacklight on November 4, 2013, http://www.youtube.com/watch?v=GEAGdwHXfLQ.

"Money & Speed: Inside the Black Box," YouTube video, 48:23, posted by VPRO Blacklight on December 13, 2012, http://www.youtube.com/watch ?v=aq1Ln1UCoEU.

Hoffman, E. P., Brown, R. H. and Kunkel, L. M. (1987). Dystrophin: the protein product of the Duchenne muscular dystrophy locus. *Cell*, **51**, 919–928.

Höglund, P., Holmberg, C., de la Chapelle, A. and Kere, J. (1994). Paternal isodisomy for chromosome 7 is compatible with normal growth and development in a patient with congenital chloride diarrhea. *Am J Hum Genet*, **55**, 747–752.

Hol, F. A., Hamel, B. C. J., Geurds, M. P. A., Hansmann, I., Nabben, F. A. E., Daniëls, O. and Mariman, E. C. M. (1995). Localization of Alagille syndrome to 20p11.2-p12 by linkage analysis of a three-generation family. *Hum Genet*, **95**, 687–690.

Holmes-Siedle, M., Ryynanen, M. and Lindenbaum, R. H. (1987). Parental decisions regarding termination of pregnancy following prenatal detection of sex chromosome abnormality. *Prenat Diagn*, **7**, 239–244.

Holmquist, G. P. (1992). Chromosome bands, their chromatic flavors and their functional features. *Am J Hum Genet*, **51**, 17–37.

Holzgreve, W., Golabi, M. and Bradley, J. (1986). Multiple congenital anomalies in a child born after prenatal diagnosis of trisomy 20 mosaicism. *Clin Genet*, **29**, 342–344.

Hoo, J.-J., Chao, M. C., Samuel, I. P. and Morgan, A. M. (1990). Proximal 15q variant as possible pitfall in the cytogenetic diagnosis of Prader-Willi syndrome. *Clin Genet*, **37**, 161–166.

Hoo, J. J., Chao, M., Szego, K., Rauer, M., Echiverri, S. C. and Harris, C. (1995). Four new cases of inverted terminal duplication: a modified hypothesis of mechanism of origin. *Am J Med Genet*, **58**, 299–304.

Hoo, J. J., Lowry, R. B., Lin, C. C. and Haslam, R. H. A. (1985). Recurrent de novo interstitial deletion of 16q in two mentally retarded sisters. *Clin Genet*, **27**, 420–425.

Hoo, J. J., Szego, K., Wong, P. and Roland, B. (1993). Evidence of chromosome 9 origin of the euchromatic variant band within 9qh. *Clin Genet*, **43**, 309–311.

Hook, E. B. (1979). Extra sex chromosomes and human behavior: the nature of the evidence regarding XYY, XXY, XXYY and XXX genotypes. In "Genetic mechanisms of sexual development" (H. L. Vallet and I. H. Porter, eds.). Academic Press, New York, pp. 437–463.

Hook, E. B. (1983). Chromosome abnormalities and spontaneous fetal death following amniocentesis: further data and associations with maternal age. *Am J Hum Genet*, **35**, 110–116.

Hook, E. B. (1986). Paternal age and genetic outcomes: implications for genetic counseling. In "Perinatal genetics" (I. H. Porter, N. H. Hatcher and A. M. Willey, eds.). Academic Press, New York.

Hook, E. B. (1987). Issues in analysis of data on paternal age and 47,+21: implications for genetic counseling for Down syndrome. *Hum Genet*, **77**, 303–306.

Hook, E. B. (1992). Chromosome abnormalities: prevalence, risks and recurrence. In "Prenatal diagnosis and screening" (D. J. H. Brock, C. H. Rodeck and M. A. Ferguson-Smith, eds.). Churchill Livingstone, Edinburgh, pp. 351–392.

Hook, E. B. (1994). Down's syndrome epidemiology and biochemical screening. In "Screening for Down's syndrome" (J. G. Grudzinskas, T. Chard, M. Chapman and H. Cuckle, eds.). Cambridge University Press, Cambridge, pp. 1–18.

Hook, E. B. and Cross, P. K. (1987a). Extra structurally abnormal chromosomes (ESAC) detected at amniocentesis: frequency in approximately 75,000 prenatal cytogenetic diagnoses and associations with maternal and paternal age. *Am J Hum Genet*, **40**, 83–101.

Hook, E. B. and Cross, P. K. (1987b). Rates of mutant and inherited structural cytogenetic abnormalities detected at amniocentesis: results on about 63,000 fetuses. *Ann Hum Genet*, **51**, 27–55.

Hook, E. B., Cross, P. K., Jackson, L. Pergament, E. and Brambati, B. (1988). Maternal age-specific rates of 47,+21 and other cytogenetic abnormalities diagnosed in the first trimester of pregnancy in chorionic villus biopsy specimens: comparison with rates expected from observations at amniocentesis. *Am J Hum Genet*, **42**, 797–807.

Hook, E. B., Mutton, D. E., Ide, R., Alberman, E. and Bobrow, M. (1995). The natural history of Down syndrome conceptuses diagnosed prenatally that are not electively terminated. *Am J Hum Genet*, **57**, 875–881.

Horn, D., Majewski, F., Hildebrandt, B. and Körner, H. (1995). Pallister-Killian syndrome: normal karyotype in prenatal chorionic villi, in postnatal lymphocytes, and in slowly growing epidermal cells, but mosaic tetrasomy 12p in skin fibroblasts. *J Med Genet*, **32**, 68–71.

Horsman, D. E., Dill, F. J., McGillivray, B. C. and Kalousek, D. K. (1987). X chromosome aneuploidy in lymphocyte cultures from women with recurrent spontaneous abortions. *Am J Med Genet*, **28**, 981–987.

Howell, R. T. (1994). "Annual Report, U. K. National External Quality Assessment Scheme in Clinical Cytogenetics 1993/94."

Howell, R. T. and Davies, T. (1994). Diagnosis of Bloom's syndrome by sister chromatid exchange evaluation in chorionic villus cultures. *Prenat Diagn*, **14**, 1071–1073.

Howell, R. T., McDermott, A., Gardner, A. and Dickinson, V. (1984). Down's syndrome with a recombinant tandem duplication of chromosome 21 derived from a maternal ring. *J Med Genet*, **21**, 310–314.

Hsia, Y. E. (1987). Genetic counseling. In "Practice of pediatrics" (V. C. Kelley, ed.). J. B. Lippincott, Philadelphia.

Hsia, Y. E., Hirschhorn, K., Silverberg, R. L. and Godmilow, L. (eds.) (1979). "Counseling in genetics." A. R. Liss, New York.

Hsu, L. Y. F. (1989). Prenatal diagnosis of 45,X/46,XY mosaicism—a review and update. *Prenat Diagn*, **9**, 31–48.

Hsu, L. Y. F., Kaffe, S., Jenkins, E. C., Alonso, L., Benn, P. A., David, K., Hirschhorn, K., Lieber, E., Shanske, A., Shapiro, L. R., Schutta, E. and Warburton, D. (1992). Proposed guidelines for diagnosis of chromosome mosaicism in amniocytes based on data derived from chromosome mosaicism and pseudomosaicism studies. *Prenat Diagn*, **12**, 555–573.

Hsu, L. Y. F., Kaffe, S. and Perlis, T. E. (1987). Trisomy 20 mosaicism in prenatal diagnosis—a review and update. *Prenat Diagn*, **7**, 581–596.

Hsu, L. Y. F., Kaffe, S. and Perlis, T. E. (1991). A revisit of trisomy 20 mosaicism in prenatal diagnosis—an overview of 103 cases. *Prenat Diagn*, **11**, 7–15.

Hsu, L. Y. F. and Perlis, T. E. (1984). United States survey on chromosome mosaicism and pseudomosaicism in prenatal diagnosis. *Prenat Diagn*, **4** (Special Issue), 97–130.

Hsu, T. C. (1979). "Human and mammalian cytogenetics. An historical perspective." Springer-Verlag, New York.

Huang, T. H.-M., Peckham, D., Batanian, J. R., Martin, M. B., Kouba, M., Caldwell, C. W. and Miles, J. H. (1994). Familial translocation t(10;14)(q26.1;q32.3): report of three offspring with 10q deletion and 14q duplication. *Clin Genet*, **46**, 299–303.

Hultén, M., Armstrong, S., Challinor, P., Gould, C., Hardy, G., Leedham, P., Lee, T. and McKeown, C. (1991). Genomic imprinting in an Angelman and Prader-Willi translocation family. *Lancet*, **338**, 638–639.

Hunter, A. G. and Allanson, J. E. (1994). Follow-up study of patients with Wiedemann-Beckwith syndrome with emphasis on the change in facial appearance over time. *Am J Med Genet,* **51**, 102–107.

Huret, J.-L., Léonard, C., Chery, M., Philippe, C., Schafei-Benaissa, E., Lefaure, G., Labrune, B. and Gilgenkrantz, S. (1995). Monosomy 21q: two cases of del(21q) and review of the literature. *Clin Genet,* **48**, 140–147.

Huson, S. M., Rodgers, C. S., Hall, C. M. and Winter, R. M. (1990). The Baller-Gerold syndrome: phenotypic and cytogenetic overlap with Roberts syndrome. *J Med Genet,* **27**, 371–375.

Ibba, R. M., Monni, G., Olla, G. and Cao, A. (1994). Umbilical artery velocity waveforms before and after chorionic villus sampling. *Prenat Diagn,* **14**, 799–802.

Ingelfinger, F. J. (1980). Arrogance. *N Engl J Med,* **303**, 1507–1511.

Ireland, M., English, C., Cross, I., Houlsby, W. T. and Burn, J. (1991). A de novo translocation t(3;17)(q26.3;q23.1) in a child with Cornelia de Lange syndrome. *J Med Genet,* **28**, 639–640.

Ireland, M., English, C., Cross, I., Lindsay, S. and Strachan, T. (1995). Partial trisomy 3q and the mild Cornelia de Lange syndrome phenotype. *J Med Genet,* **32**, 837–838.

I. S. C. N. (1995). ''An international system for human cytogenetic nomenclature'' (F. Mitelman, ed.). S. Karger, Basel.

Ishai, D., Amiel, A., Diukman, R., Cogan, O., Lichtenstein, Z., Abramovici, H. and Fejgin, M. D. (1995). Uterine cavity lavage: adding FISH to conventional cytogenetics for embryonic sexing and diagnosing common chromosomal aberrations. *Prenat Diagn,* **15**, 961–965.

Ishikiriyama, S., Tonoki, H., Shibuya, Y., Chin, S., Harada, N., Abe, K. and Niikawa, N. (1989). Waardenburg syndrome type I in a child with de novo inversion (2)(q35q37.3). *Am J Med Genet,* **33**, 505–507.

Jaafar, H., Gabriel-Robez, O., Vignon, F., Flori, E. and Rumpler, Y. (1994). Supernumerary chromosomes and spermatogenesis in a human male carrier. *Hum Genet,* **94**, 74–76.

Jabs, E. W. and Carpenter, N. (1988). Molecular cytogenetic evidence for amplification of chromosome-specific alphoid sequences at enlarged C-bands on chromosome 6. *Am J Hum Genet,* **43**, 69–74.

Jacobs, P. A. (1979). Recurrence risks for chromosome abnormalities. *Birth Defects: Orig Art Series,* **15**(5C), 71–80.

Jacobs, P. A. (1981). Mutation rates of structural chromosomal rearrangements in man. *Am J Hum Genet,* **33**, 44–54.

Jacobs, P. A., Browne, C., Gregson, N., Joyce, C. and White, H. (1992). Estimates of the frequency of chromosome abnormalities detectable in unselected newborns using moderate levels of banding. *J Med Genet,* **29**, 103–108.

Jäger, R. J., Harley, V. R., Pfeiffer, R. A., Goodfellow, P. N. and Scherer, G. (1992). A familial mutation in the testis-determining gene SRY shared by both sexes. *Hum Genet,* **90**, 350–355.

Jalal, S. M., Persons, D. L., Dewald, G. W. and Lindor, N. M. (1994). Form of 15q proximal duplication appears to be a normal euchromatic variant. *Am J Med Genet,* **52**, 495–497.

Jalal, S. M., Kukolich, M. K., Garcia, M. and Day, D. W. (1990a). Euchromatic 9q+ heteromorphism in a family. *Am J Med Genet,* **37**, 155–156.

Jalal, S. M., Schneider, N. R., Kukolich, M. K. and Wilson, G. N. (1990b). Euchromatic 16p+ heteromorphism: first report in North America. *Am J Med Genet,* **37**, 548–550.

Jalbert, P., Jalbert, H. and Sele, B. (1988). Types of imbalances in human reciprocal translocations: risks at birth. In "The cytogenetics of mammalian autosomal rearrangements" (A. Daniel, ed.). A. R. Liss, New York, pp. 267–291.

Jalbert, P., Jalbert, H., Sele, B., Mouriquand, C., Malka, J., Boucharlat, J. and Pison, H. (1975). Partial trisomy for the long arms of chromosome No. 5 due to insertion and further 'aneusomie de recombinaison.' *J Med Genet*, **12**, 418–423.

Jalbert, P., Sele, B. and Jalbert, H. (1980). Reciprocal translocations: a way to predict the mode of imbalanced segregation by pachytene-diagram drawing. A study of 151 human translocations. *Hum Genet*, **55**, 209–222.

James, R. S., Temple, I. K., Dennis, N. R. and Crolla, J. A. (1995). A search for uniparental disomy in carriers of supernumerary marker chromosomes. *Eur J Hum Genet*, **3**, 21–26.

James, R. S., Temple, I. K., Patch, C., Thompson, E. M., Hassold, T. and Jacobs, P. A. (1994). A systematic search for uniparental disomy in carriers of chromosome translocations. *Eur J Hum Genet*, **2**, 83–95.

Janke, D. (1982). Centric fission of chromosome no. 7 in three generations. *Hum Genet*, **60**, 200–201.

Jaspers, N. G. J., Taalman, R. D. F. M. and Baan, C. (1988). Patients with an inherited syndrome characterized by immunodeficiency, microcephaly, and chromosomal instability: genetic relationship to ataxia-telangiectasia. *Am J Hum Genet*, **42**, 66–73.

Jauch, A., Robson, L. and Smith, A. (1995). Investigations with fluorescence in situ hybridization (FISH) demonstrate loss of the telomeres on the reciprocal chromosome in three unbalanced translocations involving chromosome 15 in Prader-Willi and Angelman syndrome. *Hum Genet*, **96**, 345–349.

Jeffers, M. D., O'Dwyer, P., Curran, B., Leader, M. and Gillan, J. E. (1993). Partial hydatidiform mole: a common but underdiagnosed condition. A 3-year retrospective clinicopathological and DNA flow cytometric analysis. *Int J Gynecol Pathol*, **12**, 315–323.

Jenderny, J., Caliebe, A., Beyer, C. and Grote, W. (1993). Transmission of a ring chromosome 18 from a mother with 46,XX/47,XX,+r(18) mosaicism to her daughter, resulting in a 46,XX,r(18) karyotype. *J Med Genet*, **30**, 964–965.

Jenderny, J., Gebauer, J., Röhrborn, G. and Rüger, A. (1992). Sperm chromosome analysis of a man heterozygous for a pericentric inversion of chromosome 20. *Hum Genet*, **89**, 117–119.

Jenkins, D., Martin, K. and Young, I. D. (1993). Hypomelanosis of Ito associated with mosaicism for trisomy 7 and apparent 'pseudomosaicism' at amniocentesis. *J Med Genet*, **30**, 783–784.

Jewell, A. F., Simpson, G. F., Pasztor, L., Keene, C. L., Sullivan, B. A. and Schwartz, S. (1992). Prenatal diagnosis of two cases de novo dup(12p), identified by fluorescence in situ hybridization (FISH). *Am J Hum Genet (Suppl.)*, **51**, 81A.

Johansen, M., Knight, M., Maher, E. J., Smith, K. and Sargent, I. L. (1995). An investigation of methods for enriching trophoblast from maternal blood. *Prenat Diagn*, **15**, 921–931.

Johannisson, R., Löhrs, U., Wolff, H. H. and Schwinger, E. (1987). Two different XY-quadrivalent associations and impairment of fertility in men. *Cytogenet Cell Genet*, **45**, 222–230.

Johannisson, R. and Winking, H. (1994). Synaptonemal complexes of chains and rings in mice heterozygous for multiple Robertsonian translocations. *Chromosome Res*, **2**, 137–145.

Johnson, A., Wapner, R. J., Davis, G. H. and Jackson, L. G. (1990). Mosaicism in chorionic villus sampling: an association with poor perinatal outcome. *Obstet Gynecol*, **75**, 573–577.

Jones, C., Booth, C., Rita, D., Jazmines, L., Spiro, R., McCulloch, B., McCaskill, C. and Shaffer, L. G. (1995). Identification of a case of maternal uniparental disomy of chromosome 10 associated with confined placental mosaicism. *Prenat Diagn*, **15**, 843–848.

Jones, C., Slijepcevic, P., Marsh, S., Baker, E., Langdon, W. Y., Richards, R. I. and Tunnacliffe, A. (1994). Physical linkage of the fragile site *FRA11B* and a Jacobsen syndrome chromosome deletion breakpoint in 11q23.3. *Hum Mol Genet*, **3**, 2123–2130.

Jones, H. W. (1978). Problems of sex differentiation—surgical correction. *Birth Defects: Orig Art Series*, **14**(6C), pp. 63–71.

Joseph, A. and Thomas, I. M. (1982). A complex rearrangement involving three autosomes in a phenotypically normal male presenting with sterility. *J Med Genet*, **19**, 375–376.

Julian-Reynier, C., Aurran, Y., Dumaret, A., Maron, A., Chabal, F., Giraud, F. and Aymé, S. (1995). Attitudes towards Down's syndrome: follow up of a cohort of 280 cases. *J Med Genet*, **32**, 597–599.

Juyal, R. C., Greenberg, F., Mengden, G. A., Lupski, J. R., Trask, B. J., van den Engh, G., Lindsay, E. A., Christy, H., Chen, K.-S., Baldini, A., Shaffer, L. G. and Patel, P. I. (1995). Smith-Magenis syndrome deletion: a case with equivocal cytogenetic findings resolved by fluorescence in situ hybridization. *Am J Med Genet*, **58**, 286–291.

Kähkönen, M., Kokkonen, H.-L., Haapala, K., Winqvist, R. and Leisti, J. (1990). Discrepancy in cytogenetic and DNA analyses of a patient with a deletion of proximal 15q due to familial pericentric inversion and analysis of eight other patients diagnosed to have Prader-Willi syndrome. *Am J Hum Genet*, **47**, A31.

Kaiser, P. (1984). Pericentric inversions. Problems and significance for clinical genetics. *Hum Genet*, **68**, 1–47.

Kaiser, P. (1988). Pericentric inversions: their problems and clinical significance. In ''The cytogenetics of mammalian autosomal rearrangements'' (A. Daniel, ed.). A. R. Liss, New York, pp. 163–247.

Kaiser-McCaw, B. (1982). Sorting out the heterogeneity in the chromosome-instability syndromes. In ''Human genetics. Part B: medical aspects'' (B. Bonné-Tamir, ed.). A. R. Liss, New York, pp. 349–358.

Kajii, T., Ferrier, A., Niikawa, N., Takahara, H., Ohama, K. and Avirachan, S. (1980). Anatomic and chromosomal anomalies in 639 spontaneous abortuses. *Hum Genet*, **55**, 87–98.

Kalousek, D. K. (1993). The effect of confined placental mosaicism on development of the human aneuploid conceptus. *Am J Med Genet*, **45**, 13–22.

Kalousek, D. K. and Barrett, I. (1994). Genomic imprinting related to prenatal diagnosis. *Prenat Diagn*, **14**, 1191–1201.

Kalousek, D. K., Barrett, I. J. and Gärtner, A. B. (1992). Spontaneous abortion and confined chromosomal mosaicism. *Hum Genet*, **88**, 642–646.

Kalousek, D. K., Barrett, I. J. and McGillivray, B. C. (1989). Placental mosaicism and intrauterine survival of trisomies 13 and 18. *Am J Hum Genet*, **44**, 338–343.

Kalousek, D. K., Howard-Peebles, P. N., Olson, S. B., Barrett, I. J., Dorfman, A., Black, S. H., Schulman, J. D. and Wilson, R. D. (1991). Confirmation of CVS mosaicism in term placentae and high frequency of intrauterine growth retardation: association with confined placental mosaicism. *Prenat Diagn*, **11**, 743–750.

Kalousek, D. K., Langlois, S., Barrett, I., Yam, I., Wilson, D. R., Howard-Peebles, P.

N., Johnson, M. P. and Giorgiutti, E. (1993). Uniparental disomy for chromosome 16 in humans. *Am J Hum Genet*, **52**, 8–16.

Kamiguchi, Y., Rosenbusch, B., Sterzik, K. and Mikamo, K. (1993). Chromosomal analysis of unfertilized human oocytes prepared by a gradual fixation-air drying method. *Hum Genet*, **90**, 533–541.

Kaneko, N., Kawagoe, S. and Hiroi, M. (1990). Turner's syndrome—review of the literature with reference to a successful pregnancy outcome. *Gynecol Obstet Invest*, **29**, 81–87.

Karp, L. E. (1981). Sterilization of the retarded. *Am J Med Genet*, **9**, 1–3.

Karp, L. E. (1983). The terrible question. *Am J Med Genet*, **14**, 1–4.

Katzman, R. and Kawas, C. (1994). The epidemiology of dementia and Alzheimer disease. In "Alzheimer disease" (R. D. Terry, R. Katzman and K. L. Bick, eds.). Raven Press, New York, pp. 105–122.

Kausch, K., Haaf, T., Köhler, J. and Schmid, M. (1988). Complex chromosomal rearrangement in a woman with multiple miscarriages. *Am J Med Genet*, **31**, 415–420.

Keitges, E. and Palmer, C. G. (1986). Analysis of spreading of inactivation in eight X autosome translocations utilizing the high resolution RBG technique. *Hum Genet*, **72**, 231–236.

Kellner, L. H., Weiss, R. R., Weiner, Z., Neuer, M., Martin, G. M., Schulman, H. and Lipper, S. (1995). The advantages of using triple-marker screening for chromosomal abnormalities. *Am J Obstet Gynecol*, **172**, 831–836.

Kelly, P. T. (1977). "Dealing with dilemma. A manual for genetic counselors." Springer-Verlag, New York.

Kennerknecht, I., Barbi, G. and Vogel, W. (1990). Maternal transmission of ring chromosome 21. *Hum Genet*, **86**, 99–101.

Kennerknecht, I., Just, W. and Vogel, W. (1993). A triploid fetus with a diploid placenta: proposal of a mechanism. *Prenat Diagn*, **13**, 885–891.

Kennerknecht, I., von Saurma, P., Brenner, R., Just, W., Barbi, G., Sorgo, W., Heinze, E., Wolf, A. S., Schneider, V., Günther, K.-P., Teller, W. M. and Vogel, W. (1995). Agonadism in two sisters with XY gonosomal constitution, mental retardation, short stature, severely retarded bone age, and multiple extragenital malformations: a new autosomal recessive syndrome. *Am J Med Genet*, **59**, 62–67.

Keppen, L. D., Gollin, S. M., Edwards, D., Sawyer, J., Wilson, W. and Overhauser, J. (1992). Clinical phenotype and molecular analysis of a three-generation family with an interstitial deletion of the short arm of chromosome 5. *Am J Med Genet*, **44**, 356–360.

Kerber, S. and Held, K. R. (1993). Early genetic amniocentesis—4 years' experience. *Prenat Diagn*, **13**, 21–27.

Kessler, S. (ed.) (1979). "Genetic counseling. Psychological dimensions." Academic Press, New York.

Kessler, S. and Levine, E. K. (1987). Psychological aspects of genetic counseling. IV. The subjective assessment of probability. *Am J Med Genet*, **28**, 361–370.

Kher, A. S., Chattopadhyay, A., Datta, S., Kanade, S., Sreenivasan, V. K. and Bharucha, B. A. (1994). Familial mosaic Turner syndrome. *Clin Genet*, **46**, 382–383.

Khong, T. Y. and George, K. (1992). Chromosomal abnormalities associated with a single umbilical artery. *Prenat Diagn*, **12**, 965–968.

Kingston, H. M., Nicolini, U., Haslam, J. and Andrews, T. (1993). 46,XY/47,XY,+17p+ mosaicism in amniocytes associated with fetal abnormalities despite normal fetal blood karyotype. *Prenat Diagn*, **13**, 637–642.

Kircheisen, R. and Schroeder-Kurth, T. (1991). Familiäres blasenmolen-syndrom und genetische aspekte dieser gestörten trophoblastentwicklung. *Geburtshilfe Frauenheilkd*, **51**, 569–571.

Kirk, J. A., VanDevanter, D. R., Biberman, J. and Bryant, E. M. (1994). Y chromosome loss in chronic myeloid leukemia detected in both normal and malignant cells by interphase fluorescence in situ hybridization. *Genes, Chromosomes and Cancer*, **11**, 141–145.

Kleczkowska, A., Fryns, J. P. and Van den Berghe, H. (1982). Complex chromosomal rearrangements (CCR) and their genetic consequences. *J Génét Hum*, **30**, 199–214.

Kleczkowska, A., Fryns, J. P. and Van den Berghe, H. (1986). Autosomal whole arm translocations in man. A patient with t(5p7p;5q7q) type rearrangement and review of the literature. *Clin Genet*, **30**, 72–75.

Kleczkowska, A., Fryns, J. P. and Van den Berghe, H. (1987). Pericentric inversions in man: personal experience and review of the literature. *Hum Genet*, **75**, 333–338.

Kleczkowska, A., Fryns, J. P., Vinken, L. and Van den Berghe, H. (1985). Effect of balanced X/autosome translocations on sexual and physical development. A personal experience of 4 patients. *Clin Genet*, **27**, 147–152.

Klein, J., Graham, J. M., Platt, L. D. and Schreck, R. (1994). Trisomy 8 mosaicism in chorionic villus sampling: case report and counselling issues. *Prenat Diagn*, **14**, 451–454.

Kline, A. D., White, M. E., Wapner, R., Rojas, K., Biesecker, L. G., Kamholz, J., Zackai, E. H., Muenke, M., Scott, C. I. and Overhauser, J. (1993). Molecular analysis of the 18q− syndrome—and correlation with phenotype. *Am J Hum Genet*, **52**, 895–906.

Knight, L. A., Soon, G. M. and Tan, M. (1993). Extra G positive band on the long arm of chromosome 9. *J Med Genet*, **30**, 613.

Knight, S. J. L., Flannery, A. V., Hirst, M. C., Campbell, L., Christodoulou, Z., Phelps, S. R., Pointon, J., Middleton-Price, H. R., Barnicoat, A., Pembrey, M. E., Holland, J., Oostra, B. A., Bobrow, M. and Davies, K. E. (1993). Trinucleotide repeat amplification and hypermethylation of a CpG island in FRAXE mental retardation. *Cell*, **74**, 127–134.

Knight, S. J. L., Voelckel, M. A., Hirst, M. C., Flannery, A. V., Moncla, A. and Davies, K. E. (1994). Triplet repeat expansion at the *FRAXE* locus and X-linked mild mental handicap. *Am J Hum Genet*, **55**, 81–86.

Knoll, J. H. M., Rogan, P. K., Nicholls, R. D., Wu, B., Korf, B. and White, L. (1995). Allele-specific replication of 15q11q13 loci: a diagnostic test for detection of uniparental disomy. *Am J Hum Genet*, **57**, A34.

Knuutila, S., Heinonen, K., Hongell, K., Varonen, S. and Simell, O. (1984). A duplication within the critical fertility region of X chromosome in a mentally retarded woman with normal menarche. *Hereditas*, **101**, 253–255.

Knuutila, S., Larramendy, M. L., Elfving, P., El-Rifai, W., Miettinen, A. and Mitelman, F. (1995). Trisomy 7 in non-neoplastic tubular epithelial cells of the kidney. *Hum Genet*, **95**, 149–156.

Kobayashi, K., Mizuno, K., Hida, A., Komaki, R., Tomita, K., Matsushita, I., Namiki, M., Iwamoto, T., Tamura, S., Minowada, S., Nakahori, Y. and Nakagome, Y. (1994). PCR analysis of the Y chromosome long arm in azoospermic patients: evidence for a second locus required for spermatogenesis. *Hum Mol Genet*, **3**, 1965–1967.

Kobayashi, T., Narahara, K., Yokoyama, Y., Ueyama, S., Mohri, O., Fujii, T., Fujimoto,

M., Ohtsuki, S., Tsuji, K. and Seino, Y. (1991). Gardner syndrome in a boy with interstitial deletion of the long arm of chromosome 5. *Am J Med Genet*, **41**, 460–463.

Koeberl, D. D., McGillivray, B. and Sybert, V. P. (1995). Prenatal diagnosis of 45,X/46,XX mosaicism and 45,X: implications for postnatal outcome. *Am J Hum Genet*, **57**, 661–666.

Kohn, G. and Robinson, A. (1970). Tetraploidy in cells cultured from amniotic fluid. *Lancet*, **2**, 778–779.

Kojis, T. L., Gatti, R. A. and Sparkes, R. S. (1991). The cytogenetics of ataxia telangiectasia. *Cancer Genet Cytogenet*, **56**, 143–156.

Korenberg, J. R., Chen, X.-N., Schipper, R., Sun, Z., Gonsky, R., Gerwehr, S., Carpenter, N., Daumer, C., Dignan, P., Disteche, C., Graham, J. M., Hugdins, L., McGillivray, B., Miyazaki, K., Ogasawara, N., Park, J. P., Pagon, R., Pueschel, S., Sack, G., Say, B., Schuffenhauer, S., Soukup, S. and Yamanaka, T. (1994). Down syndrome phenotypes: the consequences of chromosomal imbalance. *Proc Natl Acad Sci U S A*, **91**, 4997–5001.

Korenberg, J. R., Kawashima, H., Pulst, S.-M., Ikeuchi, T., Ogasawara, N., Yamamoto, K., Schonberg, S. A., West, R., Allen, L., Magenis, E., Ikawa, K., Taniguchi, N. and Epstein, C. J. (1990). Molecular definition of a region of chromosome 21 that causes features of the Down syndrome phenotype. *Am J Hum Genet*, **47**, 236–246.

Koskinen, S., Onnelainen, T., de la Chapelle, A. and Kere, J. (1993). A rare reciprocal translocation (12;21) segregating for nine generations. *Hum Genet*, **92**, 509–512.

Kosztolányi, G. (1987). Does ''ring syndrome'' exist? An analysis of 207 case reports on patients with a ring autosome. *Hum Genet*, **75**, 174–179.

Kosztolányi, G., Méhes, K. and Hook, E. B. (1991). Inherited ring chromosomes: an analysis of published cases. *Hum Genet*, **87**, 320–324.

Kotwaliwale, S. V., Dicholkar, V. V. and Motashaw, N. D. (1991). Maternal transmission of translocation 2;21 associated with Down's syndrome. *J Med Genet*, **28**, 415–416.

Kotzot, D., Bernasconi, F., Brecevic, L., Robinson, W. P., Kiss, P., Kosztolanyi, G., Lurie, I. W., Superti-Furga, A. and Schinzel, A. (1995a). Phenotype of the Williams-Beuren syndrome associated with hemizygosity at the elastin locus. *Eur J Pediatr*, **154**, 477–482.

Kotzot, D., Schmitt, S., Bernasconi, F., Robinson, W. P., Lurie, I. W., Ilyina, H., Méhes, K., Hamel, B. C. J., Otten, B. J., Hergersberg, M., Werder, E., Schoenle, E. and Schinzel, A. (1995b). Uniparental disomy 7 in Silver-Russell syndrome and primordial growth retardation. *Hum Mol Genet*, **4**, 583–587.

Kousseff, B. G., Nichols, P., Essig, Y.-P., Miller, K., Weiss, A. and Tedesco, T. A. (1987). Complex chromosome rearrangements and congenital anomalies. *Am J Med Genet*, **26**, 771–782.

Kozma, C., Meck, J. M., Loomis, K. J. and Galindo, H. C. (1991). *De novo* duplication of 17p [dup(17)(p12→p11.2)]: report of an additional case with confirmation of the cytogenetic, phenotypic, and developmental aspects. *Am J Med Genet*, **41**, 446–450.

Krajewska-Walasek, M., Chrzanowska, K., Tylki-Szymańska, A. and Bialecka, M. (1995). A further report of Brachmann-de Lange syndrome in two sibs with normal parents. *Clin Genet*, **47**, 324–327.

Krajewska-Walasek, M., Gutkowska, A., Mospinek-Krasnopolska, M. and Chrzanowska, K. (1994). A new case of Beckwith-Wiedemann syndrome with 11p15 duplication of paternal origin [46,XY,-(21),der(21),t(11;21)(p15.2;q22.3)pat]. In "International Symposium on Genomic Imprinting." University of Florence, p. 93.

Krauss, C. M., Turksoy, R. N., Atkins, L., McLaughlin, C., Brown, L. G. and Page, D. C. (1987). Familial premature ovarian failure due to an interstitial deletion of the long arm of the X chromosome. *N Engl J Med*, **317**, 125–131.

Kremer, E. J., Pritchard, M., Lynch, M., Yu, S., Holman, K., Baker, E., Warren, S. T., Schlessinger, D., Sutherland, G. R. and Richards, R. I. (1991). Mapping of DNA instability at the fragile X to a trinucleotide repeat sequence p(CCG)n. *Science*, **252**, 1711–1714.

Krüger, G., Götz, J., Dunker, H. and Pelz, L. (1987). Isochromosome (18q) in siblings. *Clin Genet*, **32**, 249–253.

Kubota, T., Saitoh, S., Matsumoto, T., Narahara, K., Fukushima, Y., Jinno, Y. and Niikawa, N. (1994). Excess functional copy of allele at chromosomal region 11p15 may cause Wiedemann-Beckwith (EMG) syndrome. *Am J Med Genet*, **49**, 378–383.

Kuhn, E. M., Sarto, G. E., Bates, B.-J. G. and Therman, E. (1987). Gene-rich chromosome regions and autosomal trisomy. A case of chromosome 3 trisomy mosaicism. *Hum Genet*, **77**, 214–220.

Kuhnle, U., Schwarz, H. P., Löhrs, U., Stengel-Rutkowski, S., Cleve, H. and Braun, A. (1993). Familial true hermaphroditism: paternal and maternal transmission of true hermaphroditism (46,XX) and XX maleness in the absence of Y-chromosomal sequences. *Hum Genet*, **92**, 571–576.

Kulharya, A. S., Roop, H., Kukolich, M. K., Nachtman, R. G., Belmont, J. W. and Garcia-Heras, J. (1995). Mild phenotypic effects of a de novo deletion Xpter→Xp22.3 and duplication 3pter→3p23. *Am J Med Genet*, **56**, 16–21.

Kuliev, A. M., Modell, B., Jackson, L., Simpson, J. L., Brambati, B., Rhoads, G., Froster, U., Verlinsky, Y., Smidt-Jensen, S., Holzgreve, W., Ginsberg, N., Ammala, P. and Dumez, Y. (1992). Chorionic villus sampling (CVS): World Health Organization European regional office (WHO/EURO) meeting statement on the use of CVS in prenatal diagnosis. *J Assisted Reprod and Genet*, **9**, 299–302.

Kuwano, A., Mutirangura, A., Dittrich, B., Buiting, K., Horsthemke, B., Saitoh, S., Niikawa, N., Ledbetter, S. A., Greenberg, F., Chinault, A. C. and Ledbetter, D. H. (1992). Molecular dissection of the Prader-Willi/Angelman syndrome region (15q11–13) by YAC cloning and FISH analysis. *Hum Molec Genet*, **1**, 417–425.

Kuznetzova, T., Baranov, A., Ivaschenko, T., Savitsky, G. A., Lanceva, O. E., Wang, M. R., Giollant, M., Malet, P., Kascheeva, T., Vakharlovsky, V. and Baranov, V. S. (1994). X;Y translocation in a girl with short stature and some features of Turner's syndrome: cytogenetic and molecular studies. *J Med Genet*, **31**, 649–651.

Kvaløy, K., Galvagni, F. and Brown, W. R. A. (1994). The sequence organization of the long arm pseudoautosomal region of the human sex chromosomes. *Hum Mol Genet*, **3**, 771–778.

Lacombe, D., Saura, R., Taine, L. and Battin, J. (1992). Confirmation of assignment of a locus for Rubinstein-Taybi syndrome gene to 16p13.3. *Am J Med Genet*, **44**, 126–128.

Lage, J. M., Mark, S. D., Roberts, D. J., Goldstein, D. P., Bernstein, M. R. and Berkowitz, R. S. (1992). A flow cytometry study of 137 fresh hydropic placentas: correlation between types of hydatidiform moles and nuclear DNA ploidy. *Obstet Gynecol*, **79**, 403–410.

Lahn, B. T., Ma, N., Breg, W. R., Stratton, R., Surti, U. and Page, D. C. (1994). Xq-Yq interchange resulting in supernormal X-linked gene expression in severely retarded males with 46,XYq-karyotype. *Nature Genet*, **8**, 243–250.

Lamb, B. T., Sisodia, S. S., Lawler, A. M., Slunt, H. H., Kitt, C. A., Kearns, W. G., Pearson, P. L., Price, D. L. and Gearhart, J. D. (1993). Introduction and expression of the 400 kilobase *precursor amyloid protein* gene in transgenic mice. *Nature Genet*, **5**, 22–29

Lamb, J., Harris, P. C., Wilkie, A. O. M., Wood, W. G., Dauwerse, J. G. and Higgs, D. R. (1993). De novo truncation of chromosome 16p and healing with (TTAGGG)n in the α-thalassemia/mental retardation syndrome (ATR-16). *Am J Hum Genet*, **52**, 668–676.

Lamb, J., Wilkie, A. O. M., Harris, P. C., Buckle, V. J., Lindenbaum, R. H., Barton, N. J., Reeders, S. T., Weatherall, D. J. and Higgs, D. R. (1989). Detection of breakpoints in submicroscopic chromosomal translocation, illustrating an important mechanism for genetic disease. *Lancet*, **2**, 819–824.

Lancet editorial (1995). Western eyes on China's eugenics law. *Lancet*, **346**, 131.

Landenburger, G. and Delp, K. J. (1987). An approach for supportive care before, during, and after selective abortion. In "Strategies in genetic counseling: issues in perinatal care" (N. W. Paul and H. Travers, eds.). *Birth Defects: Orig Art Series*, **23**(6), pp. 84–88.

Langer, L. O., Krassikoff, N., Laxova, R., Scheer-Williams, M., Lutter, L. D., Gorlin, R. J., Jennings, C. G. and Day, D. W. (1984). The tricho-rhino-phalangeal syndrome with exostoses (or Langer-Giedion syndrome): four additional patients without mental retardation and review of the literature. *Am J Med Genet*, **19**, 81–111.

Laquerbe, A., Moustacchi, E., Fuscoe, J. C. and Papadopoulo, D. (1995). The molecular mechanism underlying formation of deletions in Fanconi anemia cells may involve a site-specific recombination. *Proc Natl Acad Sci U S A*, **92**, 831–835.

La Vecchia, C., Franceschi, S., Parazzini, F., Fasoli, M., Decarli, A., Gallus, G. and Tognoni, G. (1985). Risk factors for gestational trophoblastic disease in Italy. *Am J Epidemiol*, **121**, 457–464.

Lawler, S. D., Fisher, R. A. and Dent, J. (1991). A prospective genetic study of complete and partial hydatidiform moles. *Am J Obstet Gynecol*, **164**, 1270–1277.

Leana-Cox, J., Jenkins, L., Palmer, C. G., Plattner, R., Sheppard, L., Flejter, W. L., Zackowski, J., Tsien, F. and Schwartz, S. (1994). Molecular cytogenetic analysis of inv dup(15) chromosomes, using probes specific for the Prader-Willi/Angelman syndrome region: clinical implications. *Am J Hum Genet*, **54**, 748–756.

LeBeau, M. M. and Rowley, J. D. (1984). Heritable fragile sites in cancer. *Nature*, **308**, 607–608.

Leclercq, G., Buvat-Herbaut, M., Monnier, J. C., Vinatier, D. and Dufour, P. (1992). Syndrome de Turner et grossesse par dons d'ovocytes et fécondation *in vitro*. *J Gynecol Obstet Biol Reprod*, **21**, 635–640.

Ledbetter, D. H. (1992). Minireview: cryptic translocations and telomere integrity. *Am J Hum Genet*, **51**, 451–456.

Ledbetter, D. H. and Engel, E. (1995). Uniparental disomy in humans: development of an imprinting map and its implications for prenatal diagnosis. *Hum Mol Genet*, **4**, 1757-1764.

Ledbetter, D. H., Rich, D. C., O'Connell, P., Leppert, M. and Carey, J. C. (1989). Precise localization of NF1 to 17q11.2 by balanced translocation. *Am J Hum Genet*, **44**, 20–24.

Ledbetter, D. H., Zachary, J. M., Simpson, J. L., Golbus, M. S., Pergament, E., Jackson, L., Mahoney, M. J., Desnick, R. J., Schulman, J., Copeland, K. L., Verlinsky Y., Yang-Feng, T., Schonberg, S. A., Babu, A., Tharapel, A., Dorfmann, A., Lubs, H. A., Rhoads, G. G., Fowler, S. E. and De La Cruz, F. (1992). Cytogenetic results from the U.S. collaborative study on CVS. *Prenat Diagn*, **12**, 317–345.

Ledbetter, S. A., Kuwano, A., Dobyns, W. B. and Ledbetter, D. H. (1992). Microdeletions of chromosome 17p13 as a cause of isolated lissencephaly. *Am J Hum Genet*, **50**, 182–189.

Leichtman, D. A., Schmickel, R. D., Gelehrter, T. D., Judd, W. J., Woodbury, M. C. and Meilinger, K. L. (1978). Familial Turner syndrome. *Ann Int Med*, **89**, 473–476.

Leisti, J. T., Kaback, M. M. and Rimoin, D. L. (1975). Human X-autosome translocations: differential inactivation of the X chromosome in a kindred with an X-9 translocation. *Am J Hum Genet*, **27**, 441–453.

Lejeune, J., Gautier, M. and Turpin, R. (1959). Étude des chromosomes somatiques de neuf enfants mongoliens. *Comp Rend Acad Sci*, **248**, 1721–1722.

Lejeune, J., Lafourcade, J., Berger, R., Vialatte, J., Boeswillwald, M., Seringe, P. and Turpin, R. (1963). Trois cas de délétion partielle du bras court d'un chromosome 5. *Comp Rend Acad Sci*, **257**, 3098–3102.

Leschot, N. J., van der Velden, J., Marinkovic-Ilsen, A., Darling, S. M. and Nijenhuis, L. E. (1986). Homozygosity for a Y/22 chromosome translocation: t(Y;22)(q12; p12/13). *Clin Genet*, **29**, 251–257.

Lewin, B. (1994). Genes V. Oxford University Press, Oxford, p. 967.

Liebaers, I., Bonduelle, M., Van Assche, E., Devroey, P. and Van Steirteghem, A. (1995). Sex chromosome abnormalities after intracytoplasmic sperm injection. *Lancet*, **346**, 1095.

Liebetrau, W., Bühner, M. and Hoehn, H. (1995). Prototype sequence clues within the Fanconi anaemia group C gene. *J Med Genet*, **32**, 669–670.

Lindblom, A., Sandelin, K., Iselius, L., Dumanski, J., White, I., Nordenskjöld, M. and Larsson, C. (1994). Predisposition for breast cancer in carriers of constitutional translocation 11q;22q. *Am J Hum Genet*, **54**, 871–876.

Linden, M. G., Bender, B. G. and Robinson, A. (1995). Sex chromosome tetrasomy and pentasomy. *Pediatrics*, **96**, 672–682.

Lindenbaum, R. H., Hultén, M., McDermott, A. and Seabright, M. (1985). The prevalence of translocations in parents of children with regular trisomy 21: a possible interchromosomal effect? *J Med Genet*, **22**, 24–28.

Linder, D., McCaw, B. K. and Hecht, F. (1975). Parthenogenic origin of benign ovarian teratomas. *N Engl J Med*, **292**, 63–66.

Lindor, N. M., Karnes, P. S., Michels, V. V., Dewald, G. W., Goerss, J., Jalal, S., Jenkins, R. B., Vockley, G. and Thibodeau, S. N. (1995). Uniparental disomy in congenital disorders: a prospective study. *Am J Med Genet*, **58**, 143–146.

Lindor, N. M., Michels, V. V., Jalal, S. and Shaughnessy, W. (1995). Trisomy 9 mosaicism in a child with a tethered cord. *Clin Dysmorph*, **4**, 169–172.

Lindsay, E. A., Goldgerb, R., Jurecic, V., Morrow, B., Carlson, C., Kucherlapati, R. S., Shprintzen, R. J. and Baldini, A. (1995). Velo-cardio-facial syndrome: frequency and extent of 22q11 deletions. *Am J Med Genet*, **57**, 514–522.

Lindsay, E. A., Greenberg, F., Shaffer, L. G., Shapira, S. K., Scambler, P. J. and Baldini, A. (1995b). Submicroscopic deletions at 22q11.2: variability of the clinical picture and delineation of a commonly deleted region. *Am J Med Genet,* **56**, 191–197.

Lindsay, E. A., Grillo, A., Ferrero, G. B., Roth, E. J., Magenis, E., Grompe, M., Hultén, M., Gould, C., Baldini, A., Zoghbi, H. Y. and Ballabio, A. (1994). Microphthalmia with linear skin defects (MLS) syndrome: clinical, cytogenetic and molecular characterization. *Am J Med Genet,* **49**, 229–234.

Liou, J.-D., Chen, C.-P., Breg, W. R., Hobbins, J. C., Mahoney, M. J. and Yang-Feng, T. L. (1993). Fetal blood sampling and cytogenetic abnormalities. *Prenat Diagn,* **13**, 1–8.

Lippe, B. (1991). Turner syndrome. *Endocrinol Metabol Clin North Am,* **20**, 121–152.

Llerena, J., Murer-Orlando, M., McGuire, M., Zahed, L., Sheridan, R. J., Berry, A. C. and Bobrow, M. (1989). Spontaneous and induced chromosome breakage in chorionic villus samples: a cytogenetic approach to first trimester prenatal diagnosis of ataxia telangiectasia syndrome. *J Med Genet,* **26**, 174–178.

Lockwood, D. H. and Neu, R. L. (1993). Cytogenetic analysis of 1375 amniotic fluid specimens from pregnancies with gestational age less than 14 weeks. *Prenat Diagn,* **13**, 801–805.

Loesch, D. Z., Huggins, R., Hay, D. A., Gedeon, A. K., Mulley, J. C. and Sutherland, G. R. (1993). Genotype-phenotype relationships in fragile X syndrome: a family study. *Am J Hum Genet,* **53**, 1064–1073.

Lorda-Sanchez, I., Binkert, F., Maechler, M. and Schinzel, A. (1991). A molecular study of X isochromosomes: parental origin, centromeric structure, and mechanisms of formation. *Am J Hum Genet,* **49**, 1034–1040.

Lowery, M. C., Morris, C. A., Ewart, A., Brothman, L. J., Zhu, X. L., Leonard, C. O., Carey, J. C., Keating, M. and Brothman, A. R. (1995). Strong correlation of elastin deletions, detected by FISH, with Williams syndrome: evaluation of 235 patients. *Am J Hum Genet,* **57**, 49–53.

Lubinsky, M. S. (1986). Kouska's fallacy: the error of the divided denominator. *Lancet,* **2**, 1449–1450.

Lucente, D., Chen, H. M., Shea, D., Samec, S. N., Rutter, M., Chrast, R., Rossier, C., Buckler, A., Antonarakis, S. E. and McCormick, M. K. (1995). Localization of 102 exons to a 2.5 Mb region involved in Down syndrome. *Hum Molec Genet,* **4**, 1305-1311.

Luciani, J. M., Guichaoua, M. R., Delafontaine, D., North M. O., Gabriel-Robez O. and Rumpler, Y. (1987). Pachytene analysis in a 17;21 reciprocal translocation carrier: role of the acrocentric chromosomes in male sterility. *Hum Genet,* **77**, 246–250.

Lüdecke, H.-J., Wagner, M. J., Nardmann, J., La Pillo, B., Parrish, J. E., Willems, P. J., Haan, E. A., Frydman, M., Hamers, G. J. H., Wells, D. E. and Horsthemke, B. (1995). Molecular dissection of a contiguous gene syndrome: localization of the genes involved in the Langer-Giedion syndrome. *Hum Mol Genet,* **4**, 31–36.

Ludowese, C. J., Thompson, K. J., Sekhon, G. S. and Pauli, R. M. (1991). Absence of predictable phenotypic expression in proximal 15q duplications. *Clin Genet,* **40**, 194–201.

Lurie, I. W., Wulfsberg, E. A., Prabhakar, G., Rosenblum-Vos, L. S., Supovitz, K. R. and Cohen, M. M. (1994). Complex chromosomal rearrangements: some breakpoints may have cellular adaptive significance. *Clin Genet,* **46**, 244–247.

Lyle, R., Wright, T. J., Clark, L. N. and Hewitt, J. E. (1995). The FSHD-associated repeat, D4Z4, is a member of a dispersed family of homeobox-containing repeats, subsets of which are clustered on the short arms of the acrocentric chromosomes. *Genomics*, **28**, 389–397.

MacDermot, K. D., Jack, E., Cooke, A., Turleau, C., Lindenbaum, R. H., Pearson, J., Patel, C., Barnes, P. M., Portch, J. and Crawfurd, M. d'A. (1990). Investigation of three patients with the "ring syndrome", including familial transmission of ring 5, and estimation of reproductive risks. *Hum Genet*, **85**, 516–520.

MacDonald, I. M. and Cox, D. M. (1985). Inversion of chromosome 2(p11q13): frequency and implications for genetic counselling. *Hum Genet*, **69**, 281–283.

MacDonald, M., Hassold, T., Harvey, J., Wang, L. H., Morton, N. E. and Jacobs, P. (1994). The origin of 47,XXY and 47,XXX aneuploidy: heterogeneous mechanisms and role of aberrant recombination. *Hum Mol Genet*, **3**, 1365–1371.

Macera, M. J., Verma, R. S., Conte, R. A., Bialer, M. G. and Klein, V. R. (1995). Mechanisms of the origin of a G-positive band within the secondary constriction region of human chromosome 9. *Cytogenet Cell Genet*, **69**, 235–239.

Macintosh, M. C. M. (1994). Perception of risk. In "Screening for Down's syndrome" (J. G. Grudzinskas, T. Chard, M. Chapman and H. Cuckle, eds.). Cambridge University Press, Cambridge, pp. 19–30.

Macintosh, M. C. M., Iles, R., Teisner, B., Sharma, K., Chard, T., Grudzinskas, J. G., Ward, R. H. T. and Muller, F. (1994). Maternal serum human chorionic gonadotrophin and pregnancy-associated plasma protein A, markers for fetal Down syndrome at 8–14 weeks. *Prenat Diagn*, **14**, 203–208.

Macri, J. N., Spencer, K., Garver, K., Buchanan, P. D., Say, B., Carpenter, N. J., Muller, F. and Boué, A. (1994). Maternal serum free beta hCG screening: results of studies including 480 cases of Down syndrome. *Prenat Diagn*, **14**, 97–103.

Madan, K. (1988) Paracentric inversions and their clinical implications. In "The cytogenetics of mammalian autosomal rearrangements" (A. Daniel, ed.). A. R. Liss, New York, pp. 249–266.

Madan, K., Hompes, P. G. A., Shoemaker, J. and Ford, C. E. (1981). X-autosome translocation with a breakpoint in Xq22 in a fertile woman and her 47,XXX infertile daughter. *Hum Genet*, **59**, 290–296.

Madan, K. and Kleinhout, J. (1987). First trimester abortions associated with a translocation t(1;20)(p36;p11). *Hum Genet*, **76**, 109.

Madan, K. and Menko, F. H. (1992). Intrachromosomal insertions: a case report and a review. *Hum Genet*, **89**, 1–9.

Madan, K., Pieters, M. H. E. C., Kuyt, L. P., van Asperen, C. J., de Pater, J. M., Hamers, A. J. H., Gerssen-Schoorl, K. B. J., Hustinx, T. W. J., Breed, A. S. P. M., Van Hemel, J. O. and Smeets, D. F. C. M. (1990). Paracentric inversion inv(11)(q21q23) in the Netherlands. *Hum Genet*, **85**, 15–20.

Madan, K., Seabright, M., Lindenbaum, R. H. and Bobrow, M. (1984). Paracentric inversions in man. *J Med Genet*, **21**, 407–412.

Mangelschots, K., Van Roy, B., Speleman, F., Van Roy, N., Gheuens, J., Beuten, J., Buntinx, I., Van Thienen, M.-N., Willekens, H., Dumon, J., Ceulemans, B. and Willems, P. J. (1992). Reciprocal translocation between the proximal regions of the long arms of chromosomes 13 and 15 resulting in unbalanced offspring: characterization by fluorescence in situ hybridization and DNA analysis. *Hum Genet*, **89**, 407–413.

Mann, N. P., Fitzsimmons, J., Fitzsimmons, E. and Cooke, P. (1982). Roberts syndrome: clinical and cytogenetic aspects. *J Med Genet*, **19**, 116–119.

Mansfield, E. S. (1993). Diagnosis of Down syndrome and other aneuploidies using quantitative polymerase chain reaction and small tandem repeat polymorphisms. *Hum Mol Genet*, **2**, 43–50.

Mansour, S., Hall, C. M., Pembrey, M. E. and Young, I. D. (1995). A clinical and genetic study of campomelic dysplasia. *J Med Genet*, **32**, 415–420.

Mantel, A., Leonard, C., Husson, B., Miladi, N., Tardieu, M. and Landrieu, P. (1994). Submicroscopic deletions of 17p13.3 in type 1 lissencephaly. *Hum Genet*, **94**, 95–96.

Maraia, R., Saal, H. M. and Wangsa, D. (1991). A chromosome 17q de novo paracentric inversion in a patient with campomelic dysplasia; case report and etiologic hypothesis. *Clin Genet*, **39**, 401–408.

Maraschio, P., Cuoco, C., Gimelli, G., Zuffardi, O. and Tiepolo, L. (1988). Origin and clinical significance of inv dup(15). In "The cytogenetics of mammalian autosomal rearrangements" (A. Daniel, ed.). A. R. Liss, New York, pp. 615–634.

Maraschio, P., Tupler, R., Dainotti, E., Cortinovis, M. and Tiepolo, L. (1994). Molecular analysis of a human Y;1 translocation in an azoospermic male. *Cytogenet Cell Genet*, **65**, 256–260.

Marcantonio, S. M., Fechner, P. Y., Migeon, C. J., Perlman, E. J. and Berkovitz, G. D. (1994). Embryonic testicular regression sequence: a part of the clinical spectrum of 46,XY gonadal dysgenesis. *Am J Med Genet*, **49**, 1–5.

Marchau, F. E., Van Roy, B. C., Parizel, P. M., Lambert, J. R., De Canck, I., Leroy, J. G., Gevaert, C. M., Willems, P. J. and Dumon, J. E. (1993). Tricho-rhino-phalangeal syndrome type I (TRP I) due to an apparently balanced translocation involving 8q24. *Am J Med Genet*, **45**, 450–455.

Mark, H. F. L., Mendoza, T., Abuelo, D., Beauregard, L. J., May, J. B. and LaMarche, P. H. (1977). Reproduction in a woman with low percentage t(21q21q) mosaicism. *J Med Genet*, **14**, 221–223.

Markkanen, A., Ruutu, T., Rasi, Y., Franssila, K., Knuutila, S. and de la Chapelle, A. (1987). Constitutional translocation t(3;6)(p14;p11) in a family with hematologic malignancies. *Cancer Genet Cytogenet*, **25**, 87–96.

Maroun, L. E. (1995). Anti-interferon immunoglobulins can improve the trisomy 16 mouse phenotype. *Teratology*, **51**, 329–335.

Marteau, T., Drake, H. and Bobrow, M. (1994). Counselling following diagnosis of a fetal abnormality: the differing approaches of obstetricians, clinical geneticists, and genetic nurses. *J Med Genet*, **31**, 864–867.

Martin, A. O., Benuck, I., Traisman, H. S., Swanson, M.S., Trakas, N., Laing, K., Rosinsky, B. J., Beaird, J., Traisman, E. S., Elias, S. and Simpson, J. L. (1986). Outcome after prenatal detection of a sporadic, unstable translocation t(5;21). *J Med Genet*, **23**, 274–278.

Martin, N. J., Cartwright, D. W. and Harvey, P. J. (1985). Duplication 5q(5q22→5q33): from an intrachromosomal insertion. *Am J Med Genet*, **20**, 57–62.

Martin, R. H. (1984). Analysis of human sperm chromosome complements from a male heterozygous for a reciprocal translocation t(11;22)(q23;q11). *Clin Genet*, **25**, 357–361.

Martin, R. H. (1986). Sperm chromosome analysis in a man heterozygous for a paracentric inversion of chromosome 7 (q11q22). *Hum Genet*, **73**, 97–100.

Martin, R. H. (1988a). Abnormal spermatozoa in human translocation and inversion carriers. In "The cytogenetics of mammalian autosomal rearrangements" (A. Daniel, ed.). A. R. Liss, New York, pp. 397–417.

Martin, R. H. (1988b). Cytogenetic analysis of sperm from a male heterozygous for a 13;14 Robertsonian translocation. *Hum Genet*, **80**, 357–361.

Martin, R. H. (1991). Cytogenetic analysis of sperm from a man heterozygous for a pericentric inversion, inv(3)(p25q21). *Am J Hum Genet*, **48**, 856–861.

Martin, R. H. (1993). Analysis of sperm chromosome complements from a man heterozygous for a pericentric inversion, inv(8)(p23q22). *Cytogenet Cell Genet*, **62**, 199–202.

Martin, R. H., Chan, K., Ko, E. and Rademaker, A. W. (1994a). Detection of aneuploidy in human sperm by fluorescence in situ hybridization (FISH): different frequencies in fresh and stored sperm. *Cytogenet Cell Genet*, **65**, 95–96.

Martin, R. H., Chernos, J. E., Lowry, R. B., Pattinson, H. A., Barclay, L. and Ko, E. (1994b). Analysis of sperm chromosome complements from a man heterozygous for a pericentric inversion of chromosome 1. *Hum Genet*, **93**, 135–138.

Martin, R. H., Rademaker, A. and German, J. (1994c). Chromosomal breakage in human spermatozoa, a heterozygous effect of the Bloom syndrome mutation. *Am J Hum Genet*, **55**, 1242–1246.

Martin, R. H., Hildebrand, K., Yamamoto, J., Peterson, D., Rademaker, A. W., Taylor, P. A. and Lin, C. C. (1986b). The meiotic segregation of human sperm chromosomes in two men with accessory marker chromosomes. *Am J Med Genet*, **25**, 381–388.

Martin, R. H., Ko, E. and Hildebrand, K. (1992). Analysis of sperm chromosome complements from a man heterozygous for a Robertsonian translocation 45,XY,t(15q; 22q). *Am J Med Genet*, **43**, 855–857.

Martin, R. H., Ko, E. and Rademaker, A. (1991). Distribution of aneuploidy in human gametes: comparison between human sperm and oocytes. *Am J Med Genet*, **39**, 321–331.

Martin, R. H. and Rademaker, A. (1990). The frequency of aneuploidy among individual chromosomes in 6,821 human sperm chromosome complements. *Cytogenet Cell Genet*, **53**, 103–107.

Martínez, J. E., Tuck-Muller, C. M., Superneau, D. and Wertelecki, W. (1993). Fertility and the cri du chat syndrome. *Clin Genet*, **43**, 212–214.

Martinez-Castro, P., Ramos, M. C., Rey, J. A., Benitez, J. and Sanchez Cascos, A. (1984). Homozygosity for a Robertsonian translocation (13q14q) in three offspring of heterozygous parents. *Cytogenet Cell Genet*, **38**, 310–312.

Mascari, M. J., Gottlieb, W., Rogan, P. K., Butler, M. G., Waller, D. A., Armour, J. A. L., Jeffreys, A. J., Ladda, R. L. and Nicholls, R. D. (1992). The frequency of uniparental disomy in Prader-Willi syndrome. Implications for molecular diagnosis. *New Eng J Med*, **326**, 1599–1607.

Maserati, E., Pasquali, F., Zuffardi, O., Buttitta, P., Cuoco, C., Defant, G., Gimelli, G. and Fraccaro, M. (1991). Roberts syndrome: phenotypic variation, cytogenetic definition and heterozygote detection. *Ann Génét*, **34**, 239–246.

Masuno, M., Asano, J., Yasuda, K., Kondo, T. and Orii, T. (1993). Balanced complex rearrangement involving chromosomes 8, 9, and 12 in a normal mother, derivative chromosome 9 with recombinant chromosome 12 in her daughter with minor anomalies. *Am J Med Genet*, **45**, 65–67.

Masuno, M., Cholsong, Y., Kuwahara, T., Shimizu, N., Yamaguchi, S., Kawabata, I., Tamaya, T., Morishita, Y., Yoshimi, N. and Orii, T. (1991). Second meiotic nondisjunction of the rearranged chromosome in a familial reciprocal 5/13 translocation. *Am J Med Genet*, **41**, 32–34.

Masuno, M., Imaizumi, K., Kurosawa, K., Makita, Y., Petrij, F., Dauwerse, H. G., Breuning, M. H. and Kuroki, Y. (1994). Submicroscopic deletion of chromosome region

16p13.3 in a Japanese patient with Rubinstein-Taybi syndrome. *Am J Med Genet*, **53**, 352–354.

Mattei, M. G., Mattei, J. F., Aymé, S. and Giraud, F. (1982). X-autosome translocations: cytogenetic characteristics and their consequences. *Hum Genet*, **61**, 295–309.

McDonald-McGinn, D. M., Driscoll, D. A., Bason, L., Christensen, K., Lynch, D., Sullivan, K., Canning, D., Zavod, W., Quinn, N., Rome, J., Paris, Y., Weinberg, P., Clark, B. J., Emanuel, B. S. and Zackai, E. H. (1995). Autosomal dominant "Opitz" GBBB syndrome due to a 22q11.2 deletion. *Am J Med Genet*, **59**, 103–113.

McElreavey, K., Rappaport, R., Vilain, E., Abbas, N., Richaud, F., Lortat-Jacob, S., Berger, R., Le Coniat, M., Boucekkine, C., Kucheria, K., Temtamy, S., Nihoul-Fekete, C., Brauner, R. and Fellous, M. (1992). A minority of 46,XX true hermaphrodites are positive for the Y-DNA sequence including SRY. *Hum Genet*, **90**, 121–125.

McFadden, D. E. and Kalousek, D. K. (1989). Confirmation of prenatal diagnosis of sex chromosome mosaicism. *Am J Med Genet*, **32**, 495–497.

McFadden, D. E., Kwong, L. C., Yam, I. Y. L. and Langlois, S. (1993). Parental origin of triploidy in human fetuses: evidence for genomic imprinting. *Hum Genet*, **92**, 465–469.

McGinniss, M. J., Kazazian, H. H., Stetten, G., Petersen, M. B., Boman, H., Engel, E., Greenberg, F., Hertz, J. M., Johnson, A., Laca, Z., Mikkelsen, M., Patil, S. R., Schinzel, A. A., Tranebjaerg, L. and Antonarakis, S. E. (1992). Mechanisms of ring chromosome formation in 11 cases of human ring chromosome 21. *Am J Hum Genet*, **50**, 15–28.

Mears, A. J., Duncan, A. M. V., Budarf, M. L., Emanuel, B. S., Sellinger, B., Siegel-Bartelt, J., Greenberg, C. R. and McDermid, H. E. (1994). Molecular characterization of the marker chromosome associated with cat eye syndrome. *Am J Hum Genet*, **55**, 134–142.

Mears, A. J., El-Shanti, H., Murray, J. C., McDermid, H. E. and Patil, S. R. (1995). Minute supernumerary ring chromosome 22 associated with cat eye syndrome: further delineation of the critical region. *Am J Hum Genet*, **57**, 667–673.

Meer, B., Wolff, G. and Back, E. (1981). Segregation of a complex rearrangement of chromosomes 6, 7, 8, and 12 through three generations. *Hum Genet*, **58**, 221–225.

Mehlman, M. J., Botkin, J. R., Scarrow, A., Wooshall, A. and Kass, J. (1994). Coverage of genetic technologies under national health reform. *Am J Hum Genet*, **55**, 1054–1060.

Meijer, H., de Graaff, E., Merckx, D. M. L., Jongbloed, R. J. E., de Die-Smulders, C. E. M., Engelen, J. J. M., Fryns, J. P., Curfs, P. M. G. and Oostra, B. (1994). A deletion of 1.6kb proximal to the CCG repeat of the FMR1 gene causes the clinical phenotype of the fragile X syndrome. *Hum Mol Genet*, **3**, 615–620.

Meijers-Heijboer, E. J., Sandkuijl, L. A., Brunner, H. G., Smeets, H. J. M., Hoogeboom, A. J. M., Deelen, W. H., van Hemel, J. O., Nelen, M. R., Smeets, D. F. C. M., Niermeijer, M. F. and Halley, D. J. J. (1992). Linkage analysis with chromosome 15q11–13 markers shows genomic imprinting in familial Angelman syndrome. *J Med Genet*, **29**, 853–857.

Meindl, A., Hosenfeld, D., Brückl, W., Schuffenhauer, S., Jenderny, J., Bacskulin, A., Oppermann, H.-C., Swensson, O., Bouloux, P. and Meitinger, T. (1993). Analysis of a terminal Xp22.3 deletion in a patient with six monogenic disorders: implications for mapping of X linked ocular albinism. *J Med Genet*, **30**, 838–842.

Melnyk, A. R., Ahmed, I. and Taylor, J. C. (1995). Prenatal diagnosis of familial ring 21 chromosome. *Prenat Diagn*, **15**, 269–273.

Mendonça, B. B., Barbosa, A. S., Arnhold, I. J. P., McElreavey, K., Fellous, M. and Moreira-Filho, C. A. (1994). Gonadal agenesis in XX and XY sisters: evidence for the involvement of an autosomal gene. *Am J Med Genet*, **52**, 39–43.

Merino A., de Perdigo, A., Nombalais, F., Yvinec, M., Le Roux, M. G. and Bellec, V. (1993). Prenatal diagnosis of trisomy 9 mosaicism: two new cases. *Prenat Diagn*, **13**, 1001–1007.

Merry, D. E., Lesko, J. G., Sosnoski, D. M., Lewis, R. A., Lubinsky, M., Trask, B., van den Engh, G., Collins, F. S. and Nussbaum, R. L. (1989). Choroideremia and deafness with stapes fixation: a contiguous gene deletion syndrome in Xq21. *Am J Hum Genet*, **45**, 530–540.

Meschede, D., Froster, U. G., Bergmann, M. and Nieschlag, E. (1994). Familial pericentric inversion of chromosome 1 (p34q23) and male infertility with stage specific spermatogenic arrest. *J Med Genet*, **31**, 573–575.

Michie, S. and Marteau, T. M. (1995). Response to GIG's response to the UK Clinical Genetics Society report ''The genetic testing of children''. *J Med Genet*, **32**, 838.

Migeon, B. R. (1966). Erratum. *J Pediatr*, **69**, 178.

Migeon, B. R., Luo, S., Jani, M. and Jeppesen, P. (1994). The severe phenotype of females with tiny ring X chromosomes is associated with inability of these chromosomes to undergo X inactivation. *Am J Hum Genet*, **55**, 497–504.

Miharu, N., Best, R. G. and Young, S. R. (1994). Numerical chromosome abnormalities in spermatozoa of fertile and infertile men detected by fluorescence in situ hybridization. *Hum Genet*, **93**, 502–506.

Mikkelsen, M. (1966). Familial Down's syndrome. A cytogenetical and genealogical study of twenty-two families. *Ann Hum Genet*, **30**, 125–146.

Miller, J. F., Williamson, E., Glue, J., Gordon, Y. B., Grudzinskas, J. G. and Sykes, A. (1980). Fetal loss after implantation. A prospective study. *Lancet*, **2**, 554–556.

Miller, K., Müller, W., Winkler, L., Hadam, M. R., Ehrich, J. H. H. and Flatz, S. D. (1990). Mitotic disturbance associated with mosaic aneuploidies. *Hum Genet*, **84**, 361–364.

Miller, K., Reimer, A. and Schulze, B. (1987). Tandem duplication chromosome 21 in the offspring of a ring chromosome 21 carrier. *Ann Génét*, **30**, 180–182.

Minelli, A., Floridia, G., Rossi, E., Clementi, M., Tenconi, R., Camurri, L., Bernardi, F., Hoeller, H., Re, C. P., Maraschio, P., Wood, S., Zuffardi, O. and Danesino, C. (1993). D8S7 is consistently deleted in inverted duplications of the short arm of chromosome 8 (inv dup 8p). *Hum Genet*, **92**, 391–396.

Miniou, P., Jeanpierre, M., Blanquet, V., Sibella, V., Bonneau, D., Herbelin, C., Fischer, A., Niveleau, A. and Viegas-Péquignot, E. (1994). Abnormal methylation pattern in constitutive and facultative (X inactive chromosome) heterochromatin of ICF patients. *Hum Mol Genet*, **3**, 2093–2102.

Miny, P., Koppers, B., Dworniczak, B., Bogdanova, N., Holzgreve, W., Tercanli, S., Basaran, S., Rehder, H., Exeler, R. and Horst, J. (1995). Parental origin of the extra haploid chromosome set in triploidies diagnosed prenatally. *Am J Med Genet*, **57**, 102–106.

Mitchell, J. J., Vekemans, M., Luscombe, S., Hayden, M., Weber, B., Richter, A., Sparkes, R., Kojis, T., Watters, G. and Der Kaloustian, V. M. (1994). U-type exchange in a paracentric inversion as a possible mechanism of origin of an inverted tandem duplication of chromosome 8. *Am J Med Genet*, **49**, 384–387.

Mittwoch, U. (1992). Sex determination and sex reversal: genotype, phenotype, dogma and semantics. *Hum Genet*, **89**, 467–479.

Mittwoch, U. and Mahadevaiah, S. K. (1992). Unpaired chromosomes at meiosis: cause or effect of gametogenic insufficiency? *Cytogenet Cell Genet*, **59**, 274–279.

Monahan, P. (1992). Judgements of interest. A doctor's dilemma resolved—sterilisation of intellectually disabled females. *Australasian J Med Defence Union*, **3**, 54–55.

Moncla, A., Piras, L., Arbex, O. F., Muscatelli, F., Mattei, M.-G., Mattei, J.-F. and Fontes, M. (1993). Physical mapping of microdeletions of the chromosome 17 short arm associated with Smith-Magenis syndrome. *Hum Genet*, **90**, 657–660.

Monteleone, P. L., Volk, L. R., Sekhon, G. S., Grzegocki, J., Tietjens, M., Monteleone, J. A. and Sekhon, H. (1978). Rob(14q15q) translocation in several members of a family. *Birth Defects: Orig Art Series*, **14**(6C), pp. 303–308.

Moog, U., Engelen, J. J. M., de Die-Smulders, C. E. M., Albrechts, J. C. M., Loneus, W. H., Haagen, A. A. M., Raven, E. J. M. and Hamers, A. J. H. (1994). Partial trisomy of the short arm of chromosome 18 due to inversion duplication and direct duplication. *Clin Genet*, **46**, 423–429.

Moreau, N., Teyssier, M. and Rollet, J. (1987). A new case of (Y;1) balanced reciprocal translocation in an infertile man with Hodgkin's disease. *J Med Genet*, **24**, 379–380.

Morel, Y., Mebarki, F. and Forest, M. G. (1994). What are the indications for prenatal diagnosis in the androgen insensitivity syndrome? Facing clinical heterogeneity of phenotypes for the same genotype. *Eur J Endocrinol*, **130**, 325–326.

Mori, M. A., Huertas, H., Pinel, I., Giralt, P. and Martinez-Frias, M. L. (1985). Trisomy 13 in the child of two carriers of a 13/15 translocation. *Am J Med Genet*, **20**, 17–20.

Morichon-Delvallez, N., Couturier, J. and Frison, B. (1982). Phénotype atténué de la trisomie 4p par translocation t(X:4)(p21.2;p13). *Ann Génét*, **25**, 246–248.

Morris, A., Morton, N. E., Collins, A., Macpherson, J., Nelson, D. and Sherman, S. (1995). An *n*-allele model for progressive amplification in the *FRM1* locus. *Proc Natl Acad Sci USA*, **92**, 4833–4837.

Morris, C. A., Thomas, I. T. and Greenberg, F. (1993). Williams syndrome: autosomal dominant inheritance. *Am J Med Genet*, **47**, 478–481.

Morrow, B., Goldberg, R., Carlson, C., Das Gupta, R., Sirotkin, H., Collins, J., Dunham, I., O'Donnell, H., Scambler, P., Shprintzen, R. and Kucherlapati, R. (1995). Molecular definition of the 22q11 deletions in velo-cardio-facial syndrome. *Am J Hum Genet*, **56**, 1391–1403.

Mortimer, J. G., Chewings, W. E. and Gardner, R. J. M. (1980). A further report on a kindred with cases of 4p trisomy and monosomy. *Hum Hered*, **30**, 58–61.

Morton, N. E., Chiu, D., Holland, C., Jacobs, P. A. and Pettay, D. (1987). Chromosome anomalies as predictors of recurrence risk for spontaneous abortion. *Am J Med Genet*, **28**, 353–360.

Moss, C., Larkins, S., Stacey, M., Blight, A., Farndon, P. A. and Davison, E. V. (1993). Epidermal mosaicism and Blaschko's lines. *J Med Genet*, **30**, 752–755.

Motzkin, B., Marion, R., Goldberg, R., Shprintzen, R. and Saenger, P. (1993). Variable phenotypes in velocardiofacial syndrome with chromosomal deletion. *J Pediatr*, **123**, 406–410.

Moutou, C., Junien, C., Henry, I. and Bonaíti-Pellié, C. (1992). Beckwith-Wiedemann syndrome: a demonstration of the mechanisms responsible for the excess of transmitting females. *J Med Genet*, **29**, 217–220.

Mules, E. H. and Stamberg, J. (1984). Reproductive outcomes of paracentric inversion carriers: report of a liveborn dicentric recombinant and literature review. *Hum Genet*, **67**, 126–131.

Müller, J. and Skakkebæk, N. E. (1990). Gonadal malignancy in individuals with sex chromosome anomalies. In "Children and young adults with sex chromosome aneuploidy. Follow-up, clinical, and molecular studies" (J. A. Evans, J. L. Hamerton and A. Robinson, eds.). *Birth Defects: Orig Art Series*, **26**(4), pp. 247–255.

Mulley, J. C. and Sutherland, G. R. (1994). Diagnosis of fragile X syndrome. *Fetal Maternal Med Rev*, **6**, 1–15.

Mulley, J. C., Yu, S., Gedeon, A. K., Donnelly, A., Turner, G., Loesch, D., Chapman, C. J., Gardner, R. J. M., Richards, R. I. and Sutherland, G. R. (1992). Experience with direct molecular diagnosis of fragile X. *J Med Genet*, **29**, 368–374.

Mulley, J. C., Yu, S., Loesch, D. Z., Hay, D. A., Donnelly, A., Gedeon, A. K., Carbonell, P., López, I., Glover, G., Gabarrón, I., Yu, P. W. L., Baker, E., Haan, E. A., Hockey, A., Knight, S. J. L., Davies, K. E., Richards, R. I. and Sutherland, G. R. (1995). FRAXE and mental retardation. *J Med Genet*, **32**, 162–169.

Muneer, R. S., Himes, J. and Rennert, O. M. (1988). Complex de novo rearrangement involving four chromosomes and ten breakpoints with interstitial deletions and duplication. *Am J Med Genet*, **31**, 33–37.

Munné, S., Grifo, J., Cohen, J. and Weier, H.-U. G. (1994). Chromosome abnormalities in human arrested preimplantation embryos: a multiple-probe FISH study. *Am J Hum Genet*, **55**, 150–159.

Murphy, E.A. and Chase, G.A. (1975). "Principles of genetic counseling." Year Book Medical Publishers, Chicago.

Mutter, G. L., Stewart, C. L., Chaponot, M. L. and Pomponio, R. J. (1993). Oppositely imprinted genes H19 and insulin-like growth factor 2 are coexpressed in human androgenetic trophoblast. *Am J Hum Genet*, **53**, 1096–1102.

Nancarrow, J. K., Kremer, E., Holman, K., Eyre, H., Doggett, N. A., Le Paslier, D., Callen, D. F., Sutherland, G. R. and Richards, R. I. (1994). Implications of *FRA 16A* structure for the mechanism of chromosomal fragile site genesis. *Science*, **264**, 1938–1941.

Navarro, J., Benet, J., Martorell, M. R., Templado, C. and Egozcue, J. (1993). Segregation analysis in a man heterozygous for a pericentric inversion of chromosome 7 (p13;q36) by sperm chromosome studies. *Am J Hum Genet*, **53**, 214–219.

Navarro, J., Vidal, F., Benet, J., Templado, C., Marina, S. and Egozcue, J. (1991). XY-trivalent association and synaptic anomalies in a male carrier of a Robertsonian t(13;14) translocation. *Hum Reprod*, **6**, 376–381.

Neavel, C. B. and Soukup, S. (1994). Deletion of (11)(q24.2) in a mother and daughter with similar phenotypes. *Am J Med Genet*, **53**, 321–324.

Neri, G. (1984). A possible explanation for the low incidence of gonosomal aneuploidy among the offspring of triplo-X individuals. *Am J Med Genet*, **18**, 357–364.

Neri, G., Ricci, R., Pelino, A., Bova, R., Tedeschi, B. and Serra, A. (1983). A boy with ring chromosome 15 derived from a t(15q;15q) Robertsonian translocation in the mother: cytogenetic and biochemical findings. *Am J Med Genet*, **14**, 307–314.

Netley, C. T. (1986). Summary overview of behavioural development in individuals with neonatally identified X and Y aneuploidy. In "Prospective studies on children with sex chromosome aneuploidy" (S. G. Ratcliffe and N. Paul, eds.). *Birth Defects: Orig Art Series*, **22**(3), pp. 293–306.

Neu, R. L., Brar, H. S. and Koos, B. J. (1988). Prenatal diagnosis of inv(X)(q12q28) in a male fetus. *J Med Genet*, **25**, 52–60.

Neu, R. L., Kousseff, B. G., Hardy, D. E., Essig, Y.-P., Miller, K. L., Jervis, G. A. and

Tedesco, T. A. (1988). Trisomy 3p23→pter and monosomy 11q23→qter in an infant with two translocation carrier parents. *J Med Genet*, **25**, 631–633.

Neu, R. L., Valentine, F. A. and Gardner, L. I. (1975). Segregation of a t(14q22q) chromosome in a large kindred. *Clin Genet*, **8**, 30–36.

Neumann, A. A., Robson, L. G. and Smith, A. (1992). A 15p+ variant shown to be a t(Y;15) with fluorescence *in situ* hybridisation. *Ann Génét*, **35**, 227–230.

Niazi, M., Coleman, D. V. and Saldaña-Garcia, P. (1978). Partial trisomy 18 in a family with a translocation (18;21)(q21;q22). *J Med Genet,* **15**, 148–151.

Nicholls, R. D. (1993). Genomic imprinting and candidate genes in the Prader-Willi and Angelman syndromes. *Curr Opin Genet Dev*, **3**, 445–456.

Nicholls, R. D., Knoll, J. H. M., Butler, M. G., Karam, S. and Lalande, M. (1989). Genomic imprinting suggested by maternal heterodisomy in non-deletion Prader-Willi syndrome. *Nature*, **342**, 281–285.

Nicolaides, K., Brizot, M. de L., Patel, F. and Snijders, R. (1994). Comparison of chorionic villus sampling and amniocentesis for fetal karyotyping at 10–13 weeks' gestation. *Lancet*, **344**, 435–439.

Nicolaides, K. H., Shawwa, L., Brizot, M. and Snijders, R. J. M. (1993). Ultrasonographically detectable markers of fetal chromosomal defects. *Ultrasound Obstet Gynecol*, **3**, 56–69.

Nielsen, J. (1990). Follow-up of 25 unselected children with sex chromosome abnormalities to age 12. In ''Children and young adults with sex chromosome aneuploidy. Follow-up, clinical, and molecular studies'' (J. A. Evans, J. L. Hamerton and A. Robinson, eds.). *Birth Defects: Orig Art Series*, **26**(4), pp. 201–207.

Nielsen, J., Wohlert, M., Faaborg-Andersen, J., Eriksen, G., Hansen, K. B., Hvidman, L., Krag-Olsen, B., Moulvad, I. and Videbech, P. (1986). Chromosome examination of 20,222 newborn children: results from a 7.5-year study in Århus, Denmark. In ''Prospective studies on children with sex chromosome aneuploidy'' (S. G. Ratcliffe and N. Paul, eds.). *Birth Defects: Orig Art Series*, **22**(3), pp. 209–219.

Nielsen, J. and Wohlert, M. (1991). Chromosome abnormalities found among 34,910 newborn children: results from a 13-year incidence study in Aarhus, Denmark. *Hum Genet*, **87**, 81–83.

Nielsen, K. G., Poulsen, H., Mikkelsen, M. and Steuber, E. (1988). Multiple recurrence of trisomy 21 Down syndrome. *Hum Genet*, **78**, 103–105.

Norman, A. M., Read, A. P., Clayton-Smith, J., Andrews, T. and Donnai, D. (1992). Recurrent Wiedemann-Beckwith syndrome with inversion of chromosome (11)(p11.2p15.5). *Am J Med Genet*, **42**, 638–641.

Norris, F. M., Mercer, B. and Pertile, M. D. (1995). Interstitial insertion of NORs into Yq and 22q: two case studies. *Bull Hum Genet Soc Australasia*, **8**, 48.

North, K. N., Wu, B. L., Cao, B. N., Whiteman, D. A. H. and Korf, B. R. (1995). CHARGE association in a child with de novo inverted duplication (14)(q22→q24.3). *Am J Med Genet*, **57**, 610–614.

Nuutinen, M., Kouvalainen, K. and Knip, M. (1995). Good growth response to growth hormone in the ring 15 syndrome. *J Med Genet*, **32**, 486–487.

Nyström, A., Hedborg, F. and Ohlsson, R. (1994). Insulin-like growth factor 2 cannot be linked to a familial form of Beckwith-Wiedemann syndrome. *Eur J Pediatr*, **153**, 574–580.

Oberlé, I., Rousseau, F., Heitz, D., Kretz, C., Devys, D., Hanauer, A., Boué, J., Bertheas, M. F. and Mandel, J. L. (1991). Instability of a 550-base pair DNA segment and abnormal methylation in fragile X syndrome. *Science*, **252**, 1097–1102.

Ogata, T., Tyler-Smith, C., Purvis-Smith, S. and Turner, G. (1993). Chromosomal localisation of a gene(s) for Turner stigmata on Yp. *J Med Genet*, **30**, 918–922.

Ohashi, H., Tsukahara, M., Murano, I., Naritomi, K., Nishioka, K., Miyake, S. and Kajii, T. (1992). Pigmentary dysplasias and chromosomal mosaicism: report of 9 cases. *Am J Med Genet*, **43**, 716–721.

Olney, R. S., Khoury, M. J., Alo, C. J., Costa, P., Edmonds, L. D., Flood, T. J., Harris, J. A., Howe, H. L., Moore, C. A., Olsen, C. L., Panny, S. R. and Shaw, G. M. (1995). Increased risk for transverse digital deficiency after chorionic villus sampling: results of the United States multistate case-control study, 1988–1992. *Teratology*, **51**, 20–29.

Olson, S. B. and Magenis, R. E. (1988). Preferential paternal origin of de novo structural chromosome rearrangements. In "The cytogenetics of mammalian autosomal rearrangements" (A. Daniel, ed.). A. R. Liss, New York, pp. 583–599.

Oostra, B. A., Jacky, P. B., Brown, W. T. and Rousseau, F. (1993). Guidelines for the diagnosis of fragile X syndrome. *J Med Genet*, **30**, 410–413.

Örstavik, R. E., Tommerup, N., Eiklid, K. and Örstavik, K. H. (1995). Non-random X chromosome inactivation in an affected twin in a monozygotic twin pair discordant for Wiedemann-Beckwith syndrome. *Am J Med Genet*, **56**, 210–214.

Overhauser, J., Golbus, M. S., Schonberg, S. A. and Wasmuth, J. J. (1986). Molecular analysis of an unbalanced deletion of the short arm of chromosome 5 that produces no phenotype. *Am J Hum Genet*, **39**, 1–10.

Overhauser, J., Huang, X., Gersh, M., Wilson, W., McMahon, J., Bengtsson, U., Rojas, K., Meyer, M. and Wasmuth, J. J. (1994). Molecular and phenotypic mapping of the short arm of chromosome 5: sublocalization of the critical region for the cri-du-chat syndrome. *Hum Mol Genet*, **3**, 247–252.

Pai, G. S., Shields, S. M. and Houser, P. M. (1987). Segregation of inverted chromosome 13 in families ascertained through liveborn recombinant offspring. *Am J Med Genet*, **27**, 127–133.

Palka, G., Calabrese, G., Stuppia, L., Franchi, P. G., Morizio, E., Peila, R. and Antonucci, A. (1994). A woman with an apparent non-mosaic 45,X delivered a 46,X,der(X) liveborn female. *Clin Genet*, **45**, 93–96.

Pallister, P. D. and Opitz, J. M. (1978). The KOP translocation. *Birth Defects: Orig Art Series*, **14**(6C), 133–146.

Palmer, J. R. (1994). Advances in the epidemiology of gestational trophoblastic disease. *J Reprod Med*, **39**, 155–162.

Palomaki, G. E., Haddow, J. E., Knight, G. J., Wald, N. J., Kennard, A., Canick, J. A., Saller, D. N., Blitzer, M. G., Dickerman, L. H., Fisher, R., Hansmann, D., Hansmann, M., Luthy, D. A., Summers, A. M. and Wyatt, P. (1995). Risk-based prenatal screening for trisomy 18 using alpha-fetoprotein, unconjugated oestriol and human chorionic gonadotropin. *Prenat Diagn*, **15**, 713–723.

Pandya, P. P., Kondylios, A., Hilbert, L., Snijders, R. J. M. and Nicolaides, K. H. (1995). Chromosomal defects and outcome in 1015 fetuses with increased nuchal translucency. *Ultrasound Obstet Gynecol*, **5**, 15–19.

Pangalos, C., Avramopoulos, D., Blouin, J.-L., Raoul, O., deBlois, M.-C., Prieur, M., Schinzel, A. A., Gika, M., Abazis, D. and Antonarakis, S. E. (1994). Understanding the mechanism(s) of mosaic trisomy 21 by using DNA polymorphism analysis. *Am J Hum Genet*, **54**, 473–481.

Pangalos, C., Théophile, D., Sinet, P.-M., Marks, A., Stamboulieh-Abazis, D., Chettouh, Z., Prieur, M., Verellen, C., Rethoré, M.-O., Lejeune, J. and Delabar, J.-M. (1992a). No significant effect of monosomy for distal 21q22.3 on the Down syndrome phenotype in "mirror" duplications of chromosome 21. *Am J Hum Genet,* **51**, 1240–1250.

Pangalos, C. G., Talbot, C. C., Lewis, J. G., Adelsberger, P. A., Petersen, M. B., Serre, J.-L., Rethoré, M.-O., de Blois, M.-C., Parent, P., Schinzel, A. A., Binkert, F., Boue, J., Corbin, E., Croquette, M. F., Gilgenkrantz, S., de Grouchy, J., Bertheas, M. F., Prieur, M., Raoul, O., Serville, F., Siffroi, J. P., Thepot, F., Lejeune, J. and Antonarakis, S. E. (1992b). DNA polymorphism analysis in families with recurrence of free trisomy 21. *Am J Hum Genet,* **51**, 1015–1027.

Pankau, R., Gosch, A., Simeoni, E. and Wessel, A. (1993). Williams-Beuren syndrome in monozygotic twins with variable expression. *Am J Med Genet,* **47**, 475–477.

Papenhausen, P. R., Mueller, O. T., Johnson, V. P., Sutcliffe, M., Diamond, T. M. and Kousseff, B. G. (1995). Uniparental isodisomy of chromosome 14 in two cases: an abnormal child and a normal adult. *Am J Med Genet,* **59**, 271–275.

Papi, L., Montali, E., Marconi, G., Guazzelli, R., Bigozzi, U., Maraschio, P. and Zuffardi, O. (1989). Evidence for a human mitotic mutant with pleiotropic effect. *Ann Hum Genet,* **53**, 243–248.

Park, V., Howard-Peebles, P., Sherman, S., Taylor, A. and Wulfsberg, E. (1994). Policy statement: American College of Medical Genetics. Fragile X syndrome: diagnostic and carrier testing. *Am J Med Genet,* **53**, 380–381.

Park, V. M., Bravo, R. R. and Shulman, L. P. (1995). Double non-disjunction in maternal meiosis II giving rise to a fetus with 48,XXX,+21. *J Med Genet,* **32**, 650–653.

Parrish, J. E., Oostra, B. A., Verkerk, A. J. M. H., Richards, C. S., Reynolds, J., Spikes, A. S., Shaffer, L. G. and Nelson, D. L. (1994). Isolation of a GCC repeat showing expansion in FRAXF, a fragile site distal to FRAXA and FRAXE. *Nature Genet,* **8**, 229–235.

Patil, N., Cox, D. R., Bhat, D., Faham, M., Myers, R. M. and Peterson, A. S. (1995). A potassium channel mutation in weaver mice implicates membrane excitability in granule cell differentiation. *Nature Genet,* **11**, 126–129.

Pauli, R. M., Pagon, R. A. and Hall, J. G. (1978). Trisomy 18 in sibs and maternal chromosome 9 variant. *Birth Defects: Orig Art Series,* **14**(6C), pp. 297–301.

Pavlidis, K., McCauley, E. and Sybert, V. P. (1995). Psychosocial and sexual functioning in women with Turner syndrome. *Clin Genet,* **47**, 85–89.

Pearn, J. (1977). The subjective interpretation of medical risks. *Medikon,* **6**, 5–9, 1977.

Pearn, J. (1979). Decision-making and reproductive choice. In "Counseling in genetics" (Y. E. Hsia, K. Hirschhorn, R. L. Silverberg and L. Godmilow, eds.). A. R. Liss, New York, pp. 223–238.

Pellestor, F. (1990). Analysis of meiotic segregation in a man heterozygous for a 13;15 Robertsonian translocation and a review of the literature. *Hum Genet,* **85**, 49–54.

Pellestor, F. (1991). Frequency and distribution of aneuploidy in human female gametes. *Hum Genet,* **86**, 283–288.

Pellestor, F., Sele, B., Jalbert, H. (1987). Chromosome analysis of spermatozoa from a male heterozygous for a 13;14 Robertsonian translocation. *Hum Genet,* **76**, 116–120.

Penny, L. A., Dell'Aquila, M., Jones, M. C., Bergoffen, J., Cunniff, C., Fryns, J.-P., Grace, E., Graham, J. M., Kousseff, B., Mattina, T., Syme, J., Voullaire, L., Zelante, L., Zenger-Hain, J., Jones, O. W. and Evans, G. A. (1995). Clinical and molecular characterization of patients with distal 11q deletions. *Am J Hum Genet,* **56**, 676–683.

Penrose, L. S. (1934). The relative aetiological importance of birth order and maternal age in mongolism. *Proc Roy Soc Lond [Biol],* **115**, 431–450.

Pentao, L., Lewis, R. A., Ledbetter, D. H., Patel, P. I. and Lupski, J. R. (1992). Maternal uniparental isodisomy of chromosome 14: association with autosomal recessive rod monochromacy. *Am J Hum Genet*, **50**, 690–699.

Peoples, R., Milatovich, A. and Francke, U. (1995). Hemizygosity at the insulin-like growth factor 1 receptor (IGF1R) locus and growth failure in the ring chromosome 15 syndrome. *Cytogenet Cell Genet*, **70**, 228–234.

Persutte, W. H. and Lenke, R. R. (1995). Failure of amniotic-fluid-cell growth: is it related to fetal aneuploidy? *Lancet*, **345**, 96–97.

Pertl, B., Yau, S. C., Sherlock, J., Davies, A. F., Mathew, C. G. and Adinolfi, M. (1994). Rapid molecular method for prenatal detection of Down's syndrome. *Lancet*, **343**, 1197–1198.

Pescia, G., Tonella, A. and Jotterand-Bellomo, M. (1982). Monosomie/trisomie 4q12-q13 en mosaïque chez un enfant arrierée et dysmorphique. *Ann Génét*, **25**, 110–112.

Petersen, M. B., Adelsberger, P. A., Schinzel, A. A., Binkert, F., Hinkel, G. K. and Antonarakis, S. E. (1991). Down syndrome due to de novo Robertsonian translocation t(14q;21q): DNA polymorphism analysis suggests that the origin of the extra 21q is maternal. *Am J Hum Genet*, **49**, 529–536.

Petersen, M. B., Antonarakis, S. E., Hassold, T. J., Freeman, S. B., Sherman, S. L., Avramopoulos, D. and Mikkelsen, M. (1993). Paternal nondisjunction in trisomy 21: excess of male patients. *Hum Mol Genet*, **2**, 1691–1695.

Peterson, A., Patil, N., Robbins, C., Wang, L., Cox, D. R. and Myers, R. M. (1994). A transcript map of the Down syndrome critical region on chromosome 21. *Hum Mol Genet*, **3**, 1735–1742.

Petit, P., Hilliker, C., Van Leuven, F. and Fryns, J.-P. (1994). Mild phenotype and normal gonadal function in females with 4p trisomy due to unbalanced t(X;4)(p22.1;p14). *Clin Genet*, **46**, 304–308.

Petrella, R. and Hirschhorn, K. (1990). Trisomy 12 mosaicism detected by mid-trimester amniocentesis. *Prenat Diagn*, **10**, 781–785.

Petrij, F., Giles, R. H., Dauwerse, H. G., Saris, J. J., Hennekam, R. C. M., Masuno, M., Tommerup, N., van Ommen, G.-J. B., Goodman, R. H., Peters, D. J. M. and Breuning, M. H. (1995). Rubinstein-Taybi syndrome caused by mutations in the transcriptional co-activator CBP. *Nature*, **376**, 348–351.

Petrovic, V. (1988). A new variant of chromosome 3 with unusual staining properties. *J Med Genet*, **25**, 781–782.

Pettenati, M. J., Wheeler, M., Bartlett, D. J., Subrt, I., Rao, N., Kroovand, R. L., Burton, B. K., Kahler, S., Park, H. K., Cosper, P., Kelly, D. R. and Ranells, J. D. (1991). 45,X/47,XYY mosaicism: clinical discrepancy between prenatally and postnatally diagnosed cases. *Am J Med Genet*, **39**, 42–47.

Pettenati, M. J., Rao, N., Johnson, C., Hayworth, R., Crandall, K., Huff, O. and Thomas, I. T. (1992). Molecular cytogenetic analysis of a familial 8p23.1 deletion associated with minimal dysmorphic features, seizures, and mild mental retardation. *Hum Genet*, **89**, 602–606.

Pettenati, M. J., Rao, P. N., Phelan, M. C., Grass, F., Rao, K. W., Cosper, P., Carroll, A. J., Elder, F., Smith, J. L., Higgins, M. D., Lanman, J. T., Higgins, R. R., Butler, M. G., Luthardt, F., Keitges, E., Jackson-Cook, C., Brown, J., Schwartz, S., Van Dyke, D. L. and Palmer, C. G. (1995). Paracentric inversions in humans: a review of 446 paracentric inversions with presentation of 120 new cases. *Am J Med Genet*, **55**, 171–187.

Pettenati, M. J., Rao, P. N., Weaver, R. G., Thomas, I. T. and McMahan, M. R. (1993).

Inversion (X)(p11.4q22) associated with Norrie disease in a four generation family. *Am J Med Genet*, **45**, 577–580.

Pettenati, M. J., Weaver, R. G. and Burton, B. K. (1989). Translocation t(5;11)(q13.1; p13) associated with familial isolated aniridia. *Am J Med Genet*, **34**, 230–232.

Pettenati, M. J. and Rao, P. N. Response to Drs. Sutherland, Callen, and Gardner. *Am J Med Genet*, **59**, 391–392.

Pettigrew, A. L., Greenberg, F., Caskey, C. T. and Ledbetter, D. H. (1991). Greig syndrome associated with an interstitial deletion of 7p: confirmation of the localization of Greig syndrome to 7p13. *Hum Genet*, **87**, 452–456.

Pezzolo, A., Gimelli, G., Cohen, A., Lavaggetto, A., Romano, C., Fogu, G. and Zuffardi, O. (1993). Presence of telomeric and subtelomeric sequences at the fusion points of ring chromosomes indicates that the ring syndrome is caused by ring instability. *Hum Genet*, **92**, 23–27.

Pfeiffer, R. A. and Loidl, J. (1982). Mirror image duplications of chromosome 21. Three new cases and discussion of the mechanisms of origin. *Hum Genet*, **62**, 361–363.

Pflueger, S., Golden, J., Troiano, R., Gasparini, R. and Marini, T. (1991). Fission of familial (13;22) Robertsonian translocation resulting in fetal mosaicism. *Am J Hum Genet*, **49** (Suppl.), 283.

Phelan, M. C., Rogers, R. C., Clarkson, K. B., Bowyer, F. P., Levine, M. A., Estabrooks, L. L., Severson, M. C. and Dobyns, W. B. (1995). Albright hereditary osteodystrophy and del(2)(q37.3) in four unrelated individuals. *Am J Med Genet*, **58**, 1–7.

Phelan, M. C., Rogers, R. C. and Stevenson, R. E. (1990). Multiple, compound, and complex chromosome rearrangements. *Proc Greenwood Genet Center*, **9**, 19–37.

Phelan, M. C., Saul, R. A., Gailey, T. A. and Skinner, S. A. (1995). Prenatal diagnosis of mosaic 4p-, in a fetus with trisomy 21. *Prenat Diagn*, **15,** 274–277.

Phelan, M. C., Stevenson, R. E. and Anderson, E. V. (1993). Recombinant chromosome 9 possibly derived from breakage and reunion of sister chromatids within a paracentric inversion loop. *Am J Med Genet*, **46**, 304–308.

Philip, J., Bryndorf, T. and Christensen, B. (1994). Prenatal aneuploidy detection in interphase cells by fluorescence in situ hybridization (FISH). *Prenat Diagn*, **14**, 1203–1215.

Phillips, O. P., Cromwell, S., Rivas, M., Simpson, J. L. and Elias, S. (1995). Trisomy 21 and maternal age of menopause: does reproductive age rather than chronological age influence risk of nondisjunction? *Hum Genet*, **95**, 117–118.

Pieretti, M., Zhang, F., Fu, Y.-H., Warren, S. T., Oostra, B. A., Caskey, C. T. and Nelson, D. L. (1991). Absence of expression of the *FMR-1* gene in fragile X syndrome. *Cell*, **66**, 817–822.

Pierpont, M. E. M., Gorlin, R. J. and Moller, J. H. (1987). Chromosomal abnormalities. In "The genetics of cardiovascular disease" (M. E. M. Pierpont and J. H. Moller, eds). Martinus Nijhoff Publishing, Boston, pp. 69–94.

Pilz, D. T., Dalton, A., Long, A., Jaspan, T., Maltby, E. L. and Quarrell, O. W. J. (1995). Detecting deletions in the critical region for lissencephaly on 17p13.3 using fluorescent in situ hybridisation and a PCR assay identifying a dinucleotide repeat polymorphism. *J Med Genet*, **32**, 275–278.

Pindar, L., Whitehouse, M. and Ocraft, K. (1992). A rare case of a false-negative finding in both direct and culture of a chorionic villus sample. *Prenat Diagn*, **12**, 525–527.

Pittalis, M. C., Santarini, L. and Bovicelli, L. (1994). Prenatal diagnosis of a heterochromatic 18p+ heteromorphism. *Prenat Diagn*, **14**, 72–73.

Pivnick, E. K., Wilroy, R. S., Summitt, J. B., Tucker, B., Herrod, H. G. and Tharapel,

A. T. (1990). Adjacent-2 disjunction of a maternal t(9;22) leading to duplication 9pter→q22 and deficiency of 22pter→q11.2. *Am J Med Genet*, **37**, 92–96.

Platt, L. D., DeVore, G. R., Lopez, E., Herbert, W., Falk, R. and Alfi, O. (1986). Role of amniocentesis in ultrasound-detected fetal malformations. *Obstet Gynecol*, **68**, 153–155.

Plattner, R., Heerema, N. A., Yurov, Y. B. and Palmer, C. G. (1993). Efficient identification of marker chromosomes in 27 patients by stepwise hybridization with alpha-satellite DNA probes. *Hum Genet*, **91**, 131–140.

Polani, P., Dewhurst, J., Fergusson, I. and Kelberman, J. (1982). Meiotic chromosomes in a female with primary trisomic Down's syndrome. *Hum Genet*, **62**, 277–279.

Ponzio, G., Savin, E., Cattaneo, G., Ghiotti, M. P., Marra, A,. Zuffardi, O., Danesino, C. (1987). Translocation X;13 in a patient with retinoblastoma. *J Med Genet,* **24**, 431–434.

Potter, H. (1991). Review and hypothesis: Alzheimer disease and Down syndrome—chromosome 21 nondisjunction may underlie both disorders. *Am J Hum Genet*, **48**, 1192–1200.

Powell, C. M., Taggart, R. T., Drumheller, T. C., Wangsa, D., Qian, C., Nelson, L. M. and White, B. J. (1994). Molecular and cytogenetic studies of an X;autosome translocation in a patient with premature ovarian failure and review of the literature. *Am J Med Genet*, **52**, 19–26.

Preis, S. and Majewski, F. (1995). Monozygotic twins concordant for Rubinstein-Taybi syndrome: changing phenotype during infancy. *Clin Genet*, **48**, 72–75.

Price, H. A., Roberts, S. H. and Laurence, K. M. (1987). Homozygous paracentric inversion 12 in a mentally retarded boy: a case report and review of the literature. *Hum Genet*, **75**, 101–108.

Pronk, J. C., Gibson, R. A., Savoia, A., Wijker, M., Morgan, N. V., Melchionda, S., Ford, D., Temtany, S., Ortega, J. J., Jansen, S., Havenga, C., Cohn, R. J., de Ravel, T. J., Roberts, I., Westerveld, A., Easton, D. F., Joenje, H., Mathew, C. G. and Arwert, F. (1995). Localisation of the Fanconi anaemia complementation group A gene to chromosome 16q24.3. *Nature Genet*, **11**, 338–340.

Puck, M. H. (1981). Some considerations bearing on the doctrine of self-fulfilling prophecy in sex chromosome aneuploidy. *Am J Med Genet*, **9**, 129–137.

Punnett, H. H. (1994). Simpson-Golabi-Behmel syndrome (SGBS) in a female with an X-autosome translocation. *Am J Med Genet*, **50**, 391–393.

Purvis-Smith, S. G., Saville, T., Manass, S., Yip, M.-Y., Lam-Po-Tang, P. R. L., Duffy, B., Johnston, H., Leigh, D. and McDonald, B. (1992). Uniparental disomy 15 resulting from 'correction' of an initial trisomy 15. *Am J Hum Genet*, **50**, 1348–1350.

Quan, F., Zonana, J., Gunter, K., Peterson, K. L., Magenis, R. E. and Popovich, B. W. (1995). An atypical case of fragile X syndrome caused by a deletion that includes the FMR1 gene. *Am J Hum Genet*, **56**, 1042–1051.

Quigley, C. A., Friedman, K. J., Johnson, A., Lafreniere, R. G., Silverman, L. M., Lubahn, D. B., Brown, T. R., Wilson, E. M., Willard, H. F. and French, F. S. (1992). Complete deletion of the androgen receptor gene: definition of the null phenotype of the androgen insensitivity syndrome and determination of carrier status. *J Clin Endocrinol Metab*, **74**, 927–933.

Ramírez-Dueñas, M. de L. and Gonzalez, G. J. R. (1992). Fra(1)(p11), fra(1)(q22) and r(1)(p11q22) in a retarded girl. *Ann Génét*, **35**, 178–182.

Rani, A. S., Jyothi, A., Reddy, P. P. and Reddy, O. S. (1990). Reproduction in Down's syndrome. *Int J Gynecol Obstet*, **31**, 81–86.

Rao, P. N., Klinepeter, K., Stewart, W., Hayworth, R., Grubs, R. and Pettenati, M. J.

(1994). Molecular cytogenetic analysis of a duplication Xp in a male: further delineation of a possible sex influencing region on the X chromosome. *Hum Genet*, **94**, 149–153.

Rappold, G. A. (1993). The pseudoautosomal regions of the human sex chromosomes. *Hum Genet*, **92**, 315–324.

Ratcliffe, S. G., Butler, G. E. and Jones, M. (1990). Edinburgh study of growth and development of children with sex chromosome abnormalities. IV. In ''Children and young adults with sex chromosome aneuploidy. Follow-up, clinical, and molecular studies'' (J. A. Evans, J. L. Hamerton and A. Robinson, eds.). *Birth Defects: Orig Art Series*, **26**(4), pp. 1–44.

Ray, J. H. and German, J. (1981). The chromosome changes in Bloom's syndrome, ataxia telangiectasia, and Fanconi's anemia. In ''Genes, chromosomes, and neoplasia'' (F. E. Arrighi, P. N. Rao and E. Stubblefield, eds.). Raven Press, New York, pp. 351–378.

Reeve, A., Norman, A., Sinclair, P., Whittington-Smith, R., Hamey, Y., Donnai, D. and Read, A. (1993). True telomeric translocation in a baby with the Prader-Willi phenotype. *Am J Med Genet*, **47**, 1–6.

Reeves, R. H., Irving, N. G., Moran, T. H., Wohn, A., Kitt, C., Sisodia, S. S., Schmidt, C., Bronson, R. T. and Davisson, M. T. (1995). A mouse model for Down syndrome exhibits learning and behaviour deficits. *Nature Genet*, **11**, 177–183.

Reijo, R., Lee, T.-Y., Salo, P., Alagappan, R., Brown, L. G., Rosenberg, M., Rozen, S., Jaffe, T., Straus, D., Hovatta, O., de la Chapelle, A., Silber, S. and Page, D. C. (1995). Diverse spermatogenic defects in humans caused by Y chromosome deletions encompassing a novel RNA-binding protein gene. *Nature Genet*, **10**, 383–393.

Reik, W., Brown, K. W., Slatter, R. E., Sartori, P., Elliott, M. and Maher, E. R. (1994). Allelic methylation of *H19* and *IGF2* in the Beckwith-Wiedemann syndrome. *Hum Mol Genet*, **3**, 1297–1301.

Reik, W., Brown, K. W., Schneid, H., Le Bouc, Y., Bickmore, W. and Maher, E. R. (1995). Imprinting mutations in the Beckwith-Wiedemann syndrome suggested by an altered imprinting pattern in the *IGF2-H19* domain. *Hum Mol Genet*, **4**, 2379–2385.

Reiner, O., Carrozzo, R., Shen, Y., Wehnert, M., Faustinella, F., Dobyns, W. B., Caskey, C. T. and Ledbetter, D. H. (1993). Isolation of a Miller-Dieker lissencephaly gene containing G protein β-subunit-like repeats. *Nature*, **364**, 717–721.

Reiss, A. L., Freund, L., Abrams, M. T., Boehm, C. and Kazazian, H. (1993). Neurobehavioral effects of the fragile X premutation in adult women: a controlled study. *Am J Hum Genet*, **52**, 884–894.

Reiss, A. L., Kazazian, H. H., Krebs, C. M., McAughan, A., Boehm, C. D., Abrams, M. T. and Nelson, D. L. (1994). Frequency and stability of the fragile X mutation. *Hum Molec Genet*, **3**, 393–398.

Renaud, M., Bouchard, L., Kremp, O., Dallaire, L., Labadie, J. F., Bisson, J. and Trugeon, A. (1993). Is selective abortion for a genetic disease an issue for the medical profession? A comparative study of Quebec and France. *Prenat Diagn*, **13**, 691–706.

Rethoré, M. O., de Blois, M. C., Peeters, M., Popowski, P., Pangalos, C. and Lejeune, J. (1989). Pure partial trisomy of the short arm of chromosome 5. *Hum Genet*, **82**, 296–298.

Reyniers, E., Vits, L., DeBoulle, K., Van Roy, B., Van Velzen, D., de Graaff, E., Verkerk, A. J. M. H., Jorens, H. Z. J., Darby, J. K., Oostra, B. A. and Willems, P. J.

(1993). The full mutation in the FMR-1 gene of male fragile X patients is absent in their sperm. *Nature Genet*, **4**, 143–146.

Richards, R. I. and Sutherland, G. R. (1992). Dynamic mutations: a new class of mutations causing human disease. *Cell*, **70**, 709–712.

Richkind, K. E., Mahoney, M. J., Evans, M. I., Willner, J. and Douglass, R. (1991). Prenatal diagnosis and outcomes of five cases of mosaicism for an isochromosome of 20q. *Prenat Diagn*, **11**, 371–376.

Ridler, M. A. C., Berg, J. M., Pendrey, M. J., Saldaña, P. and Timothy, J. A. D. (1970). Familial occurrence of a small, supernumerary metacentric chromosome in phenotypically normal women. *J Med Genet*, **7**, 148–152.

Ritchie, R. J., Knight, S. J. L., Hirst, M. C., Grewal, P. K., Bobrow, M., Cross, G. S. and Davies, K. E. (1994). The cloning of *FRAXF*: trinucleotide repeat expansion and methylation at a third fragile site in distal Xqter. *Hum Mol Genet*, **3**, 2115–2121.

Ritter, C. L., Steele, M. W., Wenger, S. L. and Cohen, B. A. (1990). Chromosome mosaicism in hypomelanosis of Ito. *Am J Med Genet*, **35**, 14–17.

Rivas, F., García-Esquivel, L., Rivera, H., Jiménez, M. E., González, R. M., Cantú, J. M. (1987). Inv(4)(p16q21). A five-generation pedigree with 24 carriers and no recombinants. *Clin Genet*, **31**, 97–101.

Rivera, H., Cantú, J.M. (1986). Centric fission consequences in man. *Ann Génét*, **29**, 223–225.

Rizzu, P., Overhauser, J., Jackson, L. G. and Baldini, A. (1995). Cornelia deLange syndrome: toward the positional cloning of a locus at 3q27. *Am J Hum Genet*, **57**, A334.

Roberts, P., Williams, J. and Sills, M. A. (1989). A case of two inversion (10) recombinants in a family. *J Med Genet*, **26**, 461–464.

Roberts, S. H., Cowie, V. A. and Singh, K. R. (1986). Intrachromosomal insertion of chromosome 13 in a family with psychosis and mental subnormality. *J Ment Defic Res*, **30**, 227–232.

Roberts, S. H., Hughes, H. E., Davies, S. J. and Meredith, A. L. (1991). Bilateral split hand and split foot malformation in a boy with a de novo interstitial deletion of 7q21.3. *J Med Genet*, **28**, 479–481.

Robinson, A., Bender, B. G., Borelli, J. B., Puck, M. H., Salbenblatt, J. A. and Winter, J. S. D. (1986). Sex chromosome aneuploidy: prospective and longitudinal studies. In ''Prospective studies on children with sex chromosome aneuploidy'' (S. G. Ratcliffe and N. Paul, eds.). *Birth Defects: Orig Art Series*, **22**(3), pp. 23–71.

Robinson, A., Bender, B. G. and Linden, M. G. (1989). Decisions following the intrauterine diagnosis of sex chromosome aneuploidy. *Am J Med Genet*, **34**, 552–554.

Robinson, A., Bender, B. G. and Linden, M. G. (1992). Prognosis of prenatally diagnosed children with sex chromosome aneuploidy. *Am J Med Genet*, **44**, 365–368.

Robinson, A., Bender, B. G., Linden, M. G. and Salbenblatt, J. A. (1990). Sex chromosome aneuploidy: the Denver prospective study. In ''Children and young adults with sex chromosome aneuploidy. Follow-up, clinical, and molecular studies'' (J. A. Evans, J. L. Hamerton and A. Robinson, eds.). *Birth Defects: Orig Art Series*, **26**(4), pp. 59–115.

Robinson, W. P., Bernasconi, F., Basaran, S., Yüksel-Apak, M., Neri, G., Serville, F., Balicek, P., Haluza, R., Farah, L. M. S., Lüleci, G. and Schinzel, A. A. (1994). A somatic origin of homologous Robertsonian translocations and isochromosomes. *Am J Hum Genet*, **54**, 290–302.

Robinson, W. P., Bernasconi, F., Blouin, J. L., Basaran, S., Neri, G., Zizka, J., Antonarakis, S. E. and Schinzel, A. A. (1993a). Robertsonian translocations between homologous chromosomes are somatic events. *Am J Hum Genet*, **53** (Suppl.), A121.

Robinson, W. P., Bernasconi, F., Mutirangura, A., Ledbetter, D. H., Langlois, S., Malcolm, S., Morris, M. A. and Schinzel, A. A. (1993b). Nondisjunction of chromosome 15: origin and recombination. *Am J Hum Genet*, **53**, 740–751.

Robinson, W. P., Binkert, F., Giné, R., Vazquez, C., Müller, W., Rosenkranz, W. and Schinzel, A. (1993c). Clinical and molecular analysis of five inv dup(15) patients. *Eur J Hum Genet*, **1**, 37–50.

Robinson, W. P., Wagstaff, J., Bernasconi, F., Baccichetti, C., Artifoni, L., Franzoni, E., Suslak, L., Shih, L.-Y., Aviv, H. and Schinzel, A. A. (1993d). Uniparental disomy explains the occurrence of the Angelman or Prader-Willi syndrome in patients with an additional small inv dup(15) chromosome. *J Med Genet*, **30**, 756–760.

Robinson, W. P., Binkert, F., Bernasconi, F., Lorda-Sanchez, I., Werder, E. A. and Schinzel, A. A. (1995). Molecular studies of chromosomal mosaicism: relative frequency of chromosome gain or loss and possible role of cell selection. *Am J Hum Genet*, **56**, 444–451.

Robinson, W. P. and Lalande, M. (1995). Sex-specific meiotic recombination in the Prader-Willi/Angelman syndrome imprinted region. *Hum Mol Genet*, **4**, 801–806.

Robinson, W. P., Bottani, A., Yagang, X., Balakrishman, J., Binkert, F., Mächler, M., Prader, A. and Schinzel, A. (1991). Molecular, cytogenetic, and clinical investigations of Prader-Willi syndrome patients. *Am J Hum Genet*, **49**, 1219–1234.

Rochelson, B. L., Trunca, C., Monheit, A. G. and Baker, D. A. (1986). The use of a rapid in situ technique for third-trimester diagnosis of trisomy 18. *Am J Obstet Gynecol*, **155**, 835–836.

Rochon, L. and Vekemans, M. J. J. (1990). Triploidy arising from a first meiotic nondisjunction in a mother carrying a reciprocal translocation. *J Med Genet*, **27**, 724–726.

Rockman-Greenberg, C., Ray, M., Evans, J. A., Canning, N. and Hamerton, J. L. (1982). Homozygous Robertsonian translocations in a fetus with 44 chromosomes. *Hum Genet*, **61**, 181–184.

Rodeck, C., Tutschek, B., Sherlock, J. and Kingdom, J. (1995). Methods for the transcervical collection of fetal cells during the first trimester of pregnancy. *Prenat Diagn*, **15**, 933–942.

Rodriguez, M. T., Martin, M. J. and Abrisqueta, J. A. (1985). A complex balanced rearrangement involving four chromosomes in an azoospermic man. *J Med Genet*, **22**, 66–67.

Roland, B., Lynch, L., Berkowitz, G. and Zinberg, R. (1994). Confined placental mosaicism in CVS and pregnancy outcome. *Prenat Diagn*, **14**, 589–593.

Romain, D. R., Columbano-Green, L. M., Parfitt, R. G., Smythe, R. H., MacKenzie, N. G. and Chapman, C. J. (1988). Late replication studies and esterase D levels in a case of unbalanced X;autosome translocation, 46,X,t(X;13)(q27;q12). *J Med Genet*, **25**, 716-718.

Romain, D. R., Columbano-Green, L. M., Whyte, S., Smythe, R. H., Parfitt, R. G., Gebbie, O. B. and Chapman, C. J. (1983a). Familial paracentric inversion of 1p. *Am J Med Genet*, **14**, 629–634.

Romain, D. R., Gebbie, O. B., Parfitt, R. G., Columbano-Green, L. M., Smythe, R. H., Chapman, C. J. and Kerr, A. (1983b). Two cases of ring chromosome 11. *J Med Genet*, **20**, 380–382.

Romain, D. R., Whyte, S., Callen, D. F. and Eyre, H. J. (1991). A rare heteromorphism of chromosome 20 and reproductive loss. *J Med Genet*, **28**, 477–478.

Rosenberg, C., Janson, M., Nordeskjöld, M., Børresen, A. L. and Vianna-Morgante, A. M. (1994). Intragenic reorganization of RB1 in a complex (4;13) rearrangement demonstrated by FISH. *Cytogenet Cell Genet*, **65**, 268–271.

Rosenfeld, R. G., Frane, J., Attie, K. M., Brasel, J. A., Burstein, S., Cara, J. F., Chernausek, S., Gotlin, R. W., Kuntze, J., Lippe, B. M., Mahoney, P. C., Moore, W. V., Saenger, P. and Johanson, A. J. (1992). Six-year results of a randomized, prospective trial of human growth hormone and oxandrolone in Turner syndrome. *J Pediatr*, **121**, 49–55.

Rossi, E., Floridia, G., Casali, M., Danesino, C., Chiumello, G., Bernardi, F., Magnani, I., Papi, L., Mura, M. and Zuffardi, O. (1993). Types, stability, and phenotypic consequences of chromosome rearrangements leading to interstitial telomeric sequences. *J Med Genet*, **30**, 926–931.

Rothman, B. K. (1988). "The tentative pregnancy. Prenatal diagnosis and the future of motherhood." Pandora Press, London.

Rousseau, F., Heitz, D., Biancalana, V., Blumenfeld, S., Kretz, C., Boué, J., Tommerup, N., Van Der Hagen, C., DeLozier-Blanchet, C., Croquette, M.-F., Gilgenkrantz, S., Jalbert, P., Voelckel, M.-A., Oberlé, I. and Mandel, J.-L. (1991). Direct diagnosis by DNA analysis of the fragile X syndrome of mental retardation. *N Engl J Med*, **325**, 1673–1681.

Rousseau, F., Heitz, D., Tarleton, J., MacPherson, J., Malmgren, H., Dahl, N., Barnicoat, A., Mathew, C., Mornet, E., Tejada, I., Maddalena, A., Spiegel, R., Schinzel, A., Marcos, J. A. G., Schorderet, D. F., Schaap, T., Maccioni, L., Russo, S., Jacobs, P. A., Schwartz, C. and Mandel, J. L. (1994). A multicenter study on genotype-phenotype correlations in the fragile X syndrome, using direct diagnosis with probe StB12.3: the first 2,253 cases. *Am J Hum Genet*, **55**, 225–237.

Rousseau, F., Rouillard, P., Morel, M.-L., Khandjian, E. W. and Morgan K. (1995). Prevalence of carriers of premutation-size alleles of the *FMRI* gene—and implications for the population genetics of the fragile X syndrome. *Am J Hum Genet*, **57**, 1006–1018.

Rushton, D. I. (1981). Examination of products of conception from previable human pregnancies. *J Clin Pathol*, **34**, 819–835.

Rutgers, J. L. and Scully, R. E. (1991). The androgen insensitivity syndrome (testicular feminization): a clinicopathological study of 43 cases. *Int J Gynecol Pathol*, **10**, 126–144.

Saadallah, N. and Hultén, M. (1985). A complex three breakpoint translocation involving chromosomes 2, 4, and 9 identified by meiotic investigations of a human male ascertained for subfertility. *Hum Genet*, **71**, 312–320.

Sachs, E. S., Jahoda, M. G. J., Los, F. J., Pijpers, L. and Wladimiroff, J. W. (1990). Trisomy 21 mosaicism in gonads with unexpectedly high recurrence risks. *Am J Med Genet* (Suppl.), **7**, 186–188.

Sadler, L. S., Robinson, L. K., Verdaasdonk, K. R. and Gingell, R. (1993). The Williams syndrome: evidence for possible autosomal dominant inheritance. *Am J Med Genet*, **47**, 468–470.

Saitoh, S., Harada, N., Jinno, Y., Hashimoto, K., Imaizumi, K., Kuroki, Y., Fukushima, Y., Sugimoto, T., Renedo, M., Wagstaff, J., Lalande, M., Mutirangura, A., Kuwano., A., Ledbetter, D. H. and Niikawa, N. (1994). Molecular and clinical study of 61 Angelman syndrome patients. *Am J Med Genet*, **52**, 158–163.

Saitoh, S., Kubota, T., Ohta, T., Jinno, Y., Niikawa, N., Sugimoto, T., Wagstaff, J. and Lalande, M. (1992). Familial Angelman syndrome caused by imprinted submicroscopic deletion encompassing $GABA_A$ receptor β_3-subunit gene. *Lancet*, **339**, 366–367.

Saller, D. N. and Neiger, R. (1994). Cytogenetic abnormalities among perinatal deaths demonstrating a single umbilical artery. *Prenat Diagn*, **14**, 13–16.

Salo, P., Ignatius, J., Simola, K. O. J., Tahvanainen, E. and Kääriäinen, H. (1995). Clinical features of nine males with molecularly defined deletions of the Y chromosome long arm. *J Med Genet*, **32**, 711–715.

Salo, P., Kääriäinen, H., Petrovic, V., Peltomäki, P., Page, D. C. and de la Chapelle, A. (1995). Molecular mapping of the putative gonadoblastoma locus on the Y chromosome. *Genes, Chromosom Cancer*, **14**, 210–214.

Sander, A., Schmelzle, R. and Murray, J. (1994). Evidence for a microdeletion in 1q32–41 involving the gene responsible for Van der Woude syndrome. *Hum Mol Genet*, **3**, 575–578.

Sarno, A. P., Moorman, A. J. and Kalousek, D. K. (1993). Partial molar pregnancy with fetal survival: an unusual example of confined placental mosaicism. *Obstet Gynecol*, **82**, 716–719.

Saura, R., Traore, W., Taine, L., Wen, Z. Q., Roux, D., Maugey-Laulom, B., Ruffie, M., Vergnaud, A. and Horovitz, J. (1995). Prenatal diagnosis of trisomy 9. Six cases and a review of the literature. *Prenat Diagn*, **15**, 609–614.

Savitsky, K., Bar-Shira, A., Gilad, S., Rotman, G., Ziv, Y., Vanagaite, L., Tagle, D. A., Smith, S., Uziel, T., Sfez, S., Ashkenazi, M., Pecker, I., Frydman, M., Harnik, R., Patanjali, S. R., Simmons, A., Clines, G. A., Sartiel, A., Gatti, R. A., Chessa, L., Sanal, O., Lavin, M. F., Jaspers, N. G. J., Taylor, A. M. R., Arlett, C. F., Miki, T., Weissman, S. M., Lovett, M., Collins, F. S. and Shiloh, Y. (1995). A single ataxia telangiectasia gene with a product similar to PI-3 kinase. *Science*, **268**, 1749–1753.

Sawyer, J. R., Swanson, C. M., Wheeler, G. and Cunniff, C. (1995). Chromosome instability in ICF syndrome: formation of micronuclei from multibranched chromosomes 1 demonstrated by fluorescence in situ hybridization. *Am J Med Genet*, **56**, 203–209.

Scambler, P. J. (1993). Deletions of human chromosome 22 and associated birth defects. *Curr Opin Genet Dev*, **3**, 432–437.

Scarbrough, P. R., Hersh, J., Kukolich, M. K., Carroll, A. J., Finely, S. C., Hochberger, R., Wilkerson, S., Yen, F. F. and Althaus, B. W. (1984). Tetraploidy: a report of three live-born infants. *Am J Med Genet*, **19**, 29–37.

Schaefer, G. B., Novak, K., Steele, D., Buehler, B., Smith, S., Zaleski, D., Pickering, D., Nelson, M. and Sanger, W. (1995). Familial inverted duplication 7p. *Am J Med Genet*, **56**, 184–187.

Schanz, S. and Steinbach, P. (1989). Investigation of the "variable spreading" of X inactivation into a translocated autosome. *Hum Genet*, **82**, 244–248.

Schinzel, A. (1993a). Genomic imprinting: consequences of uniparental disomy for human disease. *Am J Med Genet*, **46**, 683–684.

Schinzel, A. (1993b). Karyotype-phenotype correlations in autosomal chromosomal aberrations. In "The phenotypic mapping of Down syndrome and other aneuploid conditions" (C. J. Epstein, ed.). Wiley-Liss, New York, pp. 19–31.

Schinzel, A. (1994). "Human cytogenetics database." Oxford University Press, Oxford.

Schinzel, A. A., Adelsberger, P. A., Binkert, F., Basaran, S. and Antonarakis, S. E.

(1992). No evidence for a paternal interchromosomal effect from analysis of the origin of nondisjunction in Down syndrome patients with concomitant familial chromosome rearrangements. *Am J Hum Genet*, **50**, 288–293.

Schinzel, A. A., Basaran, S., Bernasconi, F., Karaman, B., Yüksel-Apak, M. and Robinson, W. P. (1994a). Maternal uniparental disomy 22 has no impact on the phenotype. *Am J Hum Genet*, **54**, 21–24.

Schinzel, A. A., Brecevic, L., Bernasconi, F., Binkert, F., Berthet, F., Wuilloud, A. and Robinson, W. P. (1994b). Intrachromosomal triplication of 15q11-q13. *J Med Genet*, **31**, 798–803.

Schinzel, A. A., Robinson, W. P., Binkert, F., Torresani, T. and Werder, E. A. (1993). Exclusively paternal X chromosomes in a girl with short stature. *Hum Genet*, **92**, 175–178.

Schlessinger, D., Mandel, J.-L., Monaco, A. P., Nelson, D. L. and Willard, H. F. (1993). Report of the fourth international workshop on human X chromosome mapping 1993. *Cytogenet Cell Genet*, **64**, 148–170.

Schmidt, M. and Du Sart, D. (1992). Functional disomies of the X chromosome influence the cell selection and hence the X inactivation pattern in females with balanced X-autosome translocations: a review of 122 cases. *Am J Med Genet*, **42**, 161–169.

Schmidt, M., Du Sart, D., Kalitsis, P., Leversha, M., Dale, S., Sheffield, L. and Toniolo, D. (1991). Duplications of the X chromosome in males: evidence that most parts of the X chromosome can be active in two copies. *Hum Genet*, **86**, 519–521.

Schmitt-Ney, M., Thiele, H., Kaltwaβer, P., Bardoni, B., Cisternino, M. and Scherer, G. (1995). Two novel SRY missense mutations reducing DNA binding identified in XY females and their mosaic fathers. *Am J Hum Genet*, **56**, 862–869.

Schmutz, S. M. and Pinno, E. (1986). Morphology alone does not make an isochromosome. *Hum Genet*, **72**, 253–255.

Schnittger, S., Höfers, C., Heidemann, P., Beermann, F. and Hansmann, I. (1989). Molecular and cytogenetic analysis of an interstitial 20p deletion associated with syndromic intrahepatic ductular hypoplasia (Alagille syndrome). *Hum Genet*, **83**, 239–244.

Schorderet, D. F., Friedman, C. and Disteche, C. M. (1991). Pericentric inversion of the X chromosome: presentation of a case and review of the literature. *Ann Génét*, **34**, 98–103.

Schroder, J. and de la Chapelle, A. (1972). Fetal lymphocytes in maternal blood. *J Hematol*, **39**, 153–162.

Schröder, J., Lydecken, K. and de la Chapelle, A. (1971). Meiosis and spermatogenesis in G-trisomic males. *Hum Genet*, **13**, 15–24.

Schroeder, T. M., Auerbach, A. D. and Obe, G. (eds.) (1989). Fanconi anemia: clinical, cytogenetic and experimental aspects. Springer-Verlag, Heidelberg.

Schupf, N., Kapell, D., Lee, J. H., Ottman, R. and Mayeux, R. (1994). Increased risk of Alzheimer's disease in mothers of adults with Down's syndrome. *Lancet*, **344**, 353–356.

Schuring-Blom, G. H., Keijzer, M., Jakobs, M. E., van den Brande, D. M., Visser, H. M., Wiegant, J., Hoovers, J. M. N. and Leschot, N. J. (1993). Molecular cytogenetic analysis of term placentae suspected of mosaicism using fluorescence *in situ* hybridization. *Prenat Diagn*, **13**, 671–679.

Schwartz, S., Flannery, D. B. and Cohen, M. M. (1985). Tests appropriate for the prenatal diagnosis of ataxia telangiectasia. *Prenat Diagn*, **5**, 9–14.

Schwartz, S., Schwartz, M. F., Panny, S. R., Peterson, C. J., Waters, E. and Cohen, M. M. (1986). Inherited X-chromosome inverted tandem duplication in a male traced to a grandparental mitotic error. *Am J Hum Genet*, **38**, 741–750.

Sciorra, L. J., Hux, C., Day-Salvadore, D., Lee, M., Mandelbaum., D. E., Brady-Yasbin, S., Frybury, J., Mahoney, M. J. and Dimaio, M. S. (1992a). Trisomy 5 mosaicism detected prenatally with an affected liveborn. *Prenat Diagn*, **12**, 477–482.

Sciorra, L. J., Schlenker, E., Toke, D., Brady-Yasbin, S., Day-Salvatore, D. and Lee, M. (1992b). Low level mosaicism for a balanced 7;14 translocation in the father of an abnormal 7q+ child. *Am J Med Genet*, **42**, 296–297.

Scott, J. A., Wenger, S. L., Steele, M. W. and Chakravarti, A. (1995). Down syndrome consequent to a cryptic maternal 12p;21q chromosome translocation. *Am J Med Genet*, **56**, 67–71.

Seaver, L. H., Pierpont, J. W., Erickson, R. P., Donnerstein, R. L. and Cassidy, S. B. (1994). Pulmonary atresia associated with maternal 22q11.2 deletion: possible parent of origin effect in the conotruncal anomaly face syndrome. *J Med Genet*, **31**, 830–834.

Seller, M. J., Pal, K., Horsley, S., Davies, A. F., Berry, A. C., Meredith, R. and Mc-Cartney, A. C. E. (1995). A fetus with an X;1 balanced reciprocal translocation and eye disease. *J Med Genet*, **32**, 557–560.

Sensi, A. and Ricci, N. (1993). Mitotic errors in trisomy 21. *Nature Genet*, **5**, 215.

Serra, A. and Bova, R. (1990). Acrocentric chromosome double NOR is not a risk factor for Down syndrome. *Am J Med Genet*, **7** (Suppl.), 169–174.

Shaffer, L. G., Jackson-Cook, C. K., Stasiowski, B. A., Spence, J. E. and Brown, J. A. (1992). Parental origin determination in thirty de novo Robertsonian translocations. *Am J Med Genet*, **43**, 957–963.

Shaffer, L. G., Overhauser, J., Jackson, L. G. and Ledbetter, D. H. (1993). Genetic syndromes and uniparental disomy: a study of 16 cases of Brachmann-de Lange syndrome. *Am J Med Genet*, **47**, 383–386.

Shaham, M., Voss, R., Becker, Y., Yarkoni, S., Ornoy, A. and Kohn, G. (1982). Prenatal diagnosis of ataxia telangiectasia. *J Pediatr*, **100**, 134–137.

Shalev, E., Zalel, Y., Weiner, E., Cohen, H. and Shneur, Y. (1994). The role of cordocentesis in assessment of mosaicism found in amniotic fluid cell culture. *Acta Obstet Gynecol Scand*, **73**, 119–122.

Shaw, M. W. (1984). To be or not to be? That is the question. *Am J Hum Genet*, **36**, 1–9.

Sheehy, R. R., Brown, M. G., Warren, R. J., Schwartzman, M. and Magenis, R. E. (1987). Y-derived sequences detected in a 45,X male by in situ hybridization. *Am J Med Genet*, **27**, 831–839.

Sheppard, D. M., Fisher, R. A., Lawler, S. D. and Povey, S. (1982). Tetraploid conceptus with three paternal contributions. *Hum Genet*, **62**, 371–374.

Sheridan, R., Llerena, J., Matkins, S., Debenham, P., Cawood, A. and Bobrow, M. (1989). Fertility in a male with trisomy 21. *J Med Genet*, **26**, 294–298.

Sherman, S. L., Iselius, L., Gallano, P., Buckton, K., Collyer, S., DeMey, R., Kristoffersson, U., Lindsten, J., Mikkelsen, M., Morton, N. E., Newton, M., Nordensson, I., Petersen, M. B. and Wahlström, J. (1986). Segregation analysis of balanced pericentric inversions in pedigree data. *Clin Genet*, **30**, 87–94.

Sherman, S. L., Jacobs, P. A., Morton, N. E., Froster-Iskenius, U., Howard-Peebles, P. N., Nielsen, K. B., Partington, M. W., Sutherland, G. R., Turner, G. and Watson, M. (1985). Further segregation analysis of the fragile X syndrome with special reference to transmitting males. *Hum Genet*, **69**, 289–299.

Sherman, S. L., Morton, N. E., Jacobs, P. A. and Turner, G. (1984). The marker (X) syndrome: a cytogenetic and genetic analysis. *Ann Hum Genet*, **48**, 21–37.

Sherman, S. L., Petersen, M. B., Freeman, S. B., Hersey, J., Pettay, D., Taft, L., Frantzen, M., Mikkelsen, M. and Hassold, T. J. (1994). Non-disjunction of chromosome 21 in maternal meiosis I: evidence for a maternal age-dependent mechanism involving reduced recombination. *Hum Mol Genet*, **3**, 1529–1535.

Sherman, S. L. and Sutherland, G. R. (1986). Segregation analysis of rare autosomal fragile sites. *Hum Genet*, **72**, 123–128.

Sherman, S. L., Takaesu, N., Freeman, S. B., Grantham, M., Phillips, C., Blackston, R. D., Jacobs, P. A., Cockwell, A. E., Freeman, V., Uchida, I., Mikkelsen, M., Kurnit, D. M., Buraczynska, M., Keats, B. J. B. and Hassold, T. J. (1991). Trisomy 21: association between reduced recombination and nondisjunction. *Am J Hum Genet*, **49**, 608–620.

Shiloh, Y. (1995). Ataxia-telangiectasia: closer to unraveling the mystery. *Eur J Hum Genet*, **3**, 116–138.

Shohat, M., Legum, C., Romem, Y., Borochowitz, Z., Bach, G. and Goldman, B. (1995). Down syndrome prevention program in a population with an older maternal age. *Obstet Gynecol*, **85**, 368–373.

Shuttleworth, G. E. (1909). Mongolian imbecility. *Br Med J*, **2**, 661–665.

Sijmons, R. H., Leegte, B., van Lingen, R. A., de Pater, J. M., van der Veen, A. Y., del Canho, H., Bos, C., ten Kate, L. P. and Breed, A. S. P. M. (1993). Tetrasomy 5p mosaicism in a boy with delayed growth, hypotonia, minor anomalies, and an additional isochromosome 5p [46,XY/47,XY,+i(5p)]. *Am J Med Genet*, **47**, 559–562.

Sikkema-Raddatz, B., Sijmons, R. H., Tan-Sindhunata, M. B., van der Veen, A. Y., Brunsting, R., de Vries, B., Beekhuis, J. R., Bekedam, D. J., van Aken, B. and de Jong, B. (1995). Prenatal diagnosis in two cases of *de novo* complex balanced chromosomal rearrangements. Three-year follow-up in one case. *Prenat Diagn*, **15**, 467–473.

Silver, R. K., MacGregor, S. N., Muhlbach, L. H., Knutel, T. A. and Kambich, M. P. (1994). Congenital malformations subsequent to chorionic villus sampling: outcome analysis of 1048 consecutive procedures. *Prenat Diagn*, **14**, 421–427.

Silverman, G. A., Schneider, S. A., Massa, H. F., Flint, A., Lalande, M., Leonard, J. C., Overhauser, J, van der Engh, G. and Trask, B. J. (1995). The 18q− syndrome: analysis of chromosomes by bivariate flow karyotyping and the PCR reveals a successive set of deletion breakpoints within 18q21.1-q22.2. *Am J Hum Genet*, **56**, 926–937.

Simi, P., Ceccarelli, M., Barachini, A., Floridia, G. and Zuffardi, O. (1992). The unbalanced offspring of the male carriers of the 11q;22q translocation: nondisjunction at meiosis II in a balanced spermatocyte. *Hum Genet*, **88**, 482–483.

Simmers, R. N., Sutherland, G. R., West, A. and Richards, R. I. (1987). Fragile sites at 16q22 are not at the breakpoint of the chromosomal rearrangement in acute myelomonocytic leukemia. *Science*, **236**, 92–94.

Simmons, A. D., Goodart, S. A., Gallardo, T. D., Overhauser, J. and Lovett, M. (1995). Five novel genes from the cri-du-chat critical region isolated by direct selection. *Hum Mol Genet*, **4**, 295–302.

Simoni, G. and Sirchia, S. M. (1994). Confined placental mosaicism. *Prenat Diagn*, **14**, 1185–1189.

Simpson, J. L. (1978). True hermaphroditism: etiology and phenotypic considerations. *Birth Defects: Orig Art Series*, **14**(6C), pp. 9–35.

Simpson, J. L. and Elias, S. (1993). Isolating fetal cells from maternal blood: advances in prenatal diagnosis through molecular technology. *J Am Med Assoc*, **270**, 2357–2361.

Simpson, J. L., Lewis, D. E., Bischoff, F. Z. and Elias, S. (1995). Isolating fetal nucleated red blood cells from maternal blood: the Baylor experience—1995. *Prenat Diagn*, **15**, 907–912.

Simpson, J. L., Meyers, C. M., Martin, A. O., Elias, S. and Ober, C. (1989). Translocations are infrequent among couples having repeated spontaneous abortions but no other abnormal pregnancies. *Fertil Steril*, **51**, 811–814.

Sinclair, A. H., Berta, P., Palmer, M. S., Hawkins, J. R., Griffiths, B. L., Smith, M. J., Foster, J. W., Frischauf, A.-M., Lovell-Badge, R. and Goodfellow, P. N. (1990). A gene from the human sex-determining region encodes a protein with homology to a conserved DNA-binding motif. *Nature*, **346**, 240–244.

Singh, K. S. (1990). Trisomy 13 (Patau's syndrome): a rare case of survival into adulthood. *J Ment Defic Res*, **34**, 91–93.

Sirchia, S. M., De Andreis, C., Pariani, S., Grimoldi, M. G., Molinari, A., Buscaglia, M. and Simoni, G. (1994). Chromosome 14 maternal uniparental disomy in the euploid cell line of a fetus with mosaic 46,XX/47,XX,+14 karyotype. *Hum Genet*, **94**, 355–358.

Sivak, L. E., Esbenshade, J., Brothman, A. R., Issa, B., Lemons, R. S. and Carey, J. C. (1994). Multiple congenital anomalies in a man with (X;6) translocation. *Am J Med Genet*, **51**, 9–12.

Sjöstedt, A. W., Alatalo, M., Wahlström, J., Döbeln, U. V. and Olegard, R. (1989). Replication error, a new hypothesis to explain the origin of a supernumerary marker chromosome in a mentally retarded boy. *Hereditas*, **11**, 115–123.

Skakkebæk, N. E., Giwercman, A. and de Kretser, D. (1994). Pathogenesis and management of male infertility. *Lancet*, **343**, 1473–1479.

Slater, H., Shaw, J. H., Bankier, A., Forrest, S. M. and Dawson, G. (1995). UPD 13: no indication of maternal or paternal imprinting of genes on chromosome 13. *J Med Genet*, **32**, 493.

Slatter, R. E., Elliott, M., Welham, K., Carrera, M., Schofield, P. N., Barton, D. E. and Maher, E. R. (1994). Mosaic uniparental disomy in Beckwith-Wiedemann syndrome. *J Med Genet*, **31**, 749–753.

Slunga-Tallberg, A. and Knuutila, S. (1995). Can nucleated erythrocytes found in maternal venous blood be used in the noninvasive prenatal diagnosis of fetal chromosome abnormalities? *Eur J Hum Genet*, **3**, 264–270.

Smeets, D. F. C. M., Hamel, B. C. J., Nelen, M. R., Smeets, H. J. M., Bollen, J. H. M., Smits, A. P. T., Ropers, H.-H. and van Oost, B. A. (1992). Prader-Willi syndrome and Angelman syndrome in cousins from a family with a translocation between chromosomes 6 and 15. *N Engl J Med*, **326**, 807–811.

Smeets, D. F. C. M., Moog, U., Weemaes, C. M. R., Vaes-Peeters, G., Merkx, G. F. M., Niehof, J. P. and Hamers, G. (1994). ICF syndrome: a new case and review of the literature. *Hum Genet*, **94**, 240–246.

Smith, A., Deng, Z.-M., Beran, R., Woodage, T. and Trent, R. J. (1994). Familial unbalanced translocation t(8;15)(p23.3;q11) with uniparental disomy in Angelman syndrome. *Hum Genet*, **93**, 471–473.

Smith, A., Cohen, M., den Dulk, G. and Guirguis, A. (1989a). Chorionic villus sampling—short-term versus long-term culture in a subtle 2;18 translocation. *Prenat Diagn*, **9**, 217–220.

Smith, A., Field, B. and Learoyd, B. M. (1989b). Trisomy 18 at age 21 years. *Am J Med Genet*, **34**, 338–339.

Smith, A., Fraser, I. S. and Elliott, G. (1979). An infertile male with balanced Y;19 translocation. Review of Y;autosome translocations. *Ann Génét*, **22**, 189–194.

Smith, A., Lindeman, R., Volpato, F., Kearney, A., White, S., Haan, E. and Trent, R. J. (1991). A de novo unbalanced reciprocal translocation identified as paternal in origin in the Prader-Willi syndrome. *Hum Genet*, **86**, 534–536.

Smith, A., Robson, L., Neumann, A., Mulcahy, M., Chabros, V., Deng, Z.-M., Woodage, T. and Trent, R. J. (1993). Fluorescence *in-situ* hybridisation and molecular studies used in the characterisation of a Robertsonian translocation (13q15q) in Prader-Willi syndrome. *Clin Genet*, **43**, 5–8.

Smith, A., Watt, A. J., Cummins, M., Gardner, R. J. M. and Wilson, M. (1992). A small one-band paracentric inversion inv(4)(p15.3p16.3). *Ann Génét*, **35**, 161–163.

Smith, A. C. M., Spuhler, K., Williams, T. M., McConnell, T., Sujansky, E. and Robinson, A. (1987). Genetic risk for recombinant 8 syndrome and the transmission rate of balanced inversion 8 in the Hispanic population of the Southwestern United States. *Am J Hum Genet*, **41**, 1083–1103.

Smith, D. K., Shaw, R. W., Slack, J. and Marteau, T. M. (1995). Training obstetricians and midwives to present screening tests: evaluation of two brief interventions. *Prenat Diagn*, **15**, 317–324.

Snijders, R. J. M., Holzgreve, W., Cuckle, H. and Nicolaides, K. H. (1994a). Maternal age-specific risks for trisomies at 9–14 weeks' gestation. *Prenat Diagn*, **14**, 543–552.

Snijders, R. J. M., Shawa, L. and Nicolaides, K. H. (1994b). Fetal choroid plexus cysts and trisomy 18: assessment of risk based on ultrasound findings and maternal age. *Prenat Diagn*, **14**, 1119–1127.

Snow, K., Doud, L. K., Hagerman, R., Pergolizzi, R. G., Erster, S. H. and Thibodeau, S. N. (1993). Analysis of a CGG sequence at the FMR-1 locus in fragile X families and in the general population. *Am J Hum Genet*, **53**, 1217–1228.

Soler, A., Salami, C., Balmes, I., Carrio, A., Tejada, I., Farguell, T., Cols, N., Cararach, J. and Fortuny, A. (1981). Pericentric X chromosome in a family. *Clin Genet*, **20**, 234–235.

Sorokin, Y., Johnson, M. P., Uhlmann, W. R., Zador, I. E., Drugan, A., Koppitch, F. C., Moody, J. and Evans, M. I. (1991). Postmortem chorionic villus sampling: correlation of cytogenetic and ultrasound findings. *Am J Med Genet*, **39**, 314–316.

Speed, R. M. (1984). Meiotic configurations in female trisomy 21 foetuses. *Hum Genet*, **66**, 176–180.

Speed, R. M. (1988). The possible role of meiotic pairing anomalies in the atresia of human fetal oocytes. *Hum Genet*, **78**, 260–266.

Speed, R. M., Faed, M. J. W., Batstone, P. J., Baxby, K. and Barnetson, W. (1991). Persistence of two Y chromosomes through meiotic prophase and metaphase I in an XYY man. *Hum Genet*, **87**, 416–420.

Spence, J. E., Perciaccante, R. G., Greig, G. M., Willard, H. F., Ledbetter, D. H., Hejtmancik, J. F., Pollack, M. S., O'Brien, W. E. and Beaudet, A. L. (1988). Uniparental disomy as a mechanism for human genetic disease. *Am J Hum Genet*, **42**, 217–226.

Spinner, N. B., Rand, E. B., Fortina, P., Genin, A., Taub, R., Semeraro, A. and Piccoli, D. A. (1994). Cytologically balanced t(2;20) in a two-generation family with Alagille syndrome: cytogenetic and molecular studies. *Am J Hum Genet*, **55**, 238–243.

Spinner, N. B., Zackai, E., Cheng, S.-D. and Knoll, J. H. M. (1995). Supernumerary inv dup(15) in a patient with Angelman syndrome and a deletion of 15q11-q13. *Am J Med Genet*, **57**, 61–65.

Spurdle, A. B., Shankman, S. and Ramsay, M. (1995). XX true hermaphroditism in Southern African blacks: exclusion of SRY sequences and uniparental disomy of the X chromosome. *Am J Med Genet*, **55**, 53–56.

Staley, L. W., Hull, C. E., Mazzocco, M. M. M., Thibodeau, S. N., Snow, K., Wilson, V. L., Taylor, A., McGavran, L., Weiner, D., Riddle, J., O'Connor, R. and Hagerman, R. J. (1993). Molecular-clinical correlations in children and adults with fragile X syndrome. *Am J Dis Child*, **147**, 723–726.

Stallard, R., Krueger, S., James, R. S. and Schwartz, S. (1995). Uniparental isodisomy 13 in a normal female due to transmission of a maternal t(13q13q). *Am J Med Genet*, **57**, 14–18.

Stallard, R. and Van Dyke, D. (1986). Familial duplications of proximal 15q in normal individuals. *Am J Hum Genet*, **39**, A133.

Stamberg, J. and Thomas, G. H. (1986). Unusual supernumerary chromosomes: types encountered in a referred population, and high incidence of associated maternal chromosome abnormalities. *Hum Genet*, **72**, 140–144.

Staples, A. J., Sutherland, G. R., Haan, E. A. and Clisby, S. (1991). Epidemiology of Down syndrome in South Australia, 1960–89. *Am J Hum Genet*, **49**, 1014–1024.

Steinbach, P. (1986). Excess of mental retardation and/or congenital malformation in reciprocal translocations in man (Fryns et al., 1986). *Hum Genet*, **73**, 379.

Steinbach, P., Horstmann, W. and Scholz, W. (1980). Tandem duplication dup(X)(q13q22) in a male proband inherited from the mother showing mosaicism of X-inactivation. *Hum Genet*, **54**, 309–313.

Steinberg, C., Zackai, E. H., Eunpu, D. L., Mennuti, M. T. and Emanuel, B. S. (1984). Recurrence rate for de novo 21q21q translocation Down syndrome: a study of 112 families. *Am J Med Genet*, **17**, 523–530.

Stene, J., Stene, E. and Mikkelsen, M. (1984). Risk for chromosome abnormality at amniocentesis following a child with a non-inherited chromosome aberration. *Prenat Diagn (Special Issue)*, **4**, 81–95.

Stene, J. (1986). Comments on methods and results in: Sherman et al., "Segregation analysis of balanced pericentric inversions in pedigree data." *Clin Genet*, **30**, 95–107.

Stene, J. and Stengel-Rutkowski, S. (1982). Genetic risks for familial reciprocal translocations with special emphasis on those leading to 9p, 10p and 12p trisomies. *Ann Hum Genet*, **46**, 41–74.

Stene, J. and Stengel-Rutkowski, S. (1988). Genetic risks of familial reciprocal and Robertsonian translocation carriers. In "The cytogenetics of mammalian autosomal rearrangements" (A. Daniel, ed.). A. R. Liss, New York, pp. 3–72.

Stengel-Rutkowski, S., Stene, J. and Gallano, P. (1988). "Risk estimates in balanced parental reciprocal translocations. Monographie des Annales de Génétique." Expansion Scientifique Française, Paris.

Stengel-Rutkowski, S., Warkotsch, A., Schimanek, P., Stene, J. (1984). Familial Wolf's syndrome with a hidden 4p deletion by translocation of an 8p segment. Unbalanced inheritance from a maternal translocation (4;8)(p15.3;p22). Case report, review and risk estimates. *Clin Genet*, **25**, 500–521.

Stevens, C. A., Carey, J. C. and Shigeoka, A. O. (1990). Di George anomaly and velocardiofacial syndrome. *Pediatrics*, **85**, 526–530.

Stewart, D. A., Bailey, J. D., Netley, C. T. and Park, E. (1990). Growth, development, and behavioral outcome from mid-adolescence to adulthood in subjects with chromosome aneuploidy: the Toronto study. In "Children and young adults with sex chromosome aneuploidy. Follow-up, clinical, and molecular studies" (J. A.

Evans, J. L. Hamerton and A. Robinson, eds.). *Birth Defects: Orig Art Series*, **26**(4), pp. 131–188.

Stioui, S., Privitera, O., Brambati, B., Zuliani, G., Lalatta, F. and Simoni, G. (1992). First-trimester prenatal diagnosis of Roberts syndrome. *Prenat Diagn,* **12**, 145–149.

Stoll, C., Alembik, Y., Dott, B. and Roth, M.-P. (1990). Epidemiology of Down syndrome in 118,265 consecutive births. *Am J Med Genet*, **7** (Suppl.), 79–83.

Strain, L., Warner, J. P., Johnston, T. and Bonthron, D. T. (1995). A human parthenogenetic chimaera. *Nature Genet*, **11**, 164–169.

Strathdee, C. A., Duncan, A. M. V. and Buchwald, M. (1992a). Evidence for at least four Fanconi anaemia genes including *FACC* on chromosome 9. *Nature Genet*, **1**, 196–198.

Strathdee, C. A., Gavish, H., Shannon, W. R. and Buchwald, M. (1992b). Cloning of cDNAs for Fanconi's anaemia by functional complementation. *Nature*, **356**, 763–767.

Strathdee, G., Harrison, W., Riethman, H. C., Goodart, S. A. and Overhauser, J. (1994). Interstitial deletions are not the main mechanism leading to 18q deletions. *Am J Hum Genet*, **54**, 1085–1091.

Stratton, R. F., Dobyns, W. B., Airhart, S. D. and Ledbetter, D. H. (1984). New chromosomal syndrome: Miller-Dieker syndrome and monosomy 17p13. *Hum Genet,* **67**, 193–200.

Sturtevant, A. H. and Beadle, G. W. (1962). "An introduction to genetics." Dover, New York.

Sudha, T. and Gopinath, P. M. (1990). Homologous Robertsonian translocation (21q21q) and abortions. *Hum Genet*, **85**, 253–255.

Sujansky, E., Smith, A. C. M., Prescott, K. E., Freehauf, C. L., Clericuzio, C. and Robinson, A. (1993). Natural history of the recombinant (8) syndrome. *Am J Med Genet*, **47**, 512–525.

Sultan, C., Lumbroso, S., Poujol, N., Belon, C., Boudon, C. and Lobaccaro, J.-M. (1993). Mutations of androgen receptor gene in androgen insensitivity syndromes. *J Steroid Biochem Mol Biol*, **46**, 519–530.

Summitt, R. L., Tipton, R. E., Wilroy, R. S., Martens, P. R. and Phelan, J. P. (1978). X-autosome translocations: a review. *Birth Defects: Orig Art Series,* **14**(6C), pp. 219–247.

Sunde, L., Vejerslev, L. O., Jensen, M. P., Pedersen, S., Hertz, J. M. and Bolund, L. (1993). Genetic analysis of repeated, biparental, diploid, hydatidiform moles. *Cancer Genet Cytogenet*, **66**, 16–22.

Surti, U., Pattillo, R., O'Brien, S. and Szulman, A. (1980). Origin of choriocarcinoma cell lines. *Am J Hum Genet,* **32**, 131A.

Sutcliffe, J. S., Nelson, D. S., Zhang, F., Pieretti, M., Caskey, C. T., Saxe, D. and Warren, S. T. (1992). DNA methylation represses FMR-1 transcription in fragile X syndrome. *Hum Molec Genet*, **1**, 397–400.

Sutherland, G. R. (1988). Fragile sites and cancer breakpoints—the pessimistic view. *Cancer Genet Cytogenet*, **31**, 5–7.

Sutherland, G. R. (1991). The detection of fragile sites on human chromosomes. In "Advanced techniques in chromosome research" (K. W. Adolph, ed.). Marcel Dekker, New York, pp. 203–222.

Sutherland, G. R. (1993). Human fragile sites. In "Genetic maps. Locus maps of complex genomes" (6th edn.) (S. J. O'Brien, ed.). Cold Spring Harbor Laboratory Press, pp. 5.264–5.266.

Sutherland, G. R. and Baker, E. (1992). Characterisation of a new rare fragile site easily confused with the fragile X. *Hum Mol Genet*, **1**, 111–113.

Sutherland, G. R., Callen, D. F. and Gardner, R. J. M. (1995). Paracentric inversions do not normally generate monocentric recombinant chromosomes. *Am J Med Genet*, **59**, 390.

Sutherland, G. R. and Eyre, H. (1981). Two unusual G-band variants of the short arm of chromosome 9. *Clin Genet*, **19**, 331–334.

Sutherland, G. R., Gardiner, A. J. and Carter, R. F. (1976). Familial pericentric inversion of chromosome 19, inv(19)(p13q13) with a note on genetic counselling of pericentric inversion carriers. *Clin Genet*, **10**, 54–59.

Sutherland, G. R., Gedeon, A., Kornman, L., Donnelly, A., Byard, R. W., Mulley, J. C., Kremer, E., Lynch, M., Pritchard, M., Yu, S. and Richards, R. I. (1991). Prenatal diagnosis of fragile X syndrome by direct detection of the unstable DNA sequence. *N Engl J Med*, **325**, 1720–1722.

Sutherland, G. R., Grace, E. and Bain, A. D. (1973). Metaphase chromosomes from neonatal urine. *Hum Genet*, **17**, 273–275.

Sutherland, G. R. and Hecht, F. (1985). "Fragile sites on human chromosomes." Oxford University Press, New York.

Sutherland, G. R. and Mulley, J. C. (1990). Diagnostic molecular genetics of the fragile X. *Clin Genet*, **37**, 2–11.

Sutherland, G. R. and Simmers, R. N. (1988). No statistical association between common fragile sites and non-random chromosome breakpoints in cancer cells. *Cancer Genet Cytogenet*, **31**, 9–15.

Sutherland, G. R. and Richards, R. I. (1993). Dynamic mutations on the move. *J Med Genet*, **30**, 978–981.

Sutherland, G. R. and Richards, R. I. (1994). Dynamic mutations. *Am Scientist*, **82**, 157–163.

Sweeney, J. E., Höhmann, C. F., Oster-Granite, M. L. and Coyle, J. T. (1989). Neurogenesis of the basal forebrain in euploid and trisomy 16 mice: an animal model for developmental disorders in Down syndrome. *Neurosci*, **31**, 413–425.

Syme, R. M. and Martin, R. H. (1992). Meiotic segregation of a 21;22 Robertsonian translocation. *Hum Reprod*, **7**, 825–829.

Szamosi, T., László, A., Szollár, J. and Schuler, D. (1985). Studies in chromosome instability syndromes: progeria, lipodystrophia, Cockayne syndrome, incontinentia pigmenti and Fanconi anaemia. *Clin Genet*, **28**, 470.

Taalman, R. D. F. M., Jaspers, N. G. J., Scheres, J. M. J. C., de Wit, J. and Hustinx, T. W. J. (1983). Hypersensitivity to ionizing radiation, in vitro, as a new chromosomal breakage disorder, the Nijmegen breakage syndrome. *Mutat Res*, **112**, 23–32.

Tada, H., Ri, T., Yoshida, H., Ishimoto, K., Kaneko, M., Yamashiro, Y. and Shinohara, T. (1987). A case of Shwachman syndrome with increased spontaneous chromosome breakage. *Hum Genet*, **77**, 289–291.

Tamaren, J., Spuhler, K. and Sujansky, E. (1983). Risk of Down syndrome among second and third-degree relatives of a proband with trisomy 21. *Am J Med Genet*, **15**, 393–403.

Tamaren, J., Spuhler, K. and Sujansky, E. (1984). Response to Dr ten Kate et al. *Am J Med Genet*, **19**, 601–602.

Tarleton, J. C. and Saul, R. A. (1993). Molecular genetic advances in fragile X syndrome. *J Pediatr*, **122**, 169–185.

Tassabehji, M., Newton, V. E., Leverton, K., Turnbull, K., Seemanova, E., Kunze, J., Sperling, K., Strachan, T. and Read, A. P. (1994). PAX3 gene structure and mutations: close analogies between Waardenburg syndrome and the *Splotch* mouse. *Hum Mol Genet*, **3**, 1069–1074.

Tavormina, P. L., Shiang, R., Thompson, L. M., Zhu, Y.-Z., Wilkin, D. J., Lachman, R. S., Wilcox, W. R., Rimoin, D. L., Cohn, D. H. and Wasmuth, J. J. (1995). Thanatophoric dysplasia (types I and II) caused by distinct mutations in fibroblast growth factor receptor 3. *Nature Genet*, **9**, 321–328.

Taylor, A. M. R. and McConville, C. M. (1992). Chromosome breakage disorders. In "Prenatal diagnosis and screening" (D. J. H. Brock, C. H. Rodeck and M. A. Ferguson-Smith, eds.). Churchill Livingstone, Edinburgh, pp. 405–421.

Teebi, A. S., Murthy, D. S. K., Ismail, E. A. R. and Redha, A. A. (1992). Alagille syndrome with *de novo* del(20)(p11.2). *Am J Med Genet*, **42**, 35–38.

Temple, I. K., Cockwell, A., Hassold, T., Pettay, D. and Jacobs, P. (1991). Maternal uniparental disomy for chromosome 14. *J Med Genet*, **28**, 511–514.

Temple, I. K., Hurst, J. A., Hing, S., Butler, L. and Baraitser, M. (1990). De novo deletion of Xp22.2-pter in a female with linear skin lesions of the face and neck, microphthalmia, and anterior chamber eye abnormalities. *J Med Genet*, **27**, 56–58.

Temple, I. K., James, R. S., Crolla, J. A., Sitch, F. L., Jacobs, P. A., Howell, W. M., Betts, P., Baum, J. D. and Shield, J. P. H. (1995). An imprinted gene(s) for diabetes? *Nature Genet*, **9**, 110–112.

Ten Kate, L. P., te Meerman, G. J. and Anders, G. J. P. A. (1984). Risk of Down's syndrome among second and third-degree relatives of a proband with trisomy 21. *Am J Med Genet*, **19**, 599–600.

Terzoli, G., Lalatta, F., Lobbiani, A., Simoni, G. and Colucci, G. (1992). Fertility in a 47,XXY patient: assessment of biological paternity by deoxyribonucleic acid fingerprinting. *Fertil Steril*, **58**, 821–822.

Terzoli, G., Rossella, F., Biscaglia, M. and Simoni, G. (1990). True fetal mosaicism revealed by a single abnormal colony in amniocyte culture. *Prenat Diagn*, **10**, 273–274.

Teshima, I. E., Kalousek, D. K., Vekemans, M. J. J., Markovic, V., Cox, D. M., Dallaire, L., Gagne, R., Lin, J. C. C., Ray, M., Sergovich, F. R., Uchida, I. A., Wang, H. and Tomkins, D. J. (1992a). Chromosome mosaicism in CVS and amniocentesis samples. *Prenat Diagn*, **12**, 443–446.

Teshima, I. E., Winsor, E. J. T. and Van Allen, M. I. (1992b). Trisomy 18 and a constitutional maternal translocation (2;18). *Am J Med Genet*, **43**, 759–761.

Teyssier, M., Rafat, A. and Pugeat, M. (1993). Case of (Y;1) familial translocation. *Am J Med Genet*, **46**, 339–340.

Teyssier, M. and Moreau, N. (1985). Transmission familiale d'un chromosome 22 remainié [r(22) ou 22p0?] chez deux femmes normales. *Ann Génét*, **28**, 116–118.

Tharapel, A. T., Anderson, K. P., Simpson, J. L., Martens, P. R., Wilroy, R. S., Llerena, J. C. and Schwartz, C. E. (1993). Deletion (X)(q26.1→q28) in a proband and her mother: molecular characterization and phenotypic-karyotypic deductions. *Am J Hum Genet*, **52**, 463–471.

Tharapel, A. T., Tharapel, S. A. and Bannerman, R. M. (1985). Recurrent pregnancy losses and parental chromosome abnormalities: a review. *Br J Obstet Gynaecol*, **92**, 899–914.

Theilgaard, A. (1986). Psychologic study of XYY and XXY men. In "Prospective studies on children with sex chromosome aneuploidy" (S. G. Ratcliffe and N. Paul, eds.). *Birth Defects: Orig Art Series*, **22**(3), pp. 277–292.

Therman, E., Laxova, R. and Susman, B. (1990). The critical region on the human Xq. *Hum Genet*, **85**, 455–461.

Therman, E. and Susman, B. (1993). "Human chromosomes. Structure, behavior, and effects." Springer-Verlag, New York.

Therman, E., Susman, B. and Denniston, C. (1989). The nonrandom participation of human acrocentric chromosomes in Robertsonian translocations. *Ann Hum Genet*, **53**, 49–65.

Thomas, J. H. (1995). Genomic imprinting proposed as a surveillance mechanism for chromosome loss. *Proc Natl Acad Sci U S A*, **92**, 480–482.

Thompson, M. W. (1962). 21-trisomy in a fertile female mongol. *Can J Genet Cytol*, **4**, 352–355.

Thompson, N. M., Gulley, M. L., Rogeness, G. A., Clayton, R. J., Johnson, C., Hazelton, B., Cho, C. G. and Zellmer, V. T. (1994). Neurobehavioral characteristics of CGG amplification status in fragile X females. *Am J Med Genet*, **54**, 378–383.

Thompson, P. W. and Roberts, S. H. (1987). A new variant of chromosome 16. *Hum Genet*, **76**, 100–101.

Till, M., Rafat, A., Charrin, C., Plauchu, H. and Germain, D. (1991). Duplication of chromosome 11 centromere in fetal and maternal karyotypes: a new variant? *Prenat Diagn*, **11**, 481–482.

Tolmie, J. L., Boyd, E., Batstone, P., Ferguson-Smith, M. E., AlRoomi, L. and Connor, J. M. (1988). Siblings with chromosome mosaicism, microcephaly, and growth retardation: the phenotypic expression of a human mitotic mutant? *Hum Genet*, **80**, 197–200.

Tommerup, N. (1993). Mendelian cytogenetics. Chromosome rearrangements associated with mendelian disorders. *J Med Genet*, **30**, 713–727.

Tommerup, N., Aagaard, L., Lund, C. L., Boel, E., Baxendale, S., Bates, G. P., Lehrach, H. and Vissing, H. (1993a). A zinc-finger gene ZNF141 mapping at 4p16.3/D4S90 is a candidate gene for the Wolf-Hirschhorn (4p-) syndrome. *Hum Mol Genet*, **2**, 1571–1575.

Tommerup, N., Brandt, C. A., Pedersen, S., Bolund, L. and Kamper, J. (1993b). Sex dependant transmission of Beckwith-Wiedemann syndrome associated with a reciprocal translocation t(9;11)(p11.2;p15.5). *J Med Genet*, **30**, 958–961.

Tommerup, N., Mortensen, E., Nielsen, M. H., Wegner, R.-D., Schindler, D. and Mikkelsen, M. (1993c). Chromosomal breakage, endomitosis, endoreduplication, and hypersensitivity toward radiomimetric and alkylating agents: a possible new autosomal recessive mutation in a girl with craniosynostosis and microcephaly. *Hum Genet*, **92**, 339–346.

Tommerup, N., Schempp, W., Meinecke, P., Pedersen, S., Bolund, L., Brandt, C., Goodpasture, C., Guldberg, P., Held, K. R., Reinwein, H., Saugstad, O. D., Scherer, G., Skjeldal, O., Toder, R., Westvik, J., van der Hagen, C. B. and Wolf, U. (1993d). Assignment of an autosomal sex reversal locus (*SRA1*) and campomelic dysplasia (*CMPD1*) to 17q24.3-q25.1. *Nature Genet*, **4**, 170–173.

Tóth, A., Gaál, M. and László, J. (1984). Familial pericentric inversion of the Y chromosome. *Ann Génét*, **27**, 60–61.

Toth-Fejel, S., Magenis, R. E., Leff, S., Brown, M. G., Comegys, B., Lawce, H., Berry,

T., Kesner, D., Webb, M. J. and Olson, S. (1995). Prenatal diagnosis of chromosome 15 abnormalities in the Prader-Willi/Angelman syndrome region by traditional and molecular cytogenetics. *Am J Med Genet*, **55**, 444–452.

Troche, V. and Hernandez, E. (1986). Neoplasia arising in dysgenetic gonads. *Obstet Gynecol Surv*, **41**, 74–79.

Trunca, C., Therman, E. and Rosenwaks, Z. (1984). The phenotypic effects of small, distal Xq deletions. *Hum Genet*, **68**, 87–89.

Tsuji, K., Narahara, K., Yokoyama, Y., Grzeschik, K.-H. and Kunz, J. (1995). The breakpoint on 7p in a patient with t(6;7) and craniosynostosis is spanned by a YAC clone containing the D7S503 locus. *Hum Genet*, **95**, 303–307.

Tsukahara, M., Endo, F., Aoki, Y., Matsuo, K. and Kajii, T. (1986). Familial supernumerary nonsatellited microchromosome. *Clin Genet*, **30**, 226–229.

Tuck-Muller, C. M., Chen, H., Martínez, J. E., Shen, C.-C., Li, S., Kusyk, C., Batista, D. A. S., Bhatnagar, Y. M., Dowling, E. and Wertelecki, W. (1995). Isodicentric Y chromosome: cytogenetic, molecular and clinical studies and review of the literature. *Hum Genet*, **96**, 119–129.

Tümer, Z., Berg, A. and Mikkelsen, M. (1995). Analysis of a whole arm translocation between chromosomes 18 and 20 using fluorescence in situ hybridization: detection of a break in the centromeric α-satellite sequences. *Hum Genet*, **95**, 299–302.

Tupler, R., Barbierato, L., Larizza, D., Sampaolo, P., Piovella, F. and Maraschio, P. (1994). Balanced autosomal translocations and ovarian dysgenesis. *Hum Genet*, **94**, 171–176.

Tutschek, B., Sherlock, J., Halder, A., Delhanty, J., Rodeck, C. and Adinolfi, M. (1995). Isolation of fetal cells from transcervical samples by micromanipulation: molecular confirmation of their fetal origin and diagnosis of fetal aneuploidy. *Prenat Diagn*, **15**, 951–960.

Uchida, I.A. and Freeman, V.C.P. (1985). Trisomy 21 Down syndrome. Parental mosaicism. *Hum Genet*, **70**, 246–248.

Uchida, I.A. and Freeman, V.C.P. (1986). Trisomy 21 Down syndrome. II. Structural chromosome rearrangements in the parents. *Hum Genet*, **72**, 118–122.

Urioste, M., Martínez-Frías, M. L., Bermejo, E., Jiménez, N., Romero, D., Nieto, C. and Villa, A. (1994a). Short rib-polydactyly syndrome and pericentric inversion of chromosome 4. *Am J Med Genet*, **49**, 94–97.

Urioste, M., Visedo, G., Sanchís, A., Sentís, C., Villa, A., Ludeña, P., Hortigüela, J. L., Martínez-Frías, M. L. and Fernández-Piqueras, J. (1994b). Dynamic mosaicism involving an unstable supernumerary der(22) chromosome in cat eye syndrome. *Am J Med Genet*, **49**, 77–82.

Van Camp, G., Van Thienen, M. N., Handig, I., Van Roy, B., Rao, V. S., Milunsky, A., Read, A. P., Baldwin, C. T., Farrer, L. A., Bonduelle, M., Standaert, L., Meire, F. and Willems, P. J. (1995). Chromosome 13q deletion with Waardenburg syndrome: further evidence for a gene involved in neural crest function on 13q. *J Med Genet*, **32**, 531–536.

Van de Vooren, M. J., Planteydt, H. T., Hagemeijer, A., Peters-Slough, M. F. and Timmerman, M. J. (1984). Familial balanced insertion (5;10) and monosomy and trisomy (10)(q24.2-q25.3). *Clin Genet*, **25**, 52–58.

Van Den Berg, D. J. and Francke, U. (1993). Roberts syndrome: a review of 100 cases and a new rating system for severity. *Am J Med Genet*, **47**, 1104–1123.

Van den Ouweland, A. M. W., Deelen, W. H., Kunst, C. B., Uzielli, M.-L. G., Nelson.

D. L., Warren, S. T., Oostra, B. and Halley, D. J. J. (1994). Loss of mutation at the FMR1 locus through multiple exchanges between maternal X chromosomes. *Hum Molec Genet*, **3**, 1823–1827.

Van Der Burgt, C. J. A. M., Merkx, G. F. M., Janssen, A. H., Mulder, J. C., Suijkerbuijk, R. F. and Smeets, D. F. C. M. (1992). Partial trisomy for 5q and monosomy for 12p in a liveborn child as a result of a complex five breakpoint chromosome rearrangement in a parent. *J Med Genet*, **29**, 739–741.

Van Dyke D. L., Flejter, W. L., Worsham, M. J., Roberson, J. R., Higgins, J. V., Herr, H. M., Knuutila, S., Wang, N., Babu, V. R. and Weiss, L. (1986). A practical metaphase marker of the inactive X chromosome. *Am J Hum Genet*, **39**, 88–95.

Van Dyke, D. L. (1988). Isochromosomes and interstitial tandem direct and inverted duplications. In "The cytogenetics of mammalian autosomal rearrangements" (A. Daniel, ed.). A. R. Liss, New York, pp. 635–665.

Van Dyke, D. C. and Allen, M. (1990). Clinical management considerations in long-term survivors with trisomy 18. *Pediatrics*, **85**, 753–759.

Van Dyke, D. L., Weiss, L., Roberson, J. R. and Babu, V. R. (1983). The frequency and mutation rate of balanced autosomal rearrangements in man estimated from pre-natal genetic studies for advanced maternal age. *Am J Hum Genet*, **35**, 301–308.

Van Hemel, J. O., Schaap, C., Van Opstal, D., Mulder, M. P., Niermeijer, M. F. and Meijers, J. H. C. (1995). Recurrence of DiGeorge syndrome: prenatal detection by FISH of a molecular 22q11 deletion. *J Med Genet*, **32**, 657–658.

Van Maldergem, L., Espeel, M., Roels, F., Petit, C., Dacremont, G., Wanders, R. J. A., Verloes, A. and Gillerot, Y. (1991). X-linked recessive chondrodysplasia punctata with XY translocation in a stillborn fetus. *Hum Genet*, **87**, 661–664.

Van Opstal, D., Van Hemel, J. O., Eussen, B. H. J., Van Der Heide, A., Van Den Berg, C., In 't Veld, P. A. and Los, F. J. (1995). A chromosome 21-specific cosmid cocktail for the detection of chromosome 21 aberrations in interphase nuclei. *Prenat Diagn*, **15**, 705–711.

Varela, M., Shapira, E. and Hyman, D. B. (1991). Ullrich-Turner syndrome in mother and daughter: prenatal diagnosis of a 46,X,del(X)(p21) offspring from a 45,X mother with low-level mosaicism for the del(X)(p21) in one ovary. *Am J Med Genet*, **39**, 411–412.

Varley, J. M. (1977). Patterns of silver staining of human chromosomes. *Chromosoma*, **61**, 207–214.

Vaughan, J., Ali, Z., Bower, S., Bennett, P., Chard, T. and Moore, G. (1994). Human maternal uniparental disomy for chromosome 16 and fetal development. *Prenat Diagn*, **14**, 751–756.

Varley, J.M. (1977). Patterns of silver staining of human chromosomes. *Chromosoma*, **61**, 207–214.

Vauhkonen, A-E., Sankila, E-M., Simola, K. O. J. and de la Chapelle, A. (1985). Seg-regation and fertility analysis in an autosomal reciprocal translocation, t(1;8)(q41; q23.1). *Am J Hum Genet,* **37**, 533–542.

Vejerslev, L. O., Sunde, L., Hansen, B. F., Larsen, J. K., Christensen, I. J. and Larsen, G. (1991). Hydatidiform mole and fetus with normal karyotype: support of a separate entity. *Obstet Gynecol*, **77**, 868–874.

Vekemans, M. and Morichon-Delvallez, N. (1990). Duplication of the long arm of chro-mosome 13 secondary to a recombination in a maternal intrachromosomal inser-tion (shift). *Prenat Diagn*, **10**, 787–794.

Verkerk, A. J. M. H., deVries, B. B. A., Niermeijer, M. F., Fu, Y.-H., Nelson, D. L.,

Warren, S. T., Majoor-Krakauer, D. F., Halley, D. J. J. and Oostra, B. A. (1992). Intragenic probe used for diagnostics in fragile X families. *Am J Med Genet*, **43**, 192–196.

Verkerk, A. J. M. H., Pieretti, M., Sutcliffe, J. S., Fu, Y.-H., Kuhl, D. P. A., Pizzuti, A., Reiner, O., Richards, S., Victoria, M. F., Zhang, F., Eussen, B. E., van Ommen, G.-J. B., Blonden, L. A. J., Riggins, G. J., Chastain, J. L., Kunst, C. B., Galjaard, H., Caskey, C. T., Nelson, D. L., Oostra, B. A. and Warren, S. T. (1991). Identification of a gene *(FMR-1)* containing a CGG repeat coincident with a breakpoint cluster region exhibiting length variation in fragile X syndrome. *Cell*, **65**, 905–914.

Verlander, P. C., Lin, J. D., Udono, M. U., Zhang, Q., Gibson, R. A., Mathew, C. G. and Auerbach, A. D. (1994). Mutation analysis of the Fanconi anemia gene *FACC*. *Am J Hum Genet*, **54**, 595–601.

Verma, R.S., Rodriguez, J. and Dosik, H. (1982). The clinical significance of pericentric inversion of the human Y chromosome: A rare "third" type of heteromorphism. *J Hered*, **73**, 236–238.

Verp, M. S., Bombard, A. T., Simpson, J. L. and Elias, S. (1988). Parental decision following prenatal diagnosis of fetal chromosome abnormality. *Am J Med Genet*, **29**, 613–622.

Verp, M. S. and Simpson, J. L. (1987). Abnormal sexual differentiation and neoplasia. *Cancer Genet Cytogenet*, **25**, 191–218.

Vickers, S., Dahlitz, M., Hardy, C., Kilpatrick, M. and Webb, T. (1994). A male with a de novo translocation involving loss of 15q11q13 material and Prader-Willi syndrome. *J Med Genet*, **31**, 478–481.

Villanueva, A. L. and Rebar, R. W. (1983). Triple-X syndrome and premature ovarian failure. *Obstet Gynecol*, **62** (Suppl.), 70S-73S.

Vincent, C., Kalatzis, V., Compain, S., Levilliers, J., Slim, R., Graia, F., de Lurdes Pereira, M., Nivelon, A., Croquette, M.-F., Lacombe, D., Vigneron, J., Helias, J., Broyer, M., Callen, D. F., Haan, E. A., Weissenbach, J., Lacroix, B., Bellané-Chantelot, C., Le Paslier, D., Cohen, D. and Petit, C. (1994). A proposed new contiguous gene syndrome on 8q consists of Branchio-Oto-Renal syndrome, Duane syndrome, a dominant form of hydrocephalus and trapeze aplasia; implications for the mapping of the BOR gene. *Hum Mol Genet*, **3**, 1859–1866.

Vintzileos, A. M. and Egan, J. F. X. (1995). Adjusting the risk for trisomy 21 on the basis of second-trimester ultrasonography. *Am J Obstet Gynecol*, **172**, 837–844.

Vits, L., De Boulle, K., Reyniers, E., Handig, I., Darby, J. K., Oostra, B. and Willems, P. J. (1994). Apparent regression of the CGG repeat in FMR1 to an allele of normal size. *Hum Genet*, **94**, 523–526.

Voiculescu, I., Barbi, G., Wolff, G., Steinbach, P., Back, E. and Schempp, W. (1986). Familial pericentric inversion of chromosome 12. *Hum Genet*, **72**, 320–322.

Vockley, J., Inserra, J., Berg, R. W. and Yang-Feng, T. L. (1991). Pseudomosaicism for 4p− in amniotic fluid cell culture proven to be true mosaicism after birth. *Am J Med Genet*, **39**, 81–83.

Von Koskull, H., Ritvanen, A., Ammala, P., Gahmberg, N. and Salonen, R. (1989). Trisomy 12 mosaicism in amniocytes and dysmorphic child despite normal chromosomes in fetal blood sample. *Prenat Diagn*, **9**, 433–437.

Vortkamp, A., Gessler, M. and Grzeschik, K.-H. (1991). GLI3 zinc-finger gene interrupted by translocations in Greig syndrome families? *Nature*, **352**, 539–540.

Voss, R., Ben-Simon, E., Avital, A., Godfrey, S., Zlotogora, J., Dagan, J., Tikochinski,

Y. and Hillel, J. (1989). Isodisomy of chromosome 7 in a patient with cystic fibrosis: could uniparental disomy be common in humans. *Am J Hum Genet*, **45**, 373–380.

Wachtel, S. S. (1994). XX sex reversal in the human. In "Molecular genetics of sex determination" (S. S. Wachtel, ed.). Academic Press, New York, pp. 267–285.

Wadey, R., Daw, S., Taylor, C., Atif, U., Kamath, S., Halford, S., O'Donnell, H., Wilson, D., Goodship, J., Burn, J. and Scambler, P. (1995). Isolation of a gene encoding an integral membrane protein from the vicinity of a balanced translocation breakpoint associated with DiGeorge syndrome. *Hum Mol Genet*, **4**, 1027–1033.

Wagner, T., Wirth, J., Meyer, J., Zabel, B., Held, M., Zimmer, J., Pasantes, J., Bricarelli, F. D., Keutel, J., Hustert, E., Wolf, U., Tommerup, N., Schempp, W. and Scherer, G. (1994). Autosomal sex reversal and campomelic dysplasia are caused by mutations in and around the *SRY*-related gene *SOX9*. *Cell*, **79**, 1111–1120.

Wagstaff, J. and Hemann, M. (1995). A familial "balanced" 3;9 translocation with cryptic 8q insertion leading to deletion and duplication of 9p23 loci in siblings. *Am J Hum Genet*, **56**, 302–309.

Wagstaff, J., Knoll, J. H. M., Glatt, K. A., Shugart, Y. Y., Sommer, A. and Lalande, M. (1992). Maternal but not paternal transmission of 15q11-13-linked nondeletion Angelman syndrome leads to phenotypic expression. *Nature Genet*, **1**, 291–294.

Wagstaff, J., Shugart, Y. Y. and Lalande, M. (1993). Linkage analysis in familial Angelman syndrome. *Am J Hum Genet*, **53**, 105–112.

Wald, N. and Cuckle, H. (1992). Biochemical screening. In "Prenatal diagnosis and screening" (D. J. H. Brock and C. Rodeck, eds.). Churchill Livingstone, Edinburgh, pp. 563–577.

Walker, A. P. and Bocian, M. (1987). Partial duplication 8q12→q21.2 in two sibs with maternally derived insertional and reciprocal translocations: case reports and review of partial duplications of chromosome 8. *Am J Med Genet*, **27**, 3–22.

Wallace, B. M. N. and Hultén, M. A. (1983). Triple chromosome synapsis in oocytes from a human foetus with trisomy 21. *Ann Hum Genet*, **47**, 271–276.

Walzer, S., Bashir, A. S. and Silbert, A. R. (1990). Cognitive and behavioral factors in the learning disabilities of 47,XXY and 47,XYY boys. In "Children and young adults with sex chromosome aneuploidy. Follow-up, clinical, and molecular studies" (J. A. Evans, J. L. Hamerton and A. Robinson, eds.). *Birth Defects: Orig Art Series*, **26**(4), pp. 45–58.

Wandall, A. (1994). A stable dicentric chromosome: both centromeres develop kinetochores and attach to the spindle in monocentric and dicentric configuration. *Chromosoma*, **103**, 56–62.

Wang, F. and Li, Y. (1993). A new stable human dicentric chromosome, tdic(4;21)(p16; q22), in a woman with first trimester abortion. *J Med Genet*, **30**, 696.

Wang, H., Hunter, A. G. W., Clifford, B., McLaughlin, M. and Thompson, D. (1993). VACTERL with hydrocephalus: spontaneous chromosome breakage and rearrangement in a family showing apparent sex-linked recessive inheritance. *Am J Med Genet*, **47**, 114–117.

Wang, I., Weil, D., Levilliers, J., Affara, N. A., de la Chapelle, A. and Petit, C. (1995). Prevalence and molecular analysis of two hot spots for ectopic recombination leading to XX maleness. *Genomics*, **28**, 52–58.

Wang, J.-C. C., Passage, M. B., Yen, P. H., Shapiro, L. J. and Mohandas, T. K. (1991). Uniparental heterodisomy for chromosome 14 in a phenotypically abnormal familial balanced 13/14 Robertsonian translocation carrier. *Am J Hum Genet*, **48**, 1069–1074.

Wang, Y.-T., Bajalica, S., Han, F.-Y., Wang, Z.-C., Bui, T.-H. and Xie, Y.-G. (1994). Direct and inverted reciprocal chromosome insertions between chromosomes 7 and 14 in a woman with recurrent miscarriages. *Am J Med Genet*, **52**, 349–351.

Wapner, R. J., Simpson, J. L., Golbus, M. S., Zachary, J. M., Ledbetter, D. H., Desnick, R. J., Fowler, S. E., Jackson, L. G., Lubs, H., Mahony, R. J., Pergament, E., Rhoads, G. G., Shulman, J. D. and de la Cruz, F. (1992). Chorionic mosaicism: association with fetal loss but not with adverse perinatal outcome. *Prenat Diagn*, **12**, 347–355.

Warburton, D. (1991). De novo balanced chromosome rearrangements and extra marker chromosomes identified at prenatal diagnosis: clinical significance and distribution of breakpoints. *Am J Hum Genet*, **49**, 995–1013.

Warburton, D., Byrne, J. and Canki, N. (1991). "Chromosome anomalies and prenatal development: an atlas. Oxford monographs on medical genetics No. 20." Oxford University Press, New York.

Warburton, D. (1985). Genetic factors influencing aneuploidy frequency. In "Aneuploidy. Etiology and mechanisms" (V. L. Dellarco, P. E. Voytek, and A. Hollaender, eds.). Plenum Press, New York, pp. 133–148.

Warburton, D., Kline, J., Stein, Z., Hutzler, M., Chin, A. and Hassold, T. (1987). Does the karyotype of a spontaneous abortion predict the karyotype of a subsequent abortion?—evidence from 273 women with two karyotyped spontaneous abortions. *Am J Hum Genet*, **41**, 465–483.

Watt, J. L., Ward, K., Couzin, D. A., Stephen, G. S. and Hill, A. (1986). A paracentric inversion of 7q illustrating a possible interchromosomal effect. *J Med Genet*, **23**, 341–344.

Webb, A., Beard, J., Wright, C., Robson, S., Wolstenholme, J. and Goodship, J. (1995). A case of paternal uniparental disomy for chromosome 11. *Prenat Diagn*, **15**, 773–777.

Webb, G. C., Krumins, E. J. M., Eichenbaum, S. Z., Voullaire, L. E., Earle, E. and Choo, K. H. (1989). Non C-banding variants in some normal families might be homogeneously staining regions. *Hum Genet*, **82**, 59–62.

Webb, G. C., Voullaire, L. E. and Rogers, J. G. (1988). Duplication of a small segment of 5p due to maternal recombination within a paracentric shift. *Am J Med Genet*, **30**, 875–881.

Webb, T. (1994). Inv dup(15) supernumerary marker chromosomes. *J Med Genet*, **31**, 585–594.

Webb, T., Clayton-Smith, J., Cheng, X.-J., Knoll, J. H. M., Lalande, M., Pembrey, M. E. and Malcolm, S. (1992). Angelman syndrome with a chromosomal inversion 15 inv(p11q13) accompanied by a deletion in 15q11q13. *J Med Genet*, **29**, 921–924.

Webster, D., Arlett, C. F., Harcourt, S. A., Teo, I. A. and Henderson, L. (1982). A new syndrome of immunodeficiency and increased cellular sensitivity to DNA damaging agents. In "Ataxia-telangiectasia" (B. A. Bridges and D.G. Harnden, eds.). John Wiley & Sons, New York, pp. 379–386.

Wegner, R-D., Metzger, M., Hanefeld, F., Jaspers, N,G.J., Baan, C., Magdorf, K., Kunze, J. and Sperling, K. (1988). A new chromosomal instability disorder confirmed by complementation studies. *Clin Genet*, **33**, 20–32.

Weil, D., Portnoí, M.-F., Levilliers, J., Wang, I., Mathieu, M., Taillemite, J.-L., Meier, M., Boudailliez, B. and Petit, C. (1993). A 45,X male with an X;Y translocation: implications for the mapping of the genes responsible for Turner syndrome and X-linked chondrodysplasia punctata. *Hum Mol Genet*, **2**, 1853–1856.

Weil, D., Wang, I., Dietrich, A., Poustka, A., Weissenbach, J. and Petit, C. (1994). Highly homologous loci on the X and Y chromosomes are hot-spots for ectopic recombinations leading to XX maleness. *Nature Genet*, **7**, 414–419.

Weksberg, R. (1994). Wiedemann-Beckwith syndrome: genomic imprinting revisited. *Am J Med Genet*, **52**, 235–236.

Weksberg, R., Markovic, V. D., Shuman, C., Teshima, I. E., Hutton, E. and Shime, J. (1986). Prenatal diagnosis by chorionic villi sampling in a fetus at risk for Bloom syndrome. *Am J Hum Genet*, **39**, A268.

Weksberg, R., Smith, C., Anson-Cartwright, L. and Maloney, K. (1988). Bloom syndrome: a single complementation group defines patients of diverse ethnic origin. *Am J Hum Genet*, **42**, 816–824.

Weksberg, R., Shen, D. R., Fei, Y. L., Song, Q. L. and Squire, J. (1993a). Disruption of insulin-like growth factor 2 imprinting in Beckwith-Wiedemann syndrome. *Nature Genet*, **5**, 143–150.

Weksberg, R., Teshima, I., Williams, B. R. G., Greenberg, C. R., Pueschel, S. M., Chernos, J. E., Fowlow, S. B., Hoyme, E., Anderson, I. J., Whiteman, D. A. H., Fisher, N. and Squire, J. (1993b). Molecular characterization of cytogenetic alterations associated with the Beckwith-Wiedemann syndrome (BWS) phenotype refines the localization and suggests the gene for BWS is imprinted. *Hum Mol Genet*, **2**, 549–556.

Welborn, J. L. and Lewis, J. P. (1990). Analysis of mosaic states in amniotic fluid using the *in-situ* colony technique. *Clin Genet*, **38**, 14–20.

Wells, S., Mould, S., Robins, D., Robinson, D. and Jacobs, P. (1991). Molecular and cytogenetic analysis of a familial microdeletion of Xq. *J Med Genet*, **28**, 163–166.

Wenger, S. L., Steele, M. W., Boone, L. Y., Lenkey, S. G., Cummins, J. H. and Chen, X.-Q. (1995). "Balanced" karyotypes in six abnormal offspring of balanced reciprocal translocation normal carrier parents. *Am J Med Genet*, **55**, 47–52.

Werner, W., Herrmann, F. H. and John, B. (1982). Cytogenetic studies of a family with trisomy 21 mosaicism in two successive generations as the cause of Down's syndrome. *Hum Genet*, **60**, 202–204.

Wheeler, M., Peakman, D., Robinson, A. and Henry, G. (1988). 45,X/46,XY mosaicism: Contrast of prenatal and postnatal diagnosis. *Am J Med Genet*, **29**, 565–571.

Whiteford, M. L., Coutts, J., Al-Roomi, L., Mather, A., Lowther, G., Cooke, A., Vaughan, J. I., Moore, G. E. and Tolmie, J. L. (1995). Uniparental isodisomy for chromosome 16 in a growth-retarded infant with congenital heart disease. *Prenat Diagn*, **15**, 579–584.

Whitney, M., Thayer, M., Reifsteck, C., Olson, S., Smith, L., Jakobs, P. M., Leach, R., Naylor, S., Joenje, H. and Grompe M. (1995). Microcell mediated chromosome transfer maps the Fanconi anaemia group D gene to chromosome 3p. *Nature Genet*, **11**, 341–343.

Wilkie, A. O. M., Yang, S. P., Summers, D., Poole, M. D., Reardon, W. and Winter, R. M. (1995). Saethre-Chotzen syndrome associated with balanced translocations involving 7p21: three further families. *J Med Genet*, **32**, 174–180.

Willatt, L. R., Davison, B. C. C., Goudie, D., Alexander, J., Dyson, H. M., Jenks, P. E. and Ferguson-Smith, M. E. (1992). A male with trisomy 9 mosaicism and maternal uniparental disomy for chromosome 9 in the euploid cell line. *J Med Genet*, **29**, 742–744.

Williams, C. A., Angelman, H., Clayton-Smith, J., Driscoll, D. J., Hendrickson, J. E., Knoll, J. H. M., Magenis, R. E., Schinzel, A., Wagstaff, J., Whidden, E. M., and

Zori, R. T. (1995). Angelman syndrome: consensus for diagnostic criteria. *Am J Med Genet,* **56**, 237–238.

Williams, B. J., Ballenger, C. A., Malter, H. E., Bishop, F., Tucker, M., Zwingman, T. A. and Hassold, T. J. (1993). Non-disjunction in human sperm: results of fluorescence *in situ* hybridization studies using two and three probes. *Hum Mol Genet,* **2**, 1929–1936.

Williams, J. and Dear, P. R. F. (1987). An unbalanced t(X;10)mat translocation in a child with congenital abnormalities. *J Med Genet,* **24**, 633.

Williams, P. L. and Wendell-Smith, C. P. (1969). Basic human embryology (2nd edn.). Pitman Medical & Scientific, London.

Williamson, E. M., Miller, J. F. and Seabright, M. (1980). Pericentric inversion (13) with two different recombinants in the same family. *J Med Genet,* **17**, 309–312.

Wilson, D. I., Burn, J., Scambler, P. and Goodship, J. (1993a). DiGeorge syndrome: part of CATCH 22. *J Med Genet,* **30**, 852–856.

Wilson, L. C., Leverton, K., Oude Luttikhuis, M. E. M., Oley, C. A., Flint, J., Wolstenhome, J., Duckett, D. P., Barrow, M. A., Leonard, J. V., Read, A. P. and Trembath, R. C. (1995). Brachydactyly and mental retardation: an Albright hereditary osteodystrophy-like syndrome localized to 2q37. *Am J Hum Genet,* **56**, 400–407.

Wilson, M. G., Lin, M. S., Fujimoto, A., Herbert, W. and Kaplan, F. M. (1989). Chromosome mosaicism in 6,000 amniocenteses. *Am J Med Genet,* **32**, 506–513.

Wilson, T. A., Blethen, S. L., Vallone, A., Alenick, D. S., Nolan, P., Katz, A., Amorillo, T. P., Goldmuntz, E., Emanuel, B. S. and Driscoll, D. A. (1993b). DiGeorge anomaly with renal agenesis in infants of mothers with diabetes. *Am J Med Genet,* **47**, 1078–1082.

Winsor, E. J. T. and Van Allen, M. I. (1989). Familial marker chromosome due to 3:1 disjunction of t(9;15) in a grandparent. *Prenat Diagn,* **9**, 851–855.

Winter, J. S. D. (1990). Androgen therapy in Klinefelter syndrome during adolescence. In ''Children and young adults with sex chromosome aneuploidy. Follow-up, clinical, and molecular studies'' (J. A. Evans, J. L. Hamerton and A. Robinson, eds.). *Birth Defects: Orig Art Series,* **26**(4), pp. 235–245.

Wintle, R. F., Costa, T., Haslam, R. H. A., Teshima, I. E. and Cox, D. W. (1995). Molecular analysis redefines three human chromosome 14 deletions. *Hum Genet,* **95**, 495–500.

Witt, D. R., Lew, S. P. and Mann, J. (1988). Heritable deletion of band 16q21 with normal phenotype: relationship to late replicating DNA. *Am J Hum Genet,* **43** (Suppl.), A127.

Wolf, L. and Zarfas, D. E. (1982). Parents' attitudes towards sterilization of their mentally retarded children. *Am J Ment Defic,* **87**, 122–129.

Wolff, D. J., Raffel, L. J., Ferré, M. M. and Schwartz, S. (1991). Prenatal ascertainment of an inherited dup(18p) associated with an apparently normal phenotype. *Am J Med Genet,* **41**, 319–321.

Wolstenholme, J. (1995). An audit of trisomy 16 in man. *Prenat Diagn,* **15**, 109–121.

Wolstenholme, J., Rooney, D. E. and Davison, E. V. (1994). Confined placental mosaicism, IUGR, and adverse pregnancy outcome: a controlled retrospective U. K. collaborative survey. *Prenat Diagn,* **14**, 345–361.

Woodage, T., Prasad, M., Dixon, J. W., Selby, R. E., Romain, D. R., Columbano-Green, L. M., Graham, D., Rogan, P. K., Seip, J. R., Smith, A. and Trent, R. J. (1994). Bloom syndrome and maternal uniparental disomy for chromosome 15. *Am J Hum Genet,* **55**, 74–80.

Woods, C. G., Bankier, A., Curry, J., Sheffield, L. J., Slaney, S. F., Smith, K., Voullaire,

L. and Wellesley, D. (1994). Asymmetry and skin pigmentary anomalies in chromosome mosaicism. *J Med Genet*, **31**, 694–701.

Woods, C. G., Leversha, M. and Rogers, J. G. (1995). Severe intrauterine growth retardation with increased mitomycin C sensitivity: a further chromosome breakage syndrome. *J Med Genet*, **32**, 301–305.

Worley, K. C., Lindsay, E. A., Bailey, W., Wise, J., McCabe, E. R. B. and Baldini, A. (1995). Rapid molecular cytogenetic analysis of X-chromosomal microdeletions: fluorescence in situ hybridization (FISH) for complex glycerol kinase deficiency. *Am J Med Genet*, **57**, 615–619.

Worsham, M. J., Miller, D. A., Devries, J. M., Mitchell, A. R., Babu, V. R., Surli, V., Weiss, L. and Van Dyke, D. L. (1989). A dicentric recombinant 9 derived from a paracentric inversion: phenotype, cytogenetics, and molecular analysis of centromeres. *Am J Hum Genet*, **44**, 115–123.

Worton, R. G. and Stern, R. (1984). A Canadian collaborative study of mosaicism in amniotic fluid cell cultures. *Prenat Diagn*, **4** (Spec. Iss.), 131–144.

Wulfsberg, E. A., Curtis, J. and Jayne, C. H. (1992). Chondrodysplasia punctata: a boy with X-linked recessive chondrodysplasia punctata due to an inherited X-Y translocation with a current classification of these disorders. *Am J Med Genet*, **43**, 823–828.

Wyandt, H. E. (1988). Ring autosomes: identification, familial transmission, causes of phenotypic effects and in vitro mosaicism. In "The cytogenetics of mammalian autosomal rearrangements" (A. Daniel, ed.). A. R. Liss, New York, pp. 667–695.

Wyandt, H. E., Maher, T., Fisher, N. L., Patil, S. R., Osella, P., Luthardt, F. W., Kawada, C., Williamson, R. and Milunsky, A. (1990). Trisomy 12 mosaicism in phenotypically normal fetuses following prenatal detection. *Prenat Diagn*, **10**, 569–574.

Wyrobek, A. J. (1993). Methods and concepts in detecting abnormal reproductive outcomes of paternal origin. *Reprod Toxicol*, **7**, 3–16.

Xu, H., Wei, H., Tassone, F., Graw, S., Gardiner, K and Weissman, S. M. (1995). A search for genes from the dark band regions of human chromosome 21. *Genomics*, **27**, 1–8.

Yaspo, M.-L., Gellen, L., Mott, R., Korn, B., Nizetic, D., Poustka, A. and Lehrach, H. (1995). Model for a transcript map of human chromosome 21: isolation of new coding sequences from exon and enriched cDNA libraries. *Hum Mol Genet*, **4**, 1291–1304.

Young, I. D., Zuccollo, J. M., Maltby, E. L. and Broderick, N. J. (1992). Campomelic dysplasia associated with a de novo 2q;17q reciprocal translocation. *J Med Genet*, **29**, 251–252.

Yu, S., Mulley, J., Loesch, D., Turner, G., Donnelly, A., Gedeon, A., Hillen, D., Kremer, E., Lynch, M., Pritchard, M., Sutherland, G. R. and Richards, R. I. (1992). Fragile X syndrome: unique genetics of the heritable unstable element. *Am J Hum Genet*, **50**, 968–980.

Yu, S., Pritchard, M., Kremer, E., Lynch, M., Nancarrow, J., Baker, E., Holman, K., Mulley, J. C., Warren, S. T., Schlessinger, D., Sutherland, G. R. and Richards, R. I. (1991). Fragile X genotype characterised by an unstable region of DNA. *Science*, **252**, 1179–1181.

Yunis, J. J. and Soreng, A. L. (1984). Constitutive fragile sites and cancer. *Science*, **226**, 1199–1204.

Zachmann, M. (1994). Male pseudohermaphroditism. In "Molecular genetics of sex determination" (S. S. Wachtel, ed.). Academic Press, New York, pp. 367–397.

Zaragoza, M. V., Jacobs, P. A., James, R. S., Rogan, P., Sherman, S. and Hassold, T.

(1994). Nondisjunction of human acrocentric chromosomes: studies of 432 trisomic fetuses and liveborns. *Hum Genet*, **94**, 411–417.

Zaslav, A. L., Blumenthal, D., Fox, J. E., Thomson, K. A., Segraves, R. and Weinstein, M. E. (1993). A rare inherited euchromatic heteromorphism on chromosome 1. *Prenat Diagn*, **13**, 569–573.

Zenzes, M. T. and Casper, R. F. (1992). Cytogenetics of human oocytes, zygotes, and embryos after in vitro fertilization. *Hum Genet*, **88**, 367–375.

Zhang, F., Deleuze, J.-F., Aurias, A., Dutrillaux, A.-M., Hugon, R.-N., Alagille, D., Thomas, G. and Hadchouel, M. (1990). Interstitial deletion of the short arm of chromosome 20 in arteriohepatic dysplasia (Alagille syndrome). *J Pediatr*, **116**, 73–77.

Zhao, J., Gordon, P. L., Wilroy, R. S., Martens, P. R., Tarleton, J., Shulman, L. P., Simpson, J. L., Elias, S. and Tharapel, A. T. (1995). Characterization of an unbalanced de novo rearrangement by microsatellite polymorphism typing and by fluorescent in situ hybridization. *Am J Med Genet*, **56**, 398–402.

Zhao, Z., Lee, C.-C., Jiralerspong, S., Juyal, R. C., Lu, F., Baldini, A., Greenberg, F., Caskey, C. T. and Patel, P. I. (1995). The gene for a human microfibril-associated glycoprotein is commonly deleted in Smith-Magenis syndrome patients. *Hum Molec Genet*, **4**, 589–597.

Zheng, Y.-L., Demaria, M., Zhen, D., Vadnais, T. J. and Bianchi, D. W. (1995). Flow sorting of fetal erythroblasts using intracytoplasmic anti-fetal haemoglobin: preliminary observations on maternal samples. *Prenat Diagn*, **15**, 897–905.

Zhong, N., Yang, W., Dobkin, C. and Brown, W. T. (1995). Fragile X gene instability: anchoring AGGs and linked microsatellites. *Am J Hum Genet*, **57**, 351–361.

Zori, R. T., Lupski, J. R., Heju, Z., Greenberg, F., Killian, J. M., Gray, B. A., Driscoll, D. J., Patel, P. I. and Zackowski, J. L. (1993). Clinical, cytogenetic, and molecular evidence for an infant with Smith-Magenis syndrome born from a mother having a mosaic 17p11.2p12 deletion. *Am J Med Genet*, **46**, 504–511.

Zühlke, C., Thies, U., Braulke, I., Reis, A. and Schirren, C. (1994). Down syndrome and male fertility: PCR-derived fingerprinting, serological and andrological investigations. *Clin Genet*, **46**, 324–326.

Index